Handbook of Medical Genomics

Handbook of Medical Genomics

Editor: Barbara Pearson

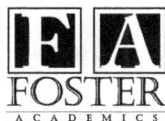

FA FOSTER
ACADEMICS

www.fosteracademics.com

www.fosteracademics.com

FA
FOSTER
ACADEMICS

Cataloging-in-Publication Data

Handbook of medical genomics / edited by Barbara Pearson.
   p. cm.
Includes bibliographical references and index.
ISBN 978-1-63242-701-4
1. Medical genetics. 2. Genomics. 3. Genomes. 4. Human genome. I. Pearson, Barbara.
RB155 .H36 2019
616.042--dc23

© Foster Academics, 2019

Foster Academics,
118-35 Queens Blvd., Suite 400,
Forest Hills, NY 11375, USA

ISBN 978-1-63242-701-4 (Hardback)

Contents

Chapter 17

Chapter 18

Chapter 19

Preface

Every book is a source of knowledge and this one is no exception. The idea that led to the conceptualization of this book was the fact that the world is advancing rapidly; which makes it crucial to document the progress in every field. I am aware that a lot of data is already available, yet, there is a lot more to learn. Hence, I accepted the responsibility of editing this book and contributing my knowledge to the community.

The diagnosis, management and counseling of individuals with hereditary disorders is under the scope of medical genomics. Mitochondrial disorders, birth defects and dysmorphology, skeletal dysplasia, mental retardation, etc. are some of the conditions studied and treated under this field. Due to the advancements in genetics, the etiologies of many endocrine, neurologic, cardiovascular, ophthalmologic, psychiatric, renal and dermatologic conditions are being explored. The sequencing of human DNA allows the identification of mutations that are linked to diseases and the genotyping of specific viruses to design treatment strategies. Genetic tests can show predisposition to various disorders such as cystic fibrosis, liver diseases, breast cancer, hemostasis disorders, etc. Genetic medicine incorporates areas such as personalized medicine, gene therapy and predictive medicine. In genetic counseling, information regarding genetic conditions, risks in other family members of developing such diseases, and diagnostic testing are provided to individuals and families. This book contains some path-breaking studies in the field of medical genomics. It unfolds the innovative aspects of genetics and genomics, which will be crucial for the progress of this field in the future. Coherent flow of topics, student-friendly language and extensive use of examples make this book an invaluable source of knowledge.

While editing this book, I had multiple visions for it. Then I finally narrowed down to make every chapter a sole standing text explaining a particular topic, so that they can be used independently. However, the umbrella subject sinews them into a common theme. This makes the book a unique platform of knowledge.

I would like to give the major credit of this book to the experts from every corner of the world, who took the time to share their expertise with us. Also, I owe the completion of this book to the never-ending support of my family, who supported me throughout the project.

Editor

Erythrocyte microRNA sequencing reveals differential expression in relapsing-remitting multiple sclerosis

Kira Groen[1,2], Vicki E. Maltby[1,2], Rodney A. Lea[2,3], Katherine A. Sanders[4], J. Lynn Fink[5], Rodney J. Scott[2,6,7], Lotti Tajouri[8] and Jeannette Lechner-Scott[1,2,9*]

Abstract

Background: There is a paucity of knowledge concerning erythrocytes in the aetiology of Multiple Sclerosis (MS) despite their potential to contribute to disease through impaired antioxidant capacity and altered haemorheological features. Several studies have identified an abundance of erythrocyte miRNAs and variable profiles associated with disease states, such as sickle cell disease and malaria. The aim of this study was to compare the erythrocyte miRNA profile of relapsing-remitting MS (RRMS) patients to healthy sex- and age-matched controls.

Methods: Erythrocytes were purified by density-gradient centrifugation and RNA was extracted. Following library preparation, samples were run on a HiSeq4000 Illumina instrument (paired-end 100 bp sequencing). Sequenced erythrocyte miRNA profiles (9 patients and 9 controls) were analysed by DESeq2. Differentially expressed miRNAs were validated by RT-qPCR using miR-152-3p as an endogenous control and replicated in a larger cohort (20 patients and 18 controls). After logarithmic transformation, differential expression was determined by two-tailed unpaired t-tests. Logistic regression analysis was carried out and receiver operating characteristic (ROC) curves were generated to determine biomarker potential.

Results: A total of 236 erythrocyte miRNAs were identified. Of twelve differentially expressed miRNAs in RRMS two showed increased expression (adj. $p < 0.05$). Only modest fold-changes were evident across differentially expressed miRNAs. RT-qPCR confirmed differential expression of miR-30b-5p (0.61 fold, $p < 0.05$) and miR-3200-3p (0.36 fold, $p < 0.01$) in RRMS compared to healthy controls. Relative expression of miR-3200-5p (0.66 fold, NS $p = 0.096$) also approached significance. MiR-3200-5p was positively correlated with cognition measured by audio-recorded cognitive screen ($r = 0.60$; $p < 0.01$). MiR-3200-3p showed greatest biomarker potential as a single miRNA (accuracy = 75.5%, $p < 0.01$, sensitivity = 72.7%, specificity = 84.0%). Combining miR-3200-3p, miR-3200-5p, and miR-30b-5p into a composite biomarker increased accuracy to 83.0% ($p < 0.05$), sensitivity to 77.3%, and specificity to 88.0%.

Conclusions: This is the first study to report differences in erythrocyte miRNAs in RRMS. While the role of miRNAs in erythrocytes remains to be elucidated, differential expression of erythrocyte miRNAs may be exploited as biomarkers and their potential contribution to MS pathology and cognition should be further investigated.

Keywords: Erythrocytes, microRNA, Relapsing-remitting multiple sclerosis, Next-generation sequencing

* Correspondence: jeannette.lechner-scott@hnehealth.nsw.gov
[1]School of Medicine and Public Health, University of Newcastle, Callaghan, NSW 2308, Australia
[2]Centre for Information Based Medicine, Level 3 West, Hunter Medical Research Institute, 1 Kookaburra Circuit, New Lambton Heights, NSW 2305, Australia
Full list of author information is available at the end of the article

Background

Multiple Sclerosis (MS) is an autoimmune disease of the central nervous system (CNS) marked by lymphocytic infiltration, demyelination, and neurodegeneration. It affects approximately 2.5 million individuals worldwide. MS is a heterogeneous disease, which is divided into three disease courses with relapsing-remitting MS (RRMS) being the most common (around 85% of the patient population) [1, 2]. Its aetiology is assumed to be the interaction between environmental risk factors and genetic predisposition [3], however the exact cause and pathophysiology remain unclear.

MS is associated with activated peripheral and CNS-resident immune cells [2] and it remains to be determined whether erythrocytes play a role in its pathology. Erythrocytes are anucleate cells responsible primarily for respiratory gas transport [4, 5], yet are also thought to play a dynamic role in health and disease [6]. The potential involvement of erythrocytes in MS has been recently reviewed [7]. Briefly, altered haemorheological features of erythrocytes have been documented in MS and may be contributing to blood-brain barrier (BBB) disruption, a hallmark of MS pathology [2]. Furthermore, erythrocytes may contribute to increased levels of oxidative stress in MS through impaired antioxidant enzyme capacity [7]. In addition to MS pathology, disease-modifying therapies (DMTs) also appear to affect erythrocytes. For instance, natalizumab has been shown to result in previously undetected circulating erythrocyte precursors [8–10]. Mitoxantrone [11], fingolimod [12], and dimethyl fumarate [13] all have the potential to cause eryptosis, erythrocyte-specific apoptosis, and interferon-β has been shown to reduce red cell distribution width, possibly altering haemorheological features [14].

More recent studies have focused on the potential use of erythrocytes as MS biomarkers, using exogenous C-peptide binding to erythrocytes [15]. Biomarkers that can accurately reflect pathological and physiological processes are crucial in diseases as complex and heterogeneous as MS. Such biomarkers are needed for diagnosis and patient stratification, but also monitoring of treatment efficacy and disease progression [16]. Current MS diagnosis and monitoring relies on procedures such as lumbar punctures and magnetic resonance imaging (MRI) of the brain and spinal cord [2]. MicroRNA (miRNA) profiles are gaining increasing interest as MS biomarkers as they can reflect a range of ongoing pathological and physiological processes simultaneously [16, 17]. MiRNAs are small (~ 22 bp) non-coding RNA molecules that control gene expression at the post-transcriptional level [18]. Studies have shown that in peripheral blood mononuclear cell (PBMC) miRNAs can accurately differentiate between MS patients and healthy controls (HCs) [19, 20]; however, PBMCs only make up

a very small percentage of whole blood elements [4]. The majority of a blood sample, erythrocytes and plasma, is discarded when assessing PBMCs. Additionally, some DMTs, such as fingolimod, are known to decrease circulating PBMC numbers [21]. Consequently, PBMC-derived miRNA profiles may not be the most suitable biomarker to monitor MS. Erythrocytes, which are abundant and can be quickly and cost-effectively purified [4], may lend themselves as a superior option.

Recent expression studies have identified an amplitude of miRNA transcripts in circulating erythrocytes [6, 22, 23]. Erythrocyte miRNA profiles were found to differ from leukocyte and reticulocyte profiles, yet largely reflect the miRNA expression of whole blood [6]. While the exact role of miRNAs in translationally inactive erythrocytes [24] is still unknown, they may be involved in intercellular communication through erythrocyte-derived extracellular vesicles (EVs) [25], or remnants of a functional erythrocyte precursor transcriptome [6, 24]. Despite uncertainty regarding the function of erythrocyte miRNAs, they have been found to differ in health and disease [6]. The use of erythrocyte-specific miRNA profiles is advantageous to whole blood miRNAs, as it eliminates variation that may arise from differences in whole blood cell composition. Erythrocytes have an average lifespan of 120 days in healthy individuals [4], but reduced lifespans have been reported in athletes [26] and some disease states [27]. Therefore, erythrocyte miRNAs may prove to present a relatively stable picture of miRNA expression, whereas translationally active cell miRNA profiles tend to only provide a snapshot of current miRNA expression, subjective to day-to-day variation [28]. However, this hypothesis demands further investigation.

Erythrocyte miRNAs may be exploited as biomarkers for MS patient stratification, diagnosis, and monitoring of treatment response and disease progression. Next-generation sequencing (NGS) technology has the potential to identify novel MS miRNA signatures in erythrocytes. The aim of this study was to characterise the erythrocyte miRNA profile of RRMS patients and compare it to HCs using NGS technologies.

Methods

Sample collection

Ethical approval was obtained from the Bond University Human Research Ethics Committee (RO-1382), the University of Newcastle Ethics Committee (H-505-0607), and the Hunter New England Health Ethics Committee (05/04/13/3.09). All participants gave written, informed consent prior to enrolment. Whole blood was collected into EDTA tubes from an initial cohort of 9 female RRMS patients and 9 female healthy controls (HCs). A further 20 female RRMS and 18 female HC samples were collected as part of the replication cohort. RRMS diagnosis was defined according to the McDonald criteria [29]. Participants who were pregnant, breastfeeding, or suffering from an autoimmune condition other than MS were excluded from the study. To minimise confounders associated with sex, only females were recruited for this pilot study. Additional patient information was obtained through MSBase, an observational database open to neurologists and health care teams [30]. Participant characteristics are summarised in Table 1.

Erythrocyte purification

Erythrocytes were purified from 10 ml whole blood by density-gradient centrifugation. Lymphoprep (Stem Cell Technologies, Canada) density-gradient media was used according to manufacturer protocol. Plasma, PBMC layer, density-gradient media, and top erythrocyte layer were aspirated. The remaining erythrocyte pellet was washed twice with Hanks-balanced salt solution (HBSS) (GE Healthcare, United Kingdom).

Purity assessment of erythrocytes

Purity of obtained erythrocytes was assessed by flow cytometry. One µl of erythrocyte pellet was stained with FITC-conjugated CD235a (Clone 2B7; erythrocytes and precursors) (BD Pharmingen, USA) and PE-conjugated CD71 (M-A712; reticulocytes) (BD Pharmingen, USA). All samples met a minimum purity cut-off of 95%.

Samples were analysed on FACS Canto II (BD Biosciences, USA) using FACS Diva Software (BD Biosciences, USA).

RNA extraction

Total RNA was extracted from 300 µl erythrocyte pellets with miRNeasy Kits (Qiagen, USA). Pellets were homogenized by vortexing samples for 1 min. Total RNA was quantified using the broad-range RNA Kit for the Qubit 2.0 (Life Technologies, USA). RNA integrity was determined with the RNA 6000 Nano kit on a 2100 Bioanalyzer (Agilent Technologies, USA).

MiRNA sequencing and analysis

Library preparation and sequencing were performed by the Diamantina Institute, University of Queensland, Brisbane, Australia. Libraries were prepared with TruSeq Small RNA Library Preparation kits (Illumina, USA). Samples were individually barcoded and then sequenced in two multiplexed pools. Samples were run on the HiSeq4000 platform (Illumina, USA) using paired-end sequencing (read length: 100 bp; coverage 1 million reads/sample). Sequencing reads were de-multiplexed using CASAVA 1.8 software package (Illumina, USA) and adapter sequences were trimmed using Trim Galore! (https://www.bioinformatics.babraham.ac.uk/projects/trim_galore/). Reads were aligned against miRBase 21 [31] using STAR [32] and NGS results were analysed by DESeq2 [33]. Significance was adjusted for false discovery rate (FDR) using the Benjamini-Hochberg procedure.

Table 1 Participant characteristics by cohort (sequencing and replication) and group (control subjects and RRMS patients)

		Sequencing Cohort		Replication Cohort	
		Control Subjects ($n = 9$)	RRMS Patients ($n = 9$)	Control Subjects ($n = 18$)	RRMS Patients ($n = 20$)
Female		100%	100%	100%	100%
Caucasian		100%	90%	94%	100%
Age (years)		34.75 (±11.45)	42.44 (±9.66)	38.92 (± 9.89)	38.39 (±9.41)
Disease Duration (years)		N/A	15.11 (±11.87)	N/A	9.29 (±.5.52)
EDSS Score			2.00 (±1.32)		2.09 (±1.53)
Age at Onset (years)			27.94 (±8.48)		28.96 (± 8.79)
Number of Relapses			5.98 (±4.91)		6.35 (± 3.33)
Days since Last Relapse			1083.00 (±1271.81)		985 (±969.75)
Treatment	Off Treatment		2		0
	Dimethyl fumarate		2		0
	Fingolimod		3		10
	Natalizumab		2		10
Time on Treatment (years)			2.46 (±2.60)		3.57 (±2.20)
Number of Relapses on Treatment			0.56 (±0.73)		1.50 (±2.12)
Most recent ARCS[a]			78.33 (±26.76)		81.35 (±20.43)

Except for percentages and absolute numbers, all data is presented as mean (± SD). *RRMS* relapsing-remitting multiple sclerosis, *EDSS* extended disability status scale, *ARCS* audio-recorded cognitive screen, *SD* standard deviation of the mean. [a]ARCS are only reported for patients who completed an ARCS within a year of sample collection (sequencing cohort $n = 3$; replication cohort $n = 17$)

Reverse transcription quantitative polymerase chain reaction (RT-qPCR) – Validation and replication

Differentially expressed erythrocyte miRNAs flagged by NGS were confirmed in the initial NGS cohort and in a replication cohort of 20 RRMS patients and 18 HCs using TaqMan Advanced miRNA Assays (Assay IDs: hsa-let-7f-5p: 478578, hsa-miR-30b-5p: 478007, hsa-miR-32-5p: 478026, hsa-96-5p: 478215, hsa-181a-5p: 477857, hsa-miR-362-5p: 478059, hsa-598-3p: 478172, hsa-652-3p: 478189, hsa-miR-660-5p: 478192, hsa-miR-1294: 478693, hsa-miR-3200-3p: 478322, hsa-miR-3200-5p: 478021; Applied Biosystems, Thermo Fisher Scientific, USA). MiR-152-3p (hsa-miR-152-3p: 477921; Applied Biosystems, Thermo Fisher Scientific, USA) was used as an endogenous normalisation control based on a previous study investigating erythrocyte miRNAs by RT-qPCR [6]. The expression of miR-152-3p did not differ between RRMS patients and healthy controls in our sequencing cohort (Additional file 1: Table S1). Additionally, miR-152-3p expression was not altered during different stages of erythroid differentiation [34], it demonstrated the least variation across 40 different human tissue samples (Applied Biosystems, unpublished data, see reference [6]), and showed great stability in a hepatic study [34]. Relative expression was calculated using the $2^{-\text{deltaCT}}$ method. All RT-qPCR experiments were performed on a ViiA 7 (Applied Biosystems, USA) instrument. IBM SPSS Statistics 24 was used for statistical analysis. Since this was a relatively small discovery-based project we chose to set a relaxed significance threshold of 0.05 so as to reduce true positive rejection rate (Type II error). Replication of significant hits using an independent replication cohort was performed the reduce the false positive rate (Type I error). Following logarithmic transformation, relative expression determined by RT-qPCR was assessed by two-tailed unpaired Student's t-tests or ANOVA, depending on the number of groups to be compared. Receiver operating characteristic (ROC) curves were generated to assess the diagnostic value of confirmed miRNAs and accuracy was determined by area under the curve (AUC). Using relative expression cut-off values that resulted in greatest sensitivity and specificity for confirmed miRNAs, logistic regression analysis was performed in IBM SPSS Statistics 24 to determine the value of composite biomarkers using multiple confirmed miRNAs. Pearson correlation coefficients between confirmed miRNA and recorded disease outcome measures (Table 1) were calculated.

MiRNA target prediction

MiRSystem was used to predict target genes of differentially expressed miRNAs as it integrates seven prediction algorithms and includes experimental validation of miRNA-mRNA interactions [35].

Results

NGS was used to determine erythrocyte miRNA profiles of 9 RRMS patients and 9 HCs. RT-qPCR was then utilised to confirm differential expression of erythrocyte miRNAs revealed by NGS in the sequencing cohort and a more uniform replication cohort of 20 RRMS patients and 18 HC samples. Participant characteristics of the sequencing and replication cohort are shown in Table 1.

Total RNA

Total erythrocyte RNA was extracted from 300 μl erythrocyte pellets (mean purity determined by flow cytometry was 99%, with < 1% leukocytes and platelets; further detail in Additional file 2: Table S2). Total erythrocyte RNA content in 10 ml whole blood was calculated by multiplying RNA yields from one aliquot by the number of aliquots obtained. Mean erythrocyte RNA yield obtained from 10 ml whole blood of MS patients ($n = 29$) was 20.12 μg ($\pm$ 17.02 μg), while the mean erythrocyte RNA content of HCs ($n = 27$) was 12.44 μg ($\pm$ 3.85 μg)/10 ml whole blood ($p < 0.05$). RNA yield did not correlated with bench time (time that passed between sample collection and processing) (MS patients: $r = 0.145$, $p = 0.553$; HC: $r = 0.169$, $p = 0.502$). Patients treated with natalizumab (32.35 μg/10 ml whole blood) had significantly greater RNA yields than patients on fingolimod (15.52 μg/10 ml whole blood, $p < 0.01$) and HCs (12.44 μg/10 ml whole blood, $p < 0.001$) (Additional file 3: Figure S1).

Next-generation sequencing results

Following TruSeq Small RNA library preparation (Illumina, USA), erythrocyte samples were sequenced by paired-end 100 bp sequencing on a HiSeq4000 (Illumina, USA) instrument, aiming for 1 million reads per sample. NGS revealed 236 known miRNAs across patient and control erythrocytes. Normalised gene counts ranged from 1 to > 21,800 (Additional file 1: Table S1). Twelve erythrocyte miRNAs were found to be differentially expressed in RRMS patients, two of which, miR-1294 (1.55-fold, FDR adj. $p < 0.05$) and let-7f-5p (1.73-fold, adj. $p < 0.05$), showed increased expression in RRMS compared to HCs. The remaining ten miRNAs, miR-181a-5p (0.45 fold, adj. $p < 0.0001$), miR-96-5p (0.43 fold, adj. $p < 0.05$), miR-32-5p (0.49 fold, adj. $p < 0.05$), miR-598-3p (0.53 fold, adj. $p < 0.05$), miR-362-5p (0.59 fold, adj. $p < 0.05$), miR-30b-5p (0.60 fold, adj. $p < 0.05$), miR-660-5p (0.64 fold, adj. $p < 0.05$), miR-652-3p (0.69 fold, adj. $p < 0.05$), and miR-3200-3p and -5p (0.85 fold, adj. $p < 0.01$), showed decreased expression in RRMS compared to HCs (Fig. 1). Four of the differentially expressed miRNAs (miR-181a-5p, miR-362-5p, miR-598-3p, and miR-96-5p) were very lowly expressed (< 100 reads) and only let-7f-5p, miR-660-5p, and miR-652-3p reached more than 800 reads per sample (Additional file 1: Table S1). No obvious clustering

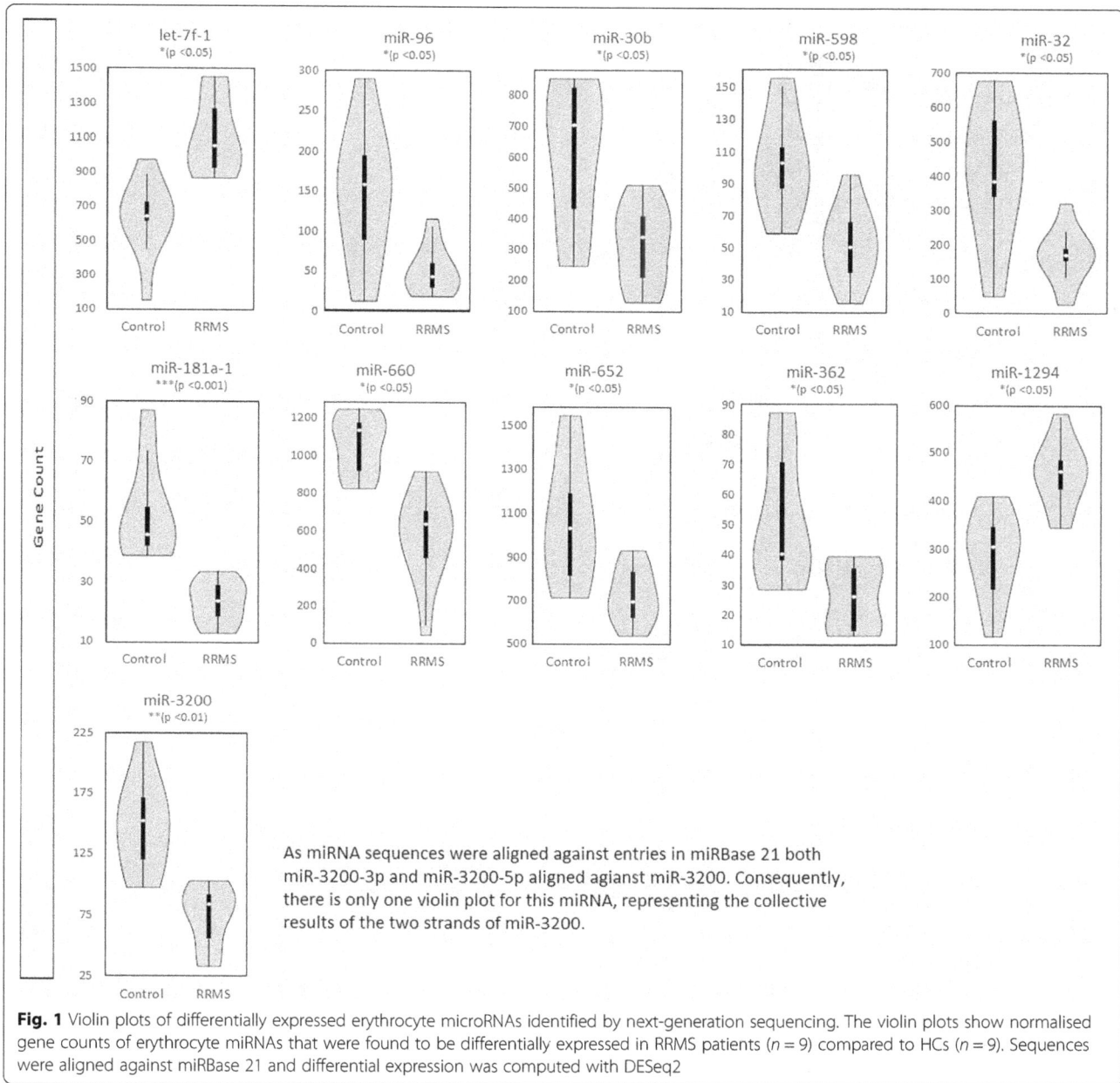

Fig. 1 Violin plots of differentially expressed erythrocyte microRNAs identified by next-generation sequencing. The violin plots show normalised gene counts of erythrocyte miRNAs that were found to be differentially expressed in RRMS patients ($n = 9$) compared to HCs ($n = 9$). Sequences were aligned against miRBase 21 and differential expression was computed with DESeq2

of patients and controls was evident when looking at global differences in miRNA expression.

Reverse transcription quantitative polymerase chain reaction results – Validation and replication

To validate NGS results, differentially expressed erythrocyte miRNAs were assessed by RT-qPCR in the original sequencing cohort and a replication cohort.

Samples that did not meet our quality control cut-off were removed from the dataset. Differential expression trends in the discovery cohort (9 RRMS patients and 5 HCs) were replicated for all miRNAs with the exception of let-7f-5p (Fig. 2). While the significance threshold ($p < 0.05$) was not reached, this may be a result of insufficient power to detect a significant change. With the aim of assessing whether differential erythrocyte miRNA expression was driven by DMTs as opposed to disease, the original sequencing cohort was segregated by DMT. No formal analysis was carried out due to lack of power, yet visual representation shows that with the exception of miR-3200-3p, miR-3200-5p, and miR-652-3p, off treatment RRMS patients' erythrocyte miRNA expression resembles that of patients on DMT (Additional file 4: Figure S2).

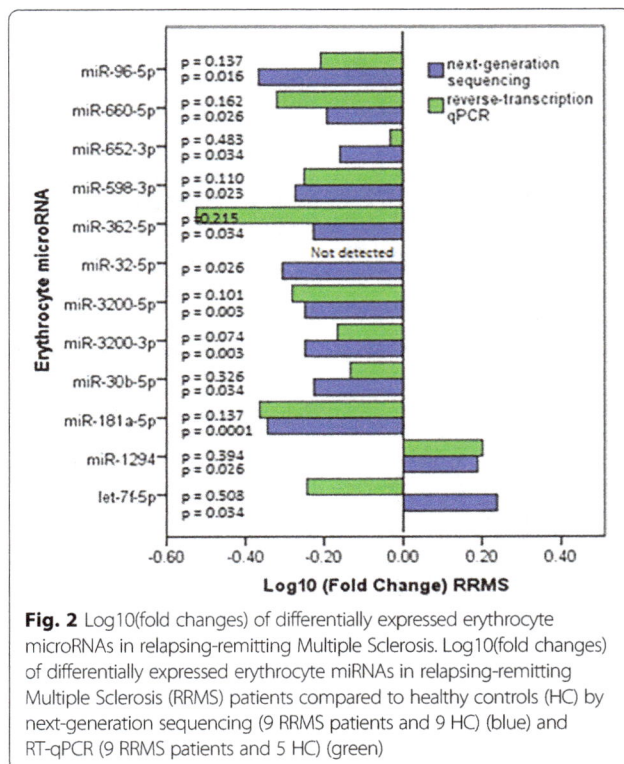

Fig. 2 Log10(fold changes) of differentially expressed erythrocyte microRNAs in relapsing-remitting Multiple Sclerosis. Log10(fold changes) of differentially expressed erythrocyte miRNAs in relapsing-remitting Multiple Sclerosis (RRMS) patients compared to healthy controls (HC) by next-generation sequencing (9 RRMS patients and 9 HC) (blue) and RT-qPCR (9 RRMS patients and 5 HC) (green)

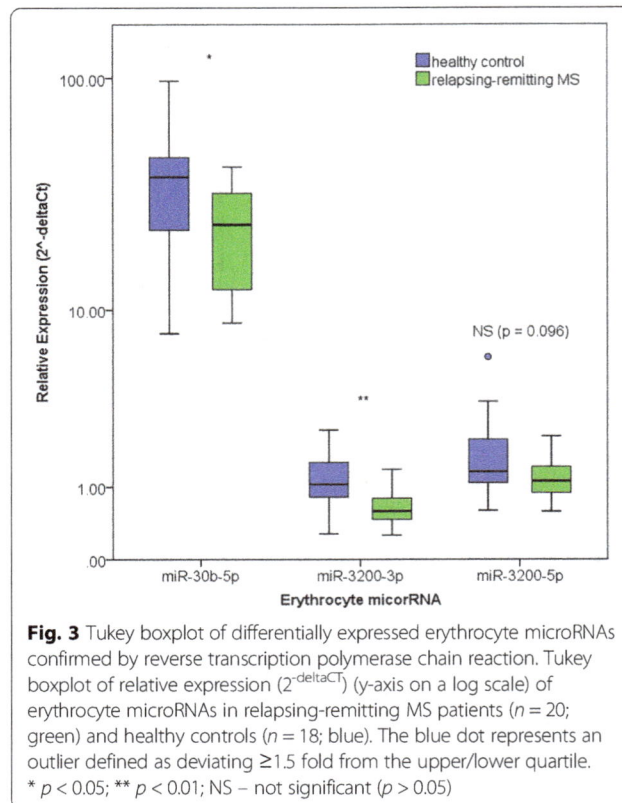

Fig. 3 Tukey boxplot of differentially expressed erythrocyte microRNAs confirmed by reverse transcription polymerase chain reaction. Tukey boxplot of relative expression ($2^{-\text{deltaCT}}$) (y-axis on a log scale) of erythrocyte microRNAs in relapsing-remitting MS patients ($n = 20$; green) and healthy controls ($n = 18$; blue). The blue dot represents an outlier defined as deviating ≥1.5 fold from the upper/lower quartile. * $p < 0.05$; ** $p < 0.01$; NS – not significant ($p > 0.05$)

RT-qPCR experiments were replicated in a larger, more uniform cohort of 20 RRMS patients and 18 HCs. Decreased expression of miR-30b-5p (0.61 fold, $p < 0.05$) and miR-3200-3p (0.36 fold, $p < 0.01$) was confirmed. Decreased expression of miR-3200-5p (0.66 fold, NS $p = 0.096$) approached significant threshold and was hence included in further analysis (Fig. 3). To assess the biomarker potential of the confirmed miRNAs, ROC curve analysis was performed for miRNAs that showed differential expression. ROC curves graphically illustrate the diagnostic potential of a binary outcome, in this case RRMS or HC, at different thresholds. This allows the determination of true and false positives for each of the thresholds, and specificity and sensitivity to be calculated.

Cut-off values that maximised both specificity and sensitivity were chosen. MiR-3200-3p showed the greatest biomarker potential being able to distinguish between RRMS patients and HCs with 75.5% accuracy ($p < 0.01$; relative expression cut-off: 0.81), 72.7% sensitivity, and 84.0% specificity. MiR-30b-5p and miR-3200-5p were able to differentiate between RRMS and HCs with 70.5% (p < 0.05) and 65.8% ($p = 0.064$) accuracy, 68.2% and 59.1% sensitivity, and 72.0% and 68.0% specificity respectively (Fig. 4; Table 2). Combining relative expression (using cut-off values in Table 2) of the three confirmed miRNAs (miR-30b-5p, miR-3200-3p, and miR-3200-5p) in a binary logistic regression with MS or HC being the dichotomous

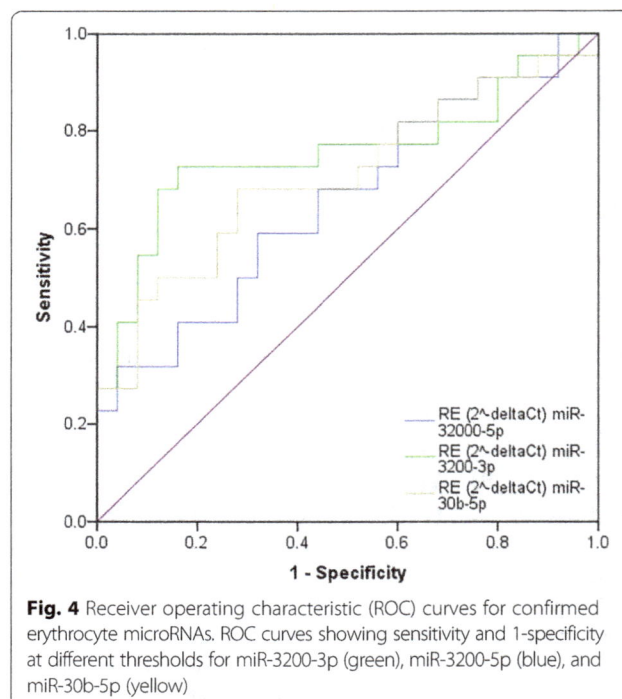

Fig. 4 Receiver operating characteristic (ROC) curves for confirmed erythrocyte microRNAs. ROC curves showing sensitivity and 1-specificity at different thresholds for miR-3200-3p (green), miR-3200-5p (blue), and miR-30b-5p (yellow)

Table 2 Receiver operating characteristic curve (ROC) results for the three confirmed erythrocyte microRNAs

MicroRNA	RE Cut-Off	Sensitivity (%)	Specificity (%)	Accuracy (%)	p-value
miR-30b-5p	34.40	68.2	72.0	70.5	0.016
miR-3200-3p	0.81	72.7	84.0	75.5	0.003
miR-3200-5p	1.20	59.1	68.0	65.8	0.064

RE relative expression ($2^{-deltaCT}$)

outcome, cases and controls could be assigned to their respective category with overall accuracy of 83.0%, 77.3% sensitivity, and 88.0% specificity (Table 3).

To determined clinical impact of differentially expressed erythrocyte miRNAs Pearson correlation coefficients between confirmed miRNAs and recorded disease outcome measures (Table 1) were calculated. Relative expression of miR-3200-5p was positively correlated with patients most recent (within a year of sample collection) cognitive assessment measured by audio-recorded cognitive screen (ARCS) [36] (Pearson correlation coefficient: 0.597; p < 0.01) (Fig. 5), as well as some of the ARCS' subdomains (Table 4). No further correlations between confirmed miRNAs and disease outcome measures, age, or bench time (elapsed time between blood collection and processing) were identified.

There were no significant differences in miRNA levels between patients on natalizumab ($n = 12$) and fingolimod ($n = 13$) across the 12 assessed erythrocyte miRNAs.

MiRNA target prediction

Given that fold changes were only modest for all differentially expressed miRNAs (Fig. 2), it is unlikely that a single miRNA is significantly affecting target gene expression. To this end, it was reasoned that several miRNAs may work in concert to target a few specific messenger RNAs (mRNAs). MiRSystem [35] was used to identify genes targeted by several of the 12 differentially expressed miRNAs identified by NGS. MiRSystem identified several genes targeted by four of the miRNAs flagged by NGS and one gene, *MIER 3* (mesoderm induction early response 1, family member 3), was targeted by five of the miRNAs identified as differentially expressed by NGS (Table 5).

Table 3 Classification of relapsing-remitting Multiple Sclerosis patients and healthy controls based on three erythrocyte miRNAs

		Predicted		Percentage Correct (%)
		RRMS	HC	
Observed	RRMS	22	3	88.0
	HC	5	17	77.3
Overall percentage				83.0

RRMS relapsing-remitting Multiple Sclerosis, HC healthy control

Discussion

This is the first study to compare the erythrocyte miRNA profile of RRMS patients to HCs. Differentially expressed erythrocyte miRNAs were identified in both the sequencing and replication cohort. Three miRNAs (miR-30b-5p, miR-3200-3p and miR-3200-5p) were found to show decreased expression in RRMS erythrocytes compared to HC erythrocytes and the combination of these miRNAs (miR-30b-5p, miR-3200-3p and miR-3200-5p) into a composite biomarker, was able to differentiate between RRMS patients and healthy controls with 77.3% sensitivity, 88.0% specificity, overall accuracy of 83.0%. Additionally, miR-3200-5p showed moderate correlation with patients' cognitive function, determined by ARCS (correlation coefficient: 0.60; $p < 0.01$).

Current MS diagnosis is based on the 2013 revisions to the McDonald criteria and clinical evidence is a crucial component of this diagnosis [29]. Diagnosis and monitoring of MS is underpinned by demyelinating lesions on MRI and supported by positive oligoclonal bands in patients' cerebrospinal fluid (CSF), requiring an invasive lumbar puncture. There is no reliable blood test that may guide diagnosis, monitoring, and selection of treatment options [1, 2]. Differential expression of miRNAs in erythrocytes, which can be easily obtained as

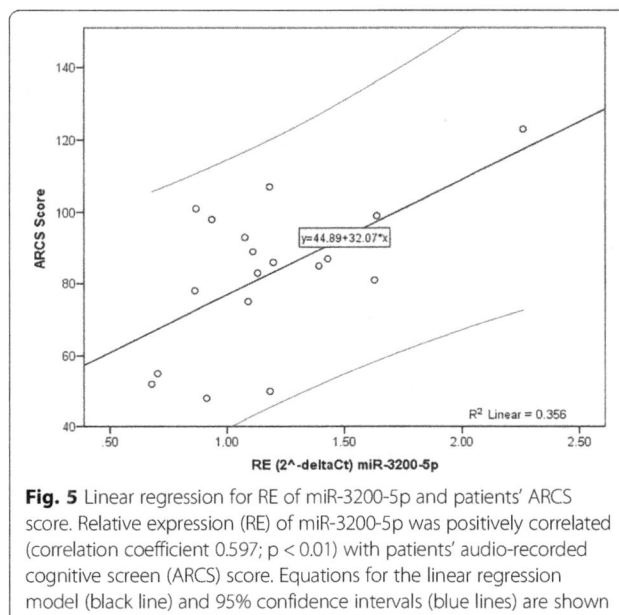

Fig. 5 Linear regression for RE of miR-3200-5p and patients' ARCS score. Relative expression (RE) of miR-3200-5p was positively correlated (correlation coefficient 0.597; p < 0.01) with patients' audio-recorded cognitive screen (ARCS) score. Equations for the linear regression model (black line) and 95% confidence intervals (blue lines) are shown

Table 4 Pearson correlation coefficients between miR-3200-5p and ARCS scores and subdomains

	Pearson Correlation Coefficient	p-value
Total ARCS	**0.597**	**0.009**
Quick ARCS	**0.592**	**0.010**
Memory Domain	0.427	0.077
Fluency Domain	**0.499**	**0.035**
Visuospatial Domain	0.314	0.205
Language Domain	0.282	0.256
Attention Domain	0.391	0.108
Speed of Writing	**0.634**	**0.005**

ARCS audio-recorded cognitive screen; significant correlations are highlighted in bold

part of other routine blood tests, indicates potential as supportive biomarkers for MS diagnosis and monitoring, reducing cost and patient discomfort associated with current paraclinical investigations. Erythrocytes are abundant in whole blood and thought to be translationally inactive; therefore, they lend themselves as stable biomarkers and should be further investigated. In order to establish the true diagnostic potential of erythrocyte miRNAs, their expression in MS needs to be compared to other differential diagnoses, this should be addressed by future studies. Differential diagnoses for MS include vascular diseases, such as systemic vasculitis, conditions of the brain and spinal cord, such as cerebellar ataxias, and tumours and structural lesions in the CNS [3]. Thus far, erythrocyte miRNAs have not been studied in diseases that make up the differential diagnoses for MS. Nonetheless, a study investigating whole blood miRNA profiles in CIS/RRMS patients and patients with neuromyelitis optica spectrum disorders (NMOSD) found differential expression of miR-30b in their discovery cohort (20 CIS/RRMS patients and 20 NMOSD patients) and replication cohort (19 RRMS/CIS patients and 18 NMOSD patients) [37]. As miR-30b was also found to be differentially expressed in this study and whole blood

miRNAs have been found to reflect erythrocyte miRNAs [6], the aforementioned finding [37] underpins the potential erythrocyte miRNAs have as diagnostic biomarkers for MS. Studies have also compared whole blood miRNA profiles between stroke patients and healthy controls, highlighting differential expression patterns [38] and focusing on let-7e-5p expression [39]. With the differential expression patterns between stroke patients and healthy controls [38, 39] differing from the differential erythrocyte miRNA expression between healthy controls and RRMS patients identified by this study, one may argue that miRNAs can differentiate between stroke and RRMS patients, however this needs to be confirmed through further investigation.

NGS of erythrocyte miRNAs of female RRMS patients and HCs revealed 236 known miRNAs across RRMS and HC samples. Several of the miRNAs flagged by NGS, including the confirmed miR-3200-3p, have also been identified in Alzheimer's Disease (AD). Satoh et al. identified decreased expression of let-7f-5p, miR-660-5p, miR-1294, and miR-3200-3p, as well as several others [40]. While not all trends match those in RRMS (Fig. 2), involvement of the same miRNAs in two distinct neurological diseases suggests their overall importance for the CNS. Satoh et al. used datasets from whole blood samples [40], not isolated erythrocytes, which raises the possibility of lymphocyte contamination. However, a previous study has shown that whole blood miRNAs largely reflect erythrocyte miRNAs [6], allowing for comparison between the two studies. Thus far, isolated erythrocyte miRNAs have not been studied in diseases other than malaria [41] and sickle cell disease [6].

One of the major symptoms of MS is cognitive impairment, which may develop in the absence of clinical relapse [2, 3]. Appropriate management of cognitive impairment is only possible if it can be detected early in the affected population [42]. Conventional neuropsychological assessment, the gold standard for detecting changes in cognition, is time-consuming, requires a

Table 5 MicroRNA target prediction results

Target Gene	Gene Description	Observed microRNA
MIER 3	mesoderm induction early response 1, family member 3	miR-181a-5p, miR-30b-5p, miR-32-5p, miR-362-5p, miR-660-5p
BCL2L11	BCL2-like 11 (apoptosis facilitator)	miR-181a-5p, miR-30b-5p, miR-32-5p, miR-362-5p
SEC24A	SEC24, family member A	miR-181a-5p, miR-30b-5p, miR-32-5p, miR-660-5p
SCN3A	sodium channel, voltage-gated type III, alpha subunit	miR-30b-5p, miR-32-5p, miR-362-5p, miR-660-5p
BCL11A	B-cell CLL/lymphoma 11A (zinc finger protein)	miR-181a-5p, miR-30b-5p, miR-32-5p, miR-362-5p
YTHDF3	YTH domain family, member 3	miR-181a-5p, miR-30b-5p, miR-362-5p, miR-660-5p
NFAT5	nuclear factor of activated T-cells 5, tonicity response	miR-181a-5p, miR-30b-5p, miR-32-5p, miR-660-5p
CPEB4	cytoplasmic polyadenylation element binding protein 4	miR-181a-5p, miR-30b-5p, miR-32-5p, miR-660-5p
LIN28		miR-181a-5p, miR-30b-5p, miR-32-5p, miR-598-3p
CNTN4	contactin 4	miR-181a-5p, miR-30b-5p, miR-32-5p, miR-362-5p

trained psychologist, and is not feasible for routine clinical practice. Consequently, other cognitive screening instruments, such as the ARCS, have been developed; nonetheless, the ARCS still requires patients to spend 35 min in a quiet room [36]. No blood-borne biomarker for cognitive impairment has been implemented in clinical practice [43]. Differential expression of miR-3200-5p was correlated with patients' most recent ARCS score (correlation coefficient: 0.597, $p < 0.01$), indicating that this miRNA may serve as a biomarker for cognitive function, reflecting global neuronal loss. The strongest correlation was observed between the subdomain speed of writing and the miRNA (correlation coefficient: 0.634, p < 0.01). Speed of writing requires patients to write out the word "table" as many times as possible in 30 s, reflecting information processing and fine motor skills [36]. The idea that circulating miRNAs may reflect cognitive impairment is not new: two small studies looked at mild cognitive impairment in the elderly and identified some miRNAs that correlated with mild cognitive impairment with high sensitivity and specificity [42, 43]. Cognitive decline is an early sign of MS and may reflect CNS damage more accurately than EDSS scores [44, 45]. Early detection for timely treatment and management are key to improve outcomes in MS, yet current cognitive screens are time and labour intensive and can be distressing for patients. The correlation between miR-3200-5p and patients' ARCS score indicates this miRNA's potential to be developed into a biomarker for cognitive impairment. Longitudinal assessment and validation in a larger cohort are necessary to confirm this hypothesis.

While a range of targets were predicted by miRSystem [35], fold changes in differentially expressed miRNAs were only minor, reducing the likelihood that a single miRNA is affecting gene expression. Nonetheless, several of the differentially expressed miRNAs were found to target the same genes, potentially amplifying dysregulation [18]. None of the predicted targets play an established role in mature erythrocytes and *MIER3* is not known to play a role in MS. The role of miRNAs in translationally inactive mature erythrocytes remains to be elucidated [24]. It has been suggested that erythrocyte miRNAs are remnants from earlier stages of erythrocyte development, where they played crucial roles in cell differentiation and maturation [6, 22]. Notwithstanding, erythrocyte miRNAs may play a more active role, functioning as intercellular communicators through erythrocyte-derived EVs. EVs are small, membrane-bound vesicles, containing proteins, nucleic acids, and lipids, which can be derived from a variety of cells, including erythrocytes [25].

None of the differentially expressed erythrocyte miRNAs were found to be highly abundant in erythrocytes (some of the most abundant miRNAs were miR-25, miR-144, miR-451, miR-182, and members of the let-7 family; Additional file 1: Table S1) and the reason for the observed differential expression remains to be clarified. Potential angles for investigation include stabilisation of certain miRNAs through associations with protein complexes, such as Argonaute proteins [22] and other non-coding RNAs [18], as well as targeted packaging and loss of certain miRNAs through EVs [25].

Recruited patients were on various DMTs (Table 1), some of which are known to alter erythrocyte phenotypes [8–13]. To account for the treatment effects, patients were recruited on a range of therapies, with the intent of identifying miRNA signatures that were disease- rather than treatment-specific. While lack of power did not allow for formal comparisons between RRMS patients on DMTs and untreated RRMS patients, visual comparison indicated that expression of miR-3200-3p, miR-3200-5p, and miR-652-3p might differ between these groups (Additional file 4: Figure S2). These differences and the effect of DMTs on erythrocyte miRNA expression needs to be further investigated and some of the findings of this study may be specific to MS patients on DMTs. Differences between DMTs were also assessed. Differential expression between natalizumab and fingolimod treated patients was evident for let-7f-5p, which showed increased expression in patients on fingolimod compared to patients on natalizumab (data not shown). While not statistically significant, this difference may explain why the trend of differential expression could not be replicated by RT-qPCR for let-7f-5p (Fig. 2). Neither of the treatment groups showed differential let-7f-5p expression compared to healthy controls (data not shown). Members of the let-7 family have been reported in other erythrocyte miRNA studies [6, 22, 23], where they are thought to be involved in erythropoiesis [46], and have also been shown to be less expressed in MS patients [47]. Cox et al. [47] used PAXGene (Qiagen, Germany) technology to analyse whole blood miRNA expression. Lack of similarity between identified miRNAs, other than let-7f, by Cox et al. and in this study, may reflect differences in cell make up, with PAXGene technology focussing mostly on leukocytes. Nevertheless, the reason for the difference in miRNA expression between treatments remains unknown and warrants further investigation.

Total RNA obtained from 10 ml whole blood varied between 9.40 and 35.35 μg (Additional file 1: Figure S1). Both reticulocytes and nucleated cells have been shown to harbour greater amounts of total RNA than erythrocytes [6]. Increased RNA yields from erythrocytes of patients treated with natalizumab may reflect increased levels of circulating erythrocyte precursors in these patients [8–10].

While low power to detect small differences in miRNA species and the recruitment of patients on different DMTs, some of which are known to alter erythrocytes [8–13], should be addressed by future studies, these preliminary results indicate that erythrocyte miRNAs should be incorporated into the growing list of MS biomarkers. Future investigations should aim to recruit larger numbers of treatment-naïve patients (including male MS patients), assess intra-individual variability, and evaluate specificity of observed differential expression to MS. In addition to healthy controls, future studies should aim to recruit pathological controls suffering from other systemic inflammatory, neurodegenerative, and autoimmune diseases.

The potential importance of erythrocyte pellets to MS and other diseases is starting to be recognized: Erythrocyte/granulocyte pellets are already being stored as part of the UK ME/CFS Biobank [48] and future investigations into erythrocytes and MS, or other autoimmune diseases, may provide a novel avenue for immunoregulatory prophylaxis and treatment options [49].

Conclusions

This is the first study to explore erythrocyte miRNAs in RRMS. We find evidence to suggest that erythrocyte miRNAs, particularly miR-30b-5p, miR-3200-3p and miR-3200-5p, may be exploited as novel MS biomarkers and miR-3200-5p may be developed into a biomarker for cognitive decline. Further investigations are warranted to substantiate these findings as erythrocytes can be easily and cost-effectively purified and novel biomarkers are required to aid diagnosis and stratification of MS patients.

Additional files

Additional file 1: Table S1. Next-generation sequencing results of erythrocyte microRNAs for 9 healthy controls and 9 relapsing-remitting Multiple Sclerosis patients.

Additional file 2: Table S2. Erythrocyte purity determined by flow cytometry ($n = 10$). Data is shown as mean percent positive events out of 20,000 events.

Additional file 3: Figure S1. Total erythrocyte RNA extracted from 10 ml whole blood by disease-modifying therapy. Mean total erythrocyte RNA yields from 10 ml whole blood for 2 patients off treatment, 2 on dimethyl fumarate, 13 on fingolimod, 12 on natalizumab and 27 healthy controls. Error bars represent standard deviation (SD). ** $p < 0.01$; *** $p < 0.001$.

Additional file 4 Figure S2. Tukey boxplot of relative expression ($2^{-deltaCt}$) of differentially expressed erythrocyte microRNAs in the sequencing cohort by disease-modifying therapy. Relative expression ($2^{-deltaCt}$) (y-axis on a logarithmic scale) of differentially expressed erythrocyte miRNAs (x-axis) by disease-modifying therapy (fingolimod: $n = 3$; natalizumab: $n = 2$; dimethyl fumarate: $n = 2$; off treatment: $n = 2$) and including healthy controls ($n = 5$). The dots represent outliers defined as deviating ≥1.5 fold from the upper/lower quartile.

Abbreviations

AD: Alzheimer's disease; ARCS: Audio-recorded cognitive screen; AUC: Area under the curve; BBB: Blood-brain barrier; CNS: Central nervous system; CSF: Cerebrospinal fluid; DMT: Disease-modifying therapy; EDSS: Extended disability status scale; EV: Extracellular vesicle; FDR: False discovery rate; HBSS: Hanks' balanced salt solution; HC: Healthy control; miRNA: microRNA; MRI: Magnetic resonance imaging; mRNA: messenger RNA; MS: Multiple Sclerosis; NGS: Next-generation sequencing; NMOSD: Neuromyelitis optica spectrum disorder; PBMC: Peripheral blood mononuclear cell; RE: Relative expression; ROC: Receiver operating characteristic; RRMS: Relapsing-remitting Multiple Sclerosis; RT-qPCR: Reverse transcription quantitative polymerase chain reaction; SD: Standard deviation of the mean

Acknowledgements

The authors would like to acknowledge PhD candidate Sharon Song and Dr. Lisa Anderson for performing the NGS experiments. We would like to acknowledge Dr. Karen Ribbons for her assistance in establishing the miRNA-ARCS correlation. Further, we would like to thank Susan Agland and Trish Collinson for assisting with sample collection and laboratory work. We would like to extend our gratitude to all MS patients and control participants that volunteered to be part of this study.

Funding

This project was funded by Bond University and an MSRA (MS Research Australia) Grant. K Groen is funded by a scholarship from the University of Newcastle and was funded by a partial scholarship from Bond University at the time of sample collection. KA Sanders was funded by a scholarship from Multiple Sclerosis Research Australia and the Trish Multiple Sclerosis Research Foundation. VE Maltby is funded by fellowships from Multiple Sclerosis Research Australia and the Canadian Institutes of Health Research.

Authors' contributions

KG and LT, who had the original idea, drafted the project proposal. KG drafted the manuscript, processed the majority of the samples, carried out the method optimisation and RT-qPCR experiments, put together figures and tables and performed statistical analysis. VEM edited the manuscript, processed some of the samples and supervised KG in the laboratory. RAL and LF carried out analysis of the NGS data and provided guidance for further statistical analysis. KAS aided sample collection and processing. All authors participated in the editing and drafting of the manuscript. JLS recruited patients through the John Hunter hospital and supervised the project with RJS. All authors read and approved the final manuscript.

Competing interests

JLS's institution receives non-directed funding, as well as honoraria for presentations and membership on advisory boards from Sanofi Aventis, Biogen Idec, Bayer Health Care, Merck Serono, Teva, Roche, and Novartis Australia.

Author details

[1]School of Medicine and Public Health, University of Newcastle, Callaghan, NSW 2308, Australia. [2]Centre for Information Based Medicine, Level 3 West, Hunter Medical Research Institute, 1 Kookaburra Circuit, New Lambton Heights, NSW 2305, Australia. [3]Institute of Health and Biomedical Innovations, Genomics Research Centre, Queensland University of Technology, Kelvin Grove, QLD 4059, Australia. [4]Centre for Anatomical and Human Sciences, Hull York Medical School, Hull HU6 7RX, UK. [5]Diamantina Institute, University of Queensland, Woolloongabba, QLD 4102, Australia. [6]Division of Molecular Genetics, Pathology North, John Hunter Hospital, New Lambton Heights, NSW 2305, Australia. [7]School of Biomedical Sciences and Pharmacy, University of Newcastle, Callaghan, NSW 2308, Australia. [8]Faculty of Health Sciences and Medicine, Bond University, QLD, Robina 4229, Australia.

[9]Department of Neurology, John Hunter Hospital, New Lambton Heights, NSW 2305, Australia.

References

1. Lublin FD, Reingold SC, Cohen JA, Cutter GR, Sorensen PS, Thompson AJ, Wolinsky JS, Balcer LJ, Banwell B, Barkhof F, et al. Defining the clinical course of multiple sclerosis: the 2013 revisions. Neurology. 2014;83(3):278–86.
2. Dendrou CA, Fugger L, Friese MA. Immunopathology of multiple sclerosis. Nat Rev Immunol. 2015;15(9):545–58.
3. Compston A, Coles A. Multiple sclerosis. Lancet. 2008;372(9648):1502–17.
4. Marieb EN, Hoehn K. Human anatomy & physiology. Boston: Pearson; 2013.
5. Klinken SP. Red blood cells. Int J Biochem Cell Bio. 2002;34(12):1513–8.
6. Chen SY, Wang Y, Telen MJ, Chi JT. The genomic analysis of erythrocyte microRNA expression in sickle cell diseases. PlosOne. 2008;3(6):e2360.
7. Groen K, Maltby VE, Sanders KA, Scott RJ, Tajouri L, Lechner-Scott J. Erythrocytes in multiple sclerosis–forgotten contributors to the pathophysiology? Mult Scler J Exp Transl Clin. 2016;2:2055217316649981.
8. Bridel C, Beauverd Y, Samii K, Lalive PH. Hematologic modifications in natalizumab-treated multiple sclerosis patients: an 18-month longitudinal study. Neurol Neuroimmunol Neuroinflamm. 2015;2(4):123.
9. Jing D, Oelschlaegel U, Ordemann R, Holig K, Ehninger G, Reichmann H, Ziemssen T, Bornhauser M. CD49d blockade by natalizumab in patients with multiple sclerosis affects steady-state hematopoiesis and mobilizes progenitors with a distinct phenotype and function. Bone Marrow Transplant. 2010;45(10):1489–96.
10. Lesesve JF, Debouverie M, Decarvalho Bittencourt M, Bene MC. CD49d blockade by natalizumab therapy in patients with multiple sclerosis increases immature B-lymphocytes. Bone Marrow Transplant. 2011;46(11):1489–91.
11. Arnold M, Bissinger R, Lang F. Mitoxantrone-induced suicidal erythrocyte death. Cell Physiol Biochem. 2014;34(5):1756–67.
12. Eberhard M, Ferlinz K, Alizzi K, Cacciato PM, Faggio C, Foller M, Lang F. FTY720-induced suicidal erythrocyte death. Cell Physiol Biochem. 2010; 26(4–5):761–6.
13. Ghashghaeinia M, Bobbala D, Wieder T, Koka S, Bruck J, Fehrenbacher B, Rocken M, Schaller M, Lang F, Ghoreschi K. Targeting glutathione by dimethylfumarate protects against experimental malaria by enhancing erythrocyte cell membrane scrambling. Am J Physiol Cell Physiol. 2010; 299(4):791–804.
14. Peng YF, Cao WY, Zhang Q, Chen D, Zhang ZX. Assessment of the relationship between red cell distribution width and multiple sclerosis. Medicine (Baltimore). 2015;94(29):e1182.
15. Lockwood SY, Summers S, Eggenberger E, Spence DM. An in vitro diagnostic for multiple sclerosis based on C-peptide binding to erythrocytes. EBioMedicine. 2016;11:249–52.
16. Bielekova B, Martin R. Development of biomarkers in multiple sclerosis. Brain. 2004;127(7):1463–78.
17. Raphael I, Webb J, Stuve O, Haskins WE, Forsthuber TG. Body fluid biomarkers in multiple sclerosis: how far we have come and how they could affect the clinic now and in the future. Expert Rev Clin Immunol. 2015;11(1):69–91.
18. Esteller M. Non-coding RNAs in human disease. Nat Rev Genet. 2011;12(12): 861–74.
19. Keller A, Leidinger P, Lange J, Borries A, Schroers H, Scheffler M, Lenhof HP, Ruprecht K, Meese E. Multiple sclerosis: microRNA expression profiles accurately differentiate patients with relapsing-remitting disease from healthy controls. PlosOne. 2009;4(10):e7440.
20. Otaegui D, Baranzini SE, Armananzas R, Calvo B, Munoz-Culla M, Khankhanian P, Inza I, Lozano JA, Castillo-Trivino T, Asensio A, et al. Differential micro RNA expression in PBMC from multiple sclerosis patients. PlosOne. 2009;4(7):e6309.
21. Chun J, Hartung HP. Mechanism of action of oral fingolimod (FTY720) in multiple sclerosis. Clin Neuropharmacol. 2010;33(2):91–101.
22. Azzouzi I, Moest H, Wollscheid B, Schmugge M, Eekels JJ, Speer O. Deep sequencing and proteomic analysis of the microRNA-induced silencing complex in human red blood cells. Exp Hematol. 2015;43(5):382–92.
23. Doss JF, Corcoran DL, Jima DD, Telen MJ, Dave SS, Chi JT. A comprehensive joint analysis of the long and short RNA transcriptomes of human erythrocytes. BMC Genomics. 2015;16(1):952.
24. Goh SH, Lee YT, Bouffard GG, Miller JL. Hembase: browser and genome portal for hematology and erythroid biology. Nucleic Acids Res. 2004; 32(suppl 1):572–4.
25. Zaborowski MP, Balaj L, Breakefield XO, Lai CP. Extracellular vesicles: composition, biological relevance, and methods of study. Bioscience. 2015; 65(8):783–97.
26. Smith J. Exercise, training and red blood cell turnover. Sports Med. 1995; 19(1):9–31.
27. Lang E, Lang F. Triggers, inhibitors, mechanisms, and significance of eryptosis: the suicidal erythrocyte death. Biomed Res Int. 2015;2015:513518.
28. Daniels SI, Sillé FCM, Goldbaum A, Yee B, Key EF, Zhang L, Smith MT, Thomas R. Improving power to detect changes in blood miRNA expression by accounting for sources of variability in experimental designs. Cancer Epidemiol Biomark Prev. 2014;23(12):2658–66.
29. Polman CH, Reingold SC, Banwell B, Clanet M, Cohen JA, Filippi M, Fujihara K, Havrdova E, Hutchinson M, Kappos L, et al. Diagnostic criteria for multiple sclerosis: 2010 revisions to the McDonald criteria. Ann Neurol. 2011;69(2): 292–302.
30. Butzkueven H, Chapman J, Cristiano E, Grand'Maison F, Hoffmann M, Izquierdo G, Jolley D, Kappos L, Leist T, Pöhlau D, et al. MSBase: an international, online registry and platform for collaborative outcomes research in multiple sclerosis. Mult Scler J. 2006;12(6):769–74.
31. Kozomara A, Griffiths-Jones S. miRBase: annotating high confidence microRNAs using deep sequencing data. Nucleic Acids Res. 2014; 42(Database issue):D68–73.
32. Dobin A, Davis CA, Schlesinger F, Drenkow J, Zaleski C, Jha S, Batut P, Chaisson M, Gingeras TR. STAR: ultrafast universal RNA-seq aligner. Bioinformatics. 2013;29(1):15–21.
33. Love MI, Huber W, Anders S. Moderated estimation of fold change and dispersion for RNA-seq data with DESeq2. Genome Biol. 2014;15(12):550.
34. Choong ML, Yang HH, McNiece I. MicroRNA expression profiling during human cord blood-derived CD34 cell erythropoiesis. Exp Hematol. 2007; 35(4):551–64.
35. Lu T-P, Lee C-Y, Tsai M-H, Chiu Y-C, Hsiao CK, Lai L-C, Chuang EY. miRSystem: an integrated system for characterizing enriched functions and pathways of MicroRNA targets. PlosOne. 2012;7(8):e42390.
36. Schofield PW, Lee SJ, Lewin TJ, Lyall G, Moyle J, Attia J, McEvoy M. The audio recorded cognitive screen (ARCS): a flexible hybrid cognitive test instrument. J Neurol Neurosurg Psychiatry. 2010;81(6):602–7.
37. Keller A, Leidinger P, Meese E, Haas J, Backes C, Rasche L, Behrens JR, Pfuhl C, Wakonig K, Giess RM, et al. Next-generation sequencing identifies altered whole blood microRNAs in neuromyelitis optica spectrum disorder which may permit discrimination from multiple sclerosis. J Neuroinflammation. 2015;12:196.
38. Tan KS, Armugam A, Sepramaniam S, Lim KY, Setyowati KD, Wang CW, Jeyaseelan K. Expression profile of MicroRNAs in young stroke patients. PlosOne. 2009;4(11):e7689.
39. Huang S, Lv Z, Guo Y, Li L, Zhang Y, Zhou L, Yang B, Wu S, Zhang Y, Xie C, et al. Identification of Blood Let-7e-5p as a Biomarker for Ischemic Stroke. PlosOne. 2016;11(10):e0163951.
40. Satoh J, Kino Y, Niida S. MicroRNA-Seq data analysis pipeline to identify blood biomarkers for Alzheimer's disease from public data. Biomark Insights. 2015;10:21–31.
41. Mantel PY, Hjelmqvist D, Walch M, Kharoubi-Hess S, Nilsson S, Ravel D, Ribeiro M, Gruring C, Ma S, Padmanabhan P, et al. Infected erythrocyte-derived extracellular vesicles alter vascular function via regulatory Ago2-miRNA complexes in malaria. Nat Commun. 2016;7:12727.
42. Kayano M, Higaki S, Satoh JI, Matsumoto K, Matsubara E, Takikawa O, Niida S. Plasma microRNA biomarker detection for mild cognitive impairment using differential correlation analysis. Biomarker Res. 2016;4:22.
43. Sheinerman KS, Tsivinsky VG, Abdullah L, Crawford F, Umansky SR. Plasma microRNA biomarkers for detection of mild cognitive impairment: biomarker validation study. Aging. 2013;5(12):925–38.
44. Feuillet L, Reuter F, Audoin B, Malikova I, Barrau K, Cherif AA, Pelletier J. Early cognitive impairment in patients with clinically isolated syndrome suggestive of multiple sclerosis. Mult Scler. 2007;13(1):124–7.
45. DeLuca GC, Yates RL, Beale H, Morrow SA. Cognitive impairment in multiple sclerosis: clinical, radiologic and pathologic insights. Brain Pathol. 2015;25(1):79–98.
46. Lawrie CH. microRNA expression in erythropoiesis and erythroid disorders. Br J Haematol. 2010;150(2):144–51.

47. Cox MB, Cairns MJ, Gandhi KS, Carroll AP, Moscovis S, Stewart GJ, Broadley S, Scott RJ, Booth DR, Lechner-Scott J. MicroRNAs miR-17 and miR-20a inhibit T cell activation genes and are under-expressed in MS whole blood. PlosOne. 2010;5(8):e12132.

48. Lacerda EM, Bowman EW, Cliff JM, Kingdon CC, King EC, Lee JS, Clark TG, Dockrell HM, Riley EM, Curran H, et al. The UK ME/CFS biobank for biomedical research on Myalgic encephalomyelitis/chronic fatigue syndrome (ME/CFS) and multiple sclerosis. Open J Bioresour. 2017;4.

49. Pishesha N, Bilate AM, Wibowo MC, Huang NJ, Li Z, Dhesycka R, Bousbaine D, Li H, Patterson HC, Dougan SK, et al. Engineered erythrocytes covalently linked to antigenic peptides can protect against autoimmune disease. Proc Natl Acad Sci U S A. 2017;114(12):3157–62.

2

Identifying the genetic causes for prenatally diagnosed structural congenital anomalies (SCAs) by whole-exome sequencing (WES)

Gordon K C Leung[1], Christopher C Y Mak[1], Jasmine L F Fung[1], Wilfred H S Wong[1], Mandy H Y Tsang[1], Mullin H C Yu[1], Steven L C Pei[1], K S Yeung[1], Gary T K Mok[1], C P Lee[2], Amelia P W Hui[2], Mary H Y Tang[2,3], Kelvin Y K Chan[2,3], Anthony P Y Liu[1], Wanling Yang[1], P C Sham[4], Anita S Y Kan[2,3*] and Brian H Y Chung[1,2,3*] (iD)

Abstract

Background: Whole-exome sequencing (WES) has become an invaluable tool for genetic diagnosis in paediatrics. However, it has not been widely adopted in the prenatal setting. This study evaluated the use of WES in prenatal genetic diagnosis in fetuses with structural congenital anomalies (SCAs) detected on prenatal ultrasound.

Method: Thirty-three families with fetal SCAs on prenatal ultrasonography and normal chromosomal microarray results were recruited. Genomic DNA was extracted from various fetal samples including amniotic fluid, chorionic villi, and placental tissue. Parental DNA was extracted from peripheral blood when available. We used WES to sequence the coding regions of parental-fetal trios and to identify the causal variants based on the ultrasonographic features of the fetus.

Results: Pathogenic mutations were identified in three families ($n = 3/33$, 9.1%), including mutations in *DNAH11*, *RAF1* and *CHD7*, which were associated with primary ciliary dyskinesia, Noonan syndrome, and CHARGE syndrome, respectively. In addition, variants of unknown significance (VUSs) were detected in six families (18.2%), in which genetic changes only partly explained prenatal features.

Conclusion: WES identified pathogenic mutations in 9.1% of fetuses with SCAs and normal chromosomal microarray results. Databases for fetal genotype-phenotype correlations and standardized guidelines for variant interpretation in prenatal diagnosis need to be established to facilitate the use of WES for routine testing in prenatal diagnosis.

Keywords: Prenatal exome, Variants of unknown clinical significance, Phenotyping

Background

Major congenital malformations occur in approximately 2–3% of all pregnancies. Fetal ultrasound is routinely used in prenatal care in developed countries, and approximately 1% of these scans reveal some form of structural congenital anomaly (SCA) [1]. Because SCAs are associated with genetic aberrations, the common practice is to offer fetal karyotyping either by chorionic villus sampling (CVS) or amniocentesis [2]. Chromosomal microarray analysis (CMA) is also used to improve the diagnostic yield of chromosomal disorders from conventional karyotype analysis [3, 4].

SCAs in the context of normal chromosome analysis (by either karyotype or CMA) remain a diagnostic challenge. Examination for dysmorphic features in the prenatal setting is particularly difficult. Without detailed clinical information on a patient's phenotype, SCAs due

* Correspondence: kansya@hku.hk; bhychung@hku.hk
[2]Department of Obstetrics and Gynaecology, Queen Mary Hospital, The University of Hong Kong, Hong Kong, Hong Kong Special Administrative Region, China
[1]Department of Paediatrics and Adolescent Medicine, LKS Faculty of Medicine, The University of Hong Kong, Room 103, 1/F, New Clinical Building, Hong Kong, Hong Kong Special Administrative Region, China
Full list of author information is available at the end of the article

to monogenic diseases often remain undiagnosed due to limitations of prenatal ultrasound or other imaging modalities. Even after comprehensive assessment of a newborn or fetal/perinatal autopsy after pregnancy termination, stillbirth, or neonatal death, many times no definitive diagnosis can be identified. This is in part due to the rarity of individual genetic syndromes and the heterogeneity of phenotypic features. All genetic conditions carry a risk of recurrence. Therefore, a genetic diagnosis is essential to provide accurate counselling regarding future pregnancies.

Currently, chromosomal microarray is the first-line prenatal diagnostic test for SCAs, as endorsed by the Society for Maternal-Fetal Medicine [5] and the American College of Obstetricians and Gynecologists [4, 6]. Wapner et al. reported the yield of karyotyping and microarray analysis in 4406 pregnancies referred for CVS or amniocentesis [3]. Chromosomal aneuploidies were identified in 8.7% of pregnancies, and when the karyotype was normal, CMA detected another clinically relevant copy number change in 6% of fetuses with structural anomalies and in 1.7% of pregnancies with advanced maternal age or positive aneuploidy screening. Our previous findings also support the use of CMA for prenatal diagnosis as either a first-line test or a further test for pregnancies with SCAs in Hong Kong [7].

WES has been used as a diagnostic tool in previously undiagnosed patients with suspected genetic disorders [8–11]. This high-throughput sequencing technique not only facilitates genetic diagnosis but also allows novel gene discovery in multiple well-defined syndromes or undiagnosed diseases [12–15]. Interpretation guidelines for assessing the pathogenicity of genetic variants in paediatric patients are now adopted in genetic laboratories or institutes [16, 17].

Although limited, several reports on the application of WES in prenatal diagnosis are available. Carss et al. presented the first cohort study of fetuses with structural abnormalities and identified genetic changes in 10% of cases using WES in 2014 [18]. Subsequent reports also showed that WES can improve the diagnostic yield in cases with cytogenetically normal findings and serve as an adjunct diagnostic tool for conventional tests [19–21]. Best et al. reviewed 31 published studies and conference abstracts on prenatal WES and reported that diagnostic rates vary from 6.2 to 80%. The study also indicated that fetuses with multiple congenital anomalies or clinical suspicion of a genetic syndrome are associated with a higher diagnostic yield [22]. The report also discussed the major challenges of using WES in the prenatal setting, such as interpretation of genetic variants. The objective of this study was to evaluate the use of WES for determining a genetic diagnosis in fetuses with prenatally diagnosed structural congenital anomalies and explore the benefits and challenges of utilizing WES in prenatal diagnosis in Hong Kong.

Methods

Ethics, consent and permissions

This study was approved by the Institutional Review Board of the University of Hong Kong/Hospital Authority Hong Kong West Cluster (HKU/HA HKW IRB) (Reference number UW14–323). Informed consent was obtained from the parents during pre-test counselling.

Patient recruitment

Thirty-three families with fetuses with SCAs, as identified by the Prenatal Diagnostic and Counselling Division in Tsan Yuk Hospital, Hong Kong, were included in the study. The remaining DNA of the fetuses after routine prenatal testing was used in subsequent analyses. DNA samples were obtained from various sources, including amniotic fluid, chorionic villi and placental tissues. Parental DNA was extracted from peripheral blood. All fetal samples were tested by normal quantitative fluorescence-polymerase chain reaction (QFPCR) and CMA, and the possibility of maternal cell contamination (MCC) was excluded.

Whole-exome sequencing

The SeqCap EZ Human Exome + UTR Kit (Roche, Germany) was used in 16 retrospective samples, and the TruSeq Rapid Exome Library Prep Kit (Illumina Inc., CA, USA) was used in 17 prospective samples for target exome enrichment. Exome enrichment was performed according to the manufacturers' protocols. Exome libraries were pooled and sequenced using Illumina platforms, with a target sequencing coverage of 100X. Raw data were analysed on the in-house bioinformatics pipeline built according to the Genome Analysis Toolkit (GATK) Best Practices Guideline for germline genetic variations [23]. The variants were then annotated using ANNOVAR [24]. Filtering was applied to rule out benign genetic variants, with a global or local (i.e., east Asian) population frequency > 0.01 [25]. Classification of pathogenic variants was performed with reference to the guideline recommended by the American College of Medical Genetics and Genomics (ACMG) [16] based on allelic frequency, family segregation, compatibility with phenotypes, in silico prediction, relevant disease databases and the literature.

Results

Thirty-three fetal samples were included, with a male to female ratio of 5:6. Sixteen samples were retrospectively archived, while 17 samples were prospectively collected. The sampling sources of genomic DNA included amniotic fluid for 22 samples, chorionic villi for four samples, placental tissues for six samples and cord blood of the fetus for one sample. MCC was not found in foetal samples by QFPCR. Thirty-three fetuses with SCAs were identified by prenatal ultrasound, including 16 (48.5%) exhibiting involvement of more than one system. The SCAs included cystic hygroma or increased nuchal translucency (NT > 3.5 mm) (N = 4) and cardiac (N = 7), central nervous system (CNS)-related (N = 25), skeletal (N = 4) and renal (N = 4) abnormalities. Other prenatal features included craniofacial dysmorphism (N = 5), flexion deformity (N = 4), situs inversus (N = 2) and ophthalmological abnormalities (N = 1).

WES was performed in 100 individuals. On average, 99.5% of the reads were mapped to the human genome (GRCh37). A total of 63.6% of the reads were mapped to the corresponding exome manifestations, and 16.6% of these reads were duplicates and were removed. The mean depth of on-target coverage was 68X. Out of the 33 families recruited, 27 families (81.8%) were sequenced as complete parental-fetal trios. One family was sequenced as a singleton, and one family was sequenced as a mother-fetus duplet. Four families were sequenced as quadruplets including a sibling with or without relevant clinical phenotypes.

For the genetic diagnosis results, we identified diagnostic mutations in three families (9.1%) (Table 1 and Fig. 1) and VUS in six families (18.2%) (Table 2). The clinical relevance of the three positive cases is described in greater detail below, while that of the fetuses with VUS is described in the Additional file 1.

PRE011 was the third pregnancy of a healthy non-consanguineous couple with two silent miscarriages. The fetus was identified to have cystic hygroma by foetal ultrasound at 12 weeks. Follow-up scans showed situs inversus, a hypoplastic left heart, a ventricular septal defect and an atretic aorta. Medical termination of the pregnancy was performed at 17 weeks of gestation. Post-mortem examination confirmed the presence of situs inversus and congenital heart defects. Trio WES showed compound heterozygous mutations in *DNAH11* (OMIM: 603339; NM_003777.3). A frameshift mutation, c.8533_8536delinsATCCG, was inherited from the father, and a missense mutation, c.13310G > A p.(Gly4437Glu), was inherited from the mother. Neither mutation was reported in unaffected individuals [26]. The frameshift mutation leads to premature termination of the protein transcript and was classified as pathogenic. The missense mutation was predicted to be deleterious by multiple bioinformatics algorithms and was therefore classified as likely pathogenic according to guideline suggested by ACMG [16]. Mutations in *DNAH11* are associated with primary ciliary dyskinesia (PCD) (OMIM: 611884), which is an autosomal recessive disorder that leads to abnormalities in the action of the cilia lining. The prenatal presentation of the fetus was compatible with PCD, but bronchiectasis and hearing problems could not be assessed in utero. Although both mutations were novel, the compatibility of the phenotypes and the loss-of-function nature of the paternal splice variant suggested that the *DNAH11* mutations were disease-causing in PRE011.

PRE032 was the first pregnancy of a healthy non-consanguineous couple. The fetus was identified to have cystic hygroma, a single umbilical artery and short long bones at 16 weeks. Follow-up scans showed additional findings of dilated left renal pelvis of 5 mm, a prominent cerebral ventricle of 9 mm, suspected partial agenesis of the corpus callosum, a right-sided aortic arch, mild cardiomegaly with a cardiothoracic ratio of 0.56, a thin rim of pericardial effusion, absence of the ductus venosus and umbilical vein drainage into the portal sinus. Medical termination of the pregnancy was performed at 22 weeks of gestation. No post-mortem examination was performed. *FGFR3* gene sequencing was performed but did not identify pathogenic mutations for skeletal dysplasia. WES identified a de novo missense mutation, c.778A > C p.(Thr260Pro), in *RAF1* (OMIM: 164760; NM_002880.3), and the mutation had not been reported. The mutation clustered with other pathogenic mutations in a conserved domain, and the same amino acid position with an alternate change was reported as pathogenic. *RAF1* is a known morbid gene associated with Noonan syndrome (OMIM: 611553). Although the mutation has not been reported previously, the ultrasound findings of the fetus were compatible with prenatal presentation of the genetic disorder. Therefore, this was also classified as pathogenic.

PRE033 was the second pregnancy of a healthy non-consanguineous couple with one silent miscarriage. The fetus was found to have cystic hygroma, pulmonary atresia with an intact ventricular septum and severe tricuspid regurgitation at 21 weeks. Medical termination of the pregnancy was performed at 22 weeks of gestation due to the presence of severe heart defects. Gross examination of the abortus showed low-set and atretic pinnae, and post-mortem examination was declined. The possibility of a Noonan-related syndrome was initially suspected, but WES showed no pathogenic mutations in associated genes. However, WES identified a de novo missense mutation, c.2957 + 1G > A, in *CHD7* (OMIM: 608892; NM_017780.3). The canonical splice site variant was predicted to lead to aberrant transcription in mRNA synthesis. Heterozygous loss-of-function mutations in *CHD7* are known to cause CHARGE syndrome in children (OMIM: 214800) [27, 28]. Although the mutation had not been reported in previous literature, the splice variant was regarded as a likely pathogenic mutation in the fetus.

Discussion

We performed WES in 33 families whose fetuses showed diverse SCAs detected by prenatal ultrasound. This demonstrates the feasibility of prenatal WES in Hong Kong. Further, we achieved a diagnostic yield of 9.1% identifying the causal mutation for the SCAs in a cohort

Table 1 List of cases with pathogenic mutation(s) identified by WES

Family number	Gene	Clinical phenotype	mutation site	allelic frequency in ExAC	parental origin	GERP score	CADD score	MutationTaster	PROVEAN	SIFT
PRE011	DNAH11	situs inversus; cardiac defects	c.13288G>A p.(Gly4430Glu)	8.14E-06	maternal	5.5199	34	Disease causing	Damaging	Damaging
			c.8533_8536delinsATCCG	not reported	paternal	N/A	36	N/A	N/A	N/A
PRE032	RAF1	multiple congenital abnormalities	c.778A>C p.(Trp260Pro)	not reported	de novo	5.73	23.6	Disease causing	Neutral	Damaging
PRE033	CHD7	cystic hygroma; pulmonary atresia (PA-IVS)	c.2957+1G>A	not reported	de novo	5.53	25.5	Disease causing	N/A	N/A

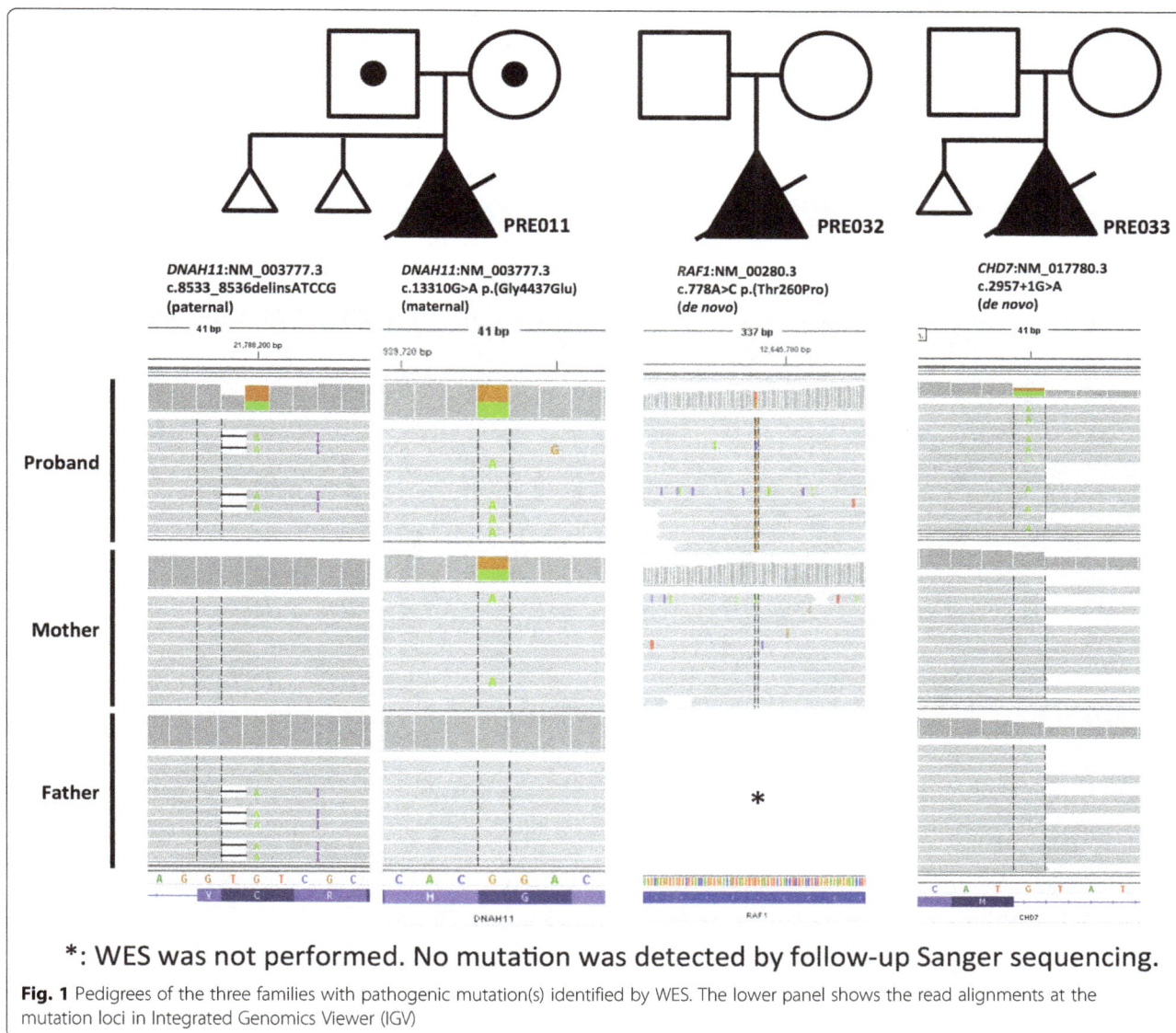

*: WES was not performed. No mutation was detected by follow-up Sanger sequencing.

Fig. 1 Pedigrees of the three families with pathogenic mutation(s) identified by WES. The lower panel shows the read alignments at the mutation loci in Integrated Genomics Viewer (IGV)

that had tested negative for chromosomal abnormalities by CMA. We also identified VUSs in 18% of the families, which are potential causal variants. Further determination of the potential pathogenicity of these variants requires postnatal follow-up with more detailed phenotyping or further biochemical testing. All three cases with pathogenic mutations identified were associated with multisystem abnormalities, indicating syndromal diagnoses that would have been difficult to establish prenatally without WES.

The application of WES for the identification of disease-causing mutations in prenatal diagnosis is often difficult compared with its application in liveborn patients. We encountered two major challenges in determining the genetic diagnoses of the fetuses with SCAs.

First, most diagnostic mutations and VUSs were not reported in the previous literature. All four mutations

from the three positive cases, and three of the eight VUSs from the six putative diagnoses were novel. In clinical genetics, gene discovery is heavily based on paediatric patients with detailed clinical phenotyping. Prenatal findings of genetic etiology could be a new area for novel discoveries, especially when mutations are perinatally fatal which decreases their likelihood of being previously reported. In order to increase the body of literature available on perinatally fatal genetic disease, comprehensive fetal phenotyping and post-mortem analysis should be encouraged, when appropriate, to aid interpretation of WES findings. Perinatal autopsy remains the gold standard for investigation of perinatal death. However, the perinatal autopsy rate is falling due, in part, to societal views on perinatal death investigation. Considering this, conversations encouraging further testing post-perinatal death

Table 2 List of cases with the possible causal genetic variant(s) identified by WES

Family number	Gene	Clinical phenotype	mutation site	allelic frequency in ExAC	parental origin	GERP score	CADD score	MutationTaster	PROVEAN	SIFT
PRE003	PACS1	ventriculomegaly; small cavum septum pellucidum	c.2413G>A;p.(Ala805Thr)	1.06E-04	maternal	4.94	16.64	Polymorphism	Neutral	Tolerated
PRE004	EEF1A2	multiple congenital abnormalities	c.862G>A;p.(Glu288Lys)	not reported	de novo	3.8199	28.1	Disease causing	Damaging	Damaging
PRE010	DIS3L2	microphthalmia; agenesis of corpus callosum	c.410A>G;p.(Tyr137Cys)	6.95E-04	maternal	5.65	11.53	Polymorphism	Neutral	Tolerated
			c.1826G>A;p.(Arg609Gln)	2.05E-05	paternal	5.42	34	Disease causing	Neutral	Damaging
PRE013	LRP2	agenesis of corpus callosum; cardiac defects	c.1593C>A;p.(Ser531Arg)	8.13E-06	maternal	5.7899	23.7	Disease causing	Neutral	Tolerated
			c.10538C>A;p.(Ser3513Tyr)	1.63E-05	paternal	5.96	28,9	Disease causing	Damaging	Damaging
PRE022	ATRX	multiple congenital abnormalities	c.1825C>G;p.(Pro609Ala)	1.07E-03	not determined	5.2199	0.004	Polymorphism	Neutral	Damaging
PRE028	MYH7	cardiac defects	c.3803G>A;p.(Arg1268His)	7.31E-05	de novo	4.9899	35	Disease causing	Damaging	Damaging

should be carefully conducted in a culturally appropriate manner.

Second, a lack of information regarding the clinical phenotypes of fetuses impeded complicates the determination of phenotype-genotype correlations. Identification of fetal features is limited by experience of obstetricians and resolution on fetal ultrasonography. In addition, assessing many late-onset features is not feasible in the prenatal setting, such as intellectual disability or global developmental delay. While this is a limitation, it is also a strength of WES. WES allows for "hypothesis free" un-biased analysis of the entire exome, as compared to the use of single gene or gene panel analyses prenatally [29]. This idea of WES as "hypothesis free" is not to indicate that it is recommended in cases with no evidence of dysmorphism but instead refers to its independence from pre-test assumptions. WES does not rely on physician hypotheses of what mutations or systems may be involved. This coverage allows for prenatal WES to be less dependent on accurate phenotype observations than testing that requires pre-test assumptions to be made [29].

One of the limitations of this study is the small cohort size. To ameliorate this, we performed a systematic review of related publications from 2014 to 2017 together with our postnatal WES cohort [30]. Publications with the keywords "Clinical exome sequencing" or "Diagnostic exome

sequencing" were included and classified into a prenatal group and a postnatal group. Only studies in which we could identify the diagnostic yield and the VUS rate were included. Incidental, secondary or other findings that were not related to the primary patient phenotypes were not considered. R statistic software version 3.4.1 with Rstudio version 1.1.383 was used to conduct the analysis. In summary, 473 fetuses and 8722 postnatal patients with diverse clinical manifestations were included. Due to the heterogeneity of the data, we used a random-effects model for the analysis. We found that the diagnostic rate of prenatal WES (0.20 with 95% CI [0.11, 0.29]) was significantly lower than that in postnatal studies (0.36 with 95% CI [0.31, 0.50]) ($p < 0.05$) (Fig. 2), while the proportion of VUSs in the prenatal group (0.46 with 95% CI [0.28, 0.64]) was slightly higher than that in the postnatal group (0.34 with 95% CI [0.24, 0.44]) (Fig. 3). Notably, the high heterogeneity ($I^2 > 80\%$) seen in this review suggested a lack of consistency in study design. Therefore, large-scale studies with a single study protocol, such as the Prenatal Assessment of Genomes and Exomes (PAGE) in the United Kingdom [18, 19] and the study by Fu et al. [31] in Guangzhou, China, are needed to establish evidence-based recommendations for WES in prenatal diagnosis, which will be critical for inclusion of WES in clinical practice.

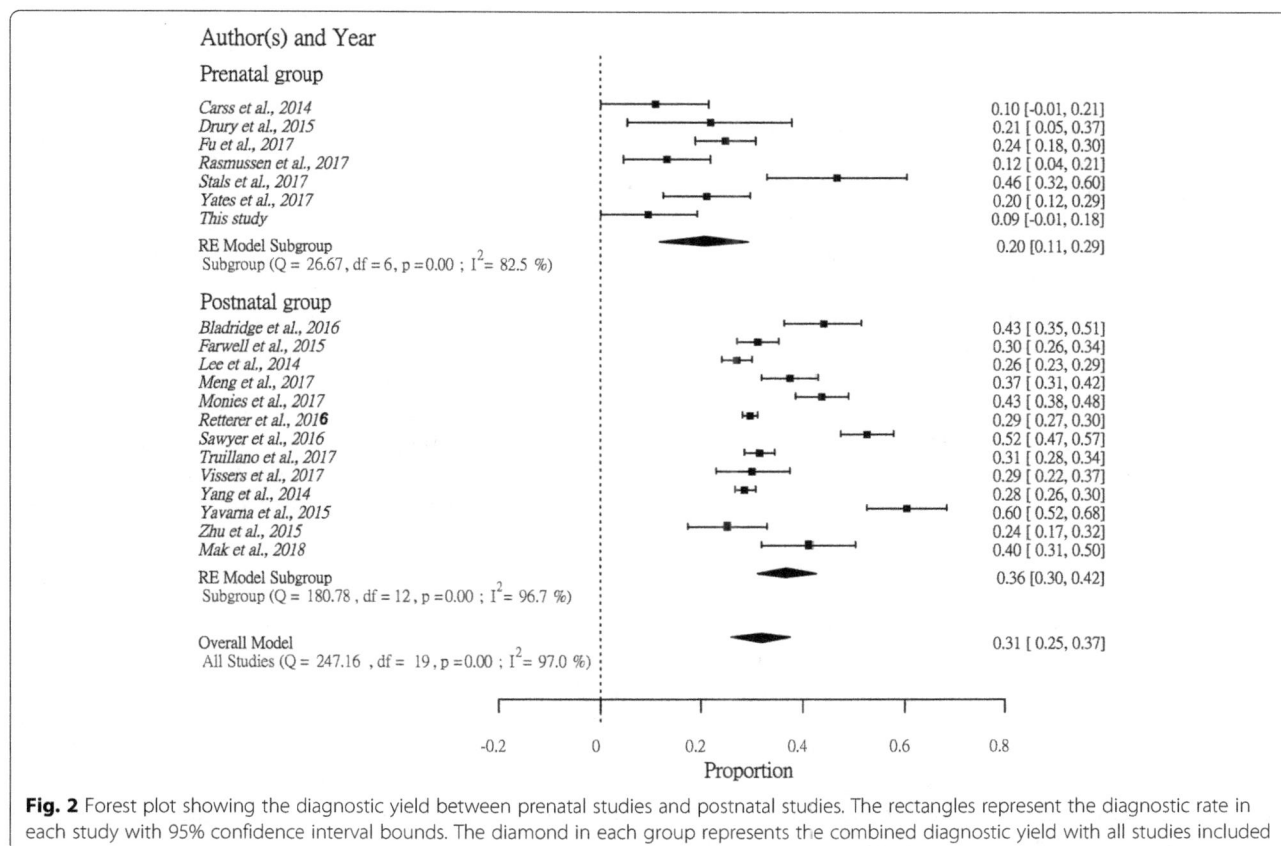

Fig. 2 Forest plot showing the diagnostic yield between prenatal studies and postnatal studies. The rectangles represent the diagnostic rate in each study with 95% confidence interval bounds. The diamond in each group represents the combined diagnostic yield with all studies included

Author(s) and Year

Prenatal group

Carss et al., 2014	0.62 [0.29, 0.96]
Drury et al., 2015	0.38 [0.04, 0.71]
Fu et al., 2017	0.35 [0.24, 0.46]
Rasmussen et al., 2017	0.46 [0.19, 0.73]
Stals et al., 2017	0.12 [-0.01, 0.24]
Yates et al., 2017	0.73 [0.61, 0.84]
This study	0.67 [0.36, 0.97]
RE Model Subgroup	0.46 [0.28, 0.64]

Subgroup (Q = 58.37, df = 6 p = 0.00 ; I^2 = 85.4 %)

Postnatal group

Bladridge et al., 2016	0.46 [0.37, 0.54]
Farwell et al., 2015	0.22 [0.17, 0.28]
Lee et al., 2014	0.52 [0.47, 0.56]
Meng et al., 2017	0.04 [0.00, 0.07]
Monies et al., 2017	0.48 [0.42, 0.54]
Retterer et al., 2015	0.46 [0.43, 0.48]
Sawyer et al., 2016	0.13 [0.08, 0.17]
Truillano et al., 2017	0.45 [0.41, 0.49]
Vissers et al., 2017	0.48 [0.38, 0.59]
Yavarna et al., 2015	0.20 [0.12, 0.27]
Zhu et al., 2015	0.47 [0.34, 0.60]
Mak et al., 2018	0.16 [0.06, 0.26]
RE Model Subgroup	0.34 [0.24, 0.44]

Subgroup (Q = 605.19, df = 11, p = 0.00 ; I^2 = 97.8 %)

Overall Model   0.37 [0.29, 0.46]
All Studies (Q = 671.52, df = 18, p =0.00 ; I^2 = 97.1 %)

-0.2   0   0.2   0.4   0.6   0.8   1

Proportion

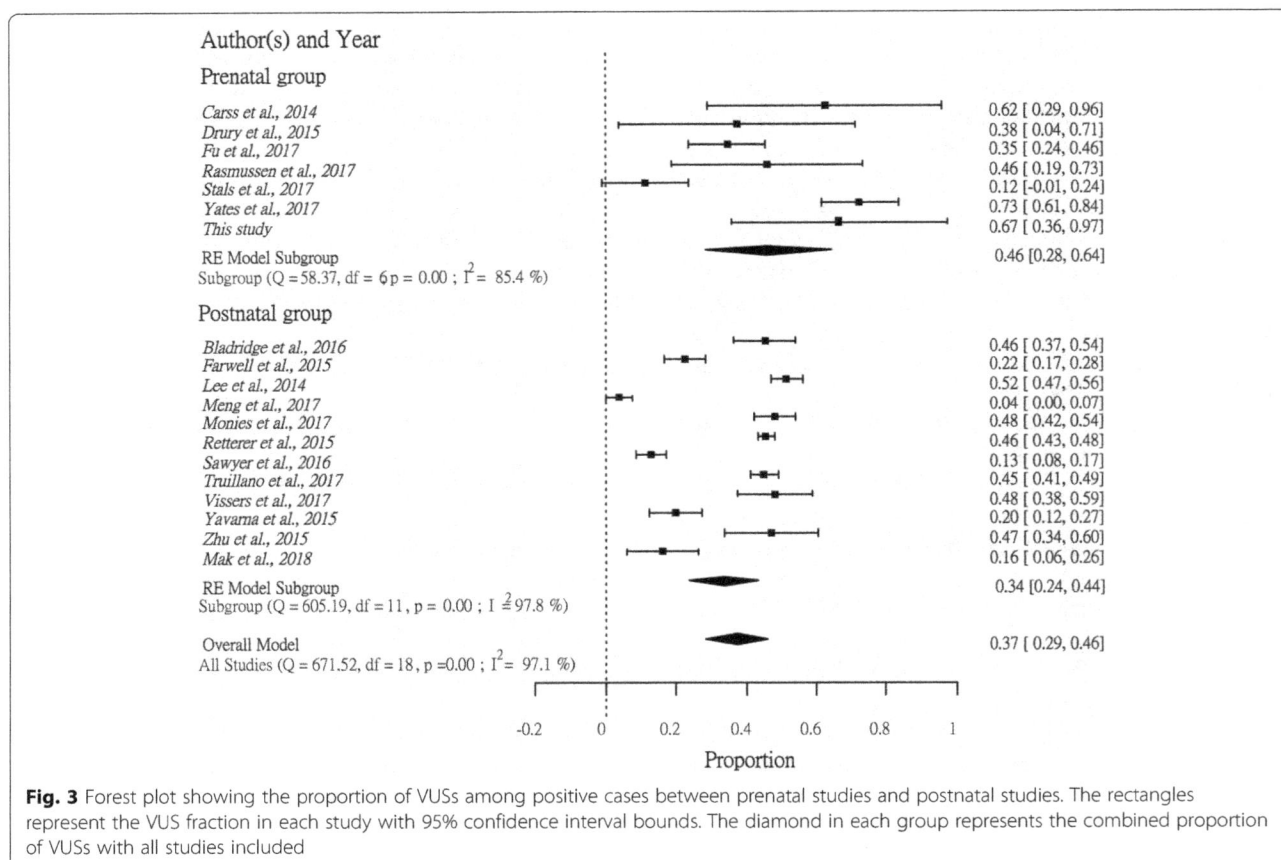

Fig. 3 Forest plot showing the proportion of VUSs among positive cases between prenatal studies and postnatal studies. The rectangles represent the VUS fraction in each study with 95% confidence interval bounds. The diamond in each group represents the combined proportion of VUSs with all studies included

It is important to address the clinical and emotional impact WES can have for families with a fetus with SCA. Our cohort included only fetuses with SCA who did not receive a diagnosis through standard testing. This lack of diagnosis with standard testing occurs in 60% of cases of SCA identified by ultrasound [22]. For these families, the lack of diagnosis and the uncertainty can be incredibly stressful. Receiving a diagnosis via WES can provide some relief from this stress and permits for more realistic and informative conversations about prognosis. Further, a firm diagnosis empowers families' decision making in a very difficult time. Physicians are also better equipped to provide postnatal treatment or palliative care in cases where a diagnosis is made [22]. Identifying a specific genetic etiology allows for accurate counseling on the risk to future children. In the case of negative results, patients who receive WES can be more confident in the specificity of their negative result than that of the standard genetic tests considering how thorough of a test WES is [29].

There has been a significant amount of focus in the literature on the potentially detrimental effect of reporting VUSs [29]. In the consideration of WES for prenatal diagnosis, emotional distress resulting from reporting

VUS is a concern. However, a study on women's experiences receiving chromosomal microarray results of unknown significance found that women with fetuses with SCA's were less concerned and traumatized by positive but uncertain results because any sort of positive result could act as confirmation that their baby had a true problem. This allowed the women interested in termination to feel more justified in their decision and less concerned about the uncertainties of ultrasound [32]. Despite this, families with a fetus with SCA receiving a result of VUS require more support as they are more likely than those with a diagnosis to feel abandoned and confused after the test [32]. These patients should also be counseled on the potential of a future diagnosis as more variants are defined over time.

A joint position statement has been recently released on the application of genome-wide sequencing for prenatal diagnosis [33]. Despite this step, international efforts are always needed to help establish standard guidelines for variant interpretation and more ethnically inclusive databases of fetal genotype-phenotype correlations. These advances will be necessary to encourage the further incorporation of WES into routine diagnostic practice in the prenatal setting.

Conclusion

In this study, it has been demonstrated that WES was feasible in prenatal diagnosis for fetuses with prenatally diagnosed SCAs. WES identified pathogenic mutations in 9.1%, and VUSs in 18.2% of fetuses with SCA with normal chromosomal microarray results. We saw that a high proportion of VUSs is one of the major challenges in prenatal exome, limited by the fetal phenotyping resolution, and the assessment of late-onset symptoms. Large cohort studies should be encouraged for a better interpretation of fetal genotype-phenotyping correlations.

Abbreviations

ACMG: American College of medical genetics and genomics; CMA: Chromosomal microarray; CVS: Chorionic villus sampling; DNA: Deoxyribonucleic acid; GATK: Genome Analysis Toolkit; MCC: Maternal cell contamination; NT: Nuchal translucency; PCD: Primary ciliary dyskinesia; QFPCR: Quantitative fluorescence-polymerase chain reaction; SCAs: Structural congenital anomalies; VUSs: Variants of unknown significance; WES: Whole-exome sequencing

Acknowledgements

We would like to thanks the clinicians and acknowledge the patients and their family members for the support in the project.

Funding

The project was funded by the Health and Medical Research Fund (ref# 02131816) offered by the Government of HKSAR.

Authors' contributions

G.K.C.L. wrote the main manuscript and performed the experiments. C.C.Y.M., J.L.F.F, M.H.Y.T., M.H.C.Y., S.L.C.P., A.S.Y.K. and G.T.K.M, assisted with the experiment, data analysis, and preparation of the manuscript. W.H.S. W. supported the statistical analysis. C.P.L., A.P.W.H., M.H.Y.T., A.S.Y.K. and B.H.Y.C. provided clinical consultation and informed consent to the patients in the study. M.H.Y.T., K.Y.K.C., A.P.Y.L., W.Y. and P.C.S. provided comments on genetic variant prioritization and bioinformatics analysis. A.S.Y.K. and B.H.Y.C. were the principal investigators who contributed to the experimental design, supervision on the project, revision of the manuscript, decision-making and approving the final version of the manuscript. All of the authors reviewed the manuscript. All authors read and approved the final manuscript.

Competing interests

The authors declare that they have no competing interests.

Author details

[1]Department of Paediatrics and Adolescent Medicine, LKS Faculty of Medicine, The University of Hong Kong, Room 103, 1/F, New Clinical Building, Hong Kong, Hong Kong Special Administrative Region, China. [2]Department of Obstetrics and Gynaecology, Queen Mary Hospital, The University of Hong Kong, Hong Kong, Hong Kong Special Administrative Region, China. [3]Prenatal Diagnostic Laboratory, Department of Obstetrics and Gynaecology, Tsan Yuk Hospital, Hong Kong, HKSAR, China. [4]Department of Psychiatry, LKS Faculty of Medicine, The University of Hong Kong, Hong Kong, HKSAR, China.

References

1. Crane JP, et al. A randomized trial of prenatal ultrasonographic screening: impact on the detection, management, and outcome of anomalous fetuses. The RADIUS Study Group. Am J Obstet Gynecol. 1994;171(2):392–9.
2. Stengel-Rutkowski S, et al. Routine G-banding in prenatal diagnosis of chromosomal disorders. Hum Genet. 1976;31(2):231–4.
3. Wapner RJ, et al. Chromosomal microarray versus karyotyping for prenatal diagnosis. N Engl J Med. 2012;367(23):2175–84.
4. American College of Obstetricians and Gynecologists. Committee opinion no. 581: the use of chromosomal microarray analysis in prenatal diagnosis. Obstet Gynecol. 2013;122(6):1374–7.
5. Dugoff L, et al. The use of chromosomal microarray for prenatal diagnosis. Am J Obstet Gynecol. 2016;215(4):B2–9.
6. American College of Obstetricians and Gynecologists. Microarrays and next-generation sequencing technology: the use of advanced genetic diagnostic tools in obstetrics and gynecology. ACOG Committee opinion no. 682. American College of Obstetricians and Gynecologists. Obstet Gynecol. 2016;128:e262–8.
7. Kan ASY, et al. Whole-genome Array CGH evaluation for replacing prenatal karyotyping in Hong Kong. PLoS One. 2014;9(2):e87988.
8. Yang Y, et al. Clinical whole-exome sequencing for the diagnosis of mendelian disorders. N Engl J Med. 2013;369(16):1502–11.
9. Ng SB, et al. Exome sequencing identifies the cause of a mendelian disorder. Nat Genet. 2010;42(1):30–5.
10. Biesecker LG, Green RC. Diagnostic clinical genome and exome sequencing. N Engl J Med. 2014;370(25):2418–25.
11. Levenson D. Whole-exome sequencing emerges as clinical diagnostic tool Testing Method Proves Useful for Diagnosing Wide Range of Genetic Disorders. Am J Med Genet A. 2014;164(1):ix–U1.
12. Bamshad MJ, et al. Exome sequencing as a tool for Mendelian disease gene discovery. Nat Rev Genet. 2011;12(11):745–55.
13. Alazami AM, et al. Accelerating novel candidate gene discovery in neurogenetic disorders via whole-exome sequencing of prescreened multiplex consanguineous families. Cell Rep. 2015;10(2):148–61.
14. Bekheirnia MR et al. Whole-exome sequencing in the molecular diagnosis of individuals with congenital anomalies of the kidney and urinary tract and identification of a new causative gene. Genet Med. 2017;19(4):412–20.
15. Need AC, et al. Clinical application of exome sequencing in undiagnosed genetic conditions. J Med Genet. 2012;49(6):353–61.
16. Richards S, et al. Standards and guidelines for the interpretation of sequence variants: a joint consensus recommendation of the American College of Medical Genetics and Genomics and the Association for Molecular Pathology. Genet Med. 2015;17(5):405–24.
17. Richards CS, et al. ACMG recommendations for standards for interpretation and reporting of sequence variations: revisions 2007. Genet Med. 2008;10(4):294–300.
18. Carss KJ, et al. Exome sequencing improves genetic diagnosis of structural fetal abnormalities revealed by ultrasound. Hum Mol Genet. 2014;23(12):3269–77.
19. Drury S, et al. Exome sequencing for prenatal diagnosis of fetuses with sonographic abnormalities. Prenat Diagn. 2015;35(10):1010–7.
20. Yates CL, et al. Whole-exome sequencing on deceased fetuses with ultrasound anomalies: expanding our knowledge of genetic disease during fetal development. Genetics in Medicine. 2017;19(10):1171–8.
21. Wapner R, et al. Whole exome sequencing in the evaluation of fetal structural anomalies: a prospective study of sequential patients. Am J Obstet Gynecol. 2017;216(1):S5–6.
22. Best S, et al. Promises, pitfalls and practicalities of prenatal whole exome sequencing. Frenat Diagn. 2018;38(1):10–19.
23. McKenna A, et al. The genome analysis toolkit: a MapReduce framework for analyzing next-generation DNA sequencing data. Genome Res. 2010;20(9):1297–303.
24. Wang K, Li M, Hakonarson H. ANNOVAR: functional annotation of genetic variants from high-throughput sequencing data. Nucleic Acids Res. 2010;38(16):e164–4.
25. Yeung KS, et al. Identification of mutations in the PI3K-AKT-mTOR signalling pathway in patients with macrocephaly and developmental delay and/or autism. Mol autism. 2017;8(1):66.
26. Lek M, et al. Analysis of protein-coding genetic variation in 60,706 humans. Nature. 2016;536(7616):285–91.
27. Janssen N, et al. Mutation update on the CHD7 gene involved in CHARGE syndrome. Hum Mutat. 2012;33(8):1149–60.

28. Zentner GE, et al. Molecular and phenotypic aspects of CHD7 mutation in CHARGE syndrome. Am J Med Genet A. 2010;152A(3):674–86.

29. Xue Y, et al. Solving the molecular diagnostic testing conundrum for Mendelian disorders in the era of next-generation sequencing: single-gene, gene panel, or exome/genome sequencing. Genet Med. 2015;17(6):444–51.

30. Mak CC, et al. Exome sequencing for paediatric-onset diseases: impact of the extensive involvement of medical geneticists in the diagnostic odyssey. NPJ Genom Med. 2018;3:19.

31. Fu F, et al. Whole exome sequencing as a diagnostic adjunct to clinical testing in fetuses with structural abnormalities. Ultrasound Obstet Gynecol. 2018;51(4):493–502.

32. Bernhardt BA, et al. Women's experiences receiving abnormal prenatal chromosomal microarray testing results. Genet Med. 2013;15(2):139–45.

33. Henson M. Joint position statement from the International Society of Prenatal Diagnosis (ISPD), the Society of Maternal Fetal Medicine (SMFM) and the perinatal Quality Foundation (PQF) on the use of genome-wide sequencing for fetal diagnosis. Prenat Diagn. 2018;38(1):6–9.

3

Longitudinal expression profiling of CD4+ and CD8+ cells in patients with active to quiescent giant cell arteritis

Elisabeth De Smit[1*†]🆔, Samuel W. Lukowski[2†], Lisa Anderson[3], Anne Senabouth[2], Kaisar Dauyey[2], Sharon Song[3], Bruce Wyse[3], Lawrie Wheeler[3], Christine Y. Chen[4], Khoa Cao[4], Amy Wong Ten Yuen[1], Neil Shuey[5], Linda Clarke[1], Isabel Lopez Sanchez[1], Sandy S. C. Hung[1], Alice Pébay[1], David A. Mackey[6], Matthew A. Brown[3], Alex W. Hewitt[1,7†] and Joseph E. Powell[2†]

Abstract

Background: Giant cell arteritis (GCA) is the most common form of vasculitis affecting elderly people. It is one of the few true ophthalmic emergencies but symptoms and signs are variable thereby making it a challenging disease to diagnose. A temporal artery biopsy is the gold standard to confirm GCA, but there are currently no specific biochemical markers to aid diagnosis. We aimed to identify a less invasive method to confirm the diagnosis of GCA, as well as to ascertain clinically relevant predictive biomarkers by studying the transcriptome of purified peripheral CD4+ and CD8+ T lymphocytes in patients with GCA.

Methods: We recruited 16 patients with histological evidence of GCA at the Royal Victorian Eye and Ear Hospital, Melbourne, Australia, and aimed to collect blood samples at six time points: acute phase, 2–3 weeks, 6–8 weeks, 3 months, 6 months and 12 months after clinical diagnosis. CD4+ and CD8+ T-cells were positively selected at each time point through magnetic-assisted cell sorting. RNA was extracted from all 195 collected samples for subsequent RNA sequencing. The expression profiles of patients were compared to those of 16 age-matched controls.

Results: Over the 12-month study period, polynomial modelling analyses identified 179 and 4 statistically significant transcripts with altered expression profiles (FDR < 0.05) between cases and controls in CD4+ and CD8+ populations, respectively. In CD8+ cells, two transcripts remained differentially expressed after 12 months; *SGTB*, associated with neuronal apoptosis, and *FCGR3A*, associated with Takayasu arteritis. We detected genes that correlate with both symptoms and biochemical markers used for predicting long-term prognosis. 15 genes were shared across 3 phenotypes in CD4 and 16 across CD8 cells. In CD8, *IL32* was common to 5 phenotypes including Polymyalgia Rheumatica, bilateral blindness and death within 12 months.

Conclusions: This is the first longitudinal gene expression study undertaken to identify robust transcriptomic biomarkers of GCA. Our results show cell type-specific transcript expression profiles, novel gene-phenotype associations, and uncover important biological pathways for this disease. In the acute phase, the gene-phenotype relationships we have identified could provide insight to potential disease severity and as such guide in initiating appropriate patient management.

Keywords: Giant cell arteritis, Disease biomarkers, RNA sequencing, Expression profiling, Transcriptome, CD4 & CD8 T lymphocytes, Magnetic-assisted cell sorting

* Correspondence: elisabethdesmit@gmail.com
†Elisabeth De Smit, Samuel W. Lukowski, Alex W. Hewitt and Joseph E. Powell contributed equally to this work.
[1]Centre for Eye Research Australia, The University of Melbourne, Royal Victorian Eye & Ear Hospital, 32 Gisborne Street, East Melbourne 3002, Australia
Full list of author information is available at the end of the article

Background

Giant Cell Arteritis (GCA) is the most common form of vasculitis in people over 50 years of age, and has a predilection for medium- and large-sized vessels of the head and neck. GCA represents one of the few true ophthalmic emergencies, and given the severe sequelae of untreated disease, a timely diagnosis is crucial [1]. GCA is a devastating disease associated with significant morbidity and mortality. If untreated, GCA can cause catastrophic complications including blindness and stroke, as well as aortic dissection and rupture.

The patho-aetiology of GCA is poorly understood. It is likely that both a genetic predisposition and possible environmental factors, the latter unconfirmed, contribute to the onset of disease [2]. GCA is a heterogenous disease and a definitive diagnosis can be difficult to establish in the acute setting. The current gold standard for diagnosis is a temporal artery biopsy, which is an invasive surgical procedure [3, 4]. There are currently no specific biomarkers to diagnose GCA, or stratify patient management.

In the acute setting, treatment with high-dose corticosteroids should be started empirically when a patient's symptoms and/or inflammatory markers suggest a diagnosis of GCA is likely [1]. Treatment should not be delayed whilst waiting for biopsy results to become available. Once diagnosed, clinicians monitor disease activity based on patients' symptoms and inflammatory markers, primarily the erythrocyte sedimentation rate (ESR) and C-reactive protein (CRP). However, these biochemical markers are non-specific and may be elevated in other inflammatory or infective diagnoses. There is a pressing need for more sensitive and specific biomarkers. This would aid in making a diagnosis, as well managing this condition more appropriately and mitigate the need for an invasive surgical procedure. Motivated by this need, we aimed to discover a biomarker so that when patients present to the emergency department with features of GCA, a blood test could be performed, allowing prompt diagnosis and initiation of appropriate treatment.

GCA is presumed to be an autoimmune disease with a highly complex immunopathogenesis. It has a strong association with HLA class II suggesting an adaptive immune response with antigen presentation to CD4+ T cells [5]. CD8+ T cells have also been described in GCA both at tissue level and peripherally [6, 7]. Transcriptional profiling in blood consists of measuring RNA abundance in circulating nucleated cells. Changes in transcript abundance can result from exposure to host- or pathogen-derived immunogenic factors. Given that T Lymphocytes are key mediators of the adaptive cellular immune response and in GCA [8], we studied the transcriptome of peripheral CD4+ and CD8+ T cells of patients with GCA. We monitored patients' expression profiling along the course of their disease to detect changes in transcripts as disease state altered and became quiescent.

Methods

Patient recruitment

Between July 2014 and June 2016, 16 patients presenting to the emergency department (ED) at the Royal Victorian Eye & Ear Hospital (RVEEH) in Melbourne (Australia), with symptoms and signs consistent with the diagnosis of GCA were enrolled in our study (Fig. 1). Ethics was approved for this study through the RVEEH (Ethics 11/998H), and all patients provided informed written consent to participate in serial sample collections, and for publication of results. We acquired blood samples from patients in the acute phase of their disease T1 (Day 0–7) but ideally prior to steroid initiation. Analysis took into account those patients who were steroid-naive at T1 and those who had already started steroid treatment, albeit in some cases less than 24 h earlier. In addition to T1, we aimed to acquire five subsequent serial samples from each patient - T2 (2–3 weeks), T3 (6–8 weeks), T4 (~ 3 months), T5 (~ 6 months) and T6 (~ 12 months) after presentation - to detect changes in their transcripts as the disease state altered and became quiescent (Additional file 1: Table S1). For each patient with GCA, we recruited an age- and gender-matched healthy control from whom two serial blood samples were collected 2–3 weeks apart. Our study design is outlined in Fig. 1.

T-cell isolation

At each visit, 36 ml of peripheral blood were collected in 4×9 ml ethylenediaminetetraacetic acid (EDTA) tubes, 18 ml of which were used to isolate each of the two T-cell populations. Once blood was collected from a patient, it was processed within 30 min. Rapid processing was conducted to avoid changes in cellular expression profiles [9]. First, the peripheral blood mononuclear cells (PBMCs) were isolated using Ficoll-Paque density centrifugation. This was followed by positive selection with magnetic antibody-coupled microbeads (MACS) (CD4 Human Microbeads (130–045-101) and CD8 Human Microbeads (130–045-201) from Miltenyi Biotec), to isolate the CD4+ and CD8+ T-cell populations from PBMCs. CD4+ cells were labelled with fluorescein isothiocyanate (CD4-Viobright FITC (130–104-515) Miltenyi Biotec) and CD8+ with allophycocyanin (CD8-APC (130–091-076) Miltenyi Biotec) antibody for purity analysis. The CD4+ and CD8+ positive fractions were eluted from the magnetically charged MS column in 1000ul of MACS BSA Stock Solution 1:20 with autoMACS Rinsing Solution (Miltenyi Biotec). A 20 μl aliquot of both CD4+ and CD8+ final cell populations was fixed in 2% paraformaldehyde (PFA) and used for analysis of the population purity on a CyAn ADP fluorescence-activated cell sorting (FACS) analyzer (Additional file 2: Fig. S1). The remainder of the positive fractions was stored at − 80 °C in lysis RLT buffer (Qiagen) to which beta-mercaptoethanol had been added as per manufacturer's guidelines for between 1 and 23 months.

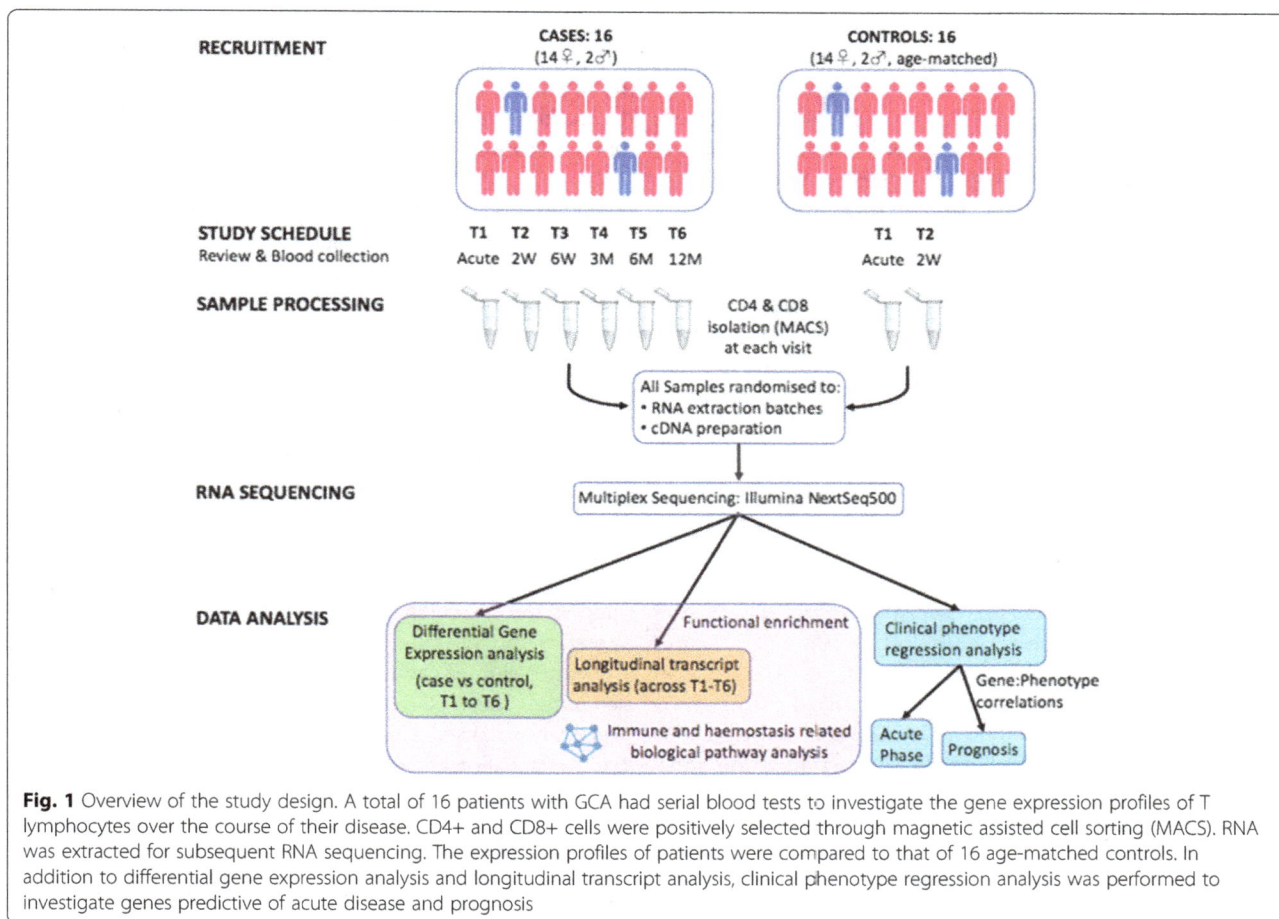

Fig. 1 Overview of the study design. A total of 16 patients with GCA had serial blood tests to investigate the gene expression profiles of T lymphocytes over the course of their disease. CD4+ and CD8+ cells were positively selected through magnetic assisted cell sorting (MACS). RNA was extracted for subsequent RNA sequencing. The expression profiles of patients were compared to that of 16 age-matched controls. In addition to differential gene expression analysis and longitudinal transcript analysis, clinical phenotype regression analysis was performed to investigate genes predictive of acute disease and prognosis

RNA extraction, cDNA processing and RNA sequencing

T cell samples underwent RNA extraction as per manufacturer's protocol (Qiagen RNeasy kit) at the Centre for Eye Research Australia (CERA) located in the Royal Victorian Eye and Ear Hospital. All T-cell lysate samples, 135 GCA patient samples and 60 control samples, were randomised to RNA extraction batches of between 20 and 24 samples to avoid batch effects. RNA samples were eluted 30 µl in RNAse free water and stored at -80 °C until all extractions were complete. Samples were tested on the NanoDrop ND-1000 spectrophotometer to check RNA quantity and quality (A260/A230 and A260/A280 between 1.8 and 2.1). Once all batches were extracted, samples were dispatched on dry ice to the Australian Translational Genomics Centre (ATGC) at Queensland University of Technology (QUT) for cDNA processing and RNA sequencing. At ATGC, RNA integrity (RIN) and quantity was confirmed with a Bioanalyzer 2100 (Agilent) before undergoing library preparation.

To avoid sequencing batch effects, all 195 samples (GCA $n = 135$, and Control $n = 60$) were re-randomised to be processed in one of three different cDNA library preparation batches (Illumina TruSeq Stranded mRNA Sample Preparation Kits). This kit purifies the polyadenylated mRNA molecules. The Illumina Truseq protocol is optimized for 0.1–4 µg of total RNA and a RIN value ≥8 is recommended. The average total RNA yield varied between samples. The average RNA concentration was 137.9 ng/µl (range 12.1 to 1130.0 ng/µl). Total RNA yield per sample averaged to 2757.7 ng (range 242.0 to 22,600.0 ng) and average RIN was 8.9 (range 7.2 to 10.0). 600 ng total RNA was used to generate cDNA libraries (30 µl) for all samples with ≥600 ng total RNA available. Samples with less than 600 ng total RNA available were used entirely. Samples were barcoded to allow large throughput at sequencing. The number of PCR cycles for cDNA amplification was adjusted as required to equalise the cDNA yield as per the protocol. Quality control of library concentrations was assessed through LabChip GX High Sensitivity DNA assay.

RNA-Seq libraries were multiplexed and sequenced (75 bp PE) in batches on an Illumina NextSeq500 high-throughput instrument. Each batch of cDNA libraries was pooled in equimolar volumes, and sequenced over three flow cells, with nine flow cells used in total. To achieve uniform sequencing across a large number of samples, the data were reviewed following each run by determining the number of mapped reads per sample. The read count per sample volume pooled was used as a metric to re-pool the cDNA libraries for additional sequencing. As such the pool of cDNA libraries for each batch was adjusted so that all samples would reach 16 million raw reads. This strategy also minimised between sample sequence run batch effects. cDNA libraries were sequenced and we obtained a median 11,017,433 mapped reads per sample and the read counts were aggregated into a single gene expression matrix. 40,744 transcripts had counts-per-million (cpm) > 1 in 50% of samples and underwent further analysis.

Computational analysis

Quality control of the sequencing data was performed on the FASTQ files. High quality reads were retained and Trimmomatic v0.36 was used to remove adapters and low quality bases. Reads were mapped to the GRCh38 human reference transcriptome using Kallisto v0.42.4 [10]. Only those with cpm > 1 in 50% of the samples were retained for further analysis. Transcript expression between libraries was normalised using the trimmed mean of M method (TMM) and corrected for batch effects using the *removeBatchEffect* function implemented in edgeR (Flowcell ID, Gender and Ethnicity) [11]. Hierarchical clustering and principal component analysis (PCA) confirmed the absence of batch effects and outlier samples (Additional file 3: Figure S2).

Differential gene expression analysis

A total of 135 GCA samples (n = 16 patients) spanning six timepoints and 60 control samples (n = 16 patients) spanning two timepoints were grouped for analysis based on their CD4 (GCA = 68, control = 30) or CD8 MACS (GCA = 67, control = 30) separation. This grouping strategy formed the basis of the differential expression design matrix, allowing pairwise comparisons between individual timepoints on a case/control or CD4/CD8 basis. Differentially expressed transcripts were considered statistically significant if their false discovery rate (FDR) was less than 0.05. Differential expression (DGE) analysis between case and control subjects was performed comparing the initial T1 case specimens versus both the T1 and T2 of control specimens. Transcripts below FDR < 0.05 and a two-fold change between cases and controls were considered significant.

Polynomial modelling of transcript expression

The longitudinal expression profile of retained transcripts across six time points was tested for significant changes using polynomial regression. Polynomial regression modelling was performed with the patient weight-normalised steroid dosage fitted as a fixed effect. Steroid dose was normalised by dividing the Daily Steroid Dose by the Patient Weight. The global model p-value was corrected for multiple testing using the Benjamini-Hochberg method (FDR) and transcripts with an adjusted p-value below the FDR threshold (< 0.05) were considered statistically significant.

Functional enrichment and pathway analysis

Functional enrichment analysis was performed using the Reactome biological pathway database via the ReactomePA software package (version 1.18) and the CPdB web server (http://cpdb.molgen.mpg.de/) [12]. Pathway analysis results with adjusted p-values below the FDR threshold (< 0.1) were considered significant.

Clinical phenotype regression analysis

Models were constructed to regress clinically relevant traits that were measured at the time of disease onset, or sample collection, against normalised gene expression levels. For quantitative clinical variables we used a linear model, and for categorical variables we used a logistic regression model. Clinical phenotypes were fitted against the expression of each of transcripts in GCA-only samples separated into CD4+ and CD8+ populations and weight-normalised daily steroid dose was included as a fixed effect. For each transcript, the adjusted p-value was calculated using the Benjamini-Hochberg method (FDR) method [13]. Transcripts with adjusted p-values below the FDR threshold (< 0.01) were retained for further analysis. The complete summary tables of tested phenotypes are available in Tables 2, 3 and 4.

Results

Patient recruitment and MACS events

Sixteen incident patients with active GCA and 16 age-matched controls were recruited. The mean age was 78.2 years in the GCA cohort and 76.6 years in the control group. Both groups had the same 14:2 female to male ratio. Table 2 provides the number of patients presenting with the common symptoms and signs associated with GCA. Additional file 4: Table S2 and Additional file 5: Table S3 describe the specific ophthalmic manifestations and long-term prognoses observed in our patient cohort. Not all patients were able to complete 12 months of participation; therefore, not all patients had six samples collected (Additional file 1: Table S1). 6 patients were steroid-naive at T1; these patients had their first sample collected in the ED prior to commencing steroid treatment. Of the other 10 patients, 3 patients had been on steroids less than 24 h, and the other 7 patients had been on steroids for between three to seven days at the time of T1.

In total, 195 MACS events, comprising 135 GCA (67 CD4 and 66 CD8 samples) and 60 control events, were performed (Additional file 1: Table S1). One patient's CD8 sample had insufficient material after isolating the PBMC layer and was therefore excluded from further analysis (Additional file 1: Table S1). Two controls were only able to provide the first time point samples. Each MACS procedure isolated between 2 and 10 million CD4+ and CD8+ cells per patient per time event. CD4+ MACS isolation resulted in greater cell counts than CD8+. The analysis on the CyAn ADP analyser revealed good population purity after MACS-positive cell selection: an average of 97% for CD4+ cells and > 94% for CD8+ cells (Additional file 2: Figure S1).

Differential expression analysis:

To determine which transcripts showed the most variation in expression over the 12-month collection period, and to identify cell type specific signatures, we analysed the expression levels of samples from GCA patients ($n = 135$) (Additional file 6: Figure S3). Figure 2 represents the expression levels of the top 40 most variable transcripts in CD4+ and CD8+ samples in GCA patients. The expression levels of control genes such as *CD4* and *CD8A/B* confirms the partitioning of CD4+ and CD8+ cells.

We investigated changes in gene expression in both CD4+ and CD8+ between cases and controls at T1. At a significance threshold of FDR < 0.05, we identified 67 down-regulated (DR) and 129 up-regulated (UR) transcripts in CD4+ samples, and 93 DR and 188 UR transcripts in CD8+ samples (Table 1). The numbers of significantly differentially expressed transcripts increased dramatically at T3 in cases compared to the controls at T1 for CD8+ samples, and resolving to a near-control profile at T6. At T3 (6–8 weeks), we detected 1927 DR and 1783 UR transcripts in CD8+ cells. Interestingly, DE transcripts in CD4+ cells reached a plateau from T2 to T4 (T2: 254 DR/228 UR; T3: 196 DR/190 UR; T4: 179 DR/200 UR).

We hypothesised that gene expression in GCA patients would return to baseline levels at approximately 12 months, corresponding to T6, marking disease quiescence. Transcripts remaining DE at T6 may be of clinical interest or mark evidence of previous disease despite current inactivity. In CD8+ cells, we identified two significant DE transcripts at T6 versus controls, *SGTB* (Small glutamine-rich tetratricopeptide repeat (TPR)-containing beta) and *FCGR3A* (Fc Fragment Of IgG Receptor IIIa),

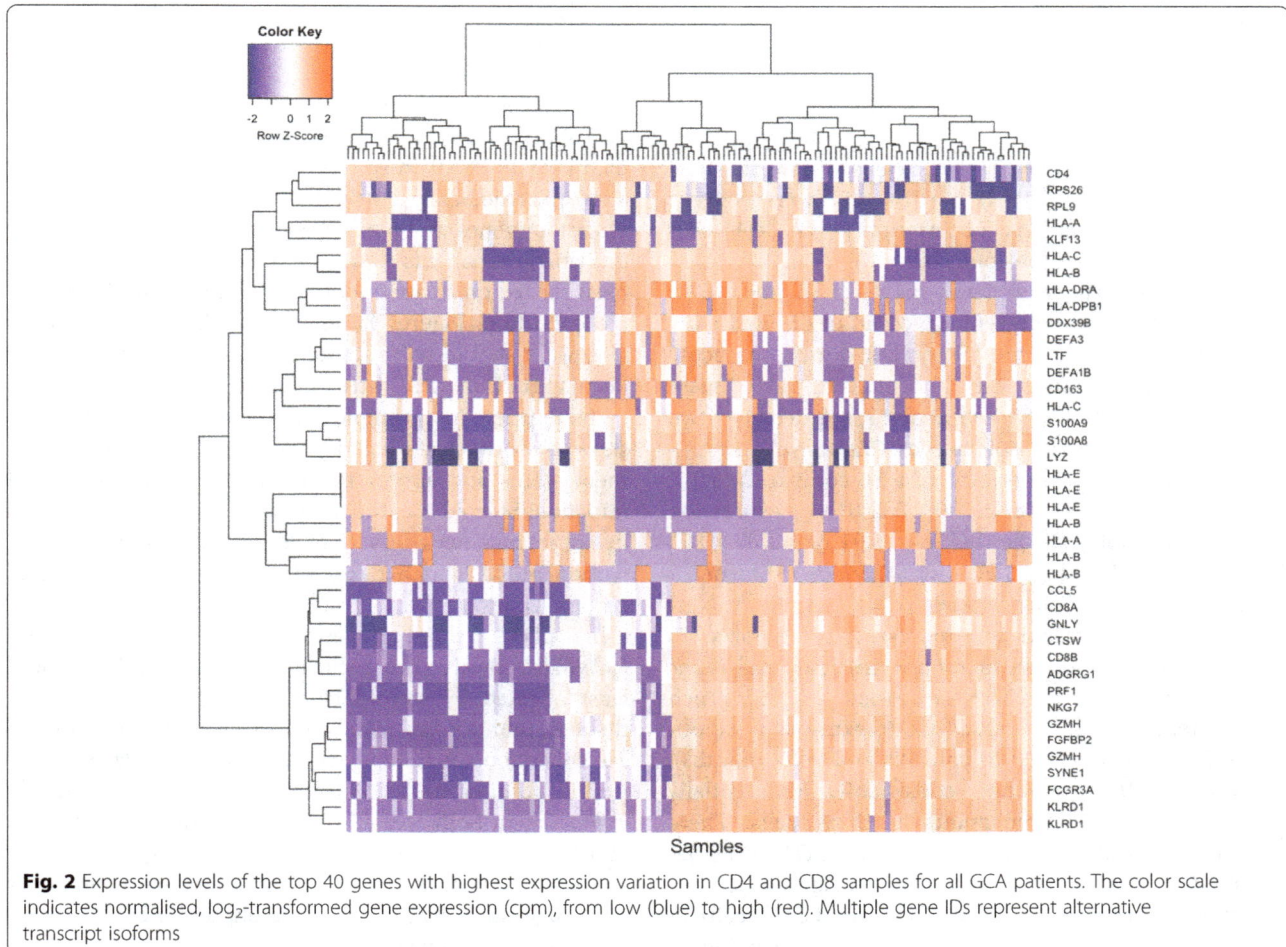

Fig. 2 Expression levels of the top 40 genes with highest expression variation in CD4 and CD8 samples for all GCA patients. The color scale indicates normalised, log$_2$-transformed gene expression (cpm), from low (blue) to high (red). Multiple gene IDs represent alternative transcript isoforms

Table 1 Number of DE genes in each comparison

Contrast	CD4		CD8	
	DR	UR	DR	UR
Control 2 vs Control 1	0	0	0	0
GCA T2 vs T1	0	0	0	0
GCA T3 vs T1	1	8	35	80
GCA T4 vs T1	2	7	1	3
GCA T5 vs T1	0	0	0	0
GCA T6 vs T1	0	0	2	0
GCA T6 vs T3	0	0	45	10
GCA T1 vs Control 1	67	129	93	188
GCA T2 vs Control 1	254	228	325	453
GCA T3 vs Control 1	196	190	1927	1783
GCA T4 vs Control 1	179	200	576	827
GCA T5 vs Control 1	1	1	101	296
GCA T6 vs Control 1	0	0	1	1
GCA T1 vs Control 2	22	58	58	156
GCA T2 vs Control 2	276	233	187	335
GCA T3 vs Control 2	194	171	1066	1227
GCA T4 vs Control 2	197	179	351	615
GCA T5 vs Control 2	2	0	55	222
GCA T6 vs Control 2	0	0	0	0

which showed $\log_2$ fold changes in expression of -0.54 ($p = 4.83 \times 10^{-7}$) and 1.99 ($p = 1.75 \times 10^{-6}$), respectively. There were no significant DE transcripts in the CD4+ cells between GCA T6 and the controls.

Differentially expressed genes between T1 and T6 in GCA patients could represent a biomarker of disease activity, marking either gene UR or DR during the acute phase of disease and then normalising as disease quiesces. From the CD8+ cell analysis, we detected two differentially expressed isoforms of *CD163* with significantly reduced expression levels. At T6 compared to T1, *CD163* isoform 1 (ENST00000359156) expression showed a $\log_2$ fold change (FC) of -6.01 ($p = 1.07 \times 10^{-6}$), whereas the $\log_2$ FC of *CD163* isoform 2 (ENST00000432237) was -9.69 ($p = 5.84 \times 10^{-8}$). Notably, *CD163* expression is suppressed in response to pro-inflammatory stimuli in monocytes [14], and is inversely correlated with *CD16* expression [14, 15], which is consistent with the increased *CD16* expression we observed in cases compared to controls at T6 (12 months). However, *CD16* was not consistently differentially expressed across all time points in CD8+ cells. There were no significant DE transcripts in the CD4+ cells between GCA T1 and T6. Reassuringly, no significant transcripts were observed in either CD4+ or CD8+ cells in the controls between T1 & T2. Tables of significant

differentially expressed transcripts are presented in Additional file 7: Table S4 (CD4) and Additional file 8: Table S5 (CD8).

Polynomial modelling of longitudinal transcript expression:

To identify important transcripts whose expression levels vary across a 12-month period of the study, we used polynomial regression to model changes in the expression levels of 40,744 transcripts separately in CD4+ and CD8+ cells across the six time points. Using this approach, we detected 179 and 4 statistically significant expression profiles (FDR < 0.05) in CD4+ and CD8+ populations, respectively. Tables of significant transcript expression models are available in Additional file 9: Table S6.

The top 12 CD4+ profiles and all 4 significant CD8+ profiles are shown in Fig. 3. In CD4+, the majority of genes demonstrated a pattern of decreased expression over the study course. Only two genes demonstrated a positive fold change and increase in expression levels over the 12 months, namely *FOXO1* involved in blood vessel development and *TRBC2* involved in complement cascade activation and phagocytosis. The four identified genes in CD8+ were *CCLN2*, *FANCA*, *PTCD2* and *THRAP3*. The first three genes demonstrate a negative $\log_2$ fold change, whilst *THRAP3* demonstrates an increased expression trend.

No substantial contribution of steroid dose to the model was observed across the 12-month time course (CD4: median beta = -0.001, median $p = 0.439$; CD8: median beta = -0.002, median $p = 0.463$). However, expression levels of certain genes at T1 may have been affected depending on whether patients were steroid-naive or had already been started on treatment at time of their first blood sample collection. Figures 3a and b highlight those patients who were steroid-naive in red and those who had already been started on steroid treatment in black. Expression of certain genes, for example *TIMD4*, *VIPR1*, and *FOXO1*, show obvious clustering depending on a patient's treatment status and appear to be affected by corticosteroid initiation. Steroid treatment, even though only initiated in some instances less than 24 h prior to blood collection at T1, has a clear effect on the expression of certain genes.

In CD4+, three genes, *LMBR1L*, *UAP1L1* and *KCNMB4*, showed least clustering at T1 and appeared least affected by steroid treatment, albeit having been through oral dose or intravenously administered prior to T1 collection. In CD8+ cells, *PTCD2* and *THRAP3* appear little affected by steroids at T1. *PTCD2* is highly expressed in both steroid-naive and patients on steroids at T1 and less so at T6, suggesting no major influence of steroids at T1. *THRAP3* shows increased expression over time suggesting that in the acute phase *THRAP3* expression might be suppressed.

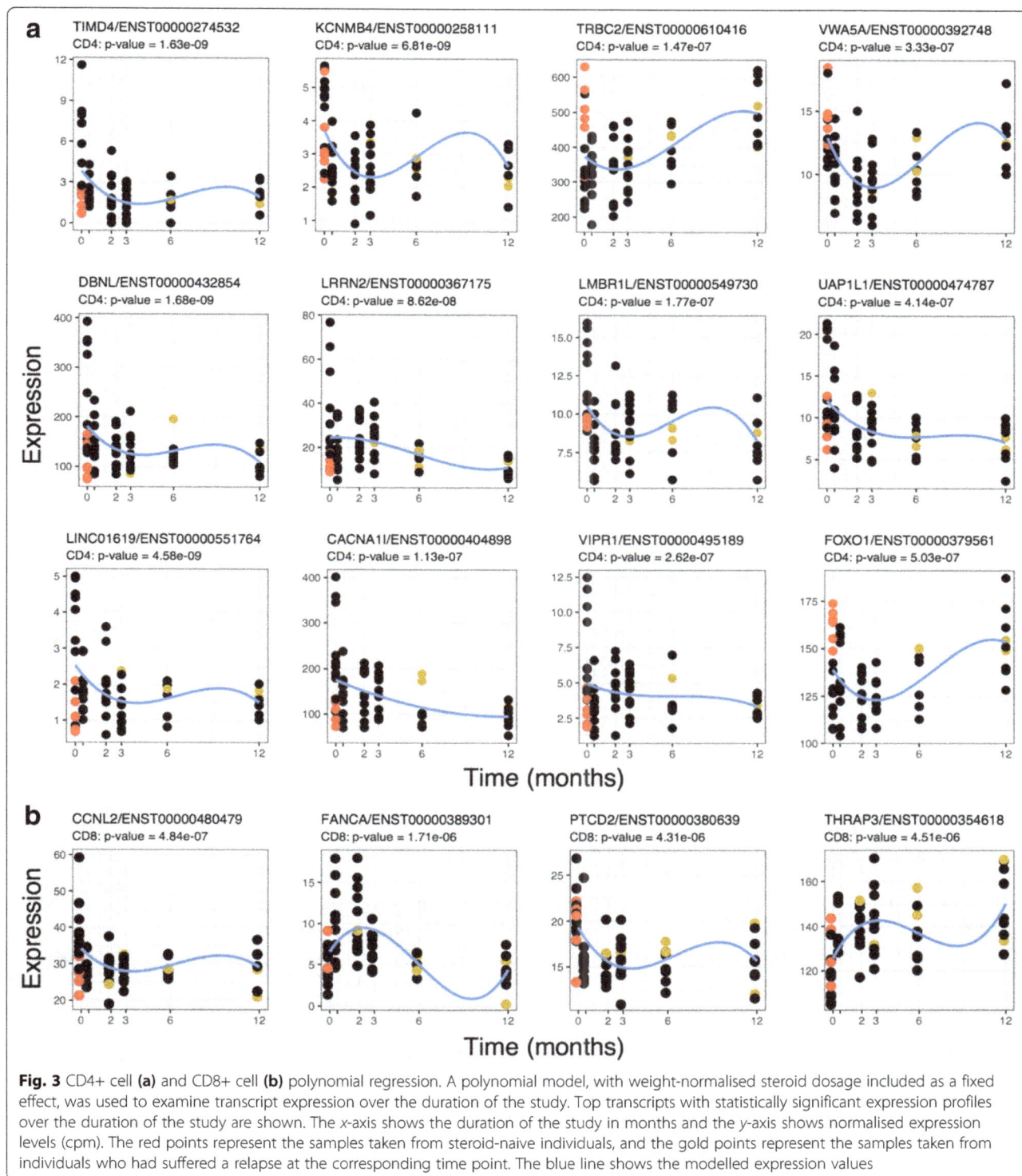

Fig. 3 CD4+ cell (**a**) and CD8+ cell (**b**) polynomial regression. A polynomial model, with weight-normalised steroid dosage included as a fixed effect, was used to examine transcript expression over the duration of the study. Top transcripts with statistically significant expression profiles over the duration of the study are shown. The x-axis shows the duration of the study in months and the y-axis shows normalised expression levels (cpm). The red points represent the samples taken from steroid-naive individuals, and the gold points represent the samples taken from individuals who had suffered a relapse at the corresponding time point. The blue line shows the modelled expression values

From our DGE analysis, we observed significant reduction in *CD163* transcript expression between T1 and T6 in the CD8 cell population analysis. Our results for the polynomial expression modelling also reflected that *CD163* was significantly reduced at T6. However, model profiles of this transcript showed that the trend over the 12-month time course was not statistically significant (FDR > 0.05). Interestingly, we noted that several *CD163* isoforms in the analyses of both CD4+ and CD8+ cell populations had compelling model profiles. For all but

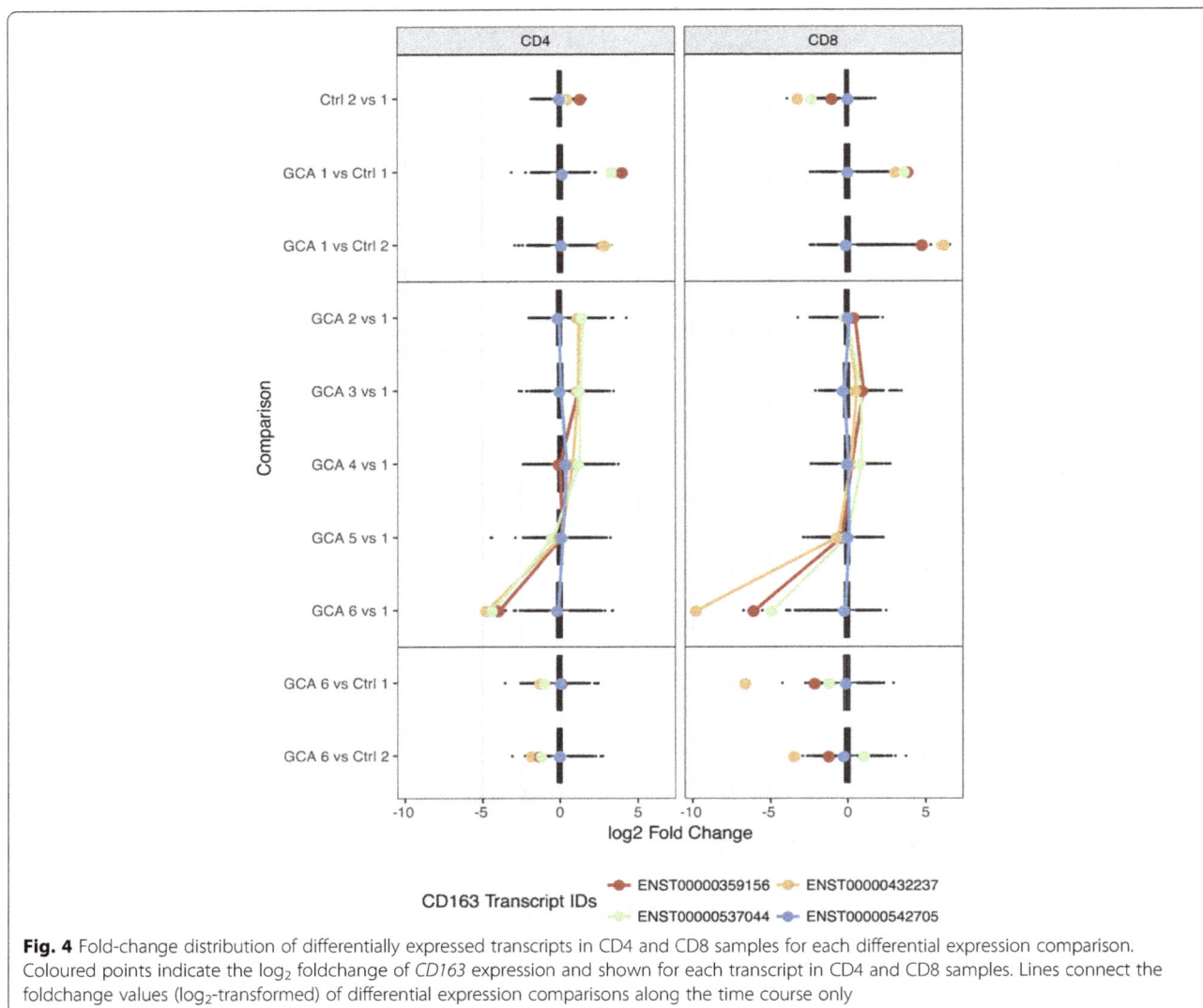

Fig. 4 Fold-change distribution of differentially expressed transcripts in CD4 and CD8 samples for each differential expression comparison. Coloured points indicate the $\log_2$ foldchange of *CD163* expression and shown for each transcript in CD4 and CD8 samples. Lines connect the foldchange values ($\log_2$-transformed) of differential expression comparisons along the time course only

one *CD163* isoform, expression levels returned to zero for all individuals at 12 months; however, these were not FDR-significant. The $\log_2$ foldchange in the expression of these transcripts over 12 months is shown in Fig. 4.

Functional enrichment and pathway analysis:

For individuals with GCA, we would expect an enrichment of immune and inflammation related pathways compared to healthy individuals. Biological pathway analysis of differentially expressed transcripts and statistically significant transcripts identified in the polynomial expression modelling analysis was performed using the curated Reactome database.

Significant DE transcripts in CD4+ samples comparing GCA to controls in the early time points showed a significant enrichment of T-cell receptor signaling (adj. p-value $= 4.25 \times 10^{-3}$; 11 genes). In CD8+ samples, we observed an enrichment of genes in pathways related to

platelet degranulation (adj. p-value $= 0.0124$; 12 genes) and activation (adj. p-value $= 0.0156$; 20 genes), as well as Fc-gamma receptor (FCGR) dependent phagocytosis (adj. p-value $= 0.0156$; 13 genes). Furthermore, CD8+ samples from first two collected samples of GCA cases showed significant enrichment of pathways related to haemostasis (adj. p-value $= 2.63 \times 10^{-6}$; 118 genes), innate immune system (adj. p-value $= 5.51 \times 10^{-6}$; 169 genes) and the adaptive immune system (adj. p-value $= 3.24 \times 10^{-4}$; 129 genes).

Transcripts with a significant association across the 12-month collection time were interrogated for enrichment of specific biological pathways. We tested all 179 CD4 and 4 CD8 significant transcripts. In the CD4 transcripts, we observed an over-representation of transcripts in the integrin cell surface interactions (adj. p-value $= 0.015$) and Caspase-mediated cleavage of cytoskeletal proteins (adj. p-value $= 0.0325$) as well as cytokine signaling (adj. p-value = 0.08) and negative regulators of RIG-I/MDA5 signaling (adj. p-value = 0.08). In the CD8 results, there were insufficient significant transcripts to perform enrichment analyses. However, a literature search revealed *THRAP3* is involved in intracellular steroid hormone receptor signaling pathways, and *FANCA* in inflammatory responses and T-cell differentiation pathways.

Clinical phenotype regression analysis:

Linear and logistic regression models were used to estimate the effect of specific clinically important phenotypes on expressed transcripts. The analyses were three-fold. The first was to determine whether there were any genes that correlated with symptoms and signs used in the acute setting (T1) (Table 2). Second, we determined whether any genes directly correlated with the biochemical markers currently used in the acute phase (T1) (Table 3). Genes resulting from these first two analyses are potential biomarkers for disease activity in the acute setting and predict relapses. Thirdly, we determined gene correlations with markers of disease severity or prognosis (Table 4). These were categorised in terms of visual outcome: whether blinded in one eye, "monocular", or both eyes, "bilateral"; relapse events; and whether the patient died during the study period. This enables us to identify genes that could provide prognostic information, ideally at the time of diagnosis (T1) but also during the course of disease (T1–6).

Correlation with clinical features in the acute setting

At the time of admission (T1), we would expect to observe some changes in gene expression to be strongly associated with clinical phenotypes related to the acute onset of disease. To identify a transcriptional signature that may be specific to active GCA, we examined the effect of clinically relevant phenotypes on gene expression

Table 3 "Acute phase" biochemical markers

	Phenotype	CD4	CD8
1	ESR	23	15
2	CRP	12	15
3	Platelets	41	7
4	WCC	75	38
5	Lymphocytes	23	63
6	Neutrophils	22	133

Number of genes significantly affected (FDR < 0.01) by biochemical markers in regression models at T1

in CD4 and CD8 samples taken at T1. Table 2 lists the eleven phenotypes and the number of statistically significant transcripts (FDR < 0.01) observed for each in CD4 or CD8 samples at T1. Genes or transcripts that are common to multiple symptoms/signs are likely to be clinically relevant, particularly at the acute onset of disease. In CD4 and CD8 samples, we identified 17 (CD4) and 27 (CD8) transcripts that were significantly associated with two or more clinical phenotypes.

In CD4 cells, *LAMTOR4* is a gene shared between jaw claudication and temporal headache, two important clinical features in acute GCA. Another gene associated with jaw claudication is *GZMB*, which is also associated with visual disturbance. *PPP1CB* and *EIF4A3* were shared by both jaw claudication and a background history of Polymyalgia Rheumatica (PMR). *EXTL3*, was expressed in both patients with jaw claudication and fatigue. We identified numerous genes associated with headache, both temporal and other types: *POFUT2* in CD4 cells, and *SLC35F6*, *HTD2*, *ZNF708*, *KLRC4-KLRK1* and *JMJD7* in CD8 cells. *EIF5A* in CD8 cells was common to both malaise and temporal headache. *SLA* and *ETS1* are genes shared by patients with a history of PMR diagnosis and those experiencing visual disturbances at T1.

Table 2 "Acute phase" symptoms, signs and relevant past medical history

	Phenotype	Number of patients with each feature at time of presentation	Number of transcripts per cell type correlating to each phenotype	
			CD4	CD8
1	Visual Disturbance	14	23	247
2	Temporal Headache	14	67	34
3	Other Headache	13	30	76
4	Scalp Tenderness	12	10	7
5	Malaise	12	8	27
6	Jaw Claudication	11	70	10
7	Fatigue	11	6	29
8	Loss of Appetite	9	59	32
9	Weight Loss	8	27	55
10	Fever	4	177	41
11	Polymyalgia Rheumatica	4	51	53

Number of patients (total n = 16) and genes significantly affected (FDR < 0.01) by clinical phenotype in regression models at T1

Table 4 "Prognostic genes"

	Phenotype	T1		T1-T6	
		CD4	CD8	CD4	CD8
1	Monocular Blindness	22	41	26	56
2	Bilateral Blindness	22	50	21	18
3	Stroke/TIA	40	4	153	70
4	Relapse Events	6	3	47	166
5	Deceased within 12 months	878	904	43	50

Number of genes significantly affected (FDR < 0.01) by outcome and prognostic phenotype markers in regression models both in the acute phase alone (T1) as well as across all time points (T1-T6)

Genes shared by three clinically important phenotypes at T1 are even more promising than those shared by two phenotypes and included 15 genes in CD4 and 16 in CD8 cells (Table 5). *SRRT* in CD4 was common to four phenotypes: death, fever, and both headache types. In CD8, *IL32* was common to five phenotypes: visual disturbance and raised neutrophils at T1, a history of PMR, and bilateral blindness and death within 12 months (Additional file 10: Table S7 & Additional file 11: Table S8 show shared genes per phenotype).

Correlation with currently used biochemical markers
We asked whether the results of several routine blood tests, including white cell count, platelet count, ESR and CRP correlated with changes in gene expression (Table 3). We observed significant clinical associations for each biochemical marker in both CD4 and CD8 samples.

Thrombocytosis - raised platelet count - is a good predictor of acute GCA [16]. Our analysis revealed associations of multiple genes common to both raised platelet count and fever in CD4 cells, namely *ATP9B, SEC23A, PDZD4, ABCA2, ELK1, CCDC88C* and *DGKZ*. In addition, ESR and CRP are biomarkers commonly used to predict the likelihood of GCA, and we found that *SAP18* in CD4 was associated with raised ESR and jaw claudication, whereas in CD8 cells *AMPD2* was associated with raised CRP and visual disturbances.

White-blood cell count (WCC), neutrophil and lymphocyte count may also be affected in GCA, although this may be due to the corticosteroid treatment rather than the inflammatory process [17]. In the CD4 cells of our patients, we found that *SPPL2B* expression was common to both those with raised WCC and jaw claudication whilst *MATR3* was associated with raised WCC and long-term monocular blindness. *NDUFS7* expression in CD4 cells was associated with an increased lymphocyte count and temporal headache in CD4, whereas in CD8 cells *AP1G2* was common to raised lymphocytes and visual disturbance. Additionally, expression of *ZNF343* and *INTS14* in CD4 cells were associated with both raised neutrophil and with scalp tenderness and event relapses respectively.

Correlation with prognostic outcome 12 months after diagnosis
We identified genes that overlap between phenotypes marking acute disease as well as those marking prognosis. For example, temporal headache at T1 as well as bilateral blindness showed significant association with CD8 expression of *TCF7* (*TH*: beta = − 0.151, adj. p-value = 6.0×10^{-4}, *BB*: beta = − 1.801, adj. p-value = 2.2×10^{-3}) and *NUCB2* (beta = 1.571, adj. p-value = 1.31×10^{-6}). The expression of such genes could provide insight into visual prognosis in those patients presenting with headache in GCA. *RPL17* in CD8 was associated between jaw claudication and relapse events, and *FTSJ1* in CD4 between jaw claudication and long-term cerebrovascular events. Many genes were shared between multiple acute phase phenotypes and mortality within 12 months (Table 5). Fig. 5 shows the network analysis of clinically correlated phenotypes with shared genes, and highlights the link between phenotypes through significant shared genes.

Discussion
Through transcriptional profiling of T-lymphocytes, we identified 4031 genes in CD4+ and CD8+ cells (CD4: 884; CD8: 3147) that are differentially expressed between patients with active GCA compared to age- and sex-matched controls. Longitudinal profiling of cases was undertaken with the aim of distinguishing genes that are up- or down-regulated during the acute phase of disease, which later normalise as the disease quiesces. We hypothesised that gene expression in GCA patients would return to normal at approximately 12 months. With polynomial modeling analysis of the significant differentially expressed genes, we identified 4 transcripts in CD8+ cells and 179 in CD4+ cells that show a change in expression profile over the course of twelve months (Fig. 2). As there were no statistically significant differentially expressed genes between both samples taken from controls subjects at separate times, the genes we report as differentially expressed likely represent true changes occurring in GCA disease activity.

Next, we determined whether the fold change in expression was secondary to the true effect of disease status rather than due to steroid treatment. It is important to take into consideration steroid influence on gene expression, especially early in the treatment course, as this would allow for the identification of a biomarker that could help diagnose GCA in the acute setting prior to treatment. As patients received high-dose corticosteroids between T2-T6, we compared gene expression of those patients who were steroid naive versus those who had already been initiated on treatment at their first sample collection. *LMBR1L, UAP1L1* and *KCNMB4* in CD4, and *PTCD2* and *THRAP3* in CD8, showed least clustering at the initial collection and seemed least affected by steroids at T1 (Fig. 3), suggesting that the expression profiles of these genes seen in patients, compared to

Table 5 Genes associated with multiple phenotypes, both acute and prognostic, in CD4 and CD8 T cells

Gene	Phenotype 1	Phenotype 2	Phenotype 3
CD4			
ATP1A1	Temporal headache	Bilateral blindness	Death within 12 months
LAMTOR4	Temporal headache	Jaw claudication	Death within 12 months
MATR3	White cell count	Monocular blindness	Death within 12 months
MLH1	Temporal headache	Bilateral blindness	Death within 12 months
NDEL1	Loss of appetite	Other headache	Death within 12 months
NDUFS7	Temporal headache	Elevated lymphocytes	Death within 12 months
PDZD4	Fever	Loss of appetite	Reduced platelets
POFUT2	Temporal headache	Other headache	Death within 12 months
RRP1	Temporal headache	Bilateral blindness	Death within 12 months
SDCCAG3	Bilateral blindness	Relapse events	Death within 12 months
SEC23A	Fever	Reduced platelets	Death within 12 months
SLC10A3	Fever	Reduced white cell count	Death within 12 months
USF2	Temporal headache	Bilateral blindness	Death within 12 months
WDR91	Loss of appetite	Elevated white cell count	Death within 12 months
ZNF343	Scalp tenderness	Reduced neutrophils	Death within 12 months
CD8			
ACADVL	Elevated neutrophils	Other headache	Death within 12 months
CD6	Elevated neutrophils	Visual disturbance	Death within 12 months
EIF5A	Malaise	Temporal headache	Death within 12 months
FDXR	Loss of appetite	Weight loss	Death within 12 months
INPPL1	Malaise	Fatigue	Elevated neutrophils
JMJD7	Temporal headache	Other headache	Death within 12 months
KIAA0513	Visual disturbance	Bilateral blindness	Death within 12 months
KLRC4-KLR1l	Temporal headache	Other headache	Death within 12 months
MTA1	Elevated neutrophils	Visual disturbance	Death within 12 months
NUCB2	Temporal headache	Bilateral blindness	Death within 12 months
PI4KA	Elevated neutrophils	Visual disturbance	Death within 12 months
PRAG1	Elevated neutrophils	Bilateral blindness	Death within 12 months
RNPS1	Malaise	Fatigue	Death within 12 months
SLC35F6	Temporal headache	Other headache	Death within 12 months
UQCRC1	Malaise	Other headache	Death within 12 months
ZNF708	Temporal headache	Other headache	Death within 12 months

controls, is likely representative of "acute disease" at T1 rather than a steroid-induced change.

Gene expression patterns seen from our polynomial modeling analysis over the 12 months might have been influenced by systemic corticosteroid treatment (Fig. 3). In CD8+ samples, differential expression of certain genes increased dramatically at around 6–8 weeks (T3) in cases compared to the controls, and in CD4+ cells, differential expression plateaued from T2-T4. Duration of steroid treatment did not have a significant effect on expression and was removed from analysis. We also adjusted for steroid dose and patient weight in our

analysis; however, the peak in expression in both cell types at these time points could be caused by a delayed or accumulation of steroid-induced effect. Nevertheless, from a diagnostic perspective, acute phase evaluation at T1 is most crucial for patient assessment and this potential delayed steroid-induced effect is not that problematic in our analysis. It does, however, make evaluation of expression levels in relation to relapse events between 0.5–12 months (T2-T6) slightly challenging.

Our results show that transcripts that remain DE at 12 months (T6) could potentially be used in clinical practice to detect evidence of previous GCA disease despite

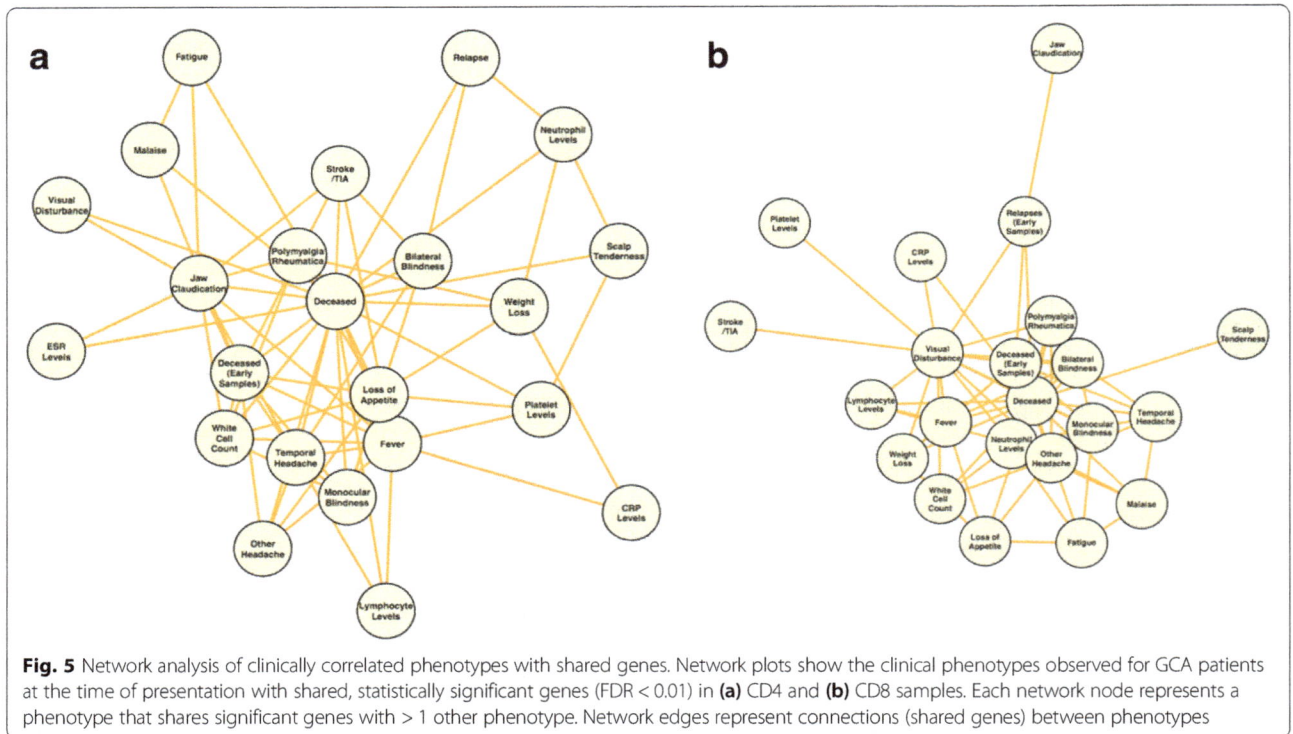

Fig. 5 Network analysis of clinically correlated phenotypes with shared genes. Network plots show the clinical phenotypes observed for GCA patients at the time of presentation with shared, statistically significant genes (FDR < 0.01) in (**a**) CD4 and (**b**) CD8 samples. Each network node represents a phenotype that shares significant genes with > 1 other phenotype. Network edges represent connections (shared genes) between phenotypes

current inactivity. In CD8+ cells, we identified two significant differentially expressed transcripts at T6 versus controls, *SGTB* and *FCGR3A*. Little is known about *SGTB* but it has been associated with neuronal apoptosis after neuroinflammation [18]. Interestingly, *FCGR3A* encodes CD16a, which forms part of the Fc receptor of the immunoglobulin complex and interacts with a number of immune-related proteins including CD4 and PTPRC, a protein required for T-cell activation. Recently, Lassaunière et al. showed that Black individuals have significantly reduced proportions of *FCGR3A* natural killer cells (95.2% vs. 96.9%) and CD8+ T lymphocytes (9.6% vs. 11.7%) compared to Caucasians [19], and this may serve as a predictive marker for a high-expressing *FCGR3A* phenotype in Caucasians, the population most affected by GCA. A recent genome-wide association study revealed that the FCGR2A/FCGR3A genes confer susceptibility to Takayasu arteritis, another chronic large-vessel vasculitis [20]. Furthermore, two recent studies investigating rejection in heart and kidney transplants, observed selective changes in endothelial/angiogenesis and natural killer cell transcripts, including *CD16A* and *FCGR3A* which showed increased expression with rejection phenotypes [21, 22]. Both studies illustrate the clinical potential of gene transcripts to illustrate transplant rejection diagnosis. A future study would need to be conducted to investigate the expression of *FCGR3A* and *CD16a* at the arterial level

(TAB) of GCA patients to determine whether increased expression at local level is representative to that found in peripheral T-cells. If so, *FCGR3A* could potentially be used as a biomarker of GCA severity in peripheral blood.

From our CD8+ cell analysis, we detected two differentially expressed isoforms of *CD163* with significantly reduced expression levels at first and last collection points. *CD163*, however, is a member of the scavenger receptor cysteine-rich (SRCR) superfamily, and is mostly expressed in monocytes and macrophages [23]. Despite an excellent T-cell population purity of > 97% isolated through MACS (Additional file 2: Figure S1), monocytes and macrophages may carry CD4+ and CD8+ cell surface markers as T lymphocytes, and may have carried over into our final positively-selected T-cell population. Irrespective of its derivative cell population, *CD163* expression may play a crucial role in the context of GCA and, as a result, provide crucial information. *CD163* is involved in dendritic cell development, a cell crucial in the pathogenesis of GCA [24]. It has been suggested that the soluble form of *CD163* (sCD163) may have an anti-inflammatory role, and be a valuable diagnostic parameter for monitoring macrophage activation in inflammatory conditions where macrophage function is affected [25]. A number of clinical studies have evaluated the role sCD163 as a disease marker in inflammatory conditions including autoimmune disease, transplantation and cancer [26–28]. Expression levels of *CD163* were reduced in our patients at T6, possibly reflecting disease quiescence. It is likely that 12 months after disease onset, the need for CD163-monocytes and macrophages to clear damaged tissue has become redundant. *CD163* featured in both our differential expression and polynomial regression analyses and therefore warrants further investigation in the context of GCA, potentially through study of peripheral or tissue monocytes and macrophages.

Another strength of this study is that, through linear and logistic regression analyses, we identified associations between specific clinically important phenotypes and expressed transcripts. We detected genes which correlated with both symptoms and signs as well as biochemical markers used in the acute setting (Table 2). Symptoms causing the most suspicion of a potential GCA diagnosis consist of jaw claudication, temporal headache (or other type), scalp tenderness and visual disturbance [1]. Genes shared by multiple phenotypes are likely to be particularly relevant to making a diagnosis and could be used as biomarkers for disease activity in the acute setting and potentially predict relapses.

Jaw claudication is often considered the most predictive symptom of GCA; for example, a patient has a nine time greater risk of a positive TAB when they experience jaw claudication [29]. In CD4 cells of our patient cohort, *LAMTOR4*, was shared between jaw claudication and temporal headache. This protein is part of the ragulator complex, which is involved in pathways regulating cell size and cell cycle arrest [30]. A gene common to both jaw claudication and visual disturbance is *GZMB*, otherwise known as Granzyme B enzyme. *GZMB* is necessary for targeting cell lysis in cell-mediated immune responses and is involved in the activation of cytokine release and cascade of caspases responsible for apoptosis execution. Its involvement has been reported in other autoimmune diseases such as type 1 diabetes and systemic lupus erythematosus [31, 32]. *PPP1CB*, linked to vascular smooth muscle contraction pathway [33], was common to patients with jaw claudication and a background history of PMR, which has been shown to increase the risk of GCA [34]. *EXTL3*, involved in the heparan sulfate biosynthesis pathway and previously associated with syphilis, was expressed in both patients with jaw claudication and fatigue [35].

Multiple genes were associated with temporal and other types of headache in our patients. These included *POFUT2* in CD4 cells and *SLC35F6, HTD2, ZNF708, KLRC4-KLRK1* and *JMJD7* in CD8 cells. These genes have been implicated in cellular defense mechanisms, innate immunity, cell proliferation and apoptosis signaling pathways [36]. One example of great clinical interest is a gene shared by patients with a history of PMR and those experiencing visual disturbances at T1. *ETS1*, controls lymphocyte differentiation and modulates cytokine and chemokine expression. Low expression levels of *ETS1*, leading to aberrant lymphocyte differentiation, have been found in systemic lupus erythematosus [37]. *ETS1* also has a potential role in the regulation of angiogenesis [38]. *ETS1* warrants further functional investigation in relation to its vascular role and as a biomarker for GCA for those patients presenting with PMR.

Three patients died during the study period. The exact cause of death for the three patients is unknown. One patient was being managed by her rural GP as lived rurally. She lived in a nursing home after losing vision in both eyes from GCA. The second patient who died was also bilaterally blind from GCA. She suffered multiple falls and died soon after. The third patient, admitted to hospital for general decline in health, was investigated for possible stroke. She had very poor appetite and died within a few weeks of admission. The bilateral visual loss likely predisposes to poor outcome, whether directly as a sign of disease severity or possibly due to increased likelihood of falls and other morbidity indirectly increasing mortality.

We determined gene correlations with markers of disease prognosis and severity (Table 3). Genes in association with poor prognostic outcome markers of GCA, such as blindness, relapses and death could provide useful predictions in the acute setting and could help determine the treatment intensity and length required for those particular patients. We identified genes that overlap between acute phase markers as well as the prognostic markers. For example, temporal headache at T1 as well as bilateral blindness showed significant association with CD8 expression of *TCF7*, which is important for adaptive T lymphocyte and innate lymphoid cell regulation [39]. Both these phenotypes were also associated with *NUCB2*, which encodes Nesfatin-1. *NUCB2* is linked to inflammation and coagulopathies, and is correlated with mortality following brain injury [40]. As *TCF7* and *NUCB2* expression are associated with temporal headache in patients with GCA, these genes could also raise suspicion of poor visual outcome in patients presenting with temporal headache with GCA diagnosis.

We identified 15 genes shared across three phenotypes in CD4 and 16 across CD8 cells (Table 5). In CD4 cells, *SRRT*, a gene associated with cell proliferation [41], was common to four phenotypes: death, fever, and both types of headaches. In CD8, *IL32*, a member of the cytokine family [42], was common to five phenotypes: a history of PMR, visual disturbance and raised neutrophils at T1, bilateral blindness and death within 12 months. *IL32* involvement has been described in vasculitides such as granulomatosis with polyangiitis and anti-neutrophil cytoplasm antibodies (ANCA) associated vasculitis [43, 44]. A previous quantitative gene expression analysis study investigating *IL32* in GCA demonstrated a strong and significant up-regulation of *IL32* in TAB specimens of patients with GCA; in particular it was highly expressed by vascular smooth muscle cells of inflamed arteries and neovessels within inflammatory infiltrates [45]. This study also evaluated circulating CD4+ Th1 lymphocytes by flow cytometry which showed that there was a greater abundance of them in GCA patients than controls and that they produced greater amounts of *IL32* [45]. From our study, expression of *IL32* in patients presenting with visual disturbance, a history of PMR in the presence of an abnormal neutrophil count, should raise suspicion of GCA diagnosis with poor prognostic outcome. Altered expression of these genes should raise suspicion of GCA diagnosis with poor outcome. Such genes warrant more investigation in the context of GCA as these correlated with not only clinical and biochemical phenotypes but also with prognoses.

The current mainstay treatment of high-dose corticosteroids is effective but is commonly associated with potentially serious complications affecting up to 89% of those with GCA [3]. Even after successful initial treatment with corticosteroids, GCA relapses in up to two-thirds of patients [46]. As shown by our study, 5 out of 16 patients experienced relapses requiring an increase in steroid dose (Additional file 1: Table S1). Unlike in other autoimmune diseases, most steroid-sparing agents and the use of adjunct agents in GCA [MB1] are not associated with a significant improvement in outcome [46, 47]. Tocilizumab, a humanized monoclonal antibody directed against the IL-6 receptor, has been found to improve both induction and maintenance of remission in patients with GCA for up to 12 months [48]. However, there is a large side effect profile from Tocilizumab. Interestingly, we did not see DGE for *IL6*.

Conclusion

GCA is a devastating disease associated with significant morbidity and mortality. We present the first longitudinal gene expression study undertaken to identify robust transcriptomic biomarkers of GCA.

Our results show cell type-specific transcript expression profiles. We have identified genes potentially implicated in the patho-aetiology of GCA which may uncover important biological pathways for this disease. In addition we have identified novel gene-phenotype associations which, in the acute phase, could act as clinical prognostic markers by providing insight into potential disease severity and therefore guide in initiating appropriate patient management.

Further functional investigation is needed to understand the pathways in which the identified genes play a role in the pathogenesis of GCA and to determine whether the DGE in this study can be translated into the clinical setting as new potential biomarkers to monitor disease activity, predict outcome and assist in finding more effective and safer treatments for GCA.

Additional files

Additional file 1: Table S1. Cases recruited and attendance for all 6 time points

Additional file 2: Figure S1. Quality control metrics for stored specimens. Representative FACS analysis for FITC bound CD4 (**A**) and APC bound CD8 cells (**B**). Panel **C** displays the FACS confirmed purity of all specimens, with case and control samples represented by red and blue triangles respectively.

Additional file 3: Figure S2. Effect of batch correction on 195 samples (2 samples of the 197 were removed). Three parameters (Flowcell ID, Gender and Ethnicity) were used to remove confounding effects in edgeR. PC1 contributes the greatest amount of variance and is largely attributed to Flowcell ID, which accounts for most of the variance in sequencing experiments.

Additional file 4: Table S2. Ophthalmic clinical summary data (GCA cases, $n = 16$).

Additional file 5: Table S3. General disease outcome and prognostic measures.

Additional file 6: Figure S3. Expression levels of the top 500 most variable transcripts in CD4 and CD8 cells, shown for each of 135 samples. Sample groups are indicated by the orange (CD4) and blue (CD8) bars at the top of the heatmap.

Additional file 7: Table S4. Differential expression results CD4.

Additional file 8: Table S5. Differential expression results CD8.

Additional file 9: Table S6. Significant polynomial modelling results.

Additional file 10: Table S7. Significant CD4 genes shared by phenotypes at T1.

Additional file 11: Table S8. Significant CD8 genes shared by phenotypes at T1.

Abbreviations
ATGC: Australian Translational Genomics Centre; CERA: Centre for Eye Research Australia; CPM: Counts-per-million; CRP: C-reactive Protein; DE: Differentially expressed; DGE: Differential gene expression; ESR: Erythrocyte Sedimentation Rate; FACS: Fluorescence-Activated Cell Sorting; FC: fold change; FDR: False Discovery Rate; GCA: Giant Cell Arteritis; IL: Interleukin; MACS: Magnetic-Assisted Cell Sorting; PBMC: Peripheral Blood Mononuclear Cells; PMR: Polymyalgia Rheumatica; RIN: RNA Integrity Number; RVEEH: Royal Victorian Eye and Ear Hospital; T1–6: Time points 1 to 6; WCC: White cell count

Acknowledgements
We thank all doctors and nurses at the Royal Victorian Eye and Ear Hospital for referring patients to us over the course of this study. We thank the Flow Cytometry Facility at the University of Melbourne Brain Centre for analysing the purity of our cell populations. Mostly, we thank all patients for their time and on-going efforts to participate in this work.

Funding
This work was supported by funding from Arthritis Australia, the Ophthalmic Research Institute of Australia, and an Australian National Health and Medical Research Council (NHMRC) grant (1083405), an NHMRC Practitioner Fellowship (AWH, 1103329), NHMRC Career Development Fellowship (JEP, 1107599) an Australian Research Council Future Fellowship (AP, FT140100047). CERA receives Operational Infrastructure Support from the Victorian Government. The funders had no role in study design, data collection and analysis, decision to publish, or preparation of the manuscript.

Authors' contributions

EDS coordinated the study, recruited patients, performed MACS experiments and RNA batch extractions. LC took patients blood samples, performed MACS and liaised with patients to organise follow-up study appointments. KC, AWTY and CC assisted in patient recruitment and MACS. NS referred patients from the neuro-ophthalmology service at the RVEEH and managed patients' medical care. ILS and SH assisted and supervised RNA extractions. LA, SS, BW, LW in MB's laboratory performed the cDNA preparations and subsequent RNA sequencing of samples across the 9 flow cells. SL, AS, KD and JP performed the bioinformatic analysis on the data generated from the RNA sequencing. DM, AP and AH organised funding for this work and designed the overall study. EDS and SL wrote the article. All authors read and approved the final manuscript.

Competing interests

The authors declare that they have no competing interests.

Author details

[1]Centre for Eye Research Australia, The University of Melbourne, Royal Victorian Eye & Ear Hospital, 32 Gisborne Street, East Melbourne 3002, Australia. [2]Institute for Molecular Bioscience, The University of Queensland, Brisbane 4072, Queensland, Australia. [3]Institute of Health and Biomedical Innovation, Queensland University of Technology, Translational Research Institute, Princess Alexandra Hospital, Brisbane 4102, Queensland, Australia. [4]Ophthalmology Department at Monash Health, Department of Surgery, School of Clinical Sciences at Monash Health, Melbourne 3168, Victoria, Australia. [5]Department of Neuro-Ophthalmology, Royal Victorian Eye and Ear Hospital, Melbourne 3002, Victoria, Australia. [6]Centre for Ophthalmology and Visual Science, The University of Western Australia, Lions Eye Institute, Perth 6009, Western Australia, Australia. [7]School of Medicine, Menzies Research Institute Tasmania, University of Tasmania, Hobart 7000, Tasmania, Australia.

References

1. De Smit E, O'Sullivan E, Mackey DA, Hewitt AW. Giant cell arteritis: ophthalmic manifestations of a systemic disease. Graefes Arch Clin Exp Ophthalmol. 2016;254:2291–306.

2. De Smit E, Clarke L, Sanfilippo PG, Merriman TR, Brown MA, Hill CL, et al. Geo-epidemiology of temporal artery biopsy-positive giant cell arteritis in Australia and New Zealand: is there a seasonal influence? RMD Open. 2017; 3:e000531.

3. Dunstan E, Lester SL, Rischmueller M, Dodd T, Black R, Ahern M, et al. Epidemiology of biopsy-proven giant cell arteritis in South Australia. Intern Med J. 2014;44:32–9.

4. Seeliger B, Sznajd J, Robson JC, Judge A, Craven A, Grayson PC, et al. Are the 1990 American College of Rheumatology vasculitis classification criteria still valid? Rheumatology. 2017; https://doi.org/10.1093/rheumatology/kex075.

5. Carmona FD, Mackie SL, Martín J-E, Taylor JC, Vaglio A, Eyre S, et al. A large-scale genetic analysis reveals a strong contribution of the HLA class II region to giant cell arteritis susceptibility. Am J Hum Genet. 2015;96:565–80.

6. Samson M, Ly KH, Tournier B, Janikashvili N, Trad M, Ciudad M, et al. Involvement and prognosis value of CD8(+) T cells in giant cell arteritis. J Autoimmun. 2016;72:73–83.

7. Weyand CM, Liao YJ, Goronzy JJ. The immunopathology of giant cell arteritis: diagnostic and therapeutic implications. J Neuroophthalmol. 2012; 32:259–65.

8. Chaussabel D, Pascual V, Banchereau J. Assessing the human immune system through blood transcriptomics. BMC Biol. 2010;8:84.

9. Lyons PA, Koukoulaki M, Hatton A, Doggett K, Woffendin HB, Chaudhry AN, et al. Microarray analysis of human leucocyte subsets: the advantages of positive selection and rapid purification. BMC Genomics. 2007;8:64.

10. Bray NL, Pimentel H, Melsted P, Pachter L. Near-optimal probabilistic RNA-seq quantification. Nat Biotechnol. 2016;34:525–7.

11. Robinson MD, McCarthy DJ, Smyth GK. edgeR: a Bioconductor package for differential expression analysis of digital gene expression data. Bioinformatics. 2010;26:139–40.

12. Kamburov A, Stelzl U, Lehrach H, Herwig R. The ConsensusPathDB interaction database: 2013 update. Nucleic Acids Res. 2013;41:D793–800.

13. Benjamini Y, Hochberg Y. On the adaptive control of the false discovery rate in multiple testing with independent statistics. J Educ Behav Stat. 2000;25:60.

14. Buechler C, Ritter M, Orsó E, Langmann T, Klucken J, Schmitz G. Regulation of scavenger receptor CD163 expression in human monocytes and macrophages by pro- and antiinflammatory stimuli. J Leukoc Biol. 2000;67:97–103.

15. Tippett E, Cheng W-J, Westhorpe C, Cameron PU, Brew BJ, Lewin SR, et al. Differential expression of CD163 on monocyte subsets in healthy and HIV-1 infected individuals. PLoS One. 2011;6:e19968.

16. El-Dairi MA, Chang L, Proia AD, Cummings TJ, Stinnett SS, Bhatti MT. Diagnostic algorithm for patients with suspected Giant cell arteritis. J Neuroophthalmol. 2015;35:246–53.

17. Abramson N, Melton B. Leukocytosis: basics of clinical assessment. Am Fam Physician. 2000;62:2053–60.

18. Cao M, Xu W, Yu J, Zheng H, Tan X, Li L, et al. Up-regulation of SGTB is associated with neuronal apoptosis after neuroinflammation induced by lipopolysaccharide. J Mol Histol. 2013;44:507–18.

19. Lassaunière R, Shalekoff S, Tiemessen CT. A novel FCGR3A intragenic haplotype is associated with increased FcγRIIIa/CD16a cell surface density and population differences. Hum Immunol. 2013;74:627–34.

20. Chen S, Wen X, Li J, Li Y, Li L, Tian X, et al. Association of FCGR2A/FCGR3A variant rs2099684 with Takayasu arteritis in the Han Chinese population. Oncotarget. 2017; https://doi.org/10.18632/oncotarget.12738.

21. Loupy A, Duong Van Huyen JP, Hidalgo L, Reeve J, Racapé M, Aubert O, et al. Gene expression profiling for the identification and classification of antibody-mediated heart rejection. Circulation. 2017;135:917–35.

22. Lefaucheur C, Viglietti D, Hidalgo LG, Ratner LE, Bagnasco SM, Batal I, et al. Complement-activating anti-HLA antibodies in kidney transplantation: allograft gene expression profiling and response to treatment. J Am Soc Nephrol. 2017; https://doi.org/10.1681/ASN.2017050589.

23. Moestrup SK, Møller HJ. CD163: a regulated hemoglobin scavenger receptor with a role in the anti-inflammatory response. Ann Med. 2004; 36:347–54.

24. Samson M, Corbera-Bellalta M, Audia S, Planas-Rigol E, Martin L, Cid MC, et al. Recent advances in our understanding of giant cell arteritis pathogenesis. Autoimmun Rev. 2017;16:833–44.

25. Ding D, Song Y, Yao Y, Zhang S. Preoperative serum macrophage activated biomarkers soluble mannose receptor (sMR) and soluble haemoglobin scavenger receptor (sCD163), as novel markers for the diagnosis and prognosis of gastric cancer. Oncol Lett. 2017;14:2982–90.

26. Rødgaard-Hansen S, St George A, Kazankov K, Bauman A, George J, Grønbæk H, et al. Effects of lifestyle intervention on soluble CD163, a macrophage activation marker, in patients with non-alcoholic fatty liver disease. Scand J Clin Lab Invest. 2017;77:498–504.

27. Pranzatelli MR, Tate ED, McGee NR. Microglial/macrophage markers CHI3L1, sCD14, and sCD163 in CSF and serum of pediatric inflammatory and non-inflammatory neurological disorders: a case-control study and reference ranges. J Neurol Sci. 2017;381:285–90.

28. Stilund M, Reuschlein A-K, Christensen T, Møller HJ, Rasmussen PV, Petersen T. Soluble CD163 as a marker of macrophage activity in newly diagnosed patients with multiple sclerosis. PLoS One. 2014;9:e98588.

29. Hayreh SS. Masticatory muscle pain: an important indicator of giant cell arteritis. Spec Care Dentist. 1998;18:60–5.

30. Stoesser GEMBL. Nucleotide sequence database (EMBL-Bank, EMBL database). Dictionary of Bioinformatics and Computational Biology. 2004;

31. Cullen SP, Brunet M, Martin SJ. Granzymes in cancer and immunity. Cell Death Differ. 2010;17:616–23.

32. Joeckel LT, Bird PI. Blessing or curse? Proteomics in granzyme research. Proteomics Clin Appl. 2014;8:351–81.

33. Takaki T, Montanger M, Serres MP, Le Berre M, Russell M, Collinson L, et al. Actomyosin drives cancer cell nuclear dysmorphia and threatens genome stability. Nat Commun. 2017;8:16013.

34. Buttgereit F, Dejaco C, Matteson EL, Dasgupta B. Polymyalgia Rheumatica and Giant cell arteritis: a systematic review. JAMA. 2016;315:2442–58.

35. Volpi S, Yamazaki Y, Brauer PM, van Rooijen E, Hayashida A, Slavotinek A, et al. EXTL3 mutations cause skeletal dysplasia, immune deficiency, and developmental delay. J Exp Med. 2017;214:623–37.

36. GeneCards. Encyclopedia of Genetics, Genomics, Proteomics and Informatics; 2008. p. 761–1.

37. Garrett-Sinha LA, Kearly A, Satterthwaite AB. The role of the transcription factor Ets1 in lupus and other autoimmune diseases. Crit Rev Immunol. 2016;36:485–510.

38. Yordy JS, Moussa O, Pei H, Chaussabel D, Li R, Watson DK. SP100 inhibits ETS1 activity in primary endothelial cells. Oncogene. 2005;24:916–31.

39. De Obaldia ME, Bhandoola A. Transcriptional regulation of innate and adaptive lymphocyte lineages. Annu Rev Immunol. 2015;33:607–42.

40. Wu G-Q, Chou X-M, Ji W-J, Yang X-G, Lan L-X, Sheng Y-J, et al. The prognostic value of plasma nesfatin-1 concentrations in patients with traumatic brain injury. Clin Chim Acta. 2016;458:124–8.

41. Ashrafi M, Sebastian A, Shih B, Greaves N, Alonso-Rasgado T, Baguneid M, et al. Whole genome microarray data of chronic wound debridement prior to application of dermal skin substitutes. Wound Repair Regen. 2016;24:870–5.

42. Kim S-H, Han S-Y, Azam T, Yoon D-Y, Dinarello CA. Interleukin-32: a cytokine and inducer of TNFalpha. Immunity. 2005;22:131–42.

43. Bae S, Kim Y-G, Choi J, Hong J, Lee S, Kang T, et al. Elevated interleukin-32 expression in granulomatosis with polyangiitis. Rheumatology. 2012;51: 1979–88.

44. Csernok E, Holle JU, Gross WL. Proteinase 3, protease-activated receptor-2 and interleukin-32: linking innate and autoimmunity in Wegener's granulomatosis. Clin Exp Rheumatol. 2008;26:S112–7.

45. Ciccia F, Alessandro R, Rizzo A, Principe S, Raiata F, Cavazza A, et al. Expression of interleukin-32 in the inflamed arteries of patients with giant cell arteritis. Arthritis Rheum. 2011;63:2097–104.

46. Labarca C, Koster MJ, Crowson CS, Makol A, Ytterberg SR, Matteson EL, et al. Predictors of relapse and treatment outcomes in biopsy-proven giant cell arteritis: a retrospective cohort study. Rheumatology. 2016;55:347–56.

47. Yates M, Loke YK, Watts RA, MacGregor AJ. Prednisolone combined with adjunctive immunosuppression is not superior to prednisolone alone in terms of efficacy and safety in giant cell arteritis: meta-analysis. Clin Rheumatol. 2014;33:227–36.

48. Roberts J, Clifford A. Update on the management of giant cell arteritis. Ther Adv Chronic Dis. 2017;8:69–79.

4

Frequency and phenotype consequence of *APOC3* rare variants in patients with very low triglyceride levels

Dana C. Crawford[1*], Nicole A. Restrepo[1], Kirsten E. Diggins[2], Eric Farber-Eger[3] and Quinn S. Wells[4]

From The 7th Translational Bioinformatics Conference
Los Angeles, CA, USA. 29 September - 01 October 2017

Abstract

Background: High levels of triglycerides (TG $\geq$ 200 mg/dL) are an emerging risk factor for cardiovascular disease. Conversely, very low levels of TG are associated with decreased risk for cardiovascular disease. Precision medicine aims to capitalize on recent findings that rare variants such as *APOC3* R19X (rs76353203) are associated with risk of disease, but it is unclear how population-based associations can be best translated in clinical settings at the individual-patient level.

Methods: To explore the potential usefulness of screening for genetic predictors of cardiovascular disease, we surveyed BioVU, the Vanderbilt University Medical Center's biorepository linked to de-identified electronic health records (EHRs), for *APOC3* 19X mutations among adult European American patients (> 45 and > 55 years of age for men and women, respectively) with the lowest percentile of TG levels. The initial search identified 262 patients with the lowest TG levels in the biorepository; among these, 184 patients with sufficient DNA and the lowest TG levels were chosen for Illumina ExomeChip genotyping.

Results: A total of two patients were identified as heterozygotes of *APOC3* R19X for a minor allele frequency (MAF) of 0.55% in this patient population. Both heterozygous patients had only a single mention of TG in the EHR (31 and 35 mg/dL, respectively), and one patient had evidence of previous cardiovascular disease.

Conclusions: In this patient population, we identified two patients who were carriers of the *APOC3* 19X null variant, but only one lacked evidence of disease in the EHR highlighting the challenges of inclusion of functional or previously associated genetic variation in clinical risk assessment.

Keywords: Precision medicine, Triglycerides, Biobank, Electronic health records, APOC3

Background

Personalized or precision medicine is meant to distinguish tailored treatment from trial and error. The concept of precision medicine is not new and has been in practice arguably since the dawn of modern medicine [1]. Health care providers have long collected detailed data on patients, ranging from basic personal histories to technical laboratory assays and diagnostic procedures, to provide specific diagnoses and treatments. These tools ordered in the precision medicine setting are constantly evolving, for example, the evolution of myocardial infarction diagnosis [2], resulting in high resolution and, in some cases, highly predictive individualized data.

Today's concept of precision medicine has evolved to specifically include the genetic profile of a patient in the prevention, diagnosis, and treatment of disease [3, 4]. Previous proxies for genetic profiles such as sex, race/ ethnicity, family history, and response to therapy are now being augmented by Clinical Laboratory Improvement Amendments-certified genotyping and sequencing

* Correspondence: dana.crawford@case.edu
[1]Department of Population and Quantitative Health Sciences, Institute for Computational Biology, Case Western Reserve University, 2103 Cornell Road, Wolstein Research Building, Suite 2-527, Cleveland, OH 44106, USA
Full list of author information is available at the end of the article

at both the targeted and whole genome level. Indeed, technological advances in high-throughput genomics coupled with their rapid decreases in costs have made generating the data almost trivial, and the emergence of electronic health records (EHRs) in part through the HITECH Act [5, 6] make it possible to effectively deliver personalized medicine to the patient.

A major challenge in the delivery of personalized medicine is not the collection of data, but the interpretation of the data. Large-scale population sequencing studies have demonstrated that potentially functional variants exist in all DNA samples sequenced, but the biological and statistical data lag in filtering the potential from truly functional, and even less data are available to direct the course of clinical action based on these genotypes. As such, major areas of active research focus on methods to translate genomic discoveries into clinical applications [7]. This broad area of investigation includes research on who to test, what to test, how to test, what to report, how to report, and how to measure its effectiveness, to name a few.

To begin to address some of these gaps in research, we have undertaken a pilot study of genotyping for a loss of function variant, *APOC3* R19X (rs76353203), in a targeted population of 184 European American adults (men > 45 and women > 55 year of age) with very low triglyceride levels in BioVU, the Vanderbilt University Medical Center (VUMC)'s biorepository linked to de-identified EHRs. Triglyceride levels (TG) are a common biomarker measured in the clinic, and patients with extreme triglyceride (TG) levels may be flagged for further evaluation for cardiovascular disease risk assessment (TG ≥200 mg/dL). Recent studies have identified a loss-of-function variant in *APOC3* (R19X or rs76353203) associated with low triglyceride levels and diminished post-prandial lipemia in heterozygous carriers [8] and improved clearance of plasma TGs after a fatty meal in homozygous carriers [9]. Although rare in the general population [10], we hypothesized that the loss-of-function allele would be at an increased frequency in this extreme population. Based on previous reports, we also hypothesized that evidence of cardiovascular disease would be absent in EHRs of these *APOC3* 19X carriers with very low TG levels.

Methods
Study population
The study population presented here is from BioVU, the VUMC's biorepository linked to de-identified EHRs. BioVU operations [11] and ethical oversight [12] have been previously described. Briefly, DNA is extracted from discarded blood drawn for routine clinical care at Vanderbilt outpatient clinics in Nashville, Tennessee and surrounding areas. The DNA samples are linked to a de-identified version of the patient's EHR. The data in this study were de-identified in accordance with provisions of Title 45, Code of Federal Regulations, part 46 (45 CFR 46); therefore, this study was considered non-human subjects research by the Vanderbilt University Internal Review Board.

Phenotyping
The de-identified EHR contains both structured (International Classification of Diseases, Ninth Revision, Clinical Modification (ICD-9-CM) billing codes; current procedural terminology (CPT) codes; problems lists; labs) and unstructured (clinical free text) data accessible for electronic phenotyping. We extracted all available labs for triglyceride levels in September 2012 for European American adults (> 45 years of age of men and > 55 years of age for women) and examined individuals whose median TG levels constituted the lowest 1% of BioVU at the time of data extraction. A total of 262 individuals were identified. Manual review of the clinical text for 30 random patients with low TG levels prior to selection for genotyping failed to identify obvious documented diagnoses or notes that may have led to very low TG levels in these patients. From these 262 individuals, 184 were selected for Illumina HumanExome BeadChip genotyping based on DNA quality and quantity, and preference was given to individuals with more than one triglyceride level reflecting consistently low TG levels.

The de-identified EHRs for the 184 patients genotyped on the Illumina HumanExome BeadChip were re-examined in July 2015 for evidence of myocardial infarction, revascularization, and other heart disease. Myocardial infarction was defined by mention of ICD-9-CM codes 410 or 410.* or a problem list mention of "MI" or "myocardial infarction." Revascularization was defined by CPT codes (Table 1). Other heart disease was defined as a problem list mention of "coronary artery disease," "CAD," "coronary heart disease," or "CHD."

Genotyping and statistical methods
Vanderbilt Technologies for Advanced Genomics (VANTAGE) genotyped 184 BioVU samples and eight International HapMap reference samples using the Illumina HumanExome BeadChip (v1.0 for 48 samples and v1.2 for 144 samples). As recommended by other research groups with Exome BeadChip experience [13], genotypes for these 192 samples were called as part of larger, ongoing Exome BeadChip projects in BioVU genotyped by VANTAGE. *APOC3* R19X (rs76353203/exm957809) was directly assayed by the Exome BeadChip, and we extracted these called genotypes for further analysis.

We also extracted genotypes for SNPs previously associated with incident myocardial infarction in European Americans [14]. Of the 46 previously associated SNPs,

Table 1 Current Procedural Terminology codes used to define revascularization among European American patients in BioVU with very low triglyceride levels

CPT code	Description
33510–33514; 33516	Coronary artery bypass grafting with venous grafting only (1–6 or more grafts)
33515	Coronary artery bypass (old code)
33517–33519; 33521–33523	Coronary artery bypass grafting with venous and arterial grafting (1–6 or more vein grafts); billed in conjunction with 33533–33536 (33517–33523 cannot be billed alone).
33520	Coronary artery bypass (old code)
33534–33536	Coronary artery bypass grafting with arterial grafting only (2–4 or more grafts)
92980–92981	Transcatheter placement of an intracoronary stent, percutaneous, with or without other therapeutic intervention, any method (single vessel and each additional vessel)
92982; 92984	Percutaneous transluminal coronary balloon angioplasty (single vessel and each additional vessel)
92995; 92996	Percutaneous transluminal coronary atherectomy, by mechanical or other method, with or without balloon angioplasty (single vessel and each additional vessel)

37 were directly assayed by the Exome BeadChip (Additional file 1: Table S1). We then calculated both unweighted and weighted genetic risk scores (GRS) based on the genotypes of these 37 SNPs. Unweighted GRS were calculated by counting the number of risk alleles per individual. Weighted GRS were calculated based on counts of risk alleles multiplied or weighted by odds ratios recently reported for European American cases of coronary artery disease in comparison with controls [15].

Results

As detailed in the Methods section, 262 European American men > 45 and women > 55 years of age had the lowest TG levels in BioVU in 2012. Slightly less than half (44%) of the patient sample was female, and the average birth decade was the 1940s. Approximately half of the patients (53.1%) with the lowest TG levels had more than one TG available in the EHR. For those with more than one TG level, the median values were calculated. The overall median TG level in this lowest 1% was 36 mg/dL.

The genotyped study population characteristics are given in Table 2. Like the 262 patients considered, the patients genotyped were majority male born in the 1940s and 1950s. The mean body mass index was 24.8 kg/m², which is considered within the normal range. The first mention of TG in the clinical record was on average 39.3 mg/dL. The median of all TG levels available for this patient population was 36 mg/dL, ranging from 13.5 to 61 mg/dL (Fig. 1).

Among the 184 patients with low TG levels in BioVU genotyped here, 14.13%, 8.15%, and 12.5% had evidence in the EHR of a myocardial infarction, revascularization, and other heart disease, respectively. Only six out of 184 patients (3.26%) had evidence of all three. The unweighted and weighted GRS for patients with events (myocardial infarction or revascularization) or evidence for other heart disease were higher compared with patients without

events or evidence for other heart disease, although these differences were not statistically significant (Table 3).

We next examined the frequency of APOC3 R19X (rs76353203) in this patient sample of extremely low TG levels. Among 182 patients successfully genotyped for this variant, two heterozygotes were identified for a sample allele frequency of 0.55%. The allele frequency for the loss-of-function allele (T) in this sample of very low TG levels is 6.9 to 27.5 fold higher compared with allele frequency estimates for American adults drawn from the general population [10, 16] and three to 10 fold lower in frequency compared with isolated populations [8, 17, 18] (Table 4).

Previous studies in outbred [10] and isolated [8, 17] populations suggest that the 19X mutation arose once on a single haplotype background. We therefore examined the diplotypes spanning APOA1/C3/A4/A5 gene cluster assayed by the Illumina HumanExome Beachip for evidence of a single haplotype background containing the 19X mutation. Of the 78 SNPs assayed (spanning

Table 2 Study population characteristics

Female, %	43.5
Decade of birth, %	
1910	0.5
1920	9.2
1930	14.7
1940	28.3
1950	37.5
1960	9.8
Mean (±SD) body mass index (kg/m²)	24.8 (±4.7)
Mean (±SD) first TG level (mg/dL)	39.3 (±18.4)

Study population characteristics (sex, decade of birth, average body mass index, and average first mention of triglyceride levels in patient's electronic health record) are given for the *genotyped* 184 patients with the lowest 1% triglyceride levels in BioVU among European American men and women > 45 and > 55 years of age, respectively

Abbreviations: SD standard deviation, *TG* triglyceride

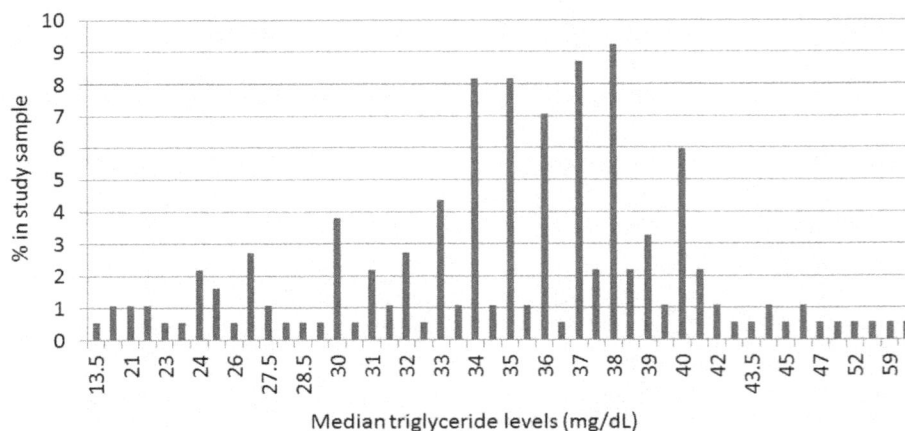

Fig. 1 Distribution of low triglyceride levels among European American adults in BioVU. A total of 184 European American adults (men > 45 years and women > 55 years) with at least one triglyceride level in the lowest 1% of BioVU were genotyped on the Illumina HumanExome BeadChip for *APOC3* R19X. The frequency (expressed as percent in the study population) is given on the y-axis and the median triglyceride levels (in mg/dL) are given on the x-axis

chr11: 116619073–116,707,837), seven SNPs overlapped with variants used to infer haplotypes in non-Hispanic whites of the Third National Health and Nutrition Examination Survey (NHANES III): rs28927680, rs964184, rs12286037, rs5110, rs675, rs5104, and rs76353203. We found that one 19X carrier was homozygous at all variants in this region that passed quality control except for 19X, and that this variant-containing haplotype background was similar to 19X backgrounds in NHANES III (G-C-C-C-A-T-T). In contrast, the second 19X carrier was heterozygous at eight sites including rs76343203. Interestingly, one of these eight heterozygous sites included rs138326449 (IVS2 + 1G > A), another *APOC3* rare variant associated with decreased levels of TG [16, 19, 20]. A query for rs138326449 in the 184 patients with very low triglycerides revealed an additional carrier for this variant. Both carriers of rs138326449 are, with the inclusion of this rare variant, heterozygous at more than one site, and one carrier has missing data (26/78 sites) at this gene cluster; therefore, his or her haplotypes could not be unambiguously inferred with confidence. Much like R19X, the frequency of rs138326449 (0.57%) is higher in

this patient population of low TG levels compared with outbred population estimates [16, 19]. A third rare *APOC3* variant (rs147210663) associated with low TG levels [16] failed genotyping in this patient population.

As expected when stratified by *APOC3* R19X genotype (Fig. 2), the mean TG level in carriers (33 mg/dL; 2.83 standard deviation) was lower compared with the non-carriers (39.51 mg/dL; 18.52 standard deviation). However, the difference was not statistically significant ($p = 0.11$) in this sample of adults with very low TG levels. Similarly, the mean TG level in IVS2 + 1G > A carriers was 32.5 mg/dL (2.12 standard deviation) for first-mentioned TG level.

Previous observational studies have suggested that TG levels are associated with risk of cardiovascular disease [21]. More recently *APOC3* 19X carrier status among other *APOC3* mutations was associated with lower risk of coronary heart disease [16]. Of the two *APOC3* 19X carriers, one had no evidence in the EHR of myocardial infarction, revascularization, or other heart disease. One *APOC3* 19X carrier had evidence in the EHR of all three. A more detailed review of the de-identified EHRs of the

Table 3 Genetic risk scores, unweighted and weighted, by case status among European American patients with very low triglyceride levels

	All patients with very low TG levels (n = 184)	Patients with no evidence of MI, revascularization, or other heart disease (n = 144)	Patients with evidence of MI (n = 26)	Patients with evidence of revascularization (n = 15)	Patients with evidence of other heart disease (n = 23)	Patients with evidence of MI, revascularization, and other heart disease (n = 6)
Unweighted GRS	38.97 (3.36)	38.78 (3.36)	39.46 (3.47)	39.07 (3.95)	39.08 (3.57)	38.00 (4.38)
Weighted GRS	41.97 (3.63)	41.77 (3.63)	42.54 (3.72)	42.08 (4.32)	42.14 (3.82)	41.02 (4.84)

We calculated unweighted and weighted genetic risk scores (GRS) based on 37 SNPs and previous association estimates in European Americans with and without coronary artery disease (Additional file 1: Table S1). Unweighted GRS were calculated as counts of risk alleles per patient, and weighted GRS were calculated using the pooled odds ratios from CARDIoGRAM [15]. Shown are the means (standard deviations) for unweighted and weighted GRS for the total study population as well as by cases status. Although unweighted and weighted GRS were higher among all patient groups with events or other heart conditions compared with patients lacking evidence of events or other heart disease, these differences were not statistically significant (unpaired t-tests; $p > 0.05$)

Table 4 *APOC3* R19X frequency, by population

Population	Sample size	Carriers identified (Overall allele frequency)	Allele frequency in European-descent populations	PubMed ID or website
European American adults with very low triglyceride levels	184	2 (0.55%)	0.55%	- (present study)
Pennsylvania Amish	2503	140 (5.6%)	5.6%	19074352
Greek isolate	1219	48 (1.9%)	1.9%	24343240
Greek isolate	1087	34 (1.42%)	1.42%	27146844
Americans regardless of health status	19,613	31 (0.08%)	0.20%	25363704
Exome Aggregation Consortium (ExAC)	60,103	83 (0.07%)	0.046%	27535533 (http://exac.broadinstitute.org/ accessed May 2017)
National Heart, Lung, and Blood Institute (NHLBI) Grand Opportunity (GO) Exome Sequencing Project (ESP)	6495	3 (0.02%)	0.035%	24941081 (http://evs.gs.washington.edu/EVS/ accessed June 2015)
Ohio and Indiana Amish	1113	0 (–)	–	25363704
1000 Genomes Project	2500	0 (–)	–	(http://useast.ensembl.org/index.html accessed June 2015)
European Americans from Baltimore	214	0 (–)	–	19074352

two *APOC3* 19X carriers was performed to identify other possible cardiovascular disease risk factors. The female 19X carrier was born in the 1940s, and her EHR contained a medical history significant for remote breast cancer treated with surgery and radiation, controlled hypertension, and overweight (BMI ~ 28 kg/m^2). This female 19X carrier had never smoked cigarettes, and there was no evidence of coronary artery disease or myocardial infarction in her EHR. A single assessment of lipids was available for this female 19X carrier: low-density lipoprotein cholesterol (LDL-C) 116 mg/dL, high density lipoprotein cholesterol (HDL-C) 52 mg/dL, and TG 35 mg/dL. The female 19X carrier had unweighted and weighted GRS of 33 and 35.39, respectively. The second *APOC3* 19X carrier was a male born in the 1920s. The male 19X carrier had a past medical history of uncontrolled hypertension, was overweight (BMI 27 kg/m^2), and was a prior smoker. The male carrier had an extensive history of cardiac disease including atrial fibrillation, coronary artery disease with prior coronary artery bypass grafting, myocardial infarction, and ischemic cardiomyopathy (ejection fraction 30%) with heart failure. The

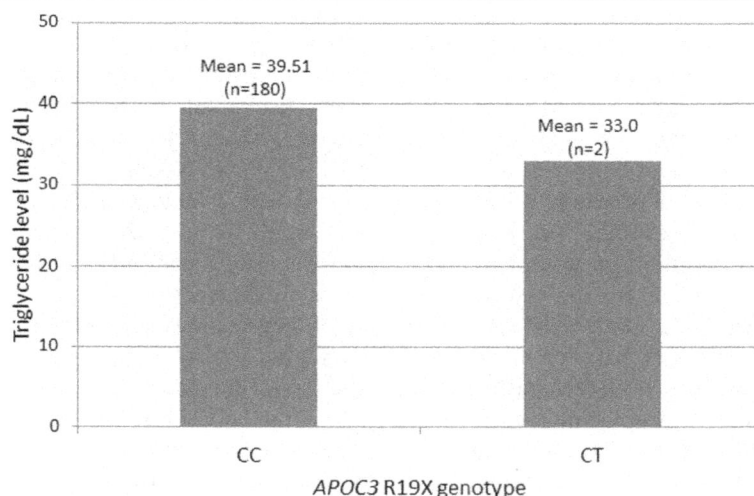

Fig. 2 Mean triglyceride levels by *APOC3* R19X genotype. A total of 184 European American adults (men > 45 years and women > 55 years) with at least one triglyceride level in the lowest 1% of BioVU were genotyped on the Illumina HumanExome BeadChip for *APOC3* R19X. Two samples failed genotyping. The means for the first mentioned triglyceride level (y-axis) were calculated for the non-carriers (CC genotype) and carriers (CT genotype) at *APOC3* R19X (x-axis). Although the mean triglyceride level in carriers (33 mg/dL; 2.83 standard deviation) was lower compared with the non-carriers (39.51 mg/dL; 18.52 standard deviation), the difference between the two is not statistically significant (two-sided t-test assuming unequal variances; *p* = 0.11)

male 19X carrier was not treated with statins due to reported intolerance, and a single measurement of lipids was available: LDL-C 69 mg/dL, HDL-C 41 mg/dL, and TG 31 mg/dL. The male 19X carrier had unweighted and weighted GRS of 32 and 34.21, respectively. Neither *APOC3* 19X carrier has died as of 2015.

The male 19X carrier was also a carrier for IVS2 + 1G > A, the only potentially compound heterozygote described in the literature to date. The other IVS2 + 1G > A carrier was a female born in the 1950s. The female IVS2 + 1G > A carrier was normal weight (BMI 23 kg/m^2) with two mentions of TG levels (34 and 23 mg/dL) in the EHR. This female IVS2 + 1G > A carrier has no evidence of myocardial infarction, revascularization, or other heart disease in the EHR.

Discussion

We evaluated 184 adult European American patients with very low TG levels extracted from EHRs for the presence of the loss-of-function allele (19X) for *APOC3* rs76353203. Overall, we identified two carrier patients, and as hypothesized, the resulting allele frequency of *APOC3* 19X was higher in this extreme patient population compared with the general population [10]. Neither carrier patient had the lowest TG levels among this patient population. A review of the EHR revealed only one of the two *APOC3* 19X carriers was free of myocardial infarction, revascularization, and other heart disease. Coincidentally, the *APOC3* 19X carrier with evidence of cardiovascular disease was also a carrier of IVS2 + 1G > A, representing to our knowledge potentially the first compound heterozygote for these mutations in the literature [16].

Based on the current literature [16], we would expect that the addition of these genomic data to the EHR would assist a physician in the assessment of the carriers' risk of future cardiovascular disease. *APOC3* R19X was originally identified in a genome-wide association study (GWAS) of TG levels in the Pennsylvania Amish where a variant in linkage disequilibrium with R19X was significantly associated with decreased TG levels [8]. Follow-up sequencing revealed the loss of function mutation in *APOC3* likely responsible for the GWAS findings [8], and subsequent studies in both isolated [17, 18] and outbred [10, 16] populations have confirmed the strong association between lower TG levels and 19X carriers. More recently, prospective epidemiologic studies have demonstrated that 19X carriers have lower rates of cardiovascular disease compared with non-carriers [16].

Interestingly, one of the two *APOC3* 19X carriers identified here has evidence in the EHR of a myocardial infarction, revascularization, and other heart disease. Also, apart from sharing low TG levels, the two 19X carriers had different cardiovascular risk profiles. While the statistical evidence for the association between lower TG levels and lower risk of coronary heart disease is strong at the population level, these data highlight the difficulty in translating a genetic association finding in the clinic for risk prediction at the patient level as envisioned for precision medicine. These data also highlight the genetic and environmental heterogeneity that drives cardiovascular disease risk. Thus, the addition of *APOC3* R19X in a clinical setting may contribute to the patient's risk assessment for cardiovascular disease, but it is not absolute and must be considered with other genetic and environmental risk factors [22].

We specifically targeted adult European Americans with low TG levels for *APOC3* R19X genotyping. The loss-of-function variant is common in isolated populations such as the Pennsylvania Amish [8] and Greek isolates [17, 18], but a study in NHANES confirmed the mutation is rare in the general population [10]. The frequency of 19X also varies by race/ethnicity. In NHANES [10] and in other studies [16], 19X is exceedingly rare in African Americans or African-descent populations compared with European-descent populations. In the present study of European Americans with low TG levels, we observed that the frequency of 19X was higher in this patient population compared with the general population, an observation consistent with the known genetic epidemiology of this loss-of-function variant. Although the carriers identified in this study had lower mean TG levels compared with non-carriers, we did not observe a statistically significant association most likely due to the fact that all patients genotyped already had low TG levels. Also, we only identified two carriers resulting in low statistical power.

The strategy of genotyping or targeting individuals with extreme phenotypes has been a popular and successful strategy in genetic epidemiology for gene discovery for many years [23]. Indeed, in the field of cardiovascular genetics, sequencing individuals with extreme LDL-C, HDL-C, and TG levels in multiple populations has identified several genetic variants and potential drug targets such as *PCSK9* [24]. An analogous strategy could be implemented in a clinical setting to augment the EHR with specific genotypes for an individual patient's risk assessment. For example, if a patient presents with an extreme lipid level, a panel of known functional variants (missense and loss-of-function) could be ordered for genotyping and added to the EHR to inform risk assessment for future cardiovascular events in that patient. A major advantage of this targeted approach is that the genetic assays would be ordered only on a fraction of the patients (e.g., patients with extreme labs) making it cost-effective compared with offering the panel to all patients regardless of lab results.

There are major disadvantages to a targeted approach to augmenting the EHR with genomic data. For most human traits and diseases, the known functional or strongly associated variants were discovered in European-descent populations [25, 26]. As such, diverse populations such as African Americans and Hispanics may not benefit from a European-centric genotyping panel. And, even among European-descent populations the catalog of genotype-phenotype associations is far from complete or strongly predictive of clinical events [27]. As technology improves to sort functional from neutral variants [28, 29], all patients may benefit from whole genome sequencing.

Conclusions

Further work is needed in developing appropriate tools for EHR integration and delivery of clinical decision support [30] for this and other clinically relevant genetic variants as envisioned in an era of precision medicine.

Abbreviations
BMI: Body mass index; CAD: Coronary artery disease; CHD: Coronary heart disease; CPT: Current procedural terminology; EHR: Electronic health record; GRS: Genetic risk score; GWAS: Genome-wide association study; HDL-C: High density lipoprotein cholesterol; ICD-9-CM: International Classification of Diseases, Ninth Revision, Clinical Modification; LDL-C: Low-density lipoprotein cholesterol; MAF: Minor allele frequency; NHANES: National Health and Nutrition Examination Survey; TG: Triglycerides; VANTAGE: Vanderbilt Technologies for Advanced Genomics; VUMC: Vanderbilt University Medical Center

Funding
The cost of publication was funded by Case Western Reserve University' Institute for Computational Biology. The dataset (s) used for the analyses described were obtained from Vanderbilt University Medical Center's BioVU which is supported by institutional funding and by the Vanderbilt CTSA grant funded by the National Center for Research Resources, Grant UL1 RR024975–01, which is now at the National Center for Advancing Translational Sciences, Grant 2 UL1 TR000445–06.

Authors' contributions
DCC designed the study. KED, EF-E, and QSW collected and prepared the data. DCC and NAR performed analyses. DCC drafted the manuscript. DCC, NAR, and QSW were major contributors in revising the manuscript critically for all important intellectual content. All authors gave approval to the final version of the manuscript and agreed to be accountable to all aspects of the work.

Competing interests
The authors declare that they have no competing interests.

Author details
[1]Department of Population and Quantitative Health Sciences, Institute for Computational Biology, Case Western Reserve University, 2103 Cornell Road, Wolstein Research Building, Suite 2-527, Cleveland, OH 44106, USA. [2]Cancer Biology, Vanderbilt University School of Medicine, Nashville, TN, USA. [3]Vanderbilt Institute for Clinical and Translational Research, Vanderbilt University Medical Center, Nashville, TN, USA. [4]Departments of Medicine and Pharmacology, Vanderbilt University Medical Center, Nashville, TN, USA.

References
1. Murray JF. Personalized medicine: been there, done that, always needs work! Am J Respir Crit Care Med. 2012;185(12):1251–2. https://doi.org/10.1164/rccm.201203-0523ED.
2. Cervellin G, Lippi G. Of MIs and men—a historical perspective on the diagnostics of acute myocardial infarction. Semin Thromb Hemost. 2014;40(5):535–43. https://doi.org/10.1055/s-0034-1383544.
3. Hamburg MA, Collins FS. The path to personalized medicine. N Engl J Med. 2010;363(4):301–4. https://doi.org/10.1056/NEJMp1006304.
4. Feero W, Guttmacher AE, Collins FS. The genome gets personal--almost. JAMA. 2008;299(11):1351–2. https://doi.org/10.1001/jama.299.11.1351.
5. Blumenthal D. Launching HITECH. N Engl J Med. 2010;362(5):382–5. https://doi.org/10.1056/NEJMp0912825.
6. Jensen PB, Jensen LJ, Brunak S. Mining electronic health records: towards better research applications and clinical care. Nat Rev Genet. 2012;13(6):395–405. https://doi.org/10.1038/nrg3208.
7. Green ED, Guyer MS. Charting a course for genomic medicine from base pairs to bedside. Nature. 2011;470(7333):204–13. https://doi.org/10.1038/nature09764.
8. Pollin TI, Damcott CM, Shen H, Ott SH, Shelton J, Horenstein RB, et al. A null mutation in human APOC3 confers a favorable plasma lipid profile and apparent Cardioprotection. Science. 2008;322(5908):1702–5. https://doi.org/10.1126/science.1161524. PMC2673993
9. Saleheen D, Natarajan P, Armean IM, Zhao W, Rasheed A, Khetarpal SA, et al. Human knockouts and phenotypic analysis in a cohort with a high rate of consanguinity. Nature. 2017;544(7649):235–9. https://doi.org/10.1038/nature22034. PMC5600291
10. Crawford DC, Dumitrescu L, Goodloe R, Brown-Gentry K, Boston J, McClellan B Jr, et al. Rare variant APOC3 R19X is associated with cardio-protective profiles in a diverse population-base survey as part of the epidemiologic architecture for genes linked to environment (EAGLE) study. Circ Cardiovasc Genet. 2014;7(6):848–53. https://doi.org/10.1161/CIRCGENETICS.113.000369. PMC4305446
11. Roden DM, Pulley JM, Basford MA, Bernard GR, Clayton EW, Balser JR, et al. Development of a large-scale De-identified DNA biobank to enable personalized medicine. Clin Pharmacol Ther. 2008;84(3):362–9. https://doi.org/10.1038/clpt.2008.89. PMC3763939
12. Pulley J, Clayton E, Bernard GR, Roden DM, Masys DR. Principles of human subjects protections applied in an opt-out, De-identified Biobank. Clin Transl Sci. 2010;3(1):42–8. https://doi.org/10.1111/j.1752-8062.2010.00175.x. PMC3075971
13. Grove ML, Yu B, Cochran BJ, Haritunians T, Bis JC, Taylor KD, et al. Best practices and joint calling of the HumanExome BeadChip: the CHARGE consortium. PLoS One. 2013;8(7):e68095. https://doi.org/10.1371/journal.pone.0068095. PMC3709915
14. Dehghan A, Bis JC, White CC, Smith AV, Morrison AC, Cupples LA, et al. Genome-wide association study for incident myocardial infarction and coronary heart disease in prospective cohort studies: the CHARGE consortium. PLoS One. 2016;11(3):e0144997. https://doi.org/10.1371/journal.pone.0144997. PMC4780701
15. Deloukas P, Kanoni S, Willenborg C, Farrall M, Assimes TL, Thompson JR, et al. Large-scale association analysis identifies new risk loci for coronary artery disease. Nat Genet. 2013;45(1):25–33. https://doi.org/10.1038/ng.2480. PMC3679547
16. TG and HDL Working Group of the Exome Sequencing Project, National Heart, Lung, and Blood Institute, Crosby J, Peloso GM, Auer PL, Crosslin DR, et al. Loss-of-function mutations in APOC3, triglycerides, and coronary disease. N Engl J Med. 2014;371(1):22–31. https://doi.org/10.1056/NEJMoa1307095. PMC4180269
17. Tachmazidou I, Dedoussis G, Southam L, Farmaki AE, Ritchie GRS, Xifara DK, et al. A rare functional cardioprotective APOC3 variant has risen in frequency in distinct population isolates. Nat Commun. 2013;4 https://doi.org/10.1038/ncomms3872. PMC3905724
18. Gilly A, Ritchie GR, Southam L, Farmaki A-E, Tsafantakis E, Dedoussis G, et al. Very low-depth sequencing in a founder population identifies a cardioprotective APOC3 signal missed by genome-wide imputation. Hum Mol Genet. 2016;25(11):2360–5. https://doi.org/10.1093/hmg/ddw088. PMC5081052
19. Timpson NJ, Walter K, Min JL, Tachmazidou I, Malerba G, Shin S-Y, et al. A rare variant in APOC3 is associated with plasma triglyceride and VLDL levels in Europeans. Nat Commun. 2014;5:4871. https://doi.org/10.1038/ncomms5871. PMC4167609

20. Drenos F, Davey Smith G, Ala-Korpela M, Kettunen J, Würtz P, Soininen P, et al. Metabolic characterization of a rare genetic variation within APOC3 and its lipoprotein lipase–independent effects. Circ Cardiovasc Genet. 2016; 9(3):231–9. https://doi.org/10.1161/circgenetics.115.001302. PMC4920206

21. Miller M, Stone NJ, Ballantyne C, Bittner V, Criqui MH, Ginsberg HN, et al. Triglycerides and cardiovascular disease: a scientific statement from the American Heart Association. Circulation. 2011;123(20):2292–333. https://doi.org/10.1161/CIR.0b013e3182160726.

22. Khera AV, Emdin CA, Drake I, Natarajan P, Bick AG, Cook NR, et al. Genetic risk, adherence to a healthy lifestyle, and coronary disease. N Engl J Med. 2016;375(24):2349–58. https://doi.org/10.1056/NEJMoa1605086. PMC5338864

23. Plomin R, Haworth CMA, Davis OSP. Common disorders are quantitative traits. Nat Rev Genet. 2009;10(12):872–8. https://doi.org/10.1038/nrg2670.

24. Cohen J, Pertsemlidis A, Kotowski IK, Graham R, Garcia CK, Hobbs HH. Low LDL cholesterol in individuals of African descent resulting from frequent nonsense mutations in PCSK9. Nat Genet. 2005;37(2):161–5. https://doi.org/10.1038/ng1509.

25. Rosenberg NA, Huang L, Jewett EM, Szpiech ZA, Jankovic I, Boehnke M. Genome-wide association studies in diverse populations. Nat Rev Genet. 2010;11(5):356–66. https://doi.org/10.1038/nrg2760. PMC3079573

26. Popejoy AB, Fullerton SM. Genomics is failing on diversity. Nature. 2016; 538(7624):161–4. https://doi.org/10.1038/538161a. PMC5089703.

27. Assimes TL, Salfati EL, Del Gobbo LC. Leveraging information from genetic risk scores of coronary atherosclerosis. Curr Opin Lipidol. 2017;28(2):104–12. https://doi.org/10.1097/mol.0000000000000400.

28. Dewey FE, Grove ME, Pan C. Clinical interpretation and implications of whole-genome sequencing. JAMA. 2014;311(10):1035–45. https://doi.org/10.1001/jama.2014.1717. PMC4119063

29. Ramos EM, Din-Lovinescu C, Berg JS, Brooks LD, Duncanson A, Dunn M, et al. Characterizing genetic variants for clinical action. Am J Med Genet C: Semin Med Genet. 2014;166(1):93–104. https://doi.org/10.1002/ajmg.c.31386. PMC4158437

30. Shirts BH, Salama JS, Aronson SJ, Chung WK, Gray SW, Hindorff LA, et al. CSER and eMERGE: current and potential state of the display of genetic information in the electronic health record. J Am Med Inform Assoc. 2015; 22(6):1231–42. https://doi.org/10.1093/jamia/ocv065. PMC5009914

5

Progression-specific genes identified in microdissected formalin-fixed and paraffin-embedded tissue containing matched ductal carcinoma in situ and invasive ductal breast cancers

Silke Schultz[1], Harald Bartsch[2], Karl Sotlar[2], Karina Petat-Dutter[2], Michael Bonin[3,4], Steffen Kahlert[5], Nadia Harbeck[5], Ulrich Vogel[6], Harald Seeger[7,8], Tanja Fehm[1,9] and Hans J. Neubauer[1*]

Abstract

Background: The transition from ductal carcinoma in situ (DCIS) to invasive breast carcinoma (IBC) is an important step during breast carcinogenesis. Understanding its molecular changes may help to identify high-risk DCIS that progress to IBC. Here, we describe a transcriptomic profiling analysis of matched formalin-fixed and paraffin-embedded (FFPE) DCIS and IBC components of individual breast tumours, containing both tumour compartments. The study was performed to validate progression-associated transcripts detected in an earlier gene profiling project using fresh frozen breast cancer tissue. In addition, FFPE tissues from patients with pure DCIS (pDCIS) were analysed to identify candidate transcripts characterizing DCIS with a high or low risk of progressing to IBC.

Methods: Fifteen laser microdissected pairs of DCIS and IBC were profiled by Illumina DASL technology and used for expression validation by qPCR. Differential expression was independently validated using further 25 laser microdissected DCIS/IBC sample pairs. Additionally, laser microdissected epithelial cells from 31 pDCIS were investigated for expression of candidate transcripts using qPCR.

Results: Multiple statistical calculation methods revealed 1784 mRNAs which are differentially expressed between DCIS and IBC ($P < 0.05$), of which 124 have also been identified in the gene profiling project using fresh frozen breast cancer tissue. Nine mRNAs that had been selected from the gene list obtained using fresh frozen tissues by applying pathway and network analysis (MMP11, GREM1, PLEKHC1, SULF1, THBS2, CSPG2, COL10A1, COL11A1, KRT14) were investigated in tissues from the same 15 microdissected specimens and the 25 independent tissue samples by qPCR. All selected transcripts were also detected in tumour cells from pDCIS. Expression of MMP11 and COL10A1 increased significantly from pDCIS to DCIS of DCIS/IBC mixed tumours.

Conclusion: We confirm differential expression of progression-associated transcripts in FFPE breast cancer samples which might mediate the transition from DCIS to IBC. MMP11 and COL10A1 may characterize pure DCIS with a high risk developing IDC.

Keywords: Breast cancer, Pure DCIS, Gene expression, Laser microdissection, Matched pairs, FFPE samples

* Correspondence: Hans.Neubauer@med.uni-tuebingen.de
[1]Department of Obstetrics and Gynaecology, Life-Science-Center, Heinrich-Heine University, Merowingerplatz 1A, 40225 Duesseldorf, Germany
Full list of author information is available at the end of the article

Background

Breast cancer is the most common malignancy among women in western countries. Its incidence has been increasing since the 1940's [1]. The prevailing concept of a multi-step model of mammary carcinogenesis is a sequence of pathologically defined stages beginning with atypical ductal hyperplasia (ADH) which is progressing to the preinvasive ductal carcinoma in situ (DCIS), a non-obligate precursor of the final stage, invasive breast carcinoma (IBC) [2, 3].

DCIS accounts for approximately one-third of all newly diagnosed breast cancer cases. It has been estimated that about 50% of untreated DCIS lesions will progress to IBC with wide variations in latency [4, 5]. Furthermore, half of the local recurrences that develop after initial surgical treatment of DCIS are invasive cancers [6]. Women diagnosed with DCIS have an estimated 4 to 12 times higher relative risk of developing invasive breast cancer [7], whereas on the other hand, some untreated DCIS will change very little within 5–20 years [8]. Given that only a minority (15–30%) of women diagnosed with pure DCIS (pDCIS) develop subsequent breast tumour within the first decade after treatment with lumpectomy alone, and that approximately 70% of women with pDCIS are treated with lumpectomy in conjunction with radiation and antihormonal treatment, it is likely that many women with pDCIS are being overtreated [9, 10]. Thus, there is a clinical need to identify (a) prognostic biomarker(s) that accurately predict the clinical behaviour of DCIS and that support the clinician to select the most appropriate treatment regimen. Patients expected to develop indolent disease could then be treated with lumpectomy alone, whereas those expected to develop invasive disease could receive a more aggressive treatment.

The traditional grading of DCIS is based on morphologic features [11]. However, considerable heterogeneity limits classical histopathology's ability to accurately predict the risk of progression from DCIS to IBC so that it has only limited clinical value [8, 12, 13]. Invasive carcinomas have been reported to develop from DCIS of all nuclear grades [4], which supports the idea of an invasive phenotype beyond histopathological and molecular intrinsic subtypes. Understanding the molecular biology of DCIS and its transition to IBC may provide insight into tumour initiation and progression and may enable the identification of biologically and clinically significant progression-associated genes. We and others have published transcripts that are differentially expressed between matched DCIS and IBC and which may be able to predict the probability of DCIS progressing to IBC [14–18].

In the current study we used formalin-fixed, paraffin-embedded (FFPE) tissue samples from 15 patients with both DCIS and IBC (FFPE investigation). Tumour cells were – as in the first study - laser microdissected (laser capture microdissection, LCM) and extracted mRNA was expression profiled using the Whole Genome cDNA-mediated Annealing, Selection, Extension, and Ligation (DASL)-Assay - a technique developed to quantify degraded RNA samples [19]. By combining results from this FFPE investigation with data from the earlier fresh frozen investigation we identified 124 overlapping transcripts. Differential expression of nine transcripts selected based on data obtained from the initial fresh frozen experiment could be independently confirmed in an additional FFPE tissue validation set consisting of 25 independent laser microdissected DCIS/IBC sample pairs. By extending the expression validation to 31 microdissected pDCIS, two potential transcripts were identified whose expression is continuously increasing from pDCIS to DCIS of DCIS/IBC mixed tumours and further to IDC and might characterize pDCIS associated with a high-risk of progression to invasive disease.

Methods

Formalin-fixed and paraffin-embedded tumour tissue

For expression analysis paraffin blocks from 15 surgically excised primary breast cancer specimens containing both, DCIS and IBC areas, were obtained from the Department of Pathology of the University Hospital, Tuebingen, Germany. All surgical procedures had been carried out in the Department of Obstetrics and Gynaecology of the University Hospital, Tuebingen. Tissue samples were fixed in buffered formalin after surgical excision and embedded in paraffin according to standard procedures. All tissue samples were obtained with the patients' informed consents (ethical consent of the Medical Faculty Tuebingen: AZ.266/98). Cryopreserved tissue from five tumours had been studied in our earlier fresh frozen investigation [18].

For validation analysis FFPE tissues from further 25 patients with DCIS/IBC tumours and 31 patients with pDCIS were selected from the archives of the Department of Pathology, Ludwig Maximilians University, Munich. In keeping with local Ethics Committee guidelines, tissue blocks were anonymized.

The Van Nuys grading system for DCIS, in which DCIS is defined by nuclear grade [20], was applied. The predominant growth patterns were solid, cribriform, and papillary. The lesions were of nuclear grades 2 and 3. Patients with pDCIS cases were free of associated invasive components and did not have evidence of recurrence or progression to invasive disease within the 5 years prior to sample processing. It is acknowledged that DCIS may recur after long periods of time, and we cannot rule out that recurrences may be found in the pDCIS group with longer follow up, although the overall long-term recurrence rate for properly excised low grade

DCIS is less than 5%. The majority of patients underwent lumpectomy (+/− re-excision), and most of these patients received postoperative radiotherapy.

Prosigna™ breast Cancer prognostic gene signature assay

The Prosigna™ Assay measures the expression of 58 genes including reference genes to classify the tumour sample into one of the four intrinsic subtypes and to give information about the risk of recurrence (ROR). For determination of the ROR category of each tumour sample the ROR score is separated into three risk groups: low (ROR score 0–40), intermediate (ROR score 40–60) and high (ROR score 60–100, [21]. The assay was used according to the manufacturer's conditions. Briefly, 250 ng total RNA of FFPE samples was captured by barcoded reporter probes and hybridized overnight (65 °C) to the surface of the Prosigna™ test cartridge. After immobilization of the RNA-probe-complex the expression of the genes was determined by counting the barcodes using the nCounter® Analysis System (NanoString Technologies®).

Laser capture microdissection (LCM)

Laser capture microdissection of FFPE tissue was performed in order to enrich for tumour cells for subsequent molecular analysis. In brief, serial FFPE sections were cut at 5–8 µm and mounted on special 2-µm-thick membrane slides (MMI AG, Glattbrugg, Switzerland), dried for 10 min at 50 °C and stored at − 20 °C until further

deparaffinization and staining. To preserve RNA integrity, these two steps were kept as short as possible. To protect the RNA from contamination and nuclease degradation, the whole system (including microtome and water bath) was cleaned with RNaseZap (Ambion, Austin, USA) or heated to 180 °C for 4 h, and only RNase-free reagents were used. To avoid cross contamination, the microtome blade, DEPC water and chemicals were renewed before processing each new FFPE block. Deparaffinization was achieved by immersion of the slide-mounted section in xylene (2 × 10 min) and pure ethanol (2 × 2 min). The sections were then rehydrated for 1 min and stained with hematoxylin QS counterstain (Linaris GmbH, Dossenheim, Germany) for 10 s. Finally, the specimen were briefly washed in RNase-free water, dehydrated in pure ethanol for 3 min and air-dried for 30 min.

LCM was performed with the MMI µCut system (MMI AG, Glattbrugg, Switzerland). A representative section before and after the LCM procedures is shown in Fig. 1. Depending on the extent of intervening stroma, areas ranging from 1 to 20 µm² (approx. 10,000 to 200,000 cells) were dissected, placed into 30 µl lysis buffer (High pure miRNA isolation kit, Roche, Mannheim, Germany) and stored at − 80 °C until further use.

RNA extraction

Total RNA was isolated with the High pure miRNA isolation kit (Roche, Mannheim, Germany) according to

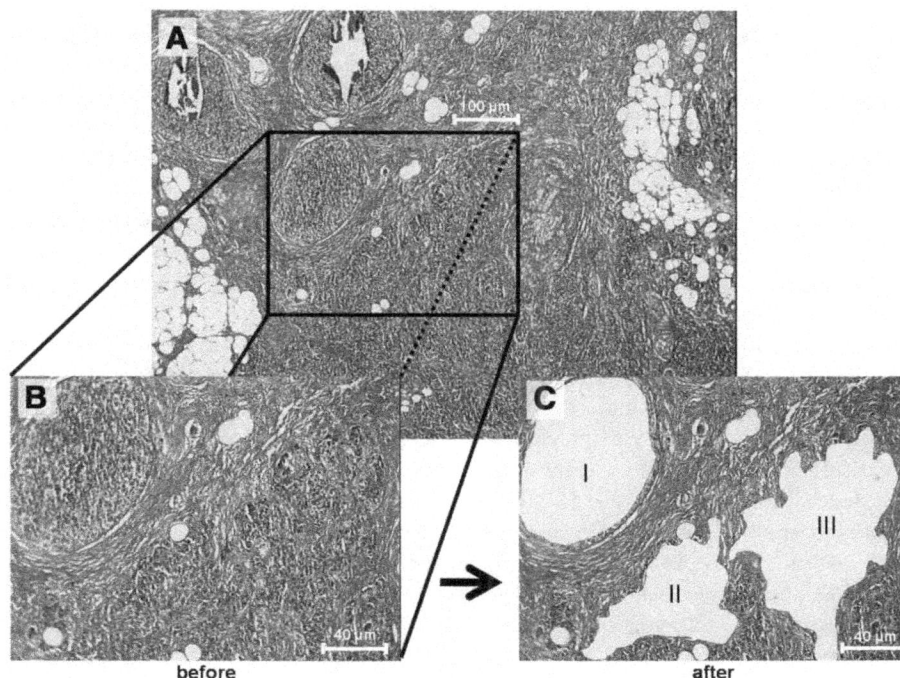

Fig. 1 Laser capture microdissection. Depicted are images of stained tissue section before (**a**, **b**) and after (**c**) LCM in a representative breast cancer. I = DCIS area after LCM, II & III = IBC areas after LCM. Magnification A) 4×; B and C) 10×. Size Bar A) 100 µm; B and C) 40 µm

the one-column protocol. In brief, harvested cells were lysed in lysis buffer and digested with proteinase K (1 mg/ml) overnight (55 °C). Then binding buffer and binding enhancer were added. The mixture was transferred to a High pure filter tube and centri-fuged (30 s, 13,000 xg). After washing, total RNA was eluted and quantified with NanoDrop Spectrophotometer ND-1000 (NanoDrop Tech., Wilmington, USA). Approximately 20–100 ng of total RNA was retrieved by RNA extraction.

Whole genome DASL assay

About 200 ng mRNA was hybridized to the Whole-Genome Gene Expression DASL-Array (Illumina Inc., San Diego, USA) according to the manufacturer's instructions. This system uses priming with random hexamers instead of oligo(dT) priming to achieve higher detection rates with RNA extracted from FFPE tissue [22]. After cDNA synthesis and biotinylation, the resultant cDNA was connected with assay-specific oligonucleotides to bind to paramagnetic beads. Following PCR using fluorescence-labelled primers, the amplification products were hybridized to the Whole-Genome Expression BeadChip and scanned by BeadArray Reader (Illumina Inc., San Diego, USA). The GEO database accession number for this dataset is GSE72205. Eleven of the 31 selected pDCIS have also been investigated by DASL-Array and results are included in the GSE data set.

Statistical analysis of microarray data

Statistical analysis of the results of the FF investigation was performed as described previously [18]. To analyse the DASL array data the intensities of replicate beads and quality control were averaged with Genome Studio V2009.1 software (Illumina, San Diego, CA). No background correction or normalization was performed at this stage [23]. Summarized intensities together with standard errors, number of beads per bead type and detection p-values were exported. All subsequent data analysis steps were performed on the software platform R 2.12.0 and Bioconductor 2.6.1 [24] with the packages 'beadarray' [25, 26], 'limma' [27], 'RankProd' [28] and 'GOstats' [29]. Initially, the expression data from all chips were normalized with VSN [30]. Non-informative probes were removed from the data set. The differences in mRNA expression levels between DCIS and IBC were analysed by three different approaches. First, linear modelling was used as a parametric approach. The factors *tumour stage* (DCIS/IBC) and *patient* were used to design a linear model capturing the influence of the different factors on gene expression levels. The coefficients describing the expression profiles of the remaining probes were calculated and the standard errors were determined using an empirical Bayesian approach. From

the t-statistic the resulting p-values were established and corrected for multiple testing by the Benjamini-Hochberg procedure [31]. Secondly, two non-parametric tests (Wilcoxon Signed Rank and Rank Products, [28]) were applied to identify differentially expressed genes. The expression values of the DCIS samples were subtracted from the expression values of the IBC samples and the rank products were calculated as a one class case with 1000 permutations.

RNA amplification and quantitative real-time PCR (qPCR)

In order to provide enough mRNA for further investigation of the expression of several candidate genes from the limited amount of mRNA obtained from LCM tissue, total RNA (80–100 ng) was pre-amplified using the WT-Ovation™ FFPE RNA Amplification System V2 according to the manufacturer's instructions (Nugen™ Technologies, San Carlos, USA). The reactions comprise first strand cDNA synthesis, second strand cDNA synthesis and Ribo-SPIA™ amplification cycles. PCR primers were designed using the Primer3 software (http://frodo.wi.mit.edu/primer3) and ordered at biomers.net (Ulm, Germany). Primer sequences are listed in Table 1. QPCR was performed with the LightCycler® 480 System using the LightCycler® 480 SYBR Green Master I (Roche, Mannheim, Germany) and the following cycling program: 1 cycle at 95 °C for 10 min, followed by 40 amplification cycles, each cycle consisting of a denaturation step at 95 °C for 10 s, primer annealing at 58 °C for 25 s, and extension at 72 °C for 25 s. QPCR results were normalized to the expression of the housekeeping genes GAPDH (RefSeq_ID: NM_0002046.3), ACTB (RefSeq_ID: NM_007393) and YWHAZ (RefSeq_ID: NM_003406.2). Differential expression was calculated using the ΔCP method. The differential expression was further analysed by a pairwise Wilcoxon signed rank test using the JMP®-software (JMP, A Business Unit of SAS, Cary, USA). The overall alpha level was set at 0.05.

Results

Tissue selection and laser microdissection

Tissue samples were obtained from a total of 71 breast cancer patients. 15 tumours containing DCIS and IBC were selected from the FFPE tissue bank of the Institute of Pathology, University Hospital Tuebingen, Germany (Table 2). Five of these tissues correspond to cryopreserved specimen which has already been used in the fresh frozen investigation. For validation of differentially expressed transcripts, DCIS and IBC areas from additional 25 DCIS/IBC tumours, selected from the FFPE tissue bank of the Institute of Pathology, Ludwig Maximilians University Munich, Germany, were processed (Table 2). Tissue sections before and after the LCM procedures of a representative case are shown in Fig. 1. In

Table 1 Primer information: sequences and length of the amplified fragment

Gene	RefSeq_ID	Primer sequences (sense and antisense)	Size
COL10A1	NM_000493.3	5'- CCTACTCCTTATTTACGACGCAAT-3' 5'- TGAAAAGCCTTGAAAGAATGG-3'	107 bp
COL11A1	NM_001854.2	5'-TGATAATTTATGACAAAAGAACATACC-3' 5'-CCAGGTAGCCAAGACTTGAGTTTA-3'	94 bp
CSPG2	NM_004385.2	5'-GAATGGGATCCTGATGGAAC-3' 5'-AGTCCTCCATTCAGGCCTTT-3'	96 bp
GREM1	NM_013372.5	5'- TCATTTAAAAACGGCAAAGAA-3' 5'- TTCATGAAACTTGAAGCCAAA-3'	111 bp
KRT14	NM_000526.3	5'- CAGATCCCACTGGAAGATCC-3' 5'- AAGCTGTATTGATTGCCAGGA-3'	92 bp
MMP11	NM_005940.3	5'- AATCCAGGCCAAAAAGTTCA-3' 5'- CCTGGGACAGGATTGAGGTA-3'	100 bp
PLEKHC1	NM_006832.1	5'-GGCCATGTTCTAGTCTGTTGC-3' 5'-CTCTCCCTCGCACCCTTT-3'	93 bp
SULF1	NM_015170.1	5'- CAAATTAGCTGCTTGCCTGA-3' 5'- AACTTGAAATCTTTTTACAAAGCACA-3'	99 bp
THBS2	NM_003247.2	5'-AGGTTGATGAAACGTCATGTG-3' 5'-AAGTGCAGGGTTTCAGTGGT-3'	93 bp
GAPDH	NM_002046.3	5'-CTCCTCACAGTTGCCATGTA-3' 5'- GCACAGGGTACTTTATTTGATGG-3'	90 bp
ACTB	NM_007393	5'-TCCCCCAACTTGAGATGTATGAAG-3' 5'-AACTGGTCTCAAGTCAGTGTACAGG-3'	90 bp
YWHAZ	NM_003406.2	5'- TGGAGGGTCGTCTCAAGTAT-3' 5'- GCTCCGTCTCAATTTTCTCTC-3'	94 bp

order to identify potential candidate transcripts that differentiate high-risk from low-risk DCIS, the microdissected DCIS areas from 31 patients with pDCIS were used for qPCR analysis (Table 3).

The Prosigna™ Breast Cancer Prognostic Gene Signature Assay was performed for 13 out of 15 and 23 out of 25 FFPE samples and classified the majority of the IBC tumour samples of our study as luminal A subtype and determined a low risk of recurrence for them (Tables 2 and 3).

Selection of candidate genes

WG-DASL analysis in the 15 FFPE test set DCIS/IBC samples revealed 1784 transcripts that were differentially expressed between DCIS and IBC ($P < 0.05$; Additional file 1). Comparison of them with the differentially expressed transcripts from the fresh frozen investigation left 124 transcripts with analogous expression in both investigations ($P < 0.05$; Fig. 2; Additional file 2). In a previously performed network analysis using the Ingenuity® software and the significant differentially expressed transcripts obtained in the fresh frozen investigation we selected 9 genes that are involved in cellular processes such as cell-to-cell adhesion, extracellular matrix organization, metastasis, and tumour progression (Table 4): THBS2 (thrombospondin 2; RefSeq_ID: NM_003247.2), GREM1 (gremlin 1; RefSeq_ID: NM_013372.5), MMP11

(matrix-metalloproteinase 11; RefSeq_ID: NM_005940.3), COL11A1 (collagen type XI-alpha 1; RefSeq_ID: NM_001854.2), COL10A1 (collagen type X-alpha 1; RefSeq_ID: NM_000493.3), CSPG2 (chondroitin sulphate proteoglycan 2; RefSeq_ID: NM_004385.2), PLEKHC1 (pleckstrin homology domain containing member 1; RefSeq_ID: NM_006832.1), SULF1 (sulfatase 1; RefSeq_ID: NM_015170.1) and KRT14 (cytokeratin 14; RefSeq_ID: NM_000526.3). The expression of these transcripts was further investigated. In the 15 FFPE test set DCIS/IBC samples the same significant expression difference (upregulation) was obtained for COL11A1, MMP11, THBS2, CSPG2, and GREM1. Also the significant downregulation ($P < 0.05$) of KRT14 in IBC compared to DCIS could be verified. For COL10A1 ($P < 0.06$) and SULF1 (0.053) strong tendencies to upregulation in IBC were achieved. Only the differential expression of PLEKHC1 did not reach statistical significance ($P > 0.5$) in the FFPE investigation (Table 4). However, we decided to further include all 9 transcripts in the following validation experiments.

Verification of microarray data by qPCR in IBC tumour samples

To validate the WG-DASL findings, qPCR-based relative quantification was performed for the 9 selected

Table 2 Histopathological data and intrinsic subtypes of DCIS/IBC tumour samples included in the test-set (upper panel) and validation-set (lower panel; T = Tuebingen; M = Munich; n.d. = not done). The risk categories are calculated based on individual ROR (risk-of-recurrence) scores taking the lymph node status into account. For N0 patients, low-risk, ROR 0–40 (10-years distant recurrence rate < 10%), intermediate-risk, ROR 41–60 (10-years distant recurrence rate 11–20%), high-risk, ROR 61–100 (10-years distant recurrence rate > 20%). For N1 patients, low-risk, ROR 0–15, intermediate-risk, ROR 16–40, high-risk, ROR 41–100, Samples with an asterisk are similar to samples from the fresh frozen set

sample #	Age	T	Grade	N	M	ER	PR	HER2	PAM50 intrinsic subtype (ROR)	Prosigna risk category
Histopathological data and intrinsic subtypes of DCIS/IBC tumours of the test-set										
T DCIS/IBC 1	52	pT1c	G2	pN0	Mx	neg	neg	neg	luminal A (0)	low
T DCIS/IBC 2	73	pT1c	G2	pN0	M0	pos	pos	neg	luminal A (25)	low
T DCIS/IBC 3	52	pT2	G2	pN0	Mx	pos	pos	neg	luminal A (32)	low
T DCIS/IBC 4	66	pT1c	G2	pN0	Mx	pos	neg	neg	luminal A (30)	low
T DCIS/IBC 5	67	pT2	G2	pN1a	M0	pos	pos	neg	luminal A (34)	low
T DCIS/IBC 6	68	pT2	G2	pN2a	Mx	pos	pos	neg	luminal A (33)	low
T DCIS/IBC 7	45	pT2	G2	pN1a	Mx	pos	pos	neg	luminal A (27)	low
T DCIS/IBC 8*	57	pT1	G2	pN0	M0	pos	pos	pos	luminal A (55)	intermediate
T DCIS/IBC 9*	72	pT1c	G3	pN0	M0	pos	pos	neg	luminal B (80)	high
T DCIS/IBC 10	45	pT1c	G2	pN0	M0	neg	neg	neg	HER2-enriched (71)	high
T DCIS/IBC 11*	74	pT1c	G2	pN2a	M0	pos	pos	neg	HER2-enriched (93)	high
T DCIS/IBC 12*	59	pT2	G2	pN2a	M0	neg	neg	neg	basal-like (64)	high
T DCIS/IBC 13	54	pT2	G3	pN0	M0	neg	neg	neg	basal-like (59)	intermediate
T DCIS/IBC 14	49	pT2	G2	pN1a	M0	neg	neg	neg	n.d.	n.d.
T DCIS/IBC 15*	66	pT2	G2–3	pN0	M0	neg	neg	pos	n.d.	n.d.
Histopathological data and intrinsic subtypes of DCIS/IBC tumours of the validation-set										
M DCIS/IBC 1	51	pT1c	G2	pN0	M0	pos	pos	neg	luminal A (0)	low
M DCIS/IBC 2	62	pT1b	G2	pN0	Mx	pos	neg	neg	luminal A (9)	low
M DCIS/IBC 3	58	pT1b	G2	pN0	Mx	pos	pos	neg	luminal A (11)	low
M DCIS/IBC 4	45	pT1c	G1	pN0	M0	pos	pos	neg	luminal A (12)	low
M DCIS/IBC 5	62	pT1b	G2	pN0	Mx	pos	pos	neg	luminal A (20)	low
M DCIS/IBC 6	67	pT1c	G2	pN0	M0	pos	pos	neg	luminal A (26)	low
M DCIS/IBC 7	45	pT1b	G2	pN0	Mx	pos	pos	neg	luminal A (27)	low
M DCIS/IBC 8	63	pT1c	G2	pN0	M0	pos	pos	neg	luminal A (30)	low
M DCIS/IBC 9	45	pT1b	G2	pN0	Mx	pos	pos	neg	luminal A (32)	low
M DCIS/IBC 10	59	pT1c	G2	pN0	M0	pos	pos	neg	luminal A (32)	low
M DCIS/IBC 11	68	pT1b	G2	pN0	Mx	pos	pos	neg	luminal A (33)	low
M DCIS/IBC 12	54	pT1a	G2	pN0	Mx	pos	pos	neg	luminal A (33)	low
M DCIS/IBC 13	61	pT1b	G2	pN0	Mx	pos	pos	neg	luminal A (33)	low
M DCIS/IBC 14	60	pT1c	G2	pN0	Mx	pos	pos	neg	luminal A (40)	low
M DCIS/IBC 15	65	pT1c	G3	pN0	M0	pos	pos	neg	luminal A (43)	intermediate
M DCIS/IBC 16	40	pT1c	G2	pN1a	M0	pos	pos	neg	luminal A (30)	low
M DCIS/IBC 17	65	pT1c	G2	pN0	M0	pos	pos	neg	luminal A (53)	intermediate
M DCIS/IBC 18	58	pT1c	G3	pN0	Mx	pos	pos	pos	luminal A (76)	high
M DCIS/IBC 19	67	pT1c	G2	pN2a	M0	pos	pos	neg	luminal A (36)	low
M DCIS/IBC 20	42	pT1b	G3	pN1a	Mx	pos	pos	neg	luminal A (48)	intermediate
M DCIS/IBC 21	57	pT1c	G3	pN0	M0	pos	pos	neg	luminal A/B (31/58)	intermediate
M DCIS/IBC 22	51	pT1c	G3	pN0	M0	pos	pos	neg	HER2-enriched (77)	high

Table 2 Histopathological data and intrinsic subtypes of DCIS/IBC tumour samples included in the test-set (upper panel) and validation-set (lower panel; T = Tuebingen; M = Munich; n.d. = not done). The risk categories are calculated based on individual ROR (risk-of-recurrence) scores taking the lymph node status into account. For N0 patients, low-risk, ROR 0–40 (10-years distant recurrence rate < 10%), intermediate-risk, ROR 41–60 (10-years distant recurrence rate 11–20%), high-risk, ROR 61–100 (10-years distant recurrence rate > 20%). For N1 patients, low-risk, ROR 0–15, intermediate-risk, ROR 16–40, high-risk, ROR 41–100, Samples with an asterisk are similar to samples from the fresh frozen set *(Continued)*

sample #	Age	T	Grade	N	M	ER	PR	HER2	PAM50 intrinsic subtype (ROR)	Prosigna risk category
M DCIS/IBC 23	62	pT1c	G3	pN1mi	M0	pos	pos	pos	HER2-enriched (77)	high
M DCIS/IBC 24	61	pT1c	G2	pN0	M0	pos	pos	neg	n.d.	n.d.
M DCIS/IBC 25	28	pT1b	G3	pN1a	Mx	neg	pos	pos	n.d.	n.d.

Table 3 Histopathological data and intrinsic subtypes of pure DCIS tumour samples (n.d. = not done)

Histopathological data and intrinsic subtypes of pure DCIS									
sample #	Age	T	Grade	N	M	ER	PR	HER2	10-year recurrence-free survival
pDCIS 1	49	pTis	G3	pN0	M0	pos	pos	neg	low
pDCIS 2	61	pTis	G3	pN0	M0	pos	pos	neg	low
pDCIS 3	54	pTis	G3	pN0	M0	pos	pos	neg	low
pDCIS 4	44	pTis	–	pN0	M0	pos	pos	neg	low
pDICS 5	32	pTis	G3	pN0	M0	pos	pos	neg	low
pDCIS 6	65	pTis	G3	pN0	M0	neg	neg	neg	low
pDCIS 7	63	pTis	G3	pN0	M0	pos	pos	neg	low
pDCIS 8	36	pTis	G3	pN0	M0	pos	pos	neg	low
pDCIS 9	36	pTis	G3	pN0	M0	pos	pos	neg	low
pDCIS 10	63	pTis	G3	pN0	M0	pos	pos	neg	low
pDCIS 11	43	pTis	G3	pN0	M0	pos	pos	neg	low
pDCIS 12	46	pTis	G3	pN0	M0	pos	pos	neg	low
pDCIS 13	84	pTis	G2	pN0	M0	pos	pos	neg	low
pDCIS 14	55	pTis	G2	pN0	M0	pos	pos	neg	low
pDCIS 15	46	pTis	G2	pN0	M0	pos	pos	neg	low
pDCIS 16	79	pTis	G3	pN0	M0	neg	neg	pos	low
pDCIS 17	46	pT1	G3	pN0	M0	pos	pos	neg	intermediate
pDCIS 18	84	pTis	G2	pN0	M0	pos	pos	neg	low
pDCIS 19	53	pTis	G3	pN0	M0	pos	pos	neg	intermediate
pDCIS 20	46	pTis	G3	pN0	M0	neg	pos	pos	intermediate
pDCIS 21	33	pTis	G2	pN0	M0	pos	pos	neg	intermediate
pDCIS 22	71	pTis	G3	pN0	M0	pos	neg	neg	high
pDCIS 23	65	pTis	G3	pN0	M0	pos	neg	neg	high
pDCIS 24	59	pTis	G3	pN0	M0	neg	pos	pos	intermediate
pDCIS 25	65	pTis	G3	pN0	M0	neg	neg	pos	intermediate
pDCIS 26	47	pTis	G3	pN0	M0	neg	neg	pos	low
pDCIS 27	46	pTis	G3	pN0	M0	pos	neg	pos	intermediate
pDCIS 28	53	pTis	G3	pN0	M0	pos	pos	pos	intermediate
pDCIS 29	53	pT1b	G3	pN0	M0	neg	neg	neg	low
pDCIS 30	40	pTis	G3	pN0	M0	neg	neg	pos	n.d.
pDCIS 31	49	pTis	G3	pN0	M0	neg	neg	neg	n.d.

transcripts using first the same 15 LCM-isolated tissue samples that have been selected for WG-DASL profiling (test-set). In agreement with the findings of WG-DASL gene expression profiling, qPCR confirmed significant upregulation of THBS2, CSPG2, MMP11, GREM1 and COL10A1 and downregulation of KRT14 in IBC compared to the corresponding DCIS (Fig. 3a). While the difference in PLEKHC1 expression was not significant in the WG-DASL profiling experiment using the same FFPE tissues qPCR showed PLEKHC1 expression to be significantly upregulated in IBC (Fig. 3a).

Similar findings were obtained using further 25 laser microdissected DCIS and IBC pairs (validation-set). Statistically significant expression differences were found for THBS2, CSPG2, PLEKHC1, MMP11, GREM1 and KRT14 (*P* < 0.05) whereas for COL10A1 this time only a trend to increased expression in IBC was observed (Fig. 3b).

Identification of high–risk DCIS

We hypothesise that genes exhibiting a continuous increase or decrease in their expression at least from pDCIS to DCIS (of DCIS/IBC mixed tumours) and ideally further to IBC may be able to discriminate

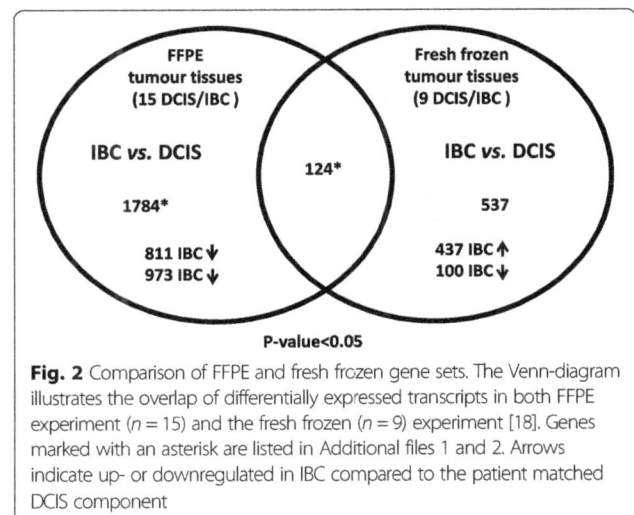

Fig. 2 Comparison of FFPE and fresh frozen gene sets. The Venn-diagram illustrates the overlap of differentially expressed transcripts in both FFPE experiment (*n* = 15) and the fresh frozen (*n* = 9) experiment [18]. Genes marked with an asterisk are listed in Additional files 1 and 2. Arrows indicate up- or downregulated in IBC compared to the patient matched DCIS component

Table 4 Selected candidate genes for validation using qPCR. The progression-associated genes were identified after analysis of the fresh frozen investigation and are significantly differentially expressed between DCIS and IBC of the same tumours. Six of them are also differentially expressed between DCIS and IBC of the investigated FFPE tumours. The differential expressions of COL10A1 of SULF1 are almost significant. Differential expression of PLEKHC1 could not be verified

Gene	RefSeq_ID	Fresh frozen investigation		FFPE investigation	
		logFC	p-value	fold change	t-test p-value
COL10A1	NM_000493.3	5.11	4.34E-05	1.86	0.06
MMP11	NM_005940.3	5.09	4.92E-06	2.31	0.0042
COL11A1	NM_001854.2	3.64	4.75E-05	1.96	0.0006
THBS2	NM_003247.2	3.50	4.34E-05	1.02	0.0479
CSPG2	NM_004385.2	3.23	0.00126	2.74	0.0033
GREM1	NM_013372.5	3.02	7.36E-05	1.85	0.0033
SULF1	NM_015170.1	2.15	0.000101	1.40	0.0553
PLEKHC1	NM_006832.1	1.84	0.000101	0.33	0.5244
KRT14	NM_000526.3	−4.00	0.00433	−1.74	0.0015

high-risk DCIS from low-risk DCIS. Therefore, the expression of the selected candidate genes was also determined in 31 laser microdissected pDCIS tissue samples. All selected target transcripts could be detected in pDCIS. For THBS2, CSPG2, GREM1 and KRT14, expression differences between pDCIS and DCIS were either not significant or did not follow a continuous trend of up- or downregulation from pDCIS to DCIS. Only the expression of COL10A1 and MMP11 was found to

progress from 'low expression' in pDCIS, to 'intermediate expression' in DCIS and 'high expression' in the corresponding IBC, the difference between pDCIS and DCIS (of DCIS/IBC mixed tumours) being significant ($P < 0.05$; Fig. 4).

Discussion

In patients with DCIS the risk of progression to IBC is the most important consideration in selecting the

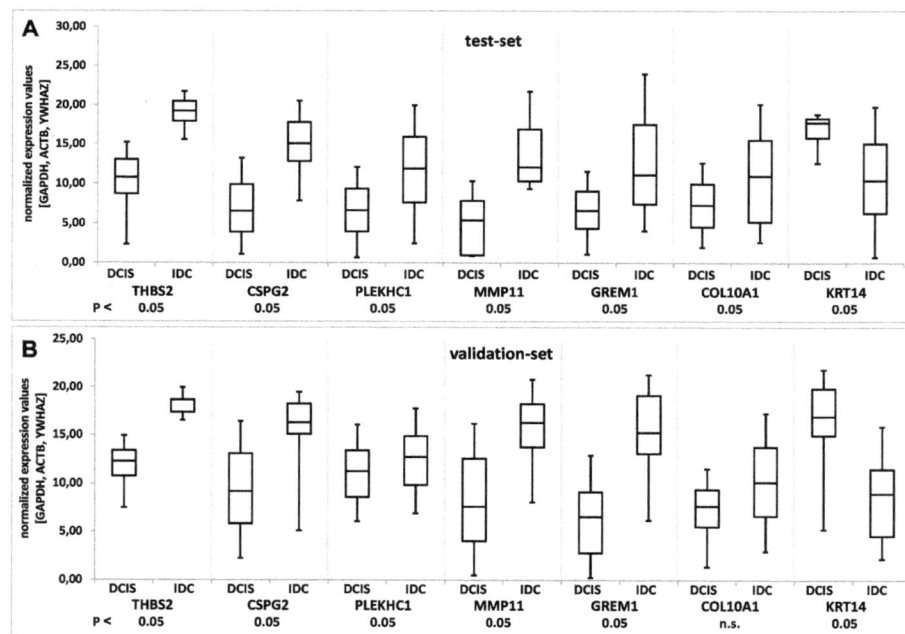

Fig. 3 Validation of differential expression of transcripts in DCIS/IBC-tumours by qPCR. **a)** Test-set: The selected progression-associated genes show a significant difference in expression between DCIS and IBC of the same tumour ($P < 0.05$). **b)** Validation-set: Except for COL10A1, all genes show significant differential expression, confirming the results of the technical validation set ($P < 0.05$). PCR values are normalized to GAPDH, ACTB and YWHAZ

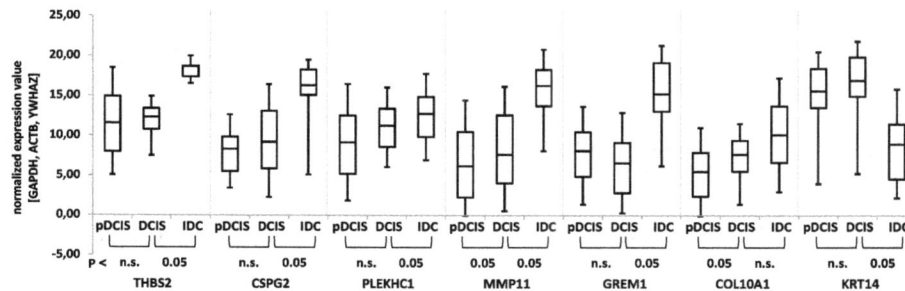

Fig. 4 Independent validation of differential expression of the gene set in pDCIS and DCIS/IBC-tumours by qPCR. Expression of MMP11 increases significantly from pDCIS to DCIS of DCIS/IBC mixed tumours and IBC ($P < 0.05$) and COL10A1 increases significantly from pDCIS to DCIS of DCIS/IBC mixed tumours ($P < 0.05$). Differences in expression of the remaining genes are not significant (n.s.). PCR values are normalized to GAPDH, ACTB and YWHAZ

appropriate management of these lesions [32]. A decisive event in breast cancer progression is the transition of tumour cells through the basement membrane into the surrounding stromal compartment. The underlying molecular events are poorly understood. Identification of genes and proteins driving this process could serve as prognostic markers and therapeutic targets. In order to address the question whether identification of molecular biomarkers for high-risk DCIS is possible we have determined transcripts, which are differentially expressed between the DCIS and IBC component found in DCIS/IBC-tumours and investigated whether such candidate transcripts are even differently represented in pDCIS that did not progress to IBC within 5 to 10 years of follow-up.

One challenge to this is, however, that for reasons of diagnostic certainty, pDCIS specimens are only rarely cryopreserved. Instead, pDCIS samples from FFPE tissue banks are widely available, but are of poorer RNA quality. Technical progress has been achieved to enable gene expression profiling of archival FFPE samples, but it still remains extremely challenging. We have applied gene expression profiling using WG-DASL Assay and qPCR to analyse epithelial cells of pDCIS, DCIS and their corresponding IBC in FFPE breast cancer tissue in the context of tumour progression. The findings were compared with results from a similar study and in which we have investigated cryopreserved breast cancer tissue containing DCIS and IBC areas [18] with the aim to independently cross-validate both expression data.

WG-DASL analysis in the 15 FFPE test set DCIS/IBC samples revealed 1784 transcripts that are differentially expressed between DCIS and IBC of which 124 showed concordant expression in cryopreserved tissues in which 537 total transcripts had been found to be differentially expressed between DCIS and IBC. The resulting overlap of 23% is quite surprising since it is known that gene expression data generated with different array platforms generally show only a marginally overlap [33]. It

suggests that our approach can provide concordant data and that the two data sets can be used for reciprocal confirmation. Further assuring is the fact that among the overlapping genes are transcripts such as MEF2C, LRRC15, BGN, BPAG1, OLFML2B, POSTN, THBS2, PLEKHC1, COL11A1 and FAP, which have already been associated with tumour progression/invasion [18, 34–38].

In order to identify a minimal gene set that may be applicable for routine clinical use by e.g. PCR to distinguish between DCIS and IBC the fresh frozen data set from Schuetz et al. [18] could be concentrated by statistical means resulting in nine transcripts. Eight of them are upregulated in IBC (THBS2, CSPG2, PLEKHC1, GREM1, MMP11, COL10A1, COL11A1, SULF1) and one is downregulated (KRT14) (Table 4; Additional file 3). Of these analogous and significant differential expression was verified for six transcripts by the DASL assay in all 15 DCIS/IBC pairs in the FFPE investigation. For two other transcripts the concordances were almost significant and only the differential expression of PLEKHC1 could not be verified (Table 4).

When validating the expression levels of the nine selected transcripts using qPCR in both the microdissected tissue specimen used for DASL gene expression profiling (test-set, $n = 15$) and in an independent set of further 25 laser microdissected DCIS/IBC pairs (validation-set) seven of them could be confirmed. Only two transcripts, SULF1 and COL11A1, did not produce conclusive PCR results. It is difficult to estimate with confidence whether this validation rate is adequate to draw conclusions, given the relatively limited number of published WG-DASL studies on FFPE tissues and the FFPE-nature and therefore highly variable quality of the starting material. We would recommend validation using a larger sample cohort. However, in summary, our results indicate that differential expression of most transcripts belonging to the minimal progression-associated gene set can be verified in an independent sample cohort.

Some of our candidate transcripts are involved in biological processes related to extracellular matrix remodelling [39]. However, these candidate genes, especially MMP11 and COL11A1, were all detected in microdissected DCIS (of DCIS/IBC mixed tumors) and in pDCIS where we could safely and completely isolate tumor cells from the surrounding stroma, therefore proving the expression of these genes in neoplastic epithelial cells. In IBC tissues, where the epithelial complexes are much smaller, we estimated to enrich the tumor cell compartment to a purity of at least 80% using LCM. Therefore we do not think that the upregulated expression we detected for these candidate genes could only be caused by ´contamination` of co-microdissected stromal cells. Immunohistochemical investigations for the in situ detection of candidate gene on the protein level would have increased the value of our findings, but were beyond the scope of the present study.

One explanation for the detection of genes which are regarded to be of stromal or fibroblast origin might be that tumour progression is thought to include processes such as epithelial-mesenchymal transition (EMT), whereby epithelial cells lose epithelial polarity, acquire a fibroblastoid phenotype and loose cell-to-cell-adhesion [40]. In support of this some of the putatively stroma-derived transcripts can be found in e.g. 'core EMT interactome gene-expression signature' in which the transcript for KRT14 is downregulated and transcripts for GREM1, PLEKHC1 and several collagens and MMPs are upregulated [41]. Also the 'EMT core signature' defined by Anastassiou et al. [41] contains GREM1 and several other genes - e.g. DCN, SPARC, INHBA, MMP13, and PDGFRB – which are represented in our FFPE data set. The role of EMT in breast cancer prognosis is still under debate; however, a number of EMT-related genes have been linked to poor outcome in breast cancer [42, 43].

In support of our data some of the differentially expressed genes represented in our progression-associated candidate set (COL10A1, COL11A1, MMP11, SULF1, and THBS2) have also been identified in another study comparing gene expression of matched DCIS/IBC pairs [14]. During breast cancer progression MMP11 expression is significantly increased in IBC compared to DCIS, supporting our data that it may be a key player driving the DCIS-to-IBC transition [39]. Vargas et al. [44] also observed genes such as COL11A1, COL5A2 and MMP13 in epithelial cells of IBC compared to DCIS.

MMP11 - also called stromelysin 3 – has already been associated with the invasion of tumour cells and is a marker of poor prognosis [18, 45, 46]. The **COL10A1** gene encodes the alpha chain of type X collagen, a short chain collagen expressed by hypertrophic chondrocytes during endochondral ossification. Its expression is

greatly increased in breast cancer tissue compared to normal breast tissue [47].

Of at least equal value for the clinical management of breast cancer would be information on the prognosis with regard to tumour progression at the DCIS stage. Therefore, one important aspect of this work is that pDCIS samples were used to verify if some of the 9 selected transcripts follow a continuous trend of up- or downregulation from pDCS to DCIS and may thus be able to discriminate between high-risk and low-risk DCIS. Besides expected inter-patient expression differences due to different origin of pDCIS and DCIS with IBC component, MMP11 and COL10A1, significantly progressed from 'low expression' in pDCIS, to 'intermediate expression' in DCIS and further to 'high expression' in the corresponding IBC, with the differences between pDCIS and DCIS of DCIS/IBC mixed tumours. The fact that the differences in COL10A1 expression did not reach significance in the independent validation cohort might be caused by the low sample numbers.

Conclusion
By validation of microarray gene expression data using LCM samples from cryopreserved and FFPE DCIS/IBC breast cancer tissues, we identified candidate progression-associated transcripts which might be important for the transition of breast epithelial cells from DCIS to IBC. In addition, the inclusion of pDCIS tissues revealed MMP11 and COL10A1 as potential indicators of high-risk DCIS.

Additional files

Additional file 1: WG-DASL analysis resulted in 1784 transcripts that were differentially expressed between DCIS and IBC in the FFPE breast cancer tissue samples ($P < 0.05$).

Additional file 2: Overlapping genes, Description: Comparison of WG-DASL results with the data from the FF investigation. 124 of the transcripts were found to show differential expression in both investigations ($P < 0.05$).

Additional file 3: Validation 5 FFPE samples analogue to FF samples, Description: A) Analogue samples FFPE-Cryo: The selected progression-associated genes are significantly differential expressed between DCIS and IBC of the same tumour ($P < 0.05$; n.s. = not significant). B) Remaining FFPE samples: Except for COL10A1, all genes are significantly differential expressed and confirm the results of the technical validation set ($P < 0.05$; n.s. = not significant). PCR values are normalized to GAPDH, ACTB and YWHAZ

Abbreviations
DASL: cDNA-mediated annealing, selection, extension and ligation; DCIS: Ductal carcinoma in situ; FF: Fresh frozen; FFPE: Formalin-fixed paraffin-embedded; IBC: Invasive duct carcinoma; LCM: Laser capture microdissection; pDCIS: Pure DCIS

Acknowledgements
We thank Sven Poths for performing the microarray hybridization and Daniel Hofmann for performing the Prosigna® analysis.

Funding

This research was supported by the German Research Foundation (DFG; FE551/3-1, SO885/1-1) and the Medical Faculty of the Heinrich-Heine University Duesseldorf (44/2013). The Microarray Facility is sponsored by the Interdisciplinary Centre of Clinical Research, Tuebingen (IZKF) and the Federal Ministry of Education and Research (grant number 01KS9602).

Authors' contributions

SS performed the RNA extraction, the molecular analysis and drafted the manuscript. KP-D and HB performed the LCM. MB was responsible for the establishment of the hybridisation methods and performed the microarray analysis. HS carried out the statistical analysis of qPCR. SK and UV provided FFPE tumour samples. TF is responsible for the storage of the tumour samples and also participated in the design of the study. HJN, NH, and KS conceived and planned the project, participated in its coordination and helped to draft the manuscript. In addition, KS and HB evaluated the tumour samples for microdissection and the Prosigna™ data. All authors read and approved the final manuscript.

Competing interests

The authors declare that they have no competing interests.

Author details

[1]Department of Obstetrics and Gynaecology, Life-Science-Center, Heinrich-Heine University, Merowingerplatz 1A, 40225 Duesseldorf, Germany. [2]Institute of Pathology, Department of Pathology, Ludwig Maximilians University, Thalkirchner Straße 36, 80337 Munich, Germany. [3]Microarray Facility, Department of Medical Genetics, Eberhard Karls University, Tuebingen, Germany. [4]IMGM Laboratories GmbH, Bunsenstr. 7a, 82152 Martinsried, Germany. [5]Department of Obstetrics and Gynaecology, Ludwig Maximilians University, Marchioninistr. 15, 81377 Munich, Germany. [6]Institute of Pathology, Eberhard Karls University, Tuebingen, Germany. [7]Department of Obstetrics and Gynaecology, Eberhard Karls University, Liebermeisterstr. 8, 72076 Tuebingen, Germany. [8]Department of Obstetrics and Gynaecology, Eberhard Karls University, Calwerstr. 7, 72076 Tuebingen, Germany. [9]Department of Obstetrics and Gynaecology, Heinrich-Heine University, Duesseldorf, Moorenstr. 5, 40225 Duesseldorf, Germany.

References

1. Lopez-Otin C. Breast and prostate Cancer: an analysis of common epidemiological, genetic, and biochemical features. Endocr Rev. 1998;19:365-96.
2. Allred DC, Mohsin SK, Fuqua SAW. Histological and biological evolution of human premalignant breast disease. Endocr Relat Cancer. 2001;8:47-61.
3. Connell PO, Fuqua SAW, Osborne CK, Clark GM, Allred DC. Analysis of loss of heterozygosity in 399 premalignant breast lesions at 15 genetic loci. J Natl Cancer Inst. 1998;90:697-703.
4. Collins LC, Tamimi RM, Baer HJ, Connolly JL, G a C, Schnitt SJ. Outcome of patients with ductal carcinoma in situ untreated after diagnostic biopsy: results from the nurses' health study. Cancer. 2005;103:1778-84.
5. Frykberg ER, FAC S. Overview of the biology and Management of Ductal Carcinoma in Situ of the breast. Cancer. 1994;74:350-61.
6. Cuzick J. Treatment of DCIS--results from clinical trials. Surg Oncol. 2003;12: 213-9.
7. Sgroi DC. Preinvasive breast cancer. Annu Rev Pathol. 2010;5:193-221.
8. Lakhani SR, Ashworth A. Microarray and histopathological analysis of tumours: the future and the past? Nat Rev Cancer. 2001;1:1-7.
9. Kerlikowske K. Characteristics associated with recurrence among women with ductal carcinoma in situ treated by lumpectomy. CancerSpectrum Knowl Environ. 2003;95:1692-702.
10. Gauthier ML, Berman HK, Miller C, Kozakeiwicz K, Chew K, Moore D, Rabban J, Chen YY, Kerlikowske K, Tlsty TD. Abrogated response to cellular stress identifies DCIS associated with subsequent tumour events and defines basal-like breast tumours. Cancer Cell. 2007;12:479-91.
11. Bethwaite P, Smith N, Delahunt B, Kenwright D. Reproducibility of new classification schemes for the pathology of ductal carcinoma in situ of the breast. J Clin Pathol. 1998;51:450-4.
12. Gradishar WJ. The future of breast cancer: the role of prognostic factors. Breast Cancer Res Treat. 2005;89(Suppl 1):S17-26.
13. Patani N, Cutuli B, Mokbel K: Current management of DCIS: a review. Breast Cancer Res Treat 2008, 111:1-10.
14. Muggerud AA, Hallett M, Johnsen H, Kleivi K, Zhou W, Tahmasebpoor S, Amini R-M, Botling J, Børresen-Dale A-L, Sørlie T, Wärnberg F. Molecular diversity in ductal carcinoma in situ (DCIS) and early invasive breast cancer. Mol Oncol. 2010;4:357-68.
15. Hannemann J, Velds A, Halfwerk JBG, Kreike B, Peterse JL, van de Vijver MJ: Classification of ductal carcinoma in situ by gene expression profiling. Breast Cancer Res 2006, 8:R61.
16. Ma X, Salunga R, Tuggle JT, Gaudet J, Enright E, Mcquary P, Payette T, Pistone M, Stecker K, Zhang BM, Zhou Y, Varnholt H, Smith B, Gadd M, Chatfield E, Kessler J, Baer TM, Erlander MG, Sgroi DC. Gene expression profiles of human breast cancer progression. Proc Natl Acad Sci U S A. 2003;100:5974-9.
17. Porter D, Lahti-domenici J, Keshaviah A, Bae YK, Argani P, Marks J, Richardson A, Cooper A, Strausberg R, Riggins GJ, Schnitt S, Gabrielson E, Gelman R, Polyak K. Molecular markers in ductal carcinoma in situ of the breast. Mol Cancer Res. 2003;1:362-75.
18. Schuetz CS, Bonin M, Clare SE, Nieselt K, Sotlar K, Walter M, Fehm T, Solomayer E, Riess O, Wallwiener D, Kurek R, Neubauer HJ. Progression-specific genes identified by expression profiling of matched ductal carcinomas in situ and invasive breast tumours, combining laser capture microdissection and oligonucleotide microarray analysis. Cancer Res. 2006;66:5278-86.
19. Bibikova M, Talantov D, Chudin E, Yeakley JM, Chen J, Doucet D, Wickham E, Atkins D, Barker D, Chee M, Wang Y, Fan J. Quantitative gene expression profiling in formalin- fixed, paraffin-embedded tissues using universal bead arrays. Am J Pathol. 2004;165:1799-807.
20. Silverstein MJ. The University of Southern California/Van Nuys prognostic index for ductal carcinoma in situ of the breast. Am J Surg. 2003;186:337-43.
21. Nielsen T, Wallden B, Schaper C, Ferree S, Liu S, Gao D, Barry G, Dowidar N, Maysuria M, Storhoff J. Analytical validation of the PAM50-based Prosigna breast Cancer prognostic gene signature assay and nCounter analysis system using formalin-fixed paraffin-embedded breast tumour specimens. BMC Cancer. 2014;14:177.
22. Farragher SM, Tanney A, Kennedy RD, Paul Harkin D. RNA expression analysis from formalin fixed paraffin embedded tissues. Histochem Cell Biol. 2008;130:435-45.
23. Dunning MJ, Barbosa-Morais NL, Lynch AG, Tavaré S, Ritchie ME. Statistical issues in the analysis of Illumina data. BMC Bioinformatics. 2008;9:85.
24. Gentleman RC, Gentleman RC, Carey VJ, Carey VJ, Bates DM, Bates DM, Bolstad B, Bolstad B, Dettling M, Dettling M, Dudoit S, Dudoit S, Ellis B, Ellis B, Gautier L, Gautier L, Ge Y, Ge Y, Gentry J, Gentry J, Hornik K, Hornik K, Hothorn T, Hothorn T, Huber W, Huber W, Iacus S, Iacus S, Irizarry R, Irizarry R, et al. Bioconductor: open software development for computational biology and bioinformatics. Genome Biol. 2004;5:R80.
25. Gautier L, Cope L, Bolstad BM, R a I. Affy - analysis of Affymetrix GeneChip data at the probe level. Bioinformatics. 2004;20:307-15.
26. Dunning MJ, Smith ML, Ritchie ME, Tavaré S. Beadarray: R classes and methods for Illumina bead-based data. Bioinformatics. 2007;23:2183-4.
27. Smyth GK. Linear models and empirical bayes methods for assessing differential expression in microarray experiments. Stat Appl Genet Mol Biol. 2004;3:Article3.
28. Hong F, Breitling R, McEntee CW, Wittner BS, Nemhauser JL, Chory J. RankProd: a bioconductor package for detecting differentially expressed genes in meta-analysis. Bioinformatics. 2006;22:2825-7.
29. Falcon S, Gentleman R. Using GOstats to test gene lists for GO term association. Bioinformatics. 2007;23:257-8.
30. Huber W, von Heydebreck A, Sültmann H, Poustka A, Vingron M: Variance stabilization applied to microarray data calibration and to the quantification of differential expression. Bioinformatics 2002, 18 Suppl 1:S96-S104.
31. Benjamini Y, Hochberg Y. Controlling the false discovery rate: a practical and powerful approach to multiple testing. J R Statist Soc. 1995;57:289-300.
32. Morrow M, Harris JR. Ductal carcinoma in situ and microinvasive carcinoma. In: Harris J, Lippman ME, Morrow M, Osborne CK, editors. Diseases of the breast. 2nd ed. Philadelphia: Lippincott Williams & Wilkins; 2004. p. 521-37.
33. Järvinen AK, Hautaniemi S, Edgren H, Auvinen P, Saarela J, Kallioniemi OP, Monni O. Are data from different gene expression microarray platforms comparable? Genomics. 2004;83:1164-8.
34. Castellana B, Escuin D, Peiró G, Garcia-Valdecasas B, Vázquez T, Pons C, Pérez-Olabarria M, Barnadas A, Lerma E. ASPN and GJB2 are implicated in the mechanisms of invasion of ductal breast carcinomas. J Cancer. 2012;3:175-83.
35. Kim H, Watkinson J, Varadan V, Anastassiou D. Multi-cancer computational analysis reveals invasion-associated variant of desmoplastic reaction involving INHBA, THBS2 and COL11A1. BMC Med Genet. 2010;3:51.

36. Gozgit JM, Pentecost BT, Sa M, Otis CN, Wu C, Arcaro KF. Use of an aggressive MCF-7 cell line variant, TMX2-28, to study cell invasion in breast cancer. Mol Cancer Res. 2006;4:905–13.

37. Knudsen ES, Ertel A, Davicioni E, Kline J, Schwartz GF, Witkiewicz AK. Progression of ductal carcinoma in situ to invasive breast cancer is associated with gene expression programs of EMT and myoepithelia. Breast Cancer Res Treat. 2012;133:1009–24.

38. Turashvili G, Bouchal J, Baumforth K, Wei W, Dziechciarkova M, Ehrmann J, Klein J, Fridman E, Skarda J, Srovnal J, Hajduch M, Murray P, Kolar Z. Novel markers for differentiation of lobular and ductal invasive breast carcinomas by laser microdissection and microarray analysis. BMC Cancer. 2007;7:55.

39. Ma X-J, Dahiya S, Richardson E, Erlander M, Sgroi DC. Gene expression profiling of the tumour microenvironment during breast cancer progression. Breast Cancer Res. 2009;11:R7.

40. Taube JH, Herschkowitz JI, Komurov K, Zhou AY, Gupta S, Yang J, Hartwell K, Onder TT, Gupta PB, Evans KW, Hollier BG, Ram PT, Lander ES, Rosen JM, R a W, S a M. Core epithelial-to-mesenchymal transition interactome gene-expression signature is associated with claudin-low and metaplastic breast cancer subtypes. Proc Natl Acad Sci U S A. 2010;107:15449–54.

41. Anastassiou D, Rumjantseva V, Cheng W, Huang J, Canoll PD, Yamashiro DJ, Kandel JJ. Human cancer cells express slug-based epithelial-mesenchymal transition gene expression signature obtained in vivo. BMC Cancer. 2011;11:529.

42. Jechlinger M, Grunert S, Tamir IH, Janda E, Lüdemann S, Waerner T, Seither P, Weith A, Beug H, Kraut N. Expression profiling of epithelial plasticity in tumour progression. Oncogene. 2003;22:7155–69.

43. Van VLJ, Dai H, Van De VMJ, Van Der KK, Marton MJ, Witteveen AT, Schreiber GJ, Kerkhoven RM, Roberts C, Bernards Â, Friend SH, Linsley PS. Gene expression profiling predicts clinical outcome of breast cancer. Nature. 2002;415:530–6.

44. Vargas AC, McCart Reed AE, Waddell N, Lane A, Reid LE, Smart CE, Cocciardi S, da Silva L, Song S, Chenevix-Trench G, Simpson PT, Lakhani SR: Gene expression profiling of tumour epithelial and stromal compartments during breast cancer progression. Breast Cancer Res Treat 2012, 135:153–165.

45. Arora S, Kaur J, Sharma C, Mathur M, Bahadur S, Shukla NK, Deo SVS, Ralhan R. Stromelysin 3, Ets-1, and vascular endothelial growth factor expression in oral precancerous and cancerous lesions: correlation with microvessel density, progression, and prognosis. Clin Cancer Res. 2005;11:2272–84.

46. Cheng C-W, Yu J-C, Wang H-W, Huang C-S, Shieh J-C, Fu Y-P, Chang C-W, Wu P-E, Shen C-Y. The clinical implications of MMP-11 and CK-20 expression in human breast cancer. Clin Chim Acta. 2010;411:234–41.

47. Chang H, Yang M, Yang Y, Hou M. MMP13 is potentially a new tumour marker for. Oncol Rep. 2009;22:1119–27.

6

RNA sequencing-based longitudinal transcriptomic profiling gives novel insights into the disease mechanism of generalized pustular psoriasis

Lingyan Wang, Xiaoling Yu, Chao Wu, Teng Zhu, Wenming Wang, Xiaofeng Zheng and Hongzhong Jin[*]

Abstract

Background: Generalized pustular psoriasis (GPP) is a rare, episodic, potentially life-threatening inflammatory disease. However, the pathogenesis of GPP, and universally accepted therapies for treating it, remain undefined.

Methods: To better understand the disease mechanism of GPP, we performed a transcriptome analysis to profile the gene expression of peripheral blood mononuclear cells (PBMCs) from patients enrolled at the time of diagnosis and receiving follow-up treatment for up to 6 months.

Results: RNA sequencing data revealed that gene expression in five GPP patients' PBMCs was profoundly altered following acitretin treatment. Differentially expressed gene (DEG) analysis suggested that genes related to psoriatic inflammation, including CXCL1, CXCL8 (IL-8), S100A8, S100A9, S100A12 and LCN2, were significantly downregulated in patients in remission from GPP. Functional enrichment and annotation analysis unveiled a cluster of DEGs significantly associated with the function of leukocytes, particularly neutrophils. Pathway analysis suggested that a variety of pro-inflammatory pathways were inhibited in patients in remission. This analysis not only reaffirmed known signaling pathways in GPP pathogenesis, but also implicated novel factors and pathways, such as cell cycle regulation pathways. Furthermore, regulator network analysis provided bioinformatics-based support for upstream molecules as potential therapeutic targets such as oncostatin M.

Conclusions: This longitudinal analysis of blood transcriptomes provides the first evidence that dysregulated gene expression in peripheral blood may significantly contribute to psoriatic inflammation in GPP patients. Novel canonical pathways and biomarkers identified in the current research may provide insights to help understand GPP pathobiology and advance novel therapeutics.

Keywords: Generalized pustular psoriasis, RNA-sequencing, Neutrophil, Peripheral blood mononuclear cell

Background

Generalized pustular psoriasis (GPP) is a potentially life-threatening, multisystemic inflammatory disease characterized by sudden, repeated episodes of high-grade fever, generalized erythematous pustular rashes, and systemic upset. GPP is often triggered by environmental factors and immune disorders, such as pregnancy, infections, drugs and hypocalcemia [1]. Although GPP has long

been considered to be a rare variant of psoriasis, some evidence suggests that it is a different entity: different clinical presentation and distinct HLA alleles have been observed in patients with GPP compared with common forms of psoriasis [2–4]. To date, the pathogenesis and pathophysiology of GPP remain largely unknown. Dysregulated expression of cytokines/chemokines, such as IL-1 and IL-36, have been suggested to play important roles in GPP [5]. In the last few years, rare variants of the genes, IL36RN, CARD14 and AP1S3 have been identified as susceptibility factors for GPP [6–8]. Nevertheless, many GPP patients do not carry mutations in any

* Correspondence: jinhongzhong@263.net
Department of Dermatology, Peking Union Medical College Hospital,
Chinese Academy of Medical Sciences and Peking Union Medical College,
Beijing, China

of these three genes, leaving the genetic basis of GPP elusive [9].

GPP is a difficult disease to treat. Therapies successful for treating plaque psoriasis are generally less effective for GPP. Since 2012, acitretin, cyclosporine or methotrexate have been the recommended first-line therapies for acute GPP. Of these, acitretin, an oral retinoid, is the preferred agent [10]. Acitretin has shown success in treating both generalized and localized pustular psoriasis, while it is less effective for plaque psoriasis [11]. Ozawa et al. [12] demonstrated that the oral retinoid has higher effectiveness in GPP patients than methotrexate, cyclosporine, psoralen and ultraviolet A irradiation. Nevertheless, the mechanism of action of acitretin still remains largely unclear, impeding its broader application. Moreover, some GPP patients do not respond to existing treatments, creating an urgent need for novel drug targets and therapeutics.

Transcriptome profiling technologies, such as microarrays and RNA sequencing (RNA-seq), are valuable tools for deciphering the regulatory network underlying disease. Recently, by performing microarray analysis with skin lesions from GPP patients, researchers have successfully identified critical genes or pathways in GPP [13, 14]. To better understand GPP pathogenesis and drug effects at the molecular level, we performed an RNA-seq-based longitudinal gene expression study of peripheral blood mononuclear cells (PBMCs) obtained from GPP patients before and during acitretin treatment. Differentially expressed genes were systematically identified and further analyzed by functional network annotation. Our study comprehensively profiled the molecular signature of GPP patients in response to drug treatment, and provides clues for potential new drug targets for GPP treatment.

Methods

Patient enrollment and sampling
This study was approved by the Medical Ethics Committee of the Peking Union Medical College Hospital. Five adult patients with GPP who responded well to acitretin treatment were included. All patients were diagnosed according to the Umezawa criteria and presented with clinically visible generalized pustules at their initial visit [15]. All patients had not undergone any systemic treatment for at least 1 month.

After receipt of written informed consent signed by the patients, 10 ml whole-blood samples were obtained from the patients at T0, T1 and T2. Blood was collected in endotoxin-free silicone-coated tubes. The PBMCs were prepared with Ficoll-Paque PLUS (GE Healthcare, Uppsala, Sweden) according to the manufacturer's instructions. The PBMCs obtained from each sample were stored at − 80 °C in sterile screw-cap tubes and thawed directly

before analysis. IL36RN mutations of all the patients were detected by using the previously described methods [16].

RNA isolation and sequencing library construction
Total RNA was extracted using Trizol (Invitrogen, Carlsbad, CA) according to the manufacturer's instructions. RNA purity was checked using a kaiaoK5500® spectrophotometer (Kaiao, Beijing, China), and its integrity and concentration were assessed using an RNA Nano 6000 Assay Kit with a Bioanalyzer 2100 system (Agilent Technologies, CA). Total RNA meeting the following conditions was used for library construction: the RNA integrity number (RIN) ≥ 7; 28S/18S rRNA ratio ≥ 1.5.

One microgram of total RNA per sample was used as initial material for library construction. Sequencing libraries with varied index labels were generated for each sample following the manufacturer's recommendations, using an NEBNext® Ultra™ RNA Library Prep Kit (NEB, Ipswich, MA). The library construction procedures were as follows. First, ribosomal RNA was removed using an Illumina Ribo-Zero™ Gold rRNA Removal Kit. RNA fragmentation was then carried out. Next, the first and second cDNA strand were sequentially synthesized. The library fragments were then purified, followed by terminal repair, dA-tailing and adapter ligation. The library fragments were purified, and UNG enzyme digestion were performed. Finally, polymerase chain reaction amplification was carried out to complete the library construction.

Library clustering and sequencing
Clustering of the index-coded samples was performed on a cBot cluster generation system using a TruSeq PE Cluster Kit v4-cBot-HS (Illumina, San Diego, CA) according to the manufacturer's instructions. After cluster generation, the libraries were sequenced on an Illumina Hiseq X10 platform (Illumina, San Diego, CA), and 125 bp paired-end reads were generated by CapitalBioTech (Beijing, China).

Quality control and read alignment
Quality control metrics were obtained for raw sequencing reads using the FastQC application [17]. Reads were mapped to the hg19 human reference genome with TopHat2 and mapped read counts were estimated by Cufflinks [18]. Transcript expression was calculated from values for fragments per kilobase of exon per million fragments mapped.

DEG analysis and statistical analysis
Differential gene expression analysis was performed using the Limma package of R language (v. 3.22.7), an R/Bioconductor software package that provides an integrated solution for both differential expression and differential splicing analyses of RNA-seq data [19]. Paired t-tests were

used to compare gene expression values between the pre- and the posttreatment samples (T1 versus T0 and T2 versus T0). The Benjamini–Hochberg method was used as an FDR adjustment for multiple testing correction. A threshold of FDR < 0.05 was used to define statistical significance. Venn diagrams showing the overlap of DEGs in different groups were constructed using an online bioinformatics tool (http://bioinformatics.psb.ugent.be/webtools/Venn/). Principle component analysis was conducted with ClustVis [20] (http://biit.cs.ut.ee/clustvis/).

Functional analysis

Metascape (http://metascape.org) was employed to perform the gene enrichment and functional annotation analyses. For the identification of pathways and regulatory networks, Canonical Pathway Analysis, Upstream Regulator Analysis, and Regulatory Effects Analysis were performed using the IPA software (Ingenuity Systems, Redwood City, CA, USA; Version: 42012434).

Reverse transcription–qPCR (RT-qPCR)

RT-qPCR was performed on 10 preselected GPP-related genes. RNA was extracted using Trizol (Invitrogen, Carlsbad, CA, USA). The sequences of the qPCR primers used in this study are shown in Additional file 1: Table S1. Each RT-qPCR reaction was performed in duplicate and the mean threshold cycle (Ct) value for each sample was used for data analysis. The $2^{-\Delta\Delta Ct}$ method was used for determining the fold-change in the expression level, and *GAPDH* was used for normalization. Paired t-test analyses were performed on the $2^{-\Delta\Delta Ct}$ values for the comparison of two groups of samples.

Results

Patient sample collection, sequencing data and differential expression analysis

Five adult patients affected with GPP were included in the current study (one male and four females, aged 36.40 ± 18.72 years). All patients fulfilled the diagnostic criteria for GPP at their initial visit [15]. Treatment was started with acitretin on an initial dose of 0.5–0.75 mg/kg/day. All five

patients achieved remission of their clinical symptoms after treatment for two weeks: pustules cleared, body temperature recovered and general symptoms improved. Once pustulation was resolved, acitretin was tapered down gradually to a final dose of 10 mg/day for long-term maintenance. Disease severity of the patients was quantified using the GPP severity score system [21]. The characteristics of these five patients are shown in Table 1.

To investigate the pathophysiological mechanisms underlying remission of GPP, transcriptome profiling was performed with PBMC samples collected at three time points: T0 (the acute phase of GPP, prior to initiation of acitretin treatment), T1 (2 weeks after treatment) and T2 (6 months after treatment). At T1, all five patients showed clearance of pustules, which is the hallmark of the end of acute psoriatic inflammation. At T2, all five patients reached stable remission. The cutaneous manifestation of one GPP patient at the different time points of sample collection is shown in Fig. 1a.

RNA-seq was performed with each sample, and approximately 80 million reads were generated per sample. Sequencing reads were aligned to the human genome and analyzed as described in the methods. Differentially expressed coding genes (DEGs) were then identified by comparing the post-treatment with the pre-treatment transcriptomes of each patient (T1 versus T0 and T2 versus T0). An adjusted p-value (FDR < 0.05) and fold change (FC) ratio ($|\log2FC| \geq 1$) were used to determine the DEGs. A heatmap of DEGs shows global transcriptome changes in individual patients after receiving treatment (Fig. 1b). A total of 2392 DEGs were identified when comparing T1 with T0 samples. Of these, 901 were upregulated (38%) and 1491 downregulated (62%). A total of 2296 DEGs were identified from the comparison of T2 and T0 samples, with approximately 40% (n = 911) upregulated and 60% (n = 1385) downregulated (Fig. 1c). As shown in Fig. 1d, 512 DEGs were common to both the T1 versus T0 and T2 versus T0 datasets (Fig. 1d). The DEGs were sorted by statistical significance (lowest false discovery rate, FDR); the top 50 upregulated and downregulated DEGs in the T1 versus T0 and T2 versus

Table 1 Characteristics of generalized pustular psoriasis patients

Patient	AoO[a]/Duration (yr)	Age range (yr)	PsA[b] [43]	PsV[c]	GPP score			IL36RN Mutation
					T0	T1	T2	
P1	21 /13	30–39	–	–	12	5	2	c.115 + 6 T > C
P2	64/3	60–69	+	+	15	7	3	c.115 + 6 T > C
P3	24/0	20–29	–	+	15	6	2	c.115 + 6 T > C and c.227C > T
P4	37/1	30–39	+	+	11	6	1	Not detected
P5	19/0	10–20	–	+	4	4	1	Not detected

[a]AoO = Age of Onset
[b]PsA = psoriatic arthritis
[c]PsV = psoriasis vulgari

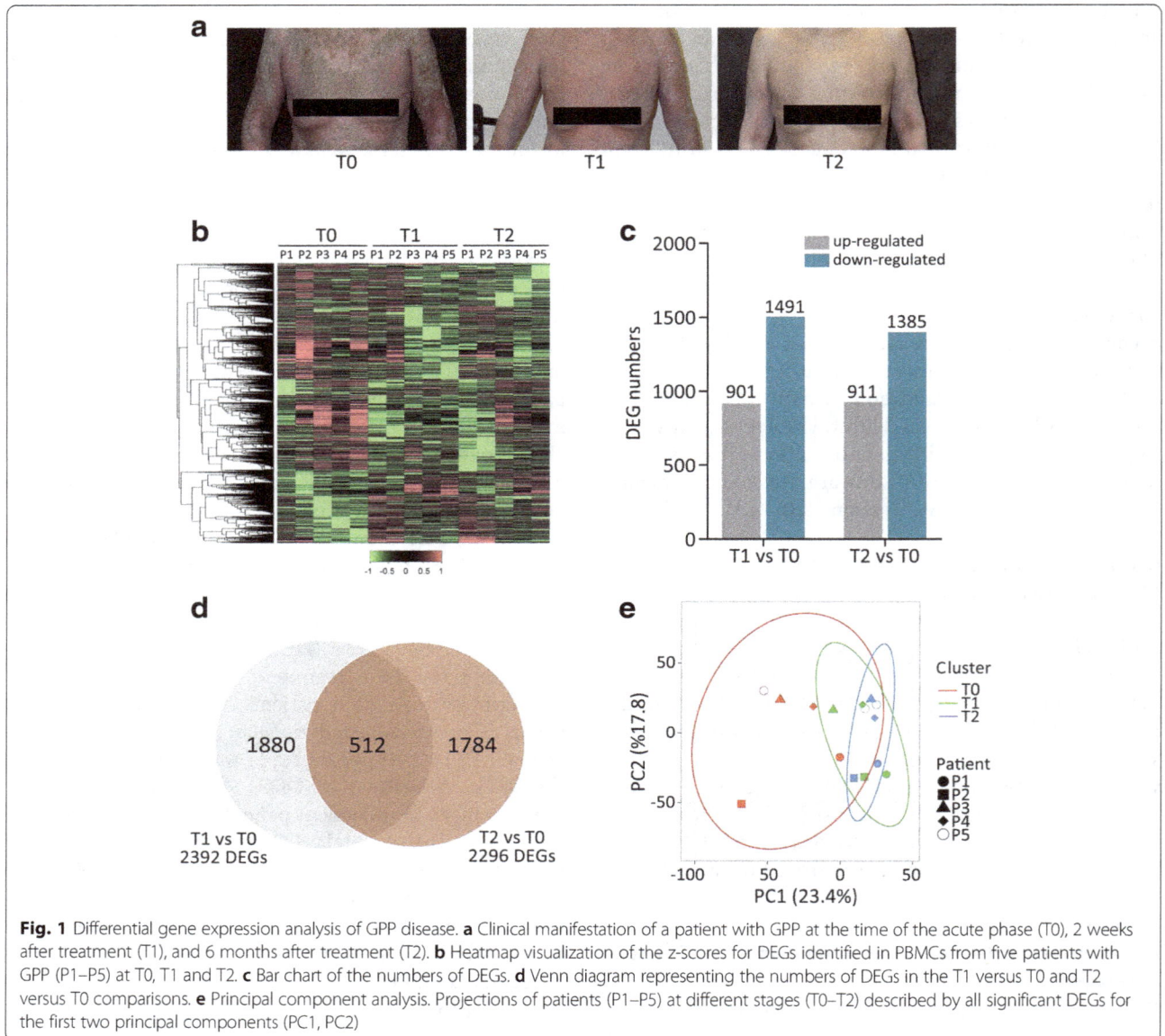

Fig. 1 Differential gene expression analysis of GPP disease. **a** Clinical manifestation of a patient with GPP at the time of the acute phase (T0), 2 weeks after treatment (T1), and 6 months after treatment (T2). **b** Heatmap visualization of the z-scores for DEGs identified in PBMCs from five patients with GPP (P1–P5) at T0, T1 and T2. **c** Bar chart of the numbers of DEGs. **d** Venn diagram representing the numbers of DEGs in the T1 versus T0 and T2 versus T0 comparisons. **e** Principal component analysis. Projections of patients (P1–P5) at different stages (T0–T2) described by all significant DEGs for the first two principal components (PC1, PC2)

T0 datasets are listed in Additional file 2: Table S2 and Additional file 3: Table S3, respectively. Next, principal component analysis (PCA) of the DEGs was conducted. We observed that the T0, T1 and T2 clusters partially overlapped, but the pre-treatment cluster (T0) was much more widely dispersed with less overlap than the two post-treatment clusters (T1 and T2) (Fig. 1e).

Functional enrichment and annotation

Functional enrichment and annotation of DEGs were performed with Metascape [22] (http://metascape.org). Metascape analysis is carried out with four gene ontology (GO) sources: GO Biological Processes, Reactome Gene Sets, Kyoto Encyclopedia of Genes and Genomes (KEGG) Pathway, and the Comprehensive Resource of Mammalian

protein complexes (CORUM). This analysis revealed that "leukocyte activation involved in immune response" was the most significantly enriched functional cluster identified at both T1 ($-\log(\text{FDR})$ = 28.0) and T2 ($-\log(\text{FDR})$ = 26.2) (Fig. 2a and b). Considering that GPP is a severe autoinflammatory disease with systemic inflammation, this result suggests that the remission of GPP is significantly associated with functional changes in peripheral blood leukocytes. DEGs were also enriched in several other clusters related to immune responses, including "cytokine signaling in immune system" (T1, $-\log(\text{FDR})$ = 12.9), "cytokine production" (T1, $-\log(\text{FDR})$ = 10.5; T2, $-\log(\text{FDR})$ = 11.2) and "positive regulation of immune response" (T1, $-\log(\text{FDR})$ = 9.2). Several clusters associated with cellular organelle biogenesis, including

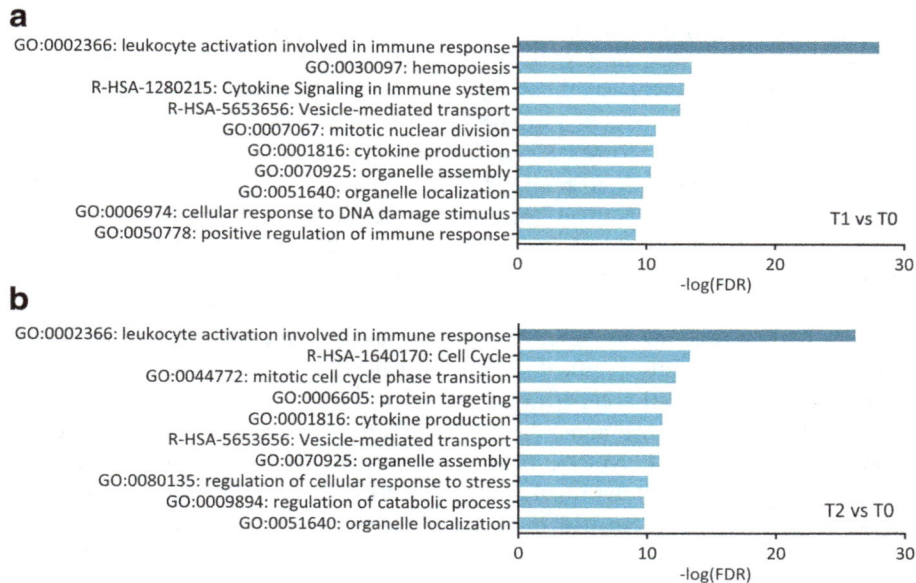

Fig. 2 Functional enrichment and annotation for DEGs. Enrichment of the top 10 clusters at **a** T1 and **b** T2 was performed using Metascape analysis, which was carried out with the four GO sources: KEGG Pathway, GO Biological Processes, Reactome Gene Sets and CORUM. *p*-Values were calculated based on the accumulative hypergeometric distribution

"vesicle-mediated transport" (T1, $-\log(\text{FDR}) = 12.6$; T2, $-\log(\text{FDR}) = 11.0$), "organelle assembly" (T1, $-\log(\text{FDR}) = 10.3$; T2, $-\log(\text{FDR}) = 11.0$) and "organelle localization" (T1, $-\log(\text{FDR}) = 9.7$; T2, $-\log(\text{FDR}) = 9.7$) were identified at both T1 and T2 (Fig. 2a and b).

To gain an in-depth understanding the relevance of circulating leukocytes in GPP, we further analyzed the DEGs in the "leukocyte activation involved in immune response" category. Metascape analysis revealed that these DEGs were significantly enriched in the category, "neutrophil activation involved in immune response" at both T1 ($-\log(\text{FDR}) = 96.8$) and T2 ($-\log(\text{FDR}) = 96.8$) (Additional file 4: Figure S1). Recently, a list has been assembled of genes known to be involved in particular aspects of neutrophil function [23]. By comparing our data with this list, we found that DEGs were identified in nearly every aspect of neutrophil biology (Table 2), suggesting that neutrophils actively function in the pathogenesis of GPP. Finally, a Molecular Complex Detection (MCODE) algorithm was further applied to identify densely connected networks in the leukocyte activation gene cluster. This analysis identified "regulated exocytosis", a process involved in neutrophil activation, as the most significantly enriched MCODE component at both T1 ($-\log P = 20.0$) and T2 ($-\log P = 16.0$) (Additional file 5: Figure S2). Collectively, our data suggest that the GPP is associated with functional change of leukocytes, especially neutrophils, in the patients' peripheral blood.

Pathway analysis

To dissect signaling pathways involved in GPP pathogenesis, we performed Canonical Pathway Analysis with the Ingenuity Pathway Analysis (IPA) software. Based on IPA GO algorithms and KnowledgeBase mining, DEGs at T1 and T2 were enriched in 83 and 74 canonical pathways, respectively (FDR < 0.05, Benjamini-Hochberg

Table 2 Differential expressed genes in involved in neutrophil function

Process	Gene Symbol
Development	CSF3R
Protein trafficking	CD63, AP3S1, AP3M2, AP1S3, AP1B1, AP1G2, AP1G1, AP2M1
Granule formation	MMP9, LTF, LCN2, HP, MMP8, DEFA1, DEFA4, ELANE, PRTN3, AZU1
Capture and rolling	PTX3
Arrest	ITGB2, CD44
Activation during transmigration	PIK3R5, MAPK14
Pattern recognition, migration	FPR1, FPR2, IFNGR1, LTB4R, TLR1, TLR5, MYD88, IRAK4, CLEC7A, NLRP3, NLRC4
Cytokine secretion	IL1B, IL8
Immune crosstalk	TNFSF13B, ARG1
phagocytosis and degranulation	NCF1, HCK, PTK2, RAB27A, RAB27B
Pyroptosis, autophagy	ATG3, GABARAPL1, CASP1
Apoptosis	HTRA2, CASP3

adjusted *p*-value) (Additional file 6: Table S4). By using an absolute z-score value above 2 as a threshold, 9 pathways were identified at T1 (Fig. 3a, top), and 13 pathways were identified at T2 (Fig. 3a, bottom). Of note, most of the signaling pathways were predicted to be inhibited after acitretin treatment. The "TREM1 Signaling" pathway were found to be inhibited at both T1 (−log(FDR) = 1.78) and T2 (−log(FDR) = 1.75). The "Interferon Signaling" (−log(FDR) = 1.3) and "Role of Pattern Recognition Receptors in Recognition of Bacteria and Viruses" (−log(FDR) = 2.2) pathways were identified at T1 and T2, respectively (Additional file 7: Figure S3, Panels A–C). These pathways are mostly implicated in innate immune responses [24, 25]. In these pathways, the expression of innate immune response genes, such as *TLR1*, *TLR5*, *TLR8*, *MYD88*, *NLRC4*, *NOD2*, *IRF7*, *IFNAR1* and *STAT1* were significantly downregulated. Moreover, IPA analysis with all DEGs identified in the current study revealed that the number of innate immunity genes was substantially more than that of adaptive

immunity genes (Additional file 8: Figure S4). These observations suggested that innate immune inflammation is predominantly involved in the inflammation seen in GPP patients. In addition, DEGs were found to be enriched in several cell cycle regulation pathways, including "Mitotic Roles of Polo-like Kinase" (−log(FDR) = 2.65) and "Cyclins and the Cell Cycle Regulation" (−log(FDR) = 1.41) (Additional file 9: Figure S5, Panels A and B), which is consistent with a previous finding showing dysregulated cell cycle gene expression in GPP patients [14].

Multiple cytokine signaling pathways that are known to play important roles in psoriasis pathogenesis were enriched in the DEGs, including the IL-1, IL-6 and IL-8 pathways (Fig. 3a). To comprehensively understand the regulation of cytokine signaling pathways in GPP, we performed a cytokine signaling-specific Canonical Pathway Analysis. The top 20 enriched cytokine signaling pathways (ranked by average −log(FDR) value) are presented by showing their −log(FDR) and z-score values in heatmap format (Fig. 3b). Judging from the z-score values, cytokine

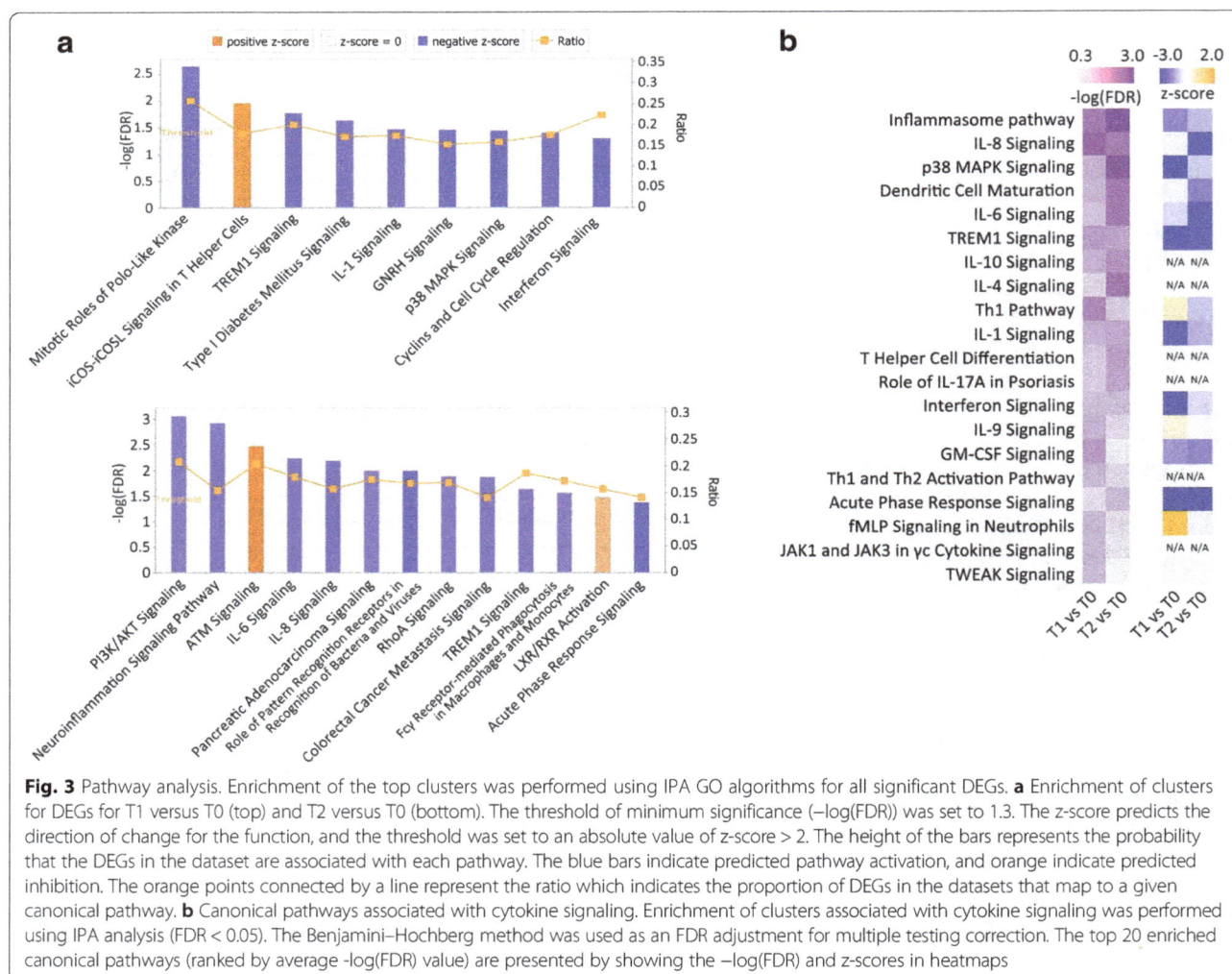

Fig. 3 Pathway analysis. Enrichment of the top clusters was performed using IPA GO algorithms for all significant DEGs. **a** Enrichment of clusters for DEGs for T1 versus T0 (top) and T2 versus T0 (bottom). The threshold of minimum significance (−log(FDR)) was set to 1.3. The z-score predicts the direction of change for the function, and the threshold was set to an absolute value of z-score > 2. The height of the bars represents the probability that the DEGs in the dataset are associated with each pathway. The blue bars indicate predicted pathway activation, and orange indicate predicted inhibition. The orange points connected by a line represent the ratio which indicates the proportion of DEGs in the datasets that map to a given canonical pathway. **b** Canonical pathways associated with cytokine signaling. Enrichment of clusters associated with cytokine signaling was performed using IPA analysis (FDR < 0.05). The Benjamini–Hochberg method was used as an FDR adjustment for multiple testing correction. The top 20 enriched canonical pathways (ranked by average -log(FDR) value) are presented by showing the −log(FDR) and z-scores in heatmaps

signaling pathways as a whole showed a generally more inhibitory pattern at T2 compared with T1, while the "Inflammasome pathway", "p38 MAPK signaling", "IL-1 signaling" and "Interferon signaling" pathways were less inhibited, suggesting that distinct cytokine signaling pathways may be regulated with different kinetics or to different extents in response to drug treatment. Notably, the "Role of IL-17A in Psoriasis" (T2, −log(FDR) = 1.67) pathway was enriched (Fig. 3b), in which downregulated *CXCL3*, *IL-8*, *S100A8*, *S100A9*, *IL17RA* and *CXCL1* expression was observed (Additional file 9: Figure S5, Panel C).

Regulatory network analysis

Next, we performed regulatory network analysis to identify gene interactions and regulatory cascades, again using IPA software. First, Upstream Regulator Analysis, which is based on expected causal effects between upstream regulators and targets, was carried out to predict upstream molecules that may be responsible for gene expression changes. The upstream regulator candidates selected for this analysis were "cytokine" and "transmembrane receptor" because cytokine signaling plays a central role in GPP pathogenesis. The top 20 upstream regulators ($p < 0.01$), ranked by absolute z-score, are shown in Fig. 4a. Remarkably, all 20 upstream regulators have negative z-scores, indicating that their downstream effects were inhibited. Of

these regulators, IL-6, IL-1B, IFN-γ, IL-21, IL-5, IL-17A, TNF, IFN-A2 and IL-15 have been reported to regulate psoriatic inflammation [26]. Moreover, therapies targeting IL-1, IL-17 and TNF have shown promise in preclinical and clinical trials, implying that our analysis may provide insight into potential drug targets for psoriasis.

To further delineate critical regulatory networks in the pathogenesis of GPP, Regulatory Effects Analysis was performed using IPA. This analysis connects upstream regulators, DEGs in our dataset, and downstream functions or diseases to generate regulatory networks. A total of 69 Regulatory Effects networks were generated ($p < 0.01$). Remarkably, all the top 10 networks, ranked by consistency score, have downstream functions of "Activation of myeloid cells" and "Activation of phagocytes". A regulatory network with the highest consistency score is shown in Fig. 4b. In this network, CSF1, F2RL1, FN1, IFN-γ, IL1R1, PI3K (complex), TLR2, TNF (family) and TRADD were identified as the upstream regulators, which target 24 downstream DEGs, resulting in an inhibitory effect on several immune cell types, including myeloid cells, phagocytes, and antigen presenting cells.

Validation of RNA-Seq results with quantitative polymerase chain reactions (qPCR)

To verify the RNA-seq results, qPCR analyses were carried out for 10 genes (Fig. 5). Eight downregulated genes

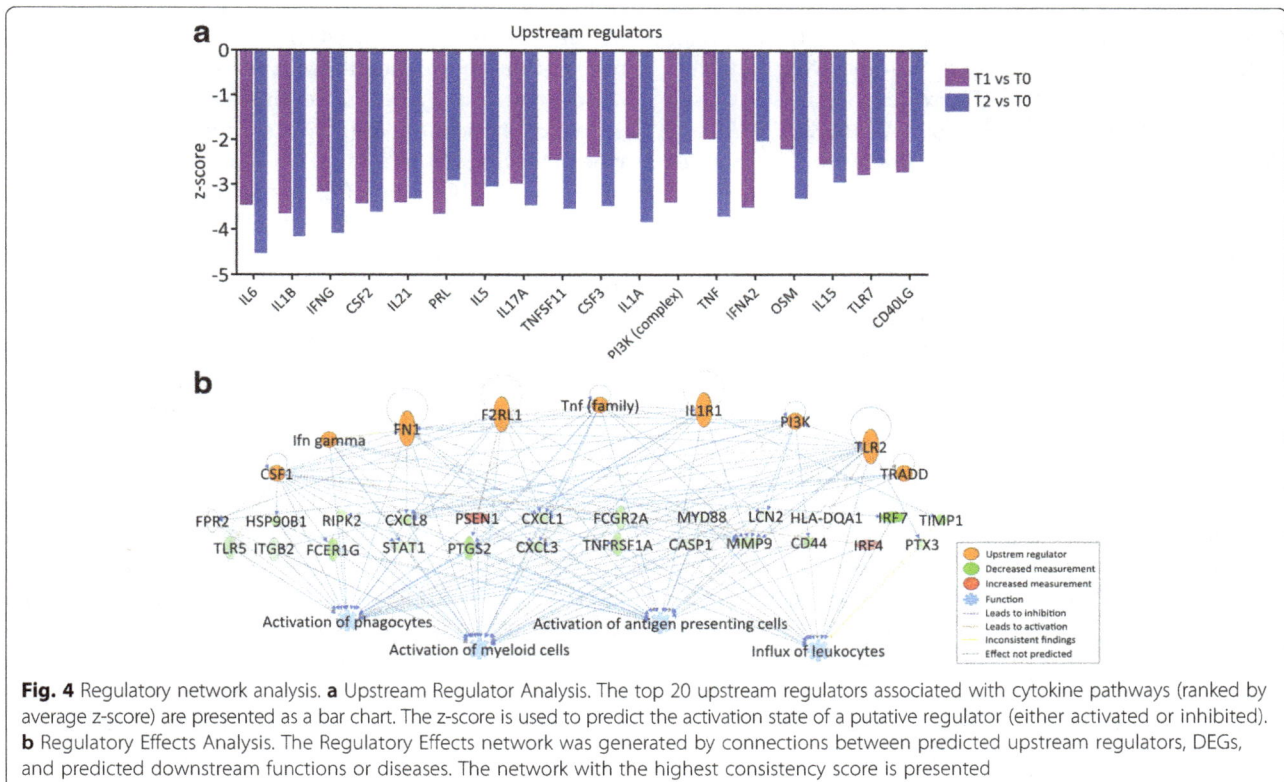

Fig. 4 Regulatory network analysis. **a** Upstream Regulator Analysis. The top 20 upstream regulators associated with cytokine pathways (ranked by average z-score) are presented as a bar chart. The z-score is used to predict the activation state of a putative regulator (either activated or inhibited). **b** Regulatory Effects Analysis. The Regulatory Effects network was generated by connections between predicted upstream regulators, DEGs, and predicted downstream functions or diseases. The network with the highest consistency score is presented

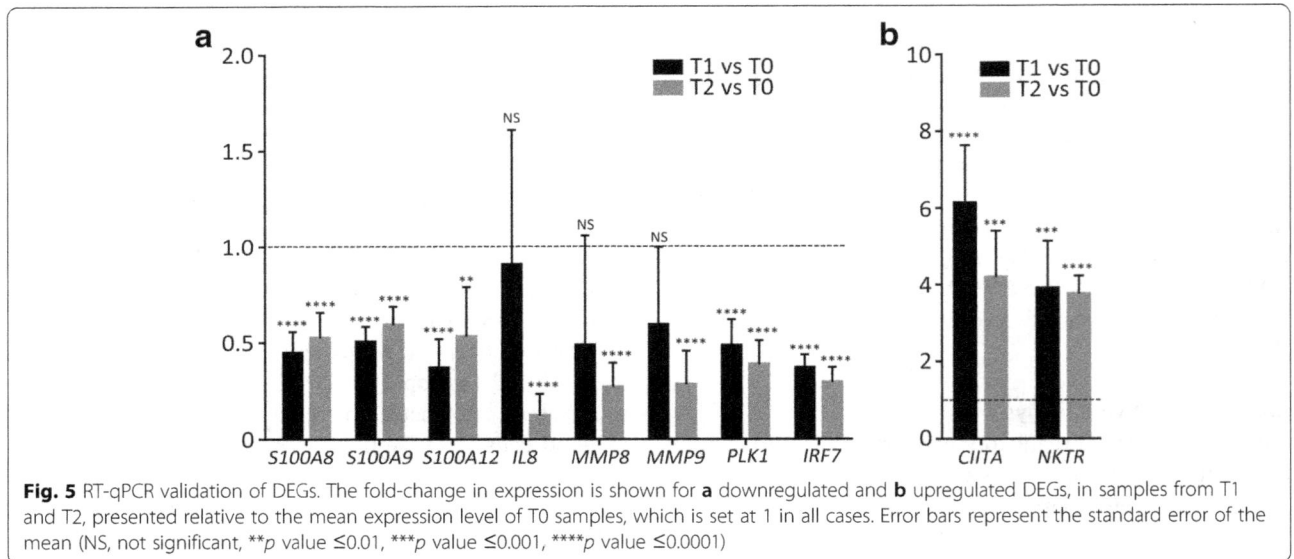

Fig. 5 RT-qPCR validation of DEGs. The fold-change in expression is shown for **a** downregulated and **b** upregulated DEGs, in samples from T1 and T2, presented relative to the mean expression level of T0 samples, which is set at 1 in all cases. Error bars represent the standard error of the mean (NS, not significant, **p value $\leq$0.01, ***p value $\leq$0.001, ****p value $\leq$0.0001)

identified by the RNA-seq analysis were tested. Of these, *S100A8*, *S100A9*, *S100A12*, *IL-8*, *MMP8* and *MMP9* encode antimicrobial peptides (AMPs) or chemoattractant molecules previously known to be involved in GPP pathogenesis, and *PLK1* and *IRF7* were identified in the current research. In addition, two highly upregulated genes, *CIITA* and *NKTR* were chosen for validation. Using the $2^{-\Delta\Delta Ct}$ method, transcript levels for each gene were measured in comparison with the housekeeping gene, *GAPDH*, and were subsequently normalized to each value in the pre-treated (T0) sample. We observed significant increases in *CIITA* and *NKTR* expression, as well as significant decreases in *S100A8*, *S100A9*, *S100A12*, *PLK1* and *IRF7*, at both T1 and T2, which is similar to the RNA-seq data. Moreover, expression of *IL-8* and *MMP8* was found to significantly decrease at T2 but was not significantly changed at T1, which is also in agreement with the RNA-seq data. One exception is the *MMP9* gene: while a significant decrease was observed at both T1 and T2 in the RNA-seq analysis, a significant decrease was only observed at T2 in the qPCR experiment.

Discussion

GPP is a severe skin disease associated with the eruption of sterile pustules and erythema. Pustular psoriasis lesions result from complex interactions among dermal or epidermal cells, resident and infiltrating immune cells, and a variety of cytokines. Previous studies have performed DEG analysis to investigate molecular abnormalities in GPP patients [13, 14]. However, these studies focused on skin lesions, and the transcriptome signature of the peripheral circulation in GPP, a systematic autoinflammatory disease, remained largely unknown. In this study, we conducted a longitudinal RNA-seq-based transcriptome analysis of

PBMCs from GPP patients before and after acitretin treatment. Our study revealed profound changes in the PBMC transcriptome, which may provide insights into GPP pathogenesis and potential biomarkers for diagnosis and therapeutics.

We found that DEGs were significantly enriched in neutrophil functions in our datasets. Neutrophils are commonly absent in the PBMC samples that are derived from healthy donors. However, a distinct subset of low-density granulocytes (LDGs) are present in PBMC preparations from patients with certain systemic inflammatory diseases [27]. For example, neutrophil-specific genes are abundant in the PBMCs from systemic lupus erythematosus (SLE) patients. This is due to the presence of LDGs in PBMCs from SLE patients [28, 29]. Besides, LDGs have also been identified in PBMCs from patients affected with psoriasis [30]. Thus, the enrichment of neutrophil-specific genes in our dataset may be resulted from elevated proportions of LDGs in GPP patients' PBMCs. It is well-known that psoriasis is a T cell-, particularly a CD4$^+$ and CD8$^+$ T cell-mediated immune disease, but the function of neutrophils is much less well understood. Recent research has suggested that neutrophils may contribute to the pathogenic functions of IL-17, possibly in conjunction with the formation of neutrophil extracellular traps, and amplify psoriatic inflammation [30–32]. In our dataset, two of the most potent chemoattractant molecules for neutrophil recruitment, CXCL1 and CXCL8 (IL-8), were significantly downregulated in patients in remission from GPP. Moreover, DEGs were identified in nearly every aspect of neutrophil biology, including protein trafficking, granule formation, capture and rolling, pattern recognition and others (Table 2). Among these DEGs, two encoding the neutrophil G protein-coupled receptors, FPR1 and FPR2, which play pattern recognition roles in chemotaxis [33], were both downregulated. It is noteworthy that FPR2 is the receptor for LL-37, an AMP that drives psoriatic inflammation [34]. Other downregulated gene transcripts related to pattern recognition in neutrophils include *IFNGR1, LTB4R, TLR1, TLR5, MYD88, NLRP3* and *NLRC4*. The downregulation of these genes may negatively control AMP-mediated neutrophil activation, thus contributing to the resolution of inflammation in GPP patients. In addition to AMP receptors, genes encoding AMPs were also downregulated. These AMPs include LCN2, S100A8, S100A9 and S100A12. Although AMPs are believed largely to be produced by keratinocytes, neutrophil-released AMPs may contribute to the initiation of psoriasis [35]. Collectively, our results suggested that AMP–neutrophil interaction may play a role in the remission of GPP.

Recently, *AP1S3* mutations were found to be associated with pustular psoriasis, and knockdown of AP1S3 resulted in the upregulation of pro-inflammatory cytokines [7, 36]. AP1S3 is involved in protein trafficking in neutrophil activation [23]. In our datasets, *AP1S3* was significantly upregulated in post-treatment patients. Thus, it is tempting to speculate that the expression level of *AP1S3*, aside from its mutation, may also contribute to GPP pathogenesis by modulating the proinflammatory response.

PLK1 is a serine/threonine-protein kinase that triggers the G2/M transition of the cell cycle and performs important functions throughout the M phase [37]. IPA revealed that the "mitotic roles of PLK kinase" pathway was significantly enriched. Surprisingly, nearly all the pivotal players in this pathway, including *PLK1, CDC20, CDC25C, CYCLIN B2* and *MLKP1*, were downregulated in GPP patients upon acitretin treatment, suggesting a cell cycle-repressing effect of the drug. Although acitretin has been reported to have an anti-proliferative effect on hyper-proliferative tissues, such as psoriasis plaques [38], the mechanism of acitretin action in GPP remains largely elusive. In support of our observation, Liang [14] et al. reported that cell cycle checkpoint genes were significantly overexpressed in patients with GPP. In concert with its anti-proliferative effect on keratinocytes, acitretin may act to tune the cell cycle in the peripheral blood cells and contribute to quenching psoriatic inflammation.

Multiple cytokine signaling pathways involved in the pathogenesis of psoriasis, including IL-1, IL-6, IL-17A and interferon signaling, were enriched in the current analysis. These results are in agreement with a previous study of transcriptome profiles in pustular psoriatic lesions [14], suggesting that PBMCs and local skin cells may share similar patterns of immune dysregulation. IL-36 signaling is considered to be one of the pathological driving forces in GPP, and missense mutations in the IL-36 receptor antagonist were found to be the genetic cause of the

disease in some patients [5]. Of note, in the current study, 3 out of 5 patients carry the c.115 + 6 T > C mutation in the *IL36RN* gene. More recently, a microarray analysis performed in psoriatic lesions from GPP patients suggested that the IL-1/IL-36 inflammatory axis appears to be central to the pathogenesis of GPP [13]. However, we did not detect changes in the transcripts of IL-36 cytokines in GPP patients under drug treatment. This discordance can be explained by the possibly distinct expression dynamics of IL-36 between blood and skin cells, or a lack of statistical power due to low sample numbers.

Upstream Regulator Analysis helps to identify critical nodes in a complex signaling network and provide potential drug targets. By this analysis, we identified multiple upstream regulators for a top-ranked network, including IL6, IL1B, IFNG, CSF2, IL21, IL17A, IFNA2, OSM and TNF, among others. TNF is known to play a central role in the inflammatory cytokine cascade, and TNF blockade in patients by biologics, such as infliximab, have shown success in GPP treatment [1]. Furthermore, IL17A is considered to be a druggable target for GPP, as evidenced by the effectiveness of IL17A blockade therapies [1]. Recently, inhibition of IL17A by secukinumab has been reported effective for a pediatric GPP patient with Deficiency of Interleukin-36-Receptor Antagonist (DITRA), implying a possible link between *IL36RN* mutation and Th17 differentiation in DITRA patients [39]. Moreover, we found that OSM, a cytokine secreted by skin-infiltrating T lymphocytes, was an upstream regulator of the network. OSM is a potent keratinocyte activator similar to TNF-α, IL-1, IL-17 and IL-22 [40]. Recently, OSM has been considered to be a drug target for multiple inflammatory diseases, such as colitis [41] and rheumatoid arthritis [42]. Based on the Upstream Regulator Analysis, we speculate that targeting the OSM pathway may have a beneficial effect on GPP.

Overall, our study provided a comprehensive gene expression profiling and molecular interaction network for GPP. GPP is likely to be genetically and physiopathologically heterogeneous among different patients. Thus, it would be beneficial to adopt specific immunointerventions for different cases. Combining the molecular profiling of a large cohort of clinical samples with in-depth bioinformatics analysis will provide further insights into strategies for GPP management and the development of tailored therapies.

Conclusions

GPP is a fatal, multisystemic inflammatory disease. Our longitude analysis provided the first comprehensive study of transcriptome dynamics in the peripheral circulation of GPP patients and showed that the alleviation of GPP primarily involves the downregulation of leukocyte activity, particularly neutrophils. Moreover, the regulatory network constructed in the current research also provide a set of molecules with therapeutic relevance. Our study illustrates how RNA-seq-based transcriptomics can shed light on mechanism of disease and drug effects at the molecular level.

Additional files

Additional file 1: Table S1. Primers used in RTqPCR validation.

Additional file 2: Table S2. The top 50 upregulated and downregulated DEGs in the T1 versus T0 dataset.

Additional file 3: Table S3. The top 50 upregulated and downregulated DEGs in the T2 versus T0 dataset.

Additional file 4: Figure S1. Functional enrichment and annotation for DEGs in the "leukocyte activation involved in immune response" category. Enrichment of the top 20 clusters at T1 (panel A) and T2 (panel B) was performed using Metascape analysis. -log(FDR) values were calculated based on the accumulative hypergeometric distribution.

Additional file 5: Figure S2. Protein-protein interaction (PPI) enrichment analysis for DEGs in the "leukocyte activation involved in immune response" category. PPI analysis for the DEGs was first carried out using the BioGrid database. The Molecular Complex Detection (MCODE) algorithm was then employed to identify densely connected network components. Based on these two analyses, a PPI network was generated for DEGs at T1 (panel A) and T2 (panel B). Pathway and process enrichment analysis was applied to each MCODE component. The three (panel A) or four (panel B) best-scoring terms (by *p*-value) were retained as the functional description of the corresponding components.

Additional file 6: Table S4. List of DEGs enriched in canonical pathways by IPA analysis.

Additional file 7: Figure S3. Gene expression heatmaps for signaling pathways inhibited at both T1 and T2. Heatmaps of expression ratios and z-scores for the "TREM1 Signaling" (panel A), "Role of Pattern Recognition Receptors in Recognition of Bacteria and Viruses" (panel B) and "Interferon Signaling" (panel C) pathways are shown. The z-scores were calculated using the IPA z-score algorithm and predicted direction of change for the function.

Additional file 8: Figure S4. The expression ratios of innate immunity and adaptive immunity genes. Ratios were calculated with IPA My List Analysis and are presented as a bar chart.

Additional file 9: Figure S5. Gene expression heatmaps for DEGs enriched in cell cycle regulation and cytokine signaling pathways. Heatmaps of expression ratios and z-scores for the "Mitotic Roles of Polo-like Kinase" (panel A), "Cyclins and the Cell Cycle Regulation" (panel B) and "Role of IL-17A in Psoriasis" (panel C) pathways. The z-scores were calculated using the IPA z-score algorithm and predicted direction of change for the function.

Abbreviations

AMP: Antimicrobial peptide; CORUM: Comprehensive Resource of Mammalian Protein Complexes; Ct: Threshold cycle; DEG: Differentially expressed gene; FDR: False discovery rate; GO: Gene ontology; GPP: Generalized pustular psoriasis; IPA: Ingenuity Pathway Analysis; KEGG: Kyoto Encyclopedia of Genes and Genomes; MCODE: Molecular Complex Detection; PBMC: Peripheral blood mononuclear cell; PCA: Principal component analysis; qPCR: Quantitative polymerase chain reaction; RNA-seq: RNA sequencing; RT-qPCR: Reverse transcription–quantitative polymerase chain reaction

Acknowledgements

We thank Nicholas Rufaut, PhD, from Liwen Bianji, Edanz Editing China (www.liwenbianji.cn/ac) for editing the English text of a draft of this manuscript. We thank Dr. Zhuo Zhou for critically reading the manuscript and making valuable suggestions.

Funding

This work was supported by the Medical and Health Science and Technology Innovation Project of the Chinese Academy of Medical Sciences (2017-12 M-3-020) and The National Natural Science Foundation of China (81773331).

Authors' contributions

LW and HJ conceived the study. HJ supervised the study. LW, XY, CW and TZ collected and prepared the blood samples. TZ, WW and XZ performed RNA extraction and qPCR analyses. LW and XY performed RNA-seq data analysis. LW, CW, TZ, WW and XZ designed and performed the bioinformatic analysis. LW and HJ drafted the manuscript. XY, CW and HJ revised the draft and made contributions to the final manuscript. All authors read and approved the final manuscript.

Competing interests

The authors declare that they have no competing interests.

References

1. Naik HB, Cowen EW. Autoinflammatory pustular neutrophilic diseases. Dermatol Clin. 2013;31(3):405–25.
2. Zachariae H, Overgaard Petersen H, Kissmeyer Nielsen F, Lamm L. HL-A antigens in pustular psoriasis. Dermatologica. 1977;154(2):73–7.
3. Ozawa A, Miyahara M, Sugai J, Iizuka M, Kawakubo Y, Matsuo I, Ohkido M, Naruse T, Ando H, Inoko H, et al. HLA class I and II alleles and susceptibility to generalized pustular psoriasis: significant associations with HLA-Cw1 and HLA-DQB1*0303. J Dermatol. 1998;25(9):573–81.
4. Bissonnette R, Suarez-Farinas M, Li X, Bonifacio KM, Brodmerkel C, Fuentes-Duculan J, Krueger JG. Based on molecular profiling of gene expression, palmoplantar Pustulosis and palmoplantar pustular psoriasis are highly related diseases that appear to be distinct from psoriasis vulgaris. PLoS One. 2016;11(5)
5. Towne JE, Sims JE. IL-36 in psoriasis. Curr Opin Pharmacol. 2012;12(4):486–90.
6. Marrakchi S, Guigue P, Renshaw BR, Puel A, Pei XY, Fraitag S, Zribi J, Bal E, Cluzeau C, Chrabieh M, et al. Interleukin-36-receptor antagonist deficiency and generalized pustular psoriasis. N Engl J Med. 2011;365(7):620–8.
7. Setta-Kaffetzi N, Simpson MA, Navarini AA, Patel VM, Lu HC, Allen MH, Duckworth M, Bachelez H, Burden AD, Choon SE, et al. AP1S3 mutations are associated with pustular psoriasis and impaired toll-like receptor 3 trafficking. Am J Hum Genet. 2014;94(5):790–7.
8. Berki DM, Liu L, Choon SE, David Burden A, Griffiths CEM, Navarini AA, Tan ES, Irvine AD, Ranki A, Ogo T, et al. Activating CARD14 mutations are associated with generalized pustular psoriasis but rarely account for familial recurrence in psoriasis vulgaris. J Invest Dermatol. 2015;135(12):2964–70.
9. Mossner R, Wilsmann-Theis D, Oji V, Gkogkolou P, Lohr S, Schulz P, Korber A, Christoph-Prinz J, Renner R, Schakel K, et al. The genetic basis for most patients with pustular skin disease remains elusive. Br J Dermatol. 2017;178(3):740–8.
10. Robinson A, Van Voorhees AS, Hsu S, Korman NJ, Lebwohl MG, Bebo BF Jr, Kalb RE. Treatment of pustular psoriasis: from the medical Board of the National Psoriasis Foundation. J Am Acad Dermatol. 2012;67(2):279–88.
11. Pang ML, Murase JE, Koo J. An updated review of acitretin–a systemic retinoid for the treatment of psoriasis. Expert Opin Drug Metab Toxicol. 2008;4(7):953–64.
12. Ozawa A, Ohkido M, Haruki Y, Kobayashi H, Ohkawara A, Ohno Y, Inaba Y, Ogawa H. Treatments of generalized pustular psoriasis: a multicenter study in Japan. J Dermatol. 1999;26(3):141–9.
13. Johnston A, Xing X, Wolterink L, Barnes DH, Yin Z, Reingold L, Kahlenberg JM, Harms PW, Gudjonsson JE. IL-1 and IL-36 are dominant cytokines in generalized pustular psoriasis. J Allergy Clin Immunol. 2017;140(1):109–20.
14. Liang Y, Xing X, Beamer MA, Swindell WR, Sarkar MK, Roberts LW, Voorhees JJ, Kahlenberg JM, Harms PW, Johnston A, et al. Six-transmembrane epithelial antigens of the prostate comprise a novel inflammatory nexus in patients with pustular skin disorders. J Allergy Clin Immunol. 2017;139(4):1217–27.
15. Umezawa Y, Ozawa A, Kawasima T, Shimizu H, Terui T, Tagami H, Ikeda S, Ogawa H, Kawada A, Tezuka T, et al. Therapeutic guidelines for the treatment of generalized pustular psoriasis (GPP) based on a proposed classification of disease severity. Arch Dermatol Res. 2003;295(Suppl 1):S43–54.

16. Zhu T, Jin H, Shu D, Li F, Wu C. Association of IL36RN mutations with clinical features, therapeutic response to acitretin, and frequency of recurrence in patients with generalized pustular psoriasis. Eur J Dermatol. 2018;28(2):217–24.

17. Patel RK, Jain M. NGS QC toolkit: a toolkit for quality control of next generation sequencing data. PLoS One. 2012;7(2):e30619.

18. Trapnell C, Roberts A, Goff L, Pertea G, Kim D, Kelley DR, Pimentel H, Salzberg SL, Rinn JL, Pachter L. Differential gene and transcript expression analysis of RNA-seq experiments with TopHat and cufflinks. Nat Protoc. 2012;7(3):562–78.

19. Ritchie ME, Phipson B, Wu D, Hu Y, Law CW, Shi W, Smyth GK. Limma powers differential expression analyses for RNA-sequencing and microarray studies. Nucleic Acids Res. 2015;43(7):e47.

20. Metsalu T, Vilo J. ClustVis: a web tool for visualizing clustering of multivariate data using principal component analysis and heatmap. Nucleic Acids Res. 2015;43(W1):W566–70.

21. Ikeda S, Takahashi H, Suga Y, Eto H, Etoh T, Okuma K, Takahashi K, Kanbara T, Seishima M, Morita A, et al. Therapeutic depletion of myeloid lineage leukocytes in patients with generalized pustular psoriasis indicates a major role for neutrophils in the immunopathogenesis of psoriasis. J Am Acad Dermatol. 2013;68(4):609–17.

22. Tripathi S, Pohl MO, Zhou Y, Rodriguez-Frandsen A, Wang G, Stein DA, Moulton HM, DeJesus P, Che J, Mulder LC, et al. Meta- and orthogonal integration of influenza "OMICs" data defines a role for UBR4 in virus budding. Cell Host Microbe. 2015;18(6):723–35.

23. Naranbhai V, Fairfax BP, Makino S, Humburg P, Wong D, Ng E, Hill AV, Knight JC. Genomic modulators of gene expression in human neutrophils. Nat Commun. 2015;6:7545.

24. Sharif O, Knapp S. From expression to signaling: roles of TREM-1 and TREM-2 in innate immunity and bacterial infection. Immunobiology. 2008;213(9–10):701–13.

25. Kameyama T, Takaoka A. Characterization of innate immune signalings stimulated by ligands for pattern recognition receptors. Methods in molecular biology (Clifton, NJ). 2014;1142:19–32.

26. Baliwag J, Barnes DH, Johnston A. Cytokines in psoriasis. Cytokine. 2015;73(2):342–50.

27. Carmona-Rivera C, Kaplan MJ. Low-density granulocytes: a distinct class of neutrophils in systemic autoimmunity. Semin Immunopathol. 2013;35(4):455–63.

28. Bennett L, Palucka AK, Arce E, Cantrell V, Borvak J, Bancherau J, Pascual V. Interferon and granulopoiesis signatures in systemic lupus erythematosus blood. J Exp Med. 2003;197(6):711–23.

29. Villanueva E, Yalavarthi S, Berthier CC, Hodgin JB, Khandpur R, Lin AM, Rubin CJ, Zhao W, Olsen SH, Klinker M, et al. Netting neutrophils induce endothelial damage, infiltrate tissues, and expose immunostimulatory molecules in systemic lupus erythematosus. J Immunol. 2011;187(1):538–52.

30. Lin AM, Rubin CJ, Khandpur R, Wang JY, Riblett M, Yalavarthi S, Villanueva EC, Shah P, Kaplan MJ, Bruce AT. Mast cells and neutrophils release IL-17 through extracellular trap formation in psoriasis. J Immunol. 2011;187(1):490–500.

31. Taylor PR, Roy S, Jr LS, sun Y, Howell SJ, cobb BA, li X, Pearlman E. Autocrine IL-17A–IL-17RC neutrophil activation in fungal infections is regulated by IL-6, IL-23, RORγt and Dectin-2. Nat Immunol. 2014;15(2):143–51.

32. Reich K, Papp KA, Matheson RT, Tu JH, Bissonnette R, Bourcier M, Gratton D, Kunynetz RA, Poulin Y, Rosoph LA, et al. Evidence that a neutrophil-keratinocyte crosstalk is an early target of IL-17A inhibition in psoriasis. Exp Dermatol. 2015;24(7):529–35.

33. Chen K, Bao Z, Gong W, Tang P, Yoshimura T, Wang JM. Regulation of inflammation by members of the formyl-peptide receptor family. J Autoimmun. 2017;85:64–77.

34. Elssner A, Duncan M, Gavrilin M, Wewers MD. A novel P2X7 receptor activator, the human cathelicidin-derived peptide LL37, induces IL-1 beta processing and release. J Immunol. 2004;172(8):4987–94.

35. Zenz R, Eferl R, Kenner L, Florin L, Hummerich L, Mehic D, Scheuch H, Angel P, Tschachler E, Wagner EF. Psoriasis-like skin disease and arthritis caused by inducible epidermal deletion of Jun proteins. Nature. 2005;437(7057):369–75.

36. Mahil SK, Twelves S, Farkas K, Setta-Kaffetzi N, Burden AD, Gach JE, Irvine AD, Kepiro L, Mockenhaupt M, Oon HH, et al. AP1S3 mutations cause skin autoinflammation by disrupting keratinocyte autophagy and up-regulating IL-36 production. J Invest Dermatol. 2016;136(11):2251–9.

37. Otto T, Sicinski P. Cell cycle proteins as promising targets in cancer therapy. Nat Rev Cancer. 2017;17(2):93–115.

38. Sarkar R, Chugh S, Garg VK. Acitretin in dermatology. Indian J Dermatol Venereol Leprol. 2013;79(6):759–71.

39. Cordoro KM, Ucmak D, Hitraya-Low M, Rosenblum MD, Liao W. Response to interleukin (IL)-17 inhibition in an adolescent with severe manifestations of IL-36 receptor antagonist deficiency (DITRA). JAMA dermatology. 2017;153(1):106–8.

40. Boniface K, Diveu C, Morel F, Pedretti N, Froger J, Ravon E, Garcia M, Venereau E, Preisser L, Guignouard E, et al. Oncostatin M secreted by skin infiltrating T lymphocytes is a potent keratinocyte activator involved in skin inflammation. J Immunol. 2007;178(7):4615–22.

41. West NR, Hegazy AN, Owens BMJ, Bullers SJ, Linggi B, Buonocore S, Coccia M, Gortz D, This S, Stockenhuber K, et al. Oncostatin M drives intestinal inflammation and predicts response to tumor necrosis factor-neutralizing therapy in patients with inflammatory bowel disease. Nat Med. 2017;23(5):579–89.

42. Su CM, Chiang YC, Huang CY, Hsu CJ, Fong YC, Tang CH. Osteopontin promotes Oncostatin M production in human osteoblasts: implication of rheumatoid arthritis therapy. J Immunol. 2015;195(7):3355–64.

43. Moll JM, Wright V. Psoriatic arthritis. Semin Arthritis Rheum. 1973;3(1):55–78.

7

Strategies to minimize false positives and interpret novel microdeletions based on maternal copy-number variants in 87,000 noninvasive prenatal screens

Kristjan Eerik Kaseniit[†], Gregory J Hogan[†], Kevin M D'Auria, Carrie Haverty and Dale Muzzey[*]◉

Abstract

Background: Noninvasive prenatal screening (NIPS) of common aneuploidies using cell-free DNA from maternal plasma is part of routine prenatal care and is widely used in both high-risk and low-risk patient populations. High specificity is needed for clinically acceptable positive predictive values. Maternal copy-number variants (mCNVs) have been reported as a source of false-positive aneuploidy results that compromises specificity.

Methods: We surveyed the mCNV landscape in 87,255 patients undergoing NIPS. We evaluated both previously reported and novel algorithmic strategies for mitigating the effects of mCNVs on the screen's specificity. Further, we analyzed the frequency, length, and positional distribution of CNVs in our large dataset to investigate the curation of novel fetal microdeletions, which can be identified by NIPS but are challenging to interpret clinically.

Results: mCNVs are common, with 65% of expecting mothers harboring an autosomal CNV spanning more than 200 kb, underscoring the need for robust NIPS analysis strategies. By analyzing empirical and simulated data, we found that general, outlier-robust strategies reduce the rate of mCNV-caused false positives but not as appreciably as algorithms specifically designed to account for mCNVs. We demonstrate that large-scale tabulation of CNVs identified via routine NIPS could be clinically useful: together with the gene density of a putative microdeletion region, we show that the region's relative tolerance to duplications versus deletions may aid the interpretation of microdeletion pathogenicity.

Conclusions: Our study thoroughly investigates a common source of NIPS false positives and demonstrates how to bypass its corrupting effects. Our findings offer insight into the interpretation of NIPS results and inform the design of NIPS algorithms suitable for use in screening in the general obstetric population.

Keywords: Noninvasive prenatal screening, Copy-number variant, Microdeletion, Variant interpretation

Background

Noninvasive prenatal screening (NIPS) aims to detect fetal chromosomal abnormalities early in pregnancy by quantifying cell-free DNA (cfDNA) in maternal plasma [1]. Due to its high sensitivity and specificity, clinical ease, low cost, and minimal risk of complications, NIPS has been widely adopted for the general obstetric population, including high- and average-risk pregnancies [2].

High specificity is critical in fetal aneuploidy screening, because professional guidelines recommend that all patients with positive aneuploidy results be offered follow-up invasive testing [2, 3], a procedure associated with an increased risk of pregnancy loss [4].

When performing NIPS by whole genome sequencing (WGS) of cfDNA, a sample is considered aneuploid for a given region if it has a statistically significant deviation in the number of sequenced fragments ("depth") relative to the average depth of disomic background samples and/or regions. Because most cfDNA originates from the mother, copy-number variants in the maternal genome (mCNVs)

* Correspondence: research@counsyl.com
[†]Kristjan Eerik Kaseniit and Gregory J Hogan contributed equally to this work.
Myriad Women's Health (previously Counsyl), 180 Kimball Way, South San Francisco, CA 94080, USA

can cause sufficiently large depth deviations to yield false positives, thereby reducing the specificity of NIPS. Indeed, the depth deviation of an mCNV relative to a fetal anomaly is so strong that even small mCNVs can have a large impact on specificity; mCNVs spanning ≥250 kb were predicted to increase the false-positive rate by 40- to 1000-fold or more [5]. Further, two recent studies of trisomies 13, 18, and 21 attributed one-third to one-half of NIPS false positives to maternal duplications [6, 7]. A 22-study meta-analysis of NIPS discordances found that 48% of false positives with an identified cause were due to mCNVs [8]. These findings underscore the need for NIPS bioinformatics pipelines to be robust to these confounding variants.

A z-score is a common statistic used in WGS-based NIPS to describe the deviation of observed from expected depth values, with a higher z-score indicating a gain in DNA suggestive of a fetal trisomy (Fig. 1a, b). The depth of a region of interest (e.g., chromosome or microdeletion) is typically measured by first subdividing the region into non-overlapping bins of equal size (e.g., 20 kb) and then calculating the average depth per bin [9]. As opposed to simply calculating a region's average depth by dividing the total mapped sequenced fragments ("reads") by its length, an average across bins provides a straightforward way to detect and omit localized anomalies such as mCNVs and alignment artifacts. If not appropriately mitigated, mCNVs cause false aneuploid calls (Fig. 1c) because they strongly deflect the depth in their encompassing bins, and this deviation affects the average bin depth and resulting z-score in a region of interest.

In addition to enhancing the search for mCNVs, partitioning reads into bins also facilitates the identification of subchromosomal fetal CNVs like microdeletions. The aneuploidy-detection algorithm can enumerate each sufficiently lengthy set of contiguous bins as a possible microdeletion, evaluate an average, compute a z-score, and yield an assertion of fetal copy number. Recent studies have shown that WGS-based NIPS data reveal novel fetal CNVs at a resolution of 7 Mb [10]; however, the clinical interpretation of such variants is not straightforward, and the utility of reporting them to patients is unestablished.

We sought to explore the impact of mCNVs on the identification and interpretation of fetal chromosomal abnormalities. Our first step was to develop an mCNV-finding algorithm to measure the frequency of mCNVs and identify patterns in their genomic locations. Next, we evaluated the impact of mCNVs on NIPS specificity, highlighting the virtues and drawbacks of different algorithmic strategies, including both adapted and novel approaches. Finally, we used the observed frequency, length, and positional distribution of mCNVs—coupled with the assumption that most mCNVs are benign—to shed light on the clinical interpretation of novel fetal microdeletions.

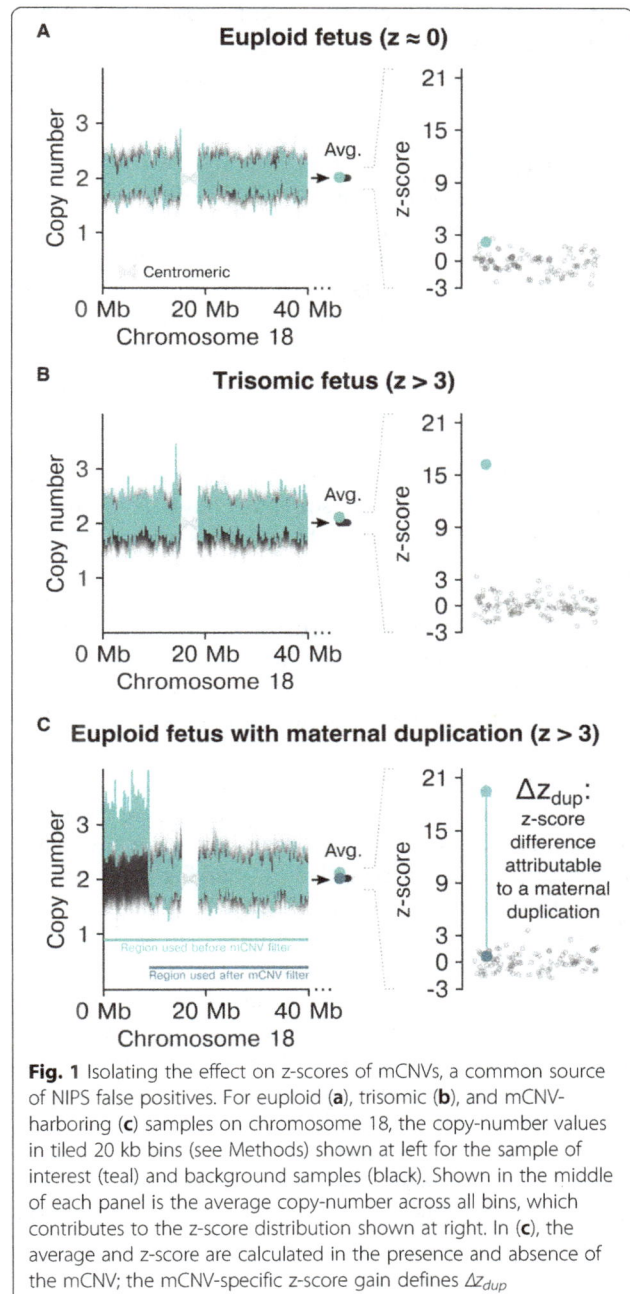

Fig. 1 Isolating the effect on z-scores of mCNVs, a common source of NIPS false positives. For euploid (**a**), trisomic (**b**), and mCNV-harboring (**c**) samples on chromosome 18, the copy-number values in tiled 20 kb bins (see Methods) shown at left for the sample of interest (teal) and background samples (black). Shown in the middle of each panel is the average copy-number across all bins, which contributes to the z-score distribution shown at right. In (**c**), the average and z-score are calculated in the presence and absence of the mCNV; the mCNV-specific z-score gain defines Δz_{dup}

Methods

Analysis of NIPS samples

The protocol for this study was reviewed and designated as exempt by Western Institutional Review Board and complied with the Health Insurance Portability and Accountability Act (HIPAA). The information associated with patient samples was de-identified in accordance with the HIPAA Privacy Rule. A waiver of informed consent was requested and approved by the IRB. A total of 87,255 de-identified samples meeting internal quality control criteria were retrospectively analyzed for the presence of mCNVs across all chromosomes. Samples without mCNVs and fetal aneuploidies comprised a subset later employed for mCNV simulations (described below).

mCNV detection

mCNVs were detected using a moving-window approach that considered copy-number values in 20 kb bins tiling each chromosome. A bin's copy-number value is a fractional number (e.g., 1.997) that reflects the bin's read depth and results from multiple normalization steps described below in the section about mCNV handling. The presence or absence of an mCNV was assessed at each bin i. First, the median copy-number value across the 10 bins i through $i + 9$ was calculated in both the sample of interest and in background samples. A z-score was computed for each sample's observed median copy-number value relative to the background average. Bins i through $i + 9$ were classified as part of an mCNV if (1) the absolute median copy-number value was <1.5 or >2.5, and (2) the absolute z-score was determined to be significant. As some genomic bins are filtered out elsewhere in the analysis pipeline (e.g., for spuriously high read depth or for "unmappable" regions with redundant sequences that complicate unique mapping of reads), gaps of up to five genomic bins within mCNVs were allowed. Consecutive mCNV calls of the same type were merged if the resulting call had a significant z-score. For example a 12-bin mCNV would be called by merging three mCNV calls starting at bins i, $i + 1$ and $i + 2$, or a 25-bin call could be made by merging calls starting at bins i and $i + 15$ (if bins $i + 10$ through $i + 14$ were a gap). The edges of merged calls were trimmed by up to 10 bins on either side, with the final mCNV boundaries determined by the pair of edges that maximized the absolute z-score of the call. Due to the trimming, calls smaller than 200 kb were possible if the trimmed set of bins yielded a large enough absolute z-score. Aside from this section, z-score refers to the aneuploidy z-score, not the z-score of the mCNV. Additional file 1: Figures S1 and S2 illustrate the efficacy of this mCNV-detection algorithm on simulated samples, which are themselves described further below.

Strategies for mCNV handling

For six NIPS bioinformatic analysis pipelines, we evaluated the specificity of whole-chromosome aneuploidies as a function of the presence of mCNVs. Each pipeline differed in key ways as described below but shared a common general analysis foundation: mapping short NGS reads from WGS of cfDNA to a reference genome, counting the number of reads per genomic bin (20 kb), applying GC-content corrections at the read level [11] and mappability corrections at the bin level [12], normalizing these reads-per-bin values at the sample and bin level, calculating

an average of these values per chromosome, and comparing the sample-specific averages of the chromosome to the averages of background samples using a z-score. The z-score is calculated based on measures of central tendency (e.g., mean or median) and dispersion (e.g., standard deviation). Each approach below differs in how these measures are calculated. The left panels of Fig. 4 illustrate the mechanics of each strategy.

The first pipeline, "Simple," is based on the initially published algorithms for NIPS [13] and does not feature any mCNV-specific nor generally robust features. The method calculates z-scores using the mean and standard deviation of the bin copy-number values without any outlier filtering.

The second pipeline, "Robust," builds on the "Simple" method, uses the median in place of the mean, and estimates the standard deviation by (1) calculating the interquartile range (IQR) of bin copy-number values, and (2) converting the IQR to an estimate of standard deviation based on the assumption that the data are normally distributed [14]. Algorithms that use robust statistical measures in some but not all steps of the z-score calculation have been previously reported [15].

The third pipeline, "Robust+Gaussian," refines the central tendency and dispersion estimations by (1) discarding the top and bottom fifth percentiles of the region's copy-number values, (2) fitting a Gaussian function to the copy-number values of a region, and (3) discarding any values more than four standard deviations away from the estimated mean. Similar methods of discarding outlying bins—without explicit mCNV detection—have been reported previously [7].

The fourth pipeline, "Z-correction," is inspired by a previously proposed compensation approach [16]. The approach assumes that mCNVs have a consistent, size-specific effect on aneuploidy z-scores and corrects for this. Our implementation uses results from the "Robust" pipeline but subtracts a z-score offset for chromosomes harboring an mCNV that is itself a function of the mCNV size. The mapping of mCNV size to z-score offset was determined via simulations (described below).

The fifth pipeline, "Value filtering," builds upon the "Robust" pipeline by filtering out any bins with copy-number value less than $c_{low} = 1.5$ or more than $c_{high} = 2.5$. The cutoff pair $c_{low} = 1.61$ and $c_{high} = 2.35$ based on the empirical bin copy-number value distribution values within and outside of mCNVs (Additional file 1: Figure S3 and S4) was also analyzed.

The sixth pipeline, "mCNV filtering," builds upon the "Robust" pipeline by identifying mCNVs and ignoring their constituent genomic bins on an individualized, per-sample basis when calculating the central tendency and dispersion.

Additional file 1: Table S1 summarizes the various algorithm strategies considered.

mCNV simulations

To supplement the mCNVs observed in our patient cohort and characterize algorithm performance for arbitrary mCNV sizes, we simulated mCNVs by scaling the bin-level copy-number values obtained from patient samples. We focused our analysis on maternal duplications as they can lead to false positives in the analysis of trisomies. For the region in which we wanted to simulate a CNV, the copy-number values were multiplied by a factor that mimics the gain observed in empirical maternal duplications; the expected ratio of bin copy numbers in maternal duplications vs. non-mCNV regions is 3/2 = 1.50, but we observed this factor to be slightly lower at 2.88/2 = 1.44 (Additional file 1: Figure S3). This approach further assumes that simulated mCNVs were inherited by the fetus. mCNVs not inherited by the fetus would have marginally decreased signal in proportion to the fetal fraction, and this would reduce their potentially compromising effect on specificity but also make them slightly more difficult to detect.

For each of the chromosomes 13, 18, and 21, at least 10,000 mCNV-harboring samples were simulated, each using as a baseline a randomly chosen sample shown to be both euploid (via the "mCNV filtering" pipeline) and void of mCNVs. Most samples (83%) were chosen for exactly one round of simulation, with the rest used in several rounds of simulations (15% in two and 2% in 3 or more simulations). The sizes of the mCNVs were selected to span a logarithmic range, and the position of each mCNV was randomly chosen. The mCNV size values used in downstream analyses were based on the simulated boundaries rather than the algorithm-detected boundaries (e.g., a 3 Mb simulated duplication identified as being 2.8 Mb by the mCNV-finding algorithm is represented in the plots and associated analyses herein based on the 3 Mb size; Additional file 1: Figure S1).

Maternal duplication impact analysis

The impact of maternal duplications on aneuploidy z-scores was evaluated in both empirical and simulated samples.

The empirical approach included only those samples observed to have an mCNV, and it estimated the median aneuploidy z-score as a function of the duplication size. If a chromosome contained multiple mCNVs, the duplication size was the sum of the observed mCNV lengths. The aneuploidy z-score has an expectation of 0 for euploid samples, and the median is not expected to deviate appreciably from 0 even if some trisomic samples are present due to their relative rarity. Hence, a systematic positive shift of the median z-score as a function of

maternal duplication size is consistent with mCNVs underlying some NIPS false positives.

The simulation-based approach directly estimated the effect of maternal duplications on z-scores and, subsequently, on specificity. We defined $\Delta z_{dup} = z_{mCNV+} - z_{mCNV-}$ as the z-score difference attributable to a maternal duplication (Fig. 1c), with z_{mCNV+} and z_{mCNV-}, respectively, representing the z-score with and without the simulated mCNV. For a given size of mCNV, positive Δz_{dup} values indicate z-scores are sensitive to the presence of maternal duplications, and no shift (Δz_{dup} of 0) means the bioinformatic analysis pipeline is not biased by mCNVs.

To calculate the specificity of NIPS as a function of mCNV size, we modeled the z-score of a euploid sample harboring an mCNV as a random variable $Z = Z_{mCNV-} + \Delta Z_{dup}$. Z_{mCNV-} represents the z-score of a sample without an mCNV. It follows a standard normal distribution $N(\mu = 0, \sigma = 1)$ and is not a function of mCNV size. By contrast, for an mCNV of size s, ΔZ_{dup} is normally distributed with mean μ_{dup} and standard deviation σ_{dup} calculated from the Δz_{dup} values of the 200 simulated samples whose mCNV sizes were closest to s. Assuming Z_{mCNV-} and ΔZ_{dup} are independent, Z is a normal random variable with mean μ_{dup} and standard deviation $(1 + \sigma_{dup}^2)^{0.5}$. Since the simulations introduced mCNVs into otherwise euploid samples, any modeled positives (i.e., $Z = Z_{mCNV-} + \Delta Z_{dup} > 3$) were false positives. Furthermore, any modeled samples with $z_{mCNV-} > 3$ were considered to be statistical false positives. Hence, the false-positive rate (FPR) attributable to mCNVs was calculated by omitting these statistical false positives:

$$FPR_{mCNV} = P(Z_{mCNV-} + \Delta Z_{dup} > 3) - P(Z_{mCNV-} > 3)$$

Specificity was simply $1 - FPR_{mCNV}$. The specificity as a function of mCNV size was estimated for each chromosome separately using simulated samples with mCNVs introduced on the chromosome of interest.

The estimate of cumulative false positives due to mCNVs per 100,000 was calculated as the weighted sum of the empirical maternal-duplication size-prevalence data (Fig. 2b) multiplied by the size-dependent specificity data from the simulation-based analysis (Fig. 4, right column).

Results

Autosomal mCNVs larger than 200 kb are detected in 65% of patients and cover the majority of the genome

As a first step toward measuring the impact of mCNVs on NIPS performance, we surveyed their frequency, size, and positional bias in 87,255 patient samples. Using a rolling-window z-score algorithm (see Methods), we identified mCNVs ≥200 kb. On average, patients had 1.07 autosomal mCNVs, and 65% of patients had at least one mCNV. There were 37% more deletions than duplications

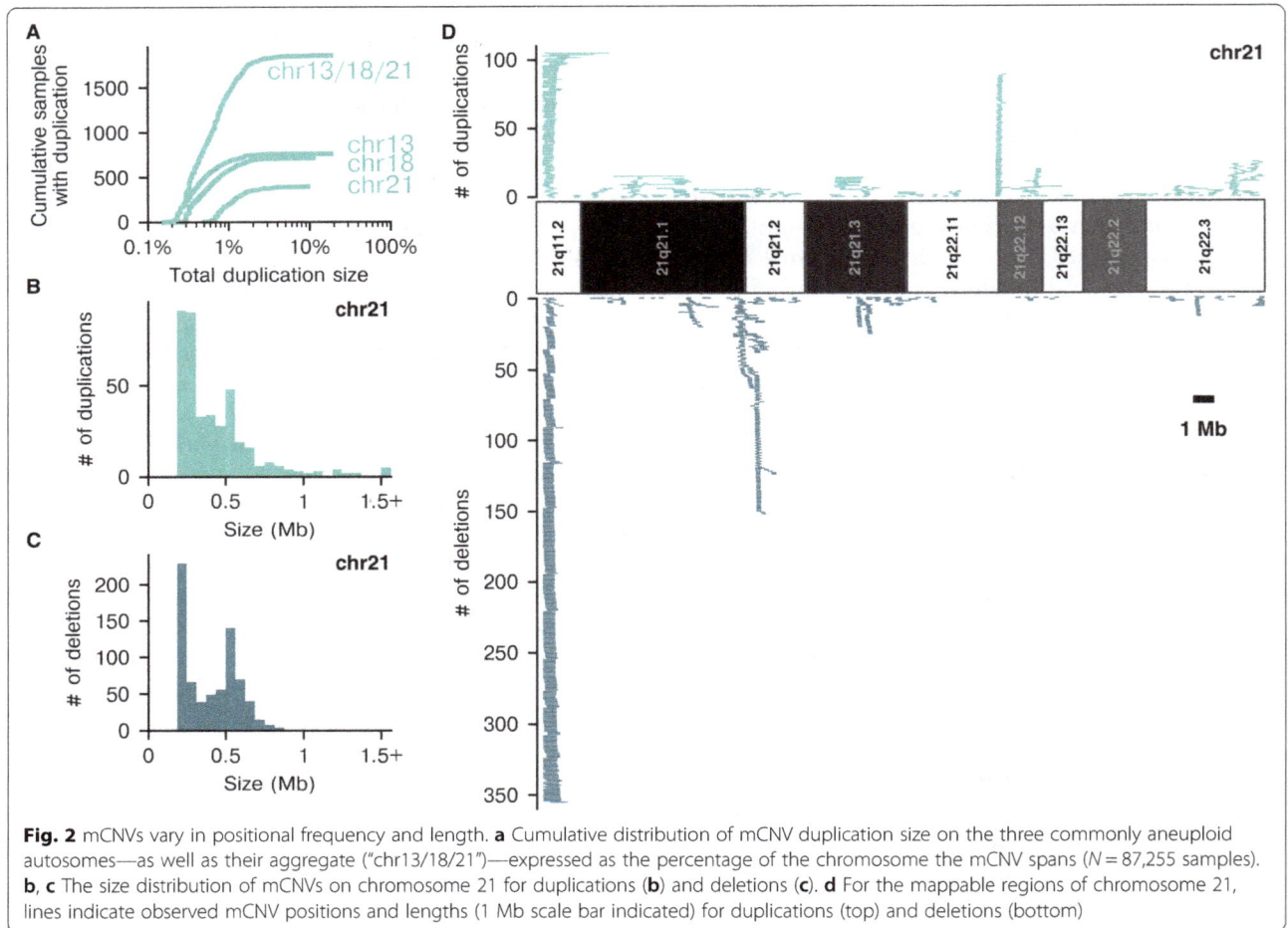

Fig. 2 mCNVs vary in positional frequency and length. **a** Cumulative distribution of mCNV duplication size on the three commonly aneuploid autosomes—as well as their aggregate ("chr13/18/21")—expressed as the percentage of the chromosome the mCNV spans (*N* = 87,255 samples). **b, c** The size distribution of mCNVs on chromosome 21 for duplications (**b**) and deletions (**c**). **d** For the mappable regions of chromosome 21, lines indicate observed mCNV positions and lengths (1 Mb scale bar indicated) for duplications (top) and deletions (bottom)

overall, but duplications were generally larger than deletions (median sizes 360 and 260 kb, respectively; Kruskal-Wallis H-test $p < 0.05$).

Chromosomes 13, 18, and 21 are commonly tested in NIPS, and mCNVs on these chromosomes pose the most direct risk for false positives. On these chromosomes, 2.1% of all patients had at least one duplication and 2.5% had at least one deletion with 4.5% having an mCNV of either type (Fig. 2a). On chromosome 21, deletions and duplications were observed at a similar frequency, yet mCNVs larger than 1 Mb were all duplications (21 duplications and no deletions, Fig. 2b, c). The high frequency of mCNVs on the commonly trisomic chromosomes illustrates why an NIPS strategy that results in no-calls for samples with mCNVs would be clinically inviable, as the rate of no-calls and invasive follow-up procedures would be unacceptably frequent.

We investigated the positional distribution of mCNVs to evaluate the previously published premise [13] that if mCNV positions were highly predictable, an algorithm could achieve robustness simply by masking out (or "blacklisting") such regions. Indeed, we observed that mCNVs were not distributed uniformly (Fig. 2d). Hotspots of mCNVs were common, with some hotspots having an equal number of duplications and deletions, and others having an imbalanced ratio of the two. However, mCNVs were not constrained to hotspot regions, as they were observed across nearly all of the mappable portion of chromosome 21, with only about 14% of the chromosome having no observed mCNVs in our dataset (approximately 7% of chromosome 13 and 9% of chromosome 18 did not have mCNVs; Additional file 1: Figure S5). Though mCNV hotspots suggest that a blacklist approach could partially mitigate the impact of mCNVs, this strategy has drawbacks: either (1) many sites are blacklisted, which would impair sensitivity for aneuploidy detection or (2) few sites are blacklisted, after which many samples would retain mCNVs within the analyzed regions that could lower specificity. This result extends to NIPS assays that apply the blacklist at a biochemical level, e.g., by only targeting certain regions for sequencing [17, 18].

The impact of mCNVs on z-scores observed in empirical data is recapitulated and supplemented with simulations

We next explored the impact of mCNVs on aneuploidy-calling fidelity as a function of mCNV size (Fig. 3). Empirically observed mCNVs rarely spanned ≥1% of a chromosome, which prohibited a statistically powered assessment of the impact of these large mCNVs. To overcome the sparsity of empirical data, we implemented simulations to systematically analyze the effects of maternal duplications on trisomy detection. To create a simulated sample harboring an mCNV of a given size and position, the bin-level copy-number data corresponding to the region of interest was scaled by an empirically derived factor in a euploid and mCNV-free sample (Fig. 3a, b). Simulated samples strongly resembled their observed counterparts, both at the level of bin profile (Fig. 3a) and the distribution of bin copy-number values (Fig. 3b). The bin copy number within simulated mCNVs was very slightly overdispersed compared to the bin copy numbers within detected patient mCNVs (Fig. 3b). The strong overlap between median z-scores for the empirical and simulated samples (Fig. 3c, thick gray and red lines, both for the "Simple" method) suggests that this dilation effect has a negligible impact on our results.

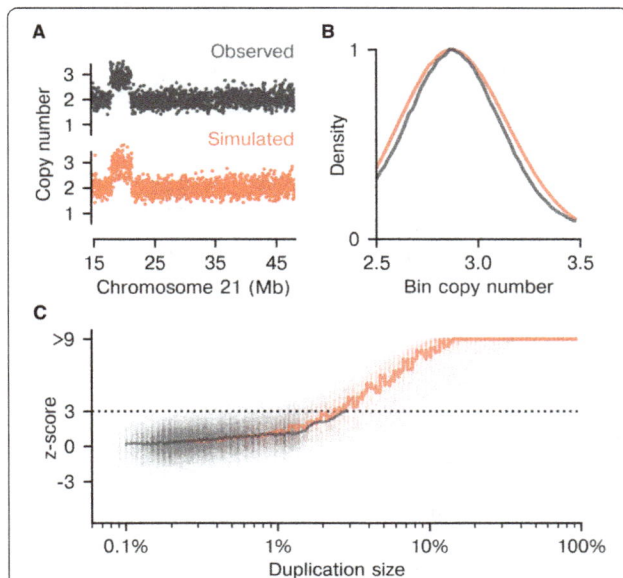

Fig. 3 Simulating mCNVs enables thorough performance analysis. **a** Simulated bin-level copy-number trace for a simulated sample containing an mCNV on chr21 (red) is highly similar to the trace for an observed sample (gray) with a similar maternal variant. **b** The probability distribution of copy-number values for bins within mCNVs is similar for simulated (red) and observed (gray) samples. **c** There is a similar upward trend in z-scores for observed (gray; $N = 38,102$ data points from 87,255 samples) and simulated (red; $N = 30,887$ data points, one per simulation) samples that have a maternal duplication of the indicated size on autosomes ("Simple" method). The solid line is a rolling median of 500 adjacent data points. Z-scores are capped at 9 in the plot only for visualization purposes

Maternal duplications exert an upward pressure on z-scores, and this effect was reproduced in our simulated data on autosomes (Fig. 3c, gray and red traces, respectively). Importantly, with the simulated data the effect was more readily observed, as the full size spectrum of potential mCNVs was modeled. Larger simulated duplications led to increasing positive shifts away from the expected median z-score of 0 for a euploid sample (Fig. 3c, red trace). The threat to the clinical performance of NIPS is that this bias toward higher z-scores contributes to false positives and lowers specificity. Indeed, the simulations suggest that the average sample harboring an mCNV spanning 2.4% or more of a chromosome would be expected to yield a false positive using the "Simple" approach (i.e., the median z-score exceeds 3).

mCNV impact on z-scores can be reduced, but not eliminated, with outlier-robust algorithms

We sought to determine which algorithmic features in an NIPS analysis pipeline minimize the effect of mCNVs on z-scores. Our simulated samples were an ideal data set for this analysis, as the samples have both a "pre-mCNV" z-score (reflecting their original status as both euploid and free of mCNVs; see Methods) and a "post-mCNV" z-score calculated after introducing a modeled maternal duplication. The difference between the post- and pre-mCNV z-scores—which we term Δz_{dup}—is a direct measure of the effect of mCNVs on z-scores. A positive Δz_{dup} means the aneuploidy z-score was increased with the introduction of a simulated mCNV.

Six analysis strategies were tested on simulated samples with maternal duplications on chromosomes 21 (Fig. 4), 13 (Additional file 1: Figure S6), or 18 (Additional file 1: Figure S7). For each test of a strategy and a chromosome, we evaluated at least 10,000 simulated samples. As described in Methods and summarized in Additional file 1: Table S1, the strategies differ both in their approaches for calculating the central tendency (e.g., mean or median) and dispersion of bin copy-number values across a chromosome and in their filtering methods that determine which bins are used in those calculations. For each method, Δz_{dup} was plotted as a function of mCNV size (Fig. 4, middle panels), and these data were sampled to estimate how specificity falls as mCNVs grow (Fig. 4, right panels; see Methods).

The "Simple" approach (Fig. 4a) summarizes the bin copy-number values of a chromosome by the mean and standard deviation, without applying any mCNV-specific or nonspecific filters. As anticipated, this method was the most susceptible to false positives due to mCNVs; at the point where duplication size exceeded 1.3% of chromosome 21 (0.42 Mb, autosomal duplications of this size or greater observed in 13% of patients), the estimated specificity dropped below 95%, and duplications spanning more

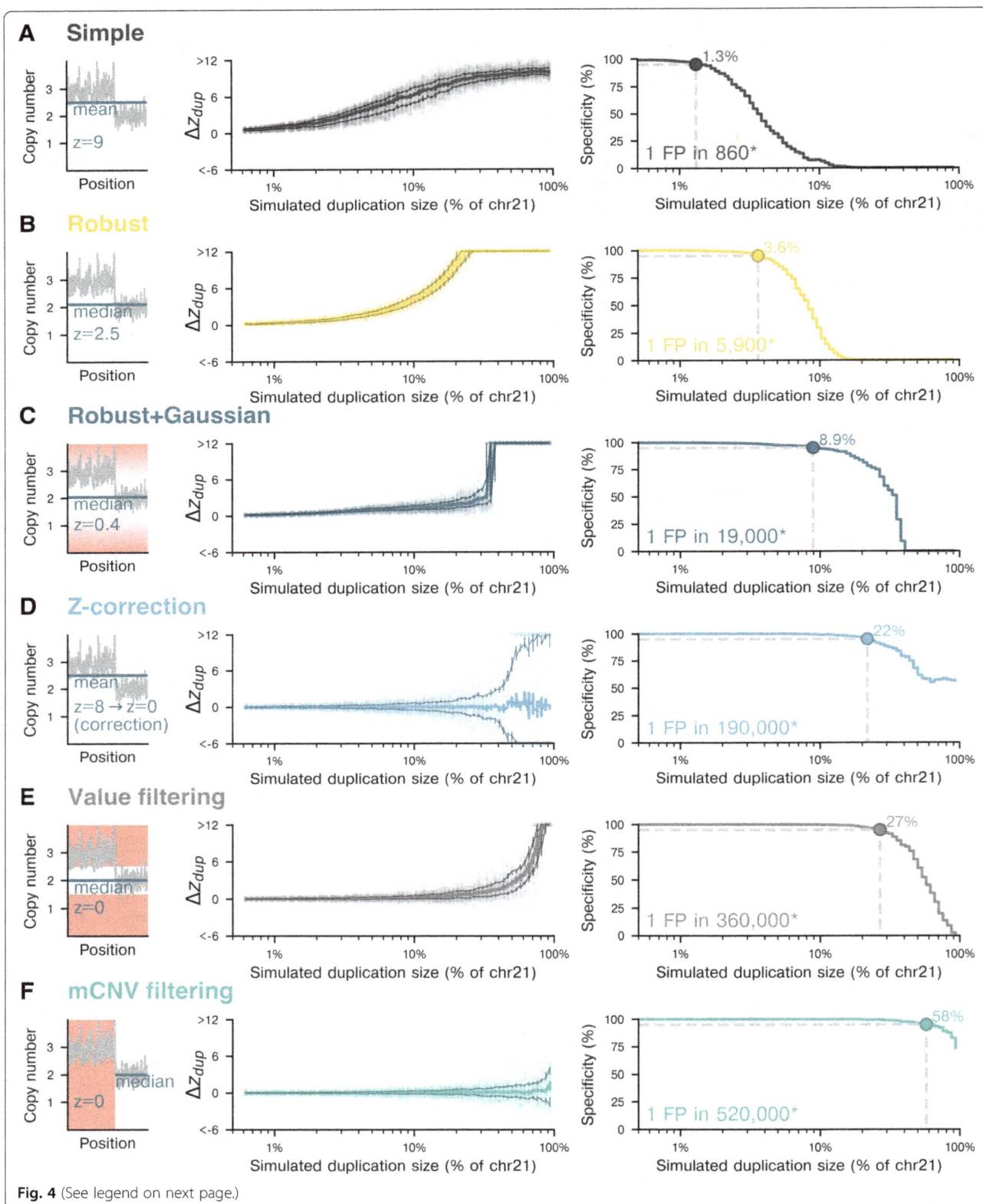

Fig. 4 (See legend on next page.)

than approximately 10% of the chromosome always caused false positive results [3]. Methods using an alternative to the z-score while still using the mean and standard deviation in the analysis—such as employing a t-test [19]—would likely be similarly susceptible to mCNVs.

The "Robust" approach (Fig. 4b) improves upon the "Simple" strategy by replacing the mean with the median and estimating the standard deviation of bin copy-number values from their interquartile range, rather than calculating the standard deviation directly. The median and IQR are less susceptible to outlying bins than the mean and standard deviation; therefore, utilizing these values is expected to increase robustness to mCNVs. Indeed, this approach had smaller z-score deflections than the "Simple" strategy for mCNVs spanning <10% of the chromosome but was still suboptimal; specificity dropped below 95% for mCNVs spanning ≥3.6% (1.2 Mb) of chromosome 21, and our patient cohort contained 1168 samples (1.3%) with duplications in that size range (Fig. 2a).

The "Robust+Gaussian" approach (Fig. 4c) adds another layer of nonspecific outlier removal to the "Robust" approach by rejecting bins that fall far outside of a Gaussian fit to the bin copy-number data. This method performed better than both the "Simple" and "Robust" methods, but was susceptible to mCNVs spanning approximately 8.9% of chromosome 21 (2.9 Mb), at which point specificity dropped below 95%. As a consequence of more stringent filtering, the Robust+Gaussian method discards more bins relative to the previous strategies. This excess bin culling would reduce sensitivity because sensitivity of WGS-based NIPS is an increasing function of the number of bins [20].

Directly accounting for mCNVs boosts specificity
We next considered strategies that specifically address mCNVs, positing that directed approaches would further boost specificity. The "Z-correction" method (Fig. 4d) first calculates a z-score for the chromosome—without removal of mCNV bins—and next subtracts a chromosome- and size-specific z-score offset determined via simulated samples analyzed with the "Robust" approach. In adjusting for mCNVs, this method assumes that the effect of mCNVs on z-score is determined by size and is reproducible across samples. This method performed better in aggregate compared to the previous approaches, as the median of Δz_{dup}

remained near 0 even for large duplications. However, Δz_{dup} values were relatively highly dispersed for simulated duplications around >3% (1 Mb) in size, meaning that an mCNV would still cause large z-score deviations for some samples. The specificity for chromosome 21 dropped below 95% at duplication sizes of approximately 22% (7.0 Mb).

The "Value filtering" approach (Fig. 4e) operates on a simple premise: neutralize mCNVs by purging bins with high (>2.5) or low (<1.5) copy-number values prior to calculating the chromosome-wide average and dispersion. This method was robust to mCNVs that were not extremely large (<95% specificity for mCNVs larger than 27% of chromosome 21, or 8.7 Mb), but showed elevated variability in Δz_{dup} for all mCNV sizes relative to other strategies. The increased noise results from filtering out bins too aggressively, leaving fewer data points—and consequently more noise—for z-score calculation. Duplications are still expected to have some bins with copy-number values less than 2.5 but elevated compared to non-duplicated regions, which is likely why large duplications caused a positive Δz_{dup}. A variant of this method using cutoff values based on empirical bin copy-number values is shown in Additional file 1: Figure S4. This method showed the most variability in the fraction of bins retained after filtering (Additional file 1:Figure S4, right panels) compared to all other methods that were analyzed, suggesting that it could have a nontrivial and variable impact on aneuploidy sensitivity for samples with mCNVs, as sensitivity depends on the number of bins available for z-score calculation [20].

Finally, the "mCNV filtering" approach (Fig. 4f) performs a sample-specific exclusion of bins included in mCNVs. Treating each sample separately, chromosomes are scanned for the presence of mCNVs (see Methods) and then mCNV-spanning bins are excised prior to all downstream calculations. This method was the most robust to mCNVs compared to the others, with specificity dropping below 95% only for maternal duplications larger than 58% of chromosome 21 (18 Mb). Because the "mCNV filtering" method removes only the data that should be removed, it decreases z-score noise, retains high specificity, and has more consistent sensitivity compared to the "Value filtering" approach due to less noise in the number of bins retained (Additional file 1: Figure S4, right panels).

mCNV filtering reduces mCNV-caused false-positive rate to fewer than 1 in 520,000

To evaluate the algorithmic strategies through a more clinically relevant lens, we calculated the expected frequency of false-positive aneuploidy calls resulting from mCNVs on chromosomes 13, 18, and 21 (see Methods). Using the measured relationship between duplication size and Δz_{dup} (Fig. 3), as well as the size and chromosome of the observed maternal duplications in over 56,000 NIPS samples (the 65% of the 87,255 sample cohort with mCNVs), we estimated the false-positive rate combined across the three chromosomes for each NIPS data-analysis strategy described earlier.

On average, mCNVs are predicted to cause a false-positive result of trisomy 13, 18, or 21 for 1 in 860 patients using the "Simple" approach. This false-positive rate is similar to the rates reported by laboratories prior to incorporating changes that mitigate the effect of mCNVs: in outcome studies, Chudova et al. reported 3 mCNV-caused false positives in 1914 patients (a rate of 1 in 640) [7], and Strom et al. reported 61 mCNV-caused false positives in 31,278 patients (a rate of 1 in 510) [6]. The "Simple" estimated false-positive rate is also consistent with aggregate statistics of NIPS specificity from meta-analyses over the time period when comparable methods were common [3].

Overall, mCNV-aware approaches ("Z-correction", "Value filtering", "mCNV filtering") had higher specificity than mCNV-unaware approaches. All mCNV-aware approaches increased the pooled specificity for the three common trisomies such that the aggregate false-positive rate was fewer than 1 in 100,000 tests. Remarkably, relative to the "Simple" approach with one false positive expected for every 860 samples, the "mCNV filtering" approach is expected to incur only one mCNV-caused false positive for every 520,000 samples, representing a 600-fold reduction.

mCNVs offer insight into clinical interpretation of novel fetal microdeletions

The high frequency and positional dispersion of CNVs across the genome (Fig. 2) was noteworthy in this ostensibly healthy pregnant population. We were curious about whether the landscape of maternal copy-number variation could inform the potential clinical impact of copy-number variation in the fetal genome. Such knowledge is important because WGS-based NIPS technology can detect novel fetal microdeletions on the order of 10 Mb [10], and it is not yet clear how to interpret the health implications of such variants.

We reasoned that the clinical consequences of a novel 10 Mb microdeletion would be less severe if there are deletions observed throughout the region in a healthy population. Therefore, we calculated the proportion of each autosomal, 10 Mb sliding window that was covered by at least three observed deletions in our mCNV dataset, termed the "deletion span" (Fig. 5a). We assumed that duplications are more likely to be benign than deletions and, therefore, calculated the corresponding duplication span for each region to serve as a proxy to control for CNV propensity. As schematized in Fig. 5a, a window with a high duplication span has several observed duplications covering most of the region, and a window with a low deletion span has deletions only in a few parts of the region. The number of observed mCNVs in a given window is not the sole determinant of the span; for example, a 10 Mb window that had a 200 kb deletion hotspot but no deletions elsewhere would have a small deletion span. Figure 5b shows span values as a function of position across chromosomes 4 and 5 (all other chromosomes in Additional file 1: Figure S8), and Fig. 5c compares deletion and duplication spans for all 10 Mb windows across autosomes. The two span measurements were significantly correlated (Pearson $r = 0.73$, $p < 0.05$), consistent with there being an intrinsic propensity for CNVs (deletions and duplications) that varies by position [21].

Based on the presumption that deletions are more likely to be pathogenic than duplications, we expected that a small deletion span, relative to the duplication span, would be a feature of pathogenic microdeletions. Therefore, we calculated the ratio of spans ("dup:del ratio") and evaluated whether pathogenic microdeletions had elevated dup:del ratios. Figure 5d shows the histogram of the dup:del ratio for autosomal 10 Mb bins; it highlights five commonly screened pathogenic microdeletions (22q11.21, 5p15, 1p36.32–33, 4p16.2–3, and 15q11.2–13.1). Four of the five pathogenic microdeletions had a dup:del ratio in the 75th percentile or greater, but 22q11.21 had a nearly 1:1 dup:del ratio (10th percentile). These data suggest that a high dup:del ratio could be a common—but not ubiquitous—feature of pathogenic microdeletions.

We investigated the density of genes in a region as a secondary feature that could distinguish whether a deletion is pathogenic. Notably, based on gene density and dup:del ratio, each of the common pathogenic microdeletions was an outlier relative to typical 10 Mb windows in the genome in one feature, the other, or both (a result robust to the mCNV-count threshold used to define a span, Additional file 1: Figure S9, as well as resamplings of the study population, Additional file 1: Figure S10). Microdeletion 22q11.21 had only an intermediate dup:del ratio, as mentioned, but its gene density is very high. Microdeletion 5p15, by contrast, had the opposite: an elevated dup:del ratio (≥99th percentile) but approximately average gene density. Finally, microdeletions 1p36, 4p16, and 15q11 all had both high gene density and elevated dup:del ratio.

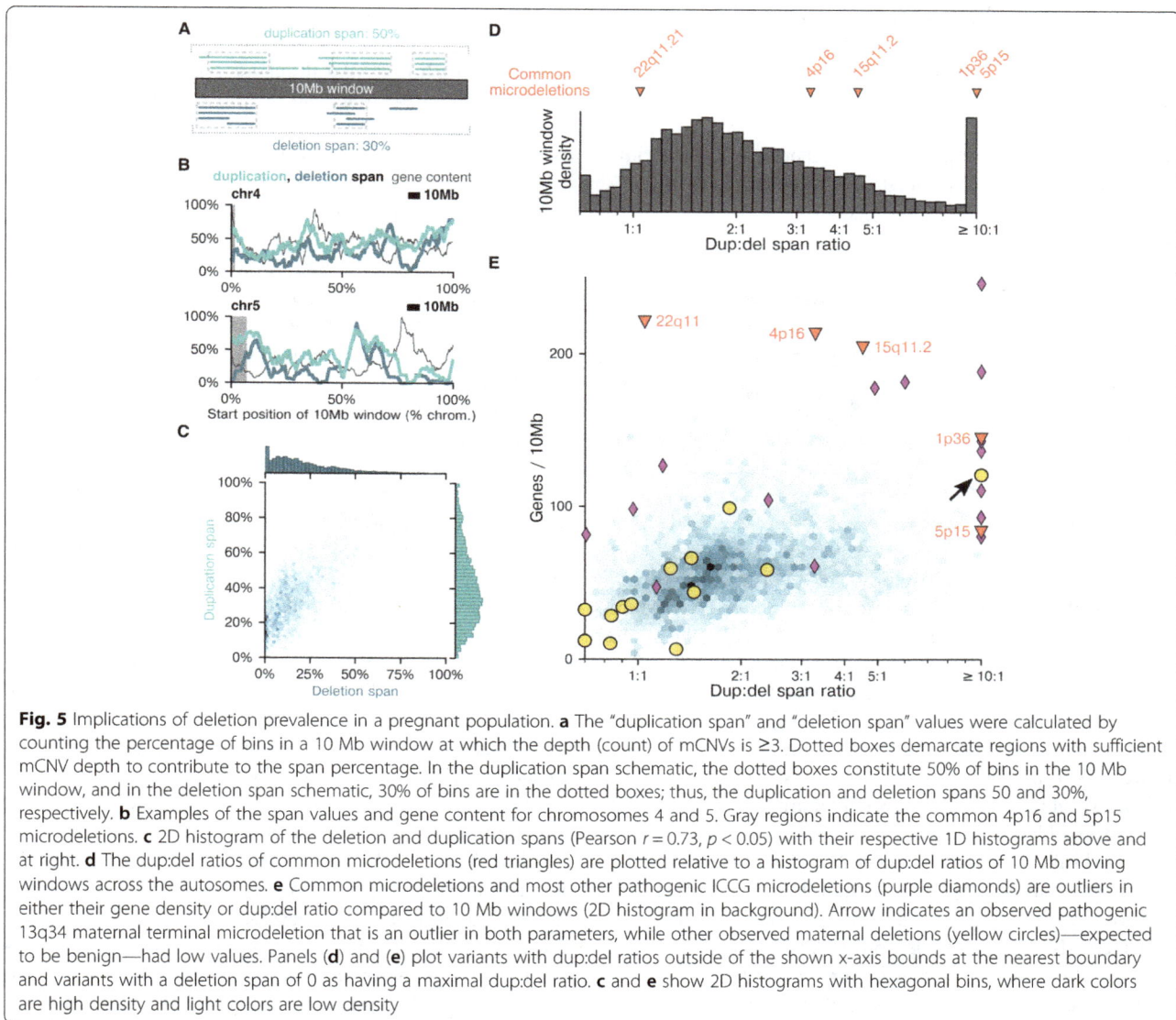

Fig. 5 Implications of deletion prevalence in a pregnant population. **a** The "duplication span" and "deletion span" values were calculated by counting the percentage of bins in a 10 Mb window at which the depth (count) of mCNVs is ≥3. Dotted boxes demarcate regions with sufficient mCNV depth to contribute to the span percentage. In the duplication span schematic, the dotted boxes constitute 50% of bins in the 10 Mb window, and in the deletion span schematic, 30% of bins are in the dotted boxes; thus, the duplication and deletion spans 50 and 30%, respectively. **b** Examples of the span values and gene content for chromosomes 4 and 5. Gray regions indicate the common 4p16 and 5p15 microdeletions. **c** 2D histogram of the deletion and duplication spans (Pearson $r = 0.73$, $p < 0.05$) with their respective 1D histograms above and at right. **d** The dup:del ratios of common microdeletions (red triangles) are plotted relative to a histogram of dup:del ratios of 10 Mb moving windows across the autosomes. **e** Common microdeletions and most other pathogenic ICCG microdeletions (purple diamonds) are outliers in either their gene density or dup:del ratio compared to 10 Mb windows (2D histogram in background). Arrow indicates an observed pathogenic 13q34 maternal terminal microdeletion that is an outlier in both parameters, while other observed maternal deletions (yellow circles)—expected to be benign—had low values. Panels (**d**) and (**e**) plot variants with dup:del ratios outside of the shown x-axis bounds at the nearest boundary and variants with a deletion span of 0 as having a maximal dup:del ratio. **c** and **e** show 2D histograms with hexagonal bins, where dark colors are high density and light colors are low density

To expand the investigation to a larger number of known pathogenic microdeletions, we additionally analyzed expert-curated pathogenic deletions [22] ≥1 Mb in length from the International Collaboration for Clinical Genomics (ICCG, formerly ISCA). Nearly all such variants were outliers in one or both metrics (purple diamonds, Fig. 5e), consistent with the findings for common microdeletions. Two known pathogenic microdeletions (2p15p16.1 and 12q14) had low dup:del ratios (~ 1:1) and relatively low gene density, but they also had low values for both the duplication span and deletion span (≤10%; Additional file 1: Table S2). As such, low span values might represent cases in which the dup:del ratio alone is equivocal for interpreting novel microdeletions.

The above analyses suggest that outlying regions in the plot of gene density versus dup:del ratio are more likely to be pathogenic when deleted. To scrutinize this

hypothesis, we tested its inverse, i.e., that deletion of non-outlying regions is benign. We observed multiple samples in our patient cohort with microdeletions ≥4 Mb, most of which we expected to be benign—or to have a mild or incompletely penetrant pathogenic phenotype—because of their presentation in expecting mothers. For all such microdeletions, we evaluated their respective gene densities, duplication spans, deletion spans, and dup:del ratios (yellow dots in Fig. 5e and Additional file 1: Figure S8; Additional file 2: Table S3). All but one of the regions directly supported our hypothesis because they were not outliers on either axis (Fig. 5e). We looked more deeply at the one variant that appeared to counter the hypothesis due to its very high dup:del ratio (yellow dot with arrow in Fig. 5e). Remarkably, this variant is a deletion of 13q34 that has recently been shown to be pathogenic, as it associates with intellectual disability and dysmorphism [23].

Therefore, rather than invalidate or weaken the hypothesis, the observed 13q34 microdeletion reinforces it.

Taken together, these observations suggest that parameterizing putative microdeletions on multiple biologically relevant axes, such as the two investigated here, could facilitate identification of pathogenic outliers and aid the clinical interpretation of novel fetal CNVs identified via NIPS.

Discussion

Here we show that mCNVs are common on the chromosomes that NIPS interrogates (4.5% of patients have mCNV on chromosome 13, 18, or 21) and can cause frequent false positives if not properly neutralized at the algorithmic level. Even NIPS tests that share a common sequencing approach (e.g., WGS of cfDNA) may nevertheless have very different test specificities based on the sophistication of their mCNV handling. Using 87,255 empirical and 30,000 simulated samples, we quantified the impact on specificity of various mCNV-mitigation strategies and observed a very wide range of values. Our novel approach, which excludes bins in mCNVs from downstream calculations, reduces the expected rate of mCNV-caused false positives nearly 600-fold relative to the algorithms used in the early iterations of WGS-based NIPS and which may still be used in practice in clinical laboratories (1 in 520,000 vs. 1 in 860; Fig. 4). Finally, as a result of characterizing the frequency, length, and position of mCNVs, our work provides initial insight into the clinical interpretation of the novel fetal microdeletions that WGS-based NIPS can detect.

Algorithmic approaches tailored to mCNVs had better specificity than strategies that had robust features but were not mCNV-specific. For example, the value-filtering approach that excludes genomic bins based on their copy-number values (Fig. 4e) performed better than a method that simply used robust statistical metrics like the median and IQR (Fig. 4b). Value filtering has drawbacks, however, as the choice of threshold results in a tradeoff between specificity and sensitivity; a permissive threshold impairs specificity by retaining some bins from mCNVs, whereas an aggressive threshold lowers sensitivity by excluding bins that may not be in mCNVs. This tradeoff is avoided with an approach that identified the location of mCNVs and removed only the relevant bins from subsequent analysis. This mCNV filtering method had the highest specificity of the options considered, with a small Δz_{dup} in aggregate across all mCNV sizes, as well as low variance in the individual Δz_{dup} values (the z-score correction method was mCNV-aware but had high variance, which is expected to lower specificity).

Though mostly tailored to retain specificity, mCNV-mitigation approaches must also not reduce sensitivity for aneuploidies. Algorithms that retain all bins ("Simple" and "Robust") were shown to be inferior due to their poor

specificity, but they may have no net impact on sensitivity because they will have higher fetal-aneuploidy sensitivity in samples with maternal duplications and lower sensitivity in samples with maternal deletions. Strategies that remove outlying bins without directly identifying mCNVs ("Robust+Gaussian" and "Value filtering") could slightly lower sensitivity for fetal aneuploidies (depending on the filtering cutoffs) because conservative filtering could superfluously remove bins not associated with mCNVs (Additional file 1: Figure S4). With the mCNV filtering approach, the small values and variance of Δz_{dup} mean that mCNVs minimally affect the z-score in either direction, suggesting that the filtering process does not compromise sensitivity. mCNV filtering could slightly boost sensitivity by avoiding false negative results in trisomic samples where the aneuploidy-inflated z-score is lowered to normal levels due to a maternal deletion.

While not directly investigated, mCNVs on non-tested chromosomes (i.e., autosomes other than chromosomes 13, 18, or 21)—or even mCNVs in other patient samples—could affect the z-score of a test chromosome [16]. WGS-based NIPS involves normalization of NGS read depth to calculate a z-score, and this normalization could include one or many chromosomes, as well as other samples in a background cohort. Robust normalization, including a large number of background samples and/or filtering out mCNVs before normalization, can mitigate spurious z-score changes due to cryptic mCNVs in the analysis pipeline.

Expert manual review of both z-scores and bin-level copy-number data across all autosomes can further safeguard against mCNV-caused false positives [24]. Based on our experience, strong collaboration between the manual reviewers and user-interface developers—as well as algorithmic flags that point out cases requiring careful scrutiny—can facilitate timely review at scale. However, we caution against an mCNV-mitigation strategy that relies solely on manual review of ideograms for putative positives [15] and foregoes a computational component that detects and assesses the impact of mCNVs. After all, most mCNVs do not cause false positives. Manual review without mCNV-specific algorithmic assistance could lower the sensitivity of the screen if trisomic samples with maternal duplications were dismissed as negatives. For instance, in addition to being cost-prohibitive and logistically challenging in a screening setting, a recently published recommendation [25] (currently used in practice [19]) supports dismissal of positive calls in samples that contain an mCNV verified by sequencing maternal white blood cell DNA. This guidance could decrease sensitivity relative to an mCNV-aware computational analysis that preserves true positive calls in aneuploid samples harboring mCNVs, where the mCNVs alone are insufficient to explain the observed z-scores.

Advances in WGS-based NIPS technology have enabled genome-wide microdeletion calling, but the challenge of interpreting positive findings could limit their clinical validity and utility. In principle, the clinical impact of a large fetal deletion stems from the cellular roles of its constituent genes and regulatory regions, but specific knowledge of these roles is often lacking. We identify the dup:del ratio as a general criterion that could advance the interpretation of large fetal CNVs; importantly, used together with gene density, each of the common microdeletions (plus the recently characterized 13q34 microdeletion [23]) was identified as an outlier. These bulk metrics might be well-suited for cases in which the genes encompassed by a novel microdeletion are not well-studied. We expect any information gained from the dup:del ratio to improve in quality with a larger patient cohort, as the observation of more mCNVs would enable use of a higher mCNV-count threshold for a bin to contribute to the duplication or deletion span. In addition, more examples of benign microdeletions observed in expecting mothers can further power the analysis.

Conclusions

With proper algorithm design and extensive testing that leverages empirical and simulated data, high specificity in NIPS is possible even in the presence of mCNVs that range widely in size. Importantly, by using the mCNV-filtering approach described here, achieving robustness to mCNVs—and the corresponding rise in positive predictive value—does not compromise detection of true aneuploidies and, thereby, preserves both high sensitivity and a low test-failure rate. While the identification and analysis of mCNVs provide biological insight into the impact of large copy-number variants, mCNV removal upstream of fetal aneuploidy assessment is important to maintain exemplary test performance, which will be especially critical as NIPS adoption increases in the wider, general obstetric population.

Additional files

Additional file 1: Table S1. Summary of the six algorithmic strategies tested. **Figure S1.** The desired versus observed mCNV size for simulations. **Figure S2.** Sensitivity of mCNV detection ascertained from simulations. **Figure S3.** Histogram of observed bin copy number estimates within mCNVs. **Figure S4.** Change in z-score due to mCNVs, the specificity attributable to false positives caused by duplications, and the proportion of available bins used for two cut-off options of the "Value filtering" method and the "mCNV filtering" method. **Figure S5.** Proportion of a chromosome covered by observed mCNVs. **Figure S6.** Change in z-score due to mCNVs and the specificity attributable to false positives caused by duplications: chromosome 13 as the basis for simulations. **Figure S7.** Change in z-score due to mCNVs and the specificity attributable to false positives caused by duplications: chromosome 18 as the basis for simulations. **Figure S8.** Duplication and deletion span values across all chromosomes. **Figure S9.** Varying the minimum required number of mCNV observations covering a genomic bin for that bin to count toward a duplication or deletion span. **Figure S10.** Bootstrapping analysis of duplication and deletion spans. **Table S2.** Properties of ICCG microdeletions and identified maternal deletions greater than 4 Mb.

Additional file 2: Table S3. Identified autosomal maternal CNVs.

Abbreviations
cfDNA: cell-free DNA; CNV: Copy-number variant; HIPAA: Health Insurance Portability and Accountability Act; ICCG: International Collaboration for Clinical Genomics (formerly ISCA); IQR: Interquartile range; kb: kilobases; Mb: Megabases; mCNV: maternal copy-number variant; NIPS: Noninvasive prenatal screening; WGS: Whole-genome sequencing

Acknowledgements
The authors are grateful to Jeffrey Tratner for support of analysis infrastructure, Katherine Johansen Taber for feedback, the R&D team at Counsyl, the reviewers of this manuscript, and the patients who underwent testing.

Funding
The study was funded by Counsyl.

Authors' contributions
KEK, GJH, KDM, CH, and DM designed the study. KEK and GJH collected and analyzed the data. KEK, GJH, and DM wrote the manuscript. All authors read and approved the final manuscript.

Competing interests
KEK, GJH, KMD, CH, and DM are employees and equity holders of Counsyl.

References
1. Norton ME, Jacobsson B, Swamy GK, Laurent LC, Ranzini AC, Brar H, et al. Cell-free DNA analysis for noninvasive examination of trisomy. N Engl J Med. 2015;372:1589–97.
2. Gregg AR, Skotko BG, Benkendorf JL, Monaghan KG, Bajaj K, Best RG, et al. Noninvasive prenatal screening for fetal aneuploidy, 2016 update: a position statement of the American College of Medical Genetics and Genomics. Genet Med. 2016;18:1056–65.
3. ACOG. Cell-free DNA screening for fetal aneuploidy. Committee Opinion No. 640. Obstet Gynecol [Internet]. 2015;126. Available from: https://journals.lww.com/greenjournal/fulltext/2015/09000/Committee_Opinion_No__640___Cell_Free_Dna.51.aspx. Accessed 8 Oct 2018.
4. Akolekar R, Beta J, Picciarelli G. Procedure-related risk of miscarriage following amniocentesis and chorionic villus sampling: a systematic review and meta-analysis. Ultrasound Obstet Gynecol [Internet]. Wiley Online Library; 2015; Available from: http://onlinelibrary.wiley.com/doi/10.1002/uog.14636/full. Accessed 8 Oct 2018.
5. Snyder MW, Simmons LE, Kitzman JO, Coe BP, Henson JM, Daza RM, et al. Copy-Number Variation and False Positive Prenatal Aneuploidy Screening Results. N Engl J Med. 2015;372:1639–45 Massachusetts Medical Society.
6. Strom CM, Maxwell MD, Owen R. Improving the Accuracy of Prenatal Screening with DNA Copy-Number Analysis. N Engl J Med. 2017;376:188–9.
7. Chudova DI, Sehnert AJ, Bianchi DW. Copy-Number Variation and False Positive Prenatal Screening Results. N Engl J Med. 2016;375:97–8.
8. Hartwig TS, Ambye L, Sørensen S, Jørgensen FS. Discordant non-invasive prenatal testing (NIPT) - a systematic review. Prenat Diagn. 2017;37:527–39.
9. Srinivasan A, Bianchi DW, Huang H, Sehnert AJ, Rava RP. Noninvasive detection of fetal subchromosome abnormalities via deep sequencing of maternal plasma. Am J Hum Genet. 2013;92:167–76.
10. Ehrich M, Tynan J, Mazloom A, Almasri E, McCullough R, Boomer T, et al. Genome-wide cfDNA screening: clinical laboratory experience with the first 10,000 cases. Genet Med. 2017;19:1332–7.
11. Benjamini Y, Speed TP. Summarizing and correcting the GC content bias in high-throughput sequencing. Nucleic Acids Res. 2012;40:e72.
12. Chandrananda D, Thorne NP, Ganesamoorthy D, Bruno DL, Benjamini Y, Speed TP, et al. Investigating and correcting plasma DNA sequencing coverage bias to enhance aneuploidy discovery. PLoS One. 2014;9:e86993.

13. Chiu RWK, Chan KCA, Gao Y, Lau VYM, Zheng W, Leung TY, et al. Noninvasive prenatal diagnosis of fetal chromosomal aneuploidy by massively parallel genomic sequencing of DNA in maternal plasma. Proc Natl Acad Sci U S A. 2008;105:20458–63.

14. Wan X, Wang W, Liu J, Tong T. Estimating the sample mean and standard deviation from the sample size, median, range and/or interquartile range. BMC Med Res Methodol. 2014;14:135.

15. Strom CM, Anderson B, Tsao D, Zhang K, Liu Y, Livingston K, et al. Improving the Positive Predictive Value of Non-Invasive Prenatal Screening (NIPS). PLoS One. 2017;12:e0167130.

16. van den Boom D, Ehrich M, Kim SK. Copy-Number Variation and False Positive Results of Prenatal Screening. N Engl J Med. 2015;373:2584.

17. Sparks AB, Wang ET, Struble CA, Barrett W, Stokowski R, McBride C, et al. Selective analysis of cell-free DNA in maternal blood for evaluation of fetal trisomy. Prenat Diagn. 2012;32:3–9.

18. Kingsley C, Wang E, Oliphant A. Commentary: Copy-Number Variation and False Positive Results of Prenatal Screening. N Engl J Med. 2015;373:2585.

19. Jiang F, Ren J, Chen F, Zhou Y, Xie J, Dan S, et al. Noninvasive Fetal Trisomy (NIFTY) test: an advanced noninvasive prenatal diagnosis methodology for fetal autosomal and sex chromosomal aneuploidies. BMC Med Genet. 2012;5:57.

20. Fan HC, Quake SR. Sensitivity of noninvasive prenatal detection of fetal aneuploidy from maternal plasma using shotgun sequencing is limited only by counting statistics. PLoS One. 2010;5:e10439.

21. Fu W, Zhang F, Wang Y, Gu X, Jin L. Identification of copy number variation hotspots in human populations. Am J Hum Genet. 2010;87:494–504.

22. Clinical Genome Resource. ISCA Curated Pathogenic/Benign Regions [Internet]. ClinGen Clinical Genome Resource. Available from: https://www.clinicalgenome.org/toolkits/array-analysis-toolkit/. Cited 31 Dec 2017.

23. Reinstein E, Liberman M, Feingold-Zadok M, Tenne T, Graham JM Jr. Terminal microdeletions of 13q34 chromosome region in patients with intellectual disability: Delineation of an emerging new microdeletion syndrome. Mol Genet Metab. 2016;118:60–3.

24. Bayindir B, Dehaspe L, Brison N, Brady P, Ardui S, Kammoun M, et al. Noninvasive prenatal testing using a novel analysis pipeline to screen for all autosomal fetal aneuploidies improves pregnancy management. Eur J Hum Genet. 2015;23:1286–93.

25. Zhou X, Sui L, Xu Y, Song Y, Qi Q, Zhang J, et al. Contribution of maternal copy number variations to false-positive fetal trisomies detected by noninvasive prenatal testing. Prenat Diagn. 2017;37:318–22.

8

Local genetic ancestry in *CDKN2B-AS1* is associated with primary open-angle glaucoma in an African American cohort extracted from de-identified electronic health records

Nicole A. Restrepo[1], Sarah M. Laper[2], Eric Farber-Eger[3] and Dana C. Crawford[1*]

From The 7th Translational Bioinformatics Conference
Los Angeles, CA, USA. 29 September - 01 October 2017

Abstract

Background: Glaucoma is a leading cause of blindness in developed countries. Primary open-angle glaucoma (POAG), the most prevalent clinical subtype of glaucoma in the United States, affects African Americans at a higher rate compared with European Americans. Risk factors identified for POAG include increased age and family history, which coupled with heritability estimates, suggest this complex condition is associated with genetic and environmental factors. To date, several genome-wide studies have identified loci significantly associated with POAG risk, but most of these studies were performed in populations of European-descent.

Methods: To identify population-specific and trans-population genetic associations for POAG, we genotyped 11,521 African Americans using the Illumina Metabochip as part of the Epidemiologic Architecture for Genes Linked to Environment (EAGLE) study accessing BioVU, the Vanderbilt University Medical Center's biorepository linked to de-identified electronic health records. Among this study population, we identified 138 cases of POAG and 1376 controls and performed Metabochip-wide tests of association. We also estimated local genetic ancestry at *CDKN2B-AS1*, a POAG-associated locus established in European-descent populations.

Results: Overall, we did not identify significant single SNP-POAG associations after adjusting for multiple testing. We did, however, detect a significant association between POAG risk and local African genetic ancestry at *CDKN2B-AS1*, where on average cases were of 90% African descent compared with controls at 58% ($p = 2 \times 10^{-6}$).

Conclusions: These data suggest that *CDKN2B-AS1* is an important locus for POAG risk among African Americans, warranting further investigation to identify the variants underlying this association.

Keywords: African Americans, Primary open-angle glaucoma, Electronic health records

* Correspondence: dana.crawford@case.edu
[1]Department of Population and Quantitative Health Sciences, Institute for Computational Biology, Case Western Reserve University, 2103 Cornell Road, Wolstein Research Building, Suite 2-527, Cleveland, OH 44106, USA
Full list of author information is available at the end of the article

Background

Glaucoma is the second leading cause of blindness in the United States, and it is the leading cause of blindness and irreversible vision loss in African Americans [1], with a prevalence approximately double that observed in European-descent populations [1–3]. The prevalence of glaucoma is similar for European, Japanese, and Indian populations with rates approaching those observed in African descent populations in the oldest age categories [4]. Although African Americans comprise the group of highest risk of developing glaucoma-related vision problems, many cases remain undiagnosed. Previous studies have suggested that nation-wide implementation of screening middle aged African Americans could decrease the rate of undiagnosed glaucoma from 50 to 27% [5]. Earlier screening and diagnosis enables patients to more effectively leverage current treatment options to reduce the risk of bilateral blindness later in life [5].

In addition to African ancestry and age [6], other known risk factors associated with the development of glaucoma include myopia [7] and high intraocular pressure [6, 8, 9]. Family history has also been associated with glaucoma risk [6, 10, 11], albeit inconsistently most likely due to the heterogeneous nature of the disease. The phenotypic heterogeneity of glaucoma has also impacted other studies attempting to establish and quantify the genetic contribution to risk in developing the disease; consequently, the majority of these studies have been conducted on more easily-measured glaucoma endophenotypes such as central corneal thickness ($h^2 = 0.35–0.72\%$) [12–14], intraocular pressure ($h^2 = 0.35–0.94\%$) [12, 14], and cup-to-disc ratio ($h^2 = 0.56–0.66\%$) [12, 15]. Pulsatility of choroidal blood flow and velocity are additional quantitative traits whose variation from normal parameters has been observed in individuals with glaucoma [16, 17], yet heritability studies have not yet found significant genetic contribution to its variability [12].

The strongest evidence for a genetic contribution related to glaucoma comes from studies of primary open-angle glaucoma (POAG), the most prevalent clinical subtype of glaucoma in the United States. Early linkage and family-based genetic association studies identified the *MYOC* (myocilin), *OPTN* (optineurin), and *WDR36* (WD repeat domain 36) [18–20] genes as the primary genes for susceptibility to POAG. Mutations in *MYOC* are known to cause hereditary early-onset POAG in multiple populations [18, 21, 22]. More recently, large-scale genome-wide association studies (GWAS) have identified variants in the *CAV1/CAV2*, *CDKN2B-AS1* and *SIX1/SIX6I* genes that influence POAG risk in European-descent and Japanese populations [23–27].

Additional genetic factors that have yet to be discovered are hypothesized to drive POAG risk and to account for the differences in incidence observed across racial/ethnic groups. For example, in a study of African Americans, the frequency of *MYOC* mutations was comparably lower (~ 1.4%) than in other populations (~ 2–4%) [28] suggesting that other genetic loci are driving risk in this group. It is possible that both population-specific and trans-population genetic variants contribute to POAG risk. To identify population-specific and trans-population genetic factors, we conducted a hypothesis-testing and hypothesis-generating genetic association study in African Americans with and without POAG drawn from a clinical cohort with electronic health records.

Methods
Study population and genotyping

The study population is a subset of the Epidemiologic Architecture for Genes Linked to Environment (EAGLE) study, a study site of the larger Population Architecture using Genomics and Epidemiology (PAGE) I study [29, 30]. In general, the PAGE study is a consortium of diverse epidemiologic and clinical cohorts with broad research goals that include the generalization of genetic associations to multiple populations [29]. To identify non-European Americans for PAGE I, EAGLE accessed the Vanderbilt University Medical Center (VUMC)'s biorepository linked to de-identified electronic health records known as BioVU [31].

VUMC's BioVU followed an opt-out model for DNA sample accrual between 2007 and 2015 [31]. That is, DNA was collected from discarded blood samples remaining after routine clinical testing and was linked to de-identified electronic health records. According to the Vanderbilt Institutional Review Board (IRB) and the Federal Office of Human Research Protections provisions, this VUMC protocol is considered nonhuman subjects research (The Code of Federal Regulations, 45 CFR 46.102 (f)) [31, 32].

As previously described [33], EAGLE selected all non-European Americans from BioVU as of 2011 for genotyping on the Metabochip (EAGLE BioVU). A total of 11,521 African Americans samples in EAGLE BioVU were genotyped [33]. From among these patients, billing and procedural codes along with text searches were used to identify POAG cases ($n = 138$) and controls ($n = 1376$). In short, controls included patients in BioVU over the age of 60 years whose records did not contain an ICD-9-CM code for any form of glaucoma nor any mention of "glaucoma" in a text search of their 'Problems List.' Manual review of all cases and a subset of controls was performed for quality assurance as previously described [34].

The Metabochip is an Illumina (San Diego, CA) custom array designed for fine-mapping of metabolic and cardiovascular traits. Fine-mapping regions cover 257 loci chosen from SNPs that reached genome-wide significance from select consortium meta-analyses [35].

The Metabochip was also designed for replication of GWAS-identified index variants for any phenotype from the GWAS Catalog (http://www.ebi.ac.uk/gwas/) as of 2009. A total of 33 GWAS-index variants representing ocular diseases (including age-related macular degeneration, POAG, normal tension glaucoma, and diabetic retinopathy) as well as related traits (myopia, ocular axial length, HbA1c, cup-to-disc ratio, intraocular pressure, and optic disc size) are directly assayed by the Metabochip (Additional file 1: Table S1).

EAGLE BioVU DNA samples were genotyped using the Metabochip following the manufacturer's protocol (Illumina, Inc.; San Diego, CA.), and 360 HapMap samples, including YRI samples, were genotyped for PAGE-wide cross-study quality control standards [36]. A description of the genotyping protocols and quality control measures has been previously published [30]. In brief, genetic variants were evaluated for deviations from Hardy Weinberg Equilibrium, which may be a result of poor genotyping. Variants with a genotyping call rate < 95% were removed from further analysis. Principal components (PC) were calculated using EIGENSOFT [37, 38]. At the sample level, DNA samples with poor sample call rate (< 95%), sex discordance, or evidence of cryptic relatedness were removed from analyses.

Statistical methods

Individuals included in this analysis were those identified as POAG cases over the age of 20 years and POAG controls over the age of 60 years. An older age threshold was applied in controls to minimize the probability of including potential future cases. African Americans are at increased risk of glaucoma over the age of 40 years, while other populations have an age-associated risk over 60 years. Age was defined as age at diagnosis in cases and age at last clinical exam in controls. T-tests and chi-square tests, where appropriate, were used to compare demographic clinical characteristics between cases and controls in Stata/SE version 14.2.

All common variants (MAF > 0.05) were tested for an association with POAG using logistic regression separately assuming a log-additive genetic model (Additional file 1: Table S2), a recessive model (Additional file 1: Table S3), and a dominant model (Additional file 1: Table S4) adjusted by age, sex, the first three PCs, and median diastolic blood pressure. Analyses were conducted using PLINKv1.90 [39]. Additionally, we tested for an association between POAG and 258 SNPs that passed quality control in the CDKN2B-AS1 region of chromosome 14. Pair-wise linkage disequilibrium (r^2) was calculated in SNAP [40] using YRI 1000 Genomes Project Pilot 1 reference data. Power calculations were performed in Quanto [41] to determine 80% power to detect an association with a case:control ratio of

1:3, assuming a log-additive model and a genome-wide significance threshold (5×10^{-8}).

Local ancestry mapping

Local ancestry for the CDKN2B-AS1 region, located on chromosome 9, was determined for the POAG cases and controls using Local Ancestry in adMixed Populations (LAMP) [42]. Input parameters included the estimated number of generations since admixture (generations = 10), estimated fraction of admixture from each population (African = 0.8, European = 0.2), and predicted recombination rate (3.4×10^{-7} bases^{-1}). The number of alleles from the ancestral populations at each SNP that was genotyped in this region was estimated, and the overall fraction of alleles from each ancestral population in this region for each patient was determined. Percent African ancestry was then tested for an association with POAG status using logistic regression using R software version 3.1.3 [43].

Global ancestry mapping

Global ancestry was calculated using fastSTRUCTURE [44] with all of the Metabochip data. Input parameters were set to default, as recommended by the authors, and the analysis was set to determine the proportion of two populations (K = 2). Admixture plots were graphed using the web graphical interface (http://pophelper.com/) of the R module "pophelper" [45].

Results

Population characteristics

A total of 138 African American POAG cases and 1376 controls passed quality control in EAGLE BioVU for the present study. We previously described [34] these cases compared with 4813 controls over the age of 40; in the present study, we compare the same cases with subset of the controls over the age of 60 years (Table 1). Here, cases were younger ($p = 0.01$) with higher cholesterol levels (183 mg/dL; $p = 0.01$), more likely to be female with higher average body mass index (30.1 kg/m^2) in comparison to controls (28.8 kg/m^2 and 169 mg/dL, respectively). Cases also presented with higher triglyceride levels compared to controls (125 mg/dL versus 97 mg/dL; $p = 0.0001$).

Local ancestry in the CDKN2B-AS1 region

We previously reported on preliminary tests of association in the CDKN2B-AS1 region [34], which was fine-mapped by the Illumina Metabochip. None of the tests of association were significant after correcting for the 258 common variants tested [34]. As we have already noted, there are multiple explanations for the lack of significant results including limited power, variability in linkage disequilibrium patterns across populations, and genetic heterogeneity. Another possible explanation for the observed null results is that the previous analysis did

Table 1 Study population characteristics of primary open-angle glaucoma cases and controls among African Americans in EAGLE BioVU

Trait	Cases (n = 138)	Controls (1376)	p-value
Median age at diagnosis or LCV (years)	62.0 (12.0)	67.3 (7.8)	0.01
% female	63.7	56.5	0.10
% hypertensive	55.1	52.5	0.50
Median BMI (kg/m^2)	30.1 (6.7)	28.8 (7.35)	0.44
Median diastolic blood pressure (mm/Hg)	74.5 (8.1)	76.0 (8.8)	0.97
Median systolic blood pressure (mm/Hg)	134.5 (14.1)	135 (14.6)	0.88
Median cholesterol (mg/dL)	183 (40.6)	169 (46.7)	0.01
Median HDL-C (mg/dL)	52.5 (25.0)	49 (17.8)	0.88
Median LDL-C (mg/dL)	103 (42.9)	93 (37.4)	0.20
Median triglycerides (mg/dL)	125 (76.3)	97 (68.1)	0.0001

Case extraction was described in Restrepo et al. [34]. Control extraction from EAGLE BioVU was also described in Restrepo et al. [34] but restricted to controls > 40 years of age (as opposed to > 60 years of age here). Values were defined or calculated for the following: Age at POAG diagnosis was determined by the date of when the POAG billing code (ICD-9-CM 365.11) was first mentioned in the records. Age at last clinic visit (LCV) was taken as the date of the last current procedure terminology (CPT) code mentioned in the records for controls. An individual was classified as hypertensive if he/she met one of three criteria: systolic blood pressure > 140 mm/Hg, diastolic blood pressure > 90 mm/Hg, or on hypertension medications all within a 2-year window of when he or she was diagnosed with POAG for cases and a 2-year window of his or her LCV date for controls. Median (and standard deviation) blood pressure (systolic and diastolic), lipids (total cholesterol, high-density lipoprotein cholesterol or HDL-C, low-density lipoprotein cholesterol or LDL-C, and triglycerides), and body mass index (height and weight) were calculated from all labs or measurements available within 2 years of POAG diagnosis or LCV. T-tests and chi-square tests, where appropriate, were used to compare demographic clinical characteristics between cases and controls. Abbreviations: standard deviation (SD)

not account for local genetic ancestry. We therefore sought to determine whether the total composition of African and European ancestry at this region could account for POAG risk.

Local ancestry for the *CDKN2B-AS1* region was determined for POAG cases and controls using LAMP [42]. The number of alleles from the ancestral populations at each SNP was estimated, and the overall fraction of alleles from each ancestral population in this region for each patient was calculated. Logistic regression was then performed between POAG case status and percent African ancestry to assess whether ancestry might alter POAG risk. The mean African ancestry for POAG cases and controls at *CDKN2B-AS1* was 0.90 and 0.58, respectively (Fig. 1), and the percent of African ancestry in the *CDKN2B-AS1* region was significantly associated with POAG at $p = 2 \times 10^{-6}$. In contrast, the average Metabo-wide global African ancestry for cases and controls was 81.5 and 79.4%, respectively, in agreement with previous estimates [46, 47].

Metabochip-wide association of POAG in African Americans

We tested all SNPs genotyped on the Illumina Metabochip for an association with POAG adjusted for age, sex, the first three principal components, and median diastolic blood pressure (Fig. 2; Additional file 1: Tables S2-S4). No SNP was significantly associated with POAG after adjusting for a strict Bonferroni correction ($p < 4.04 \times 10^{-7}$). The two most significant associations [chr1:228347779 (rs4846835) and chr1:228354829 (rs34783939)] under the log-additive genetic model are located within the protein coding gene of *GALNT2*, a member of the glycosyltransferase 2 protein family. *GALNT2* was targeted for fine-mapping by the Metabochip based on earlier reported associations with high density lipoprotein cholesterol (HDL-C) and triglyceride levels [48, 49]. It is interesting to note that *GALNT2* rs4846835 was associated with dementia and core Alzheimer's disease neuropathologic changes, albeit not at the genome-wide level [50]. Both of these variants also appear as marginally significant under a dominant genetic model (Table 3 [OR = 2.43 & 2.24 respectively]. Homozygous carriers for either of the two SNPs are rare in cases and controls at only a frequency of 1 to 2%. Variant rs4846835 heterozygotes account for 9.4% of cases and 17.5% of controls, while rs34783939 heterozygotes make up 12.3% of cases and 23.6% of controls. The variants are not in strong linkage disequilibrium with one another ($r^2 = 0.304$ in YRI, phase 1 1000 Genomes Project). It is important to note that rs34783939 is most likely multi-allelic based on later versions of the 1000 Genomes Project and other large-scale sequencing efforts.

Additional variants of interest for future studies that were marginally significant in both additive and dominant genetic modes are rs13423742 (OR$_{additive}$ = 3.04; $p = 1.14 \times 10^{-4}$), rs9479726 (OR$_{additive}$ = 0.41; $p = 1.54 \times 10^{-4}$), and rs1671152 (OR$_{additive}$ = 1.91; $p = 1.6 \times 10^{-4}$). Variant rs1671152 is a known missense variant in the glycoprotein VI (*GP6*) gene. *GP6*, a collagen receptor, is involved in platelet aggregation [54]. *GP6* RNAs are expressed in the retina and brain as shown in the FANTOM5 and GTEx datasets [55, 56]. In 1000 Genomes Project phase 3 CEU the rs1671152 (A) allele has a frequency of 0.182 while the YRI population has a frequency of 0.324, consistent with that observed in EAGLE BioVU African Americans (coded allele frequency = 0.32). The frequency of rs1671152 is twice as high in African Americans compared with European Americans suggesting it could potentially be a population-specific factor.

The intergenic SNP rs9479726 was less frequent in cases compared with controls (OR$_{additive}$ = 0.41; $1.54 \times 10{-4}$ and OR$_{dominant}$ = 0.42; 2.5×10^{-4}). None of the cases were found to be homozygous for the coded allele, while 5.7% of controls were homozygous. The 'A' allele had a

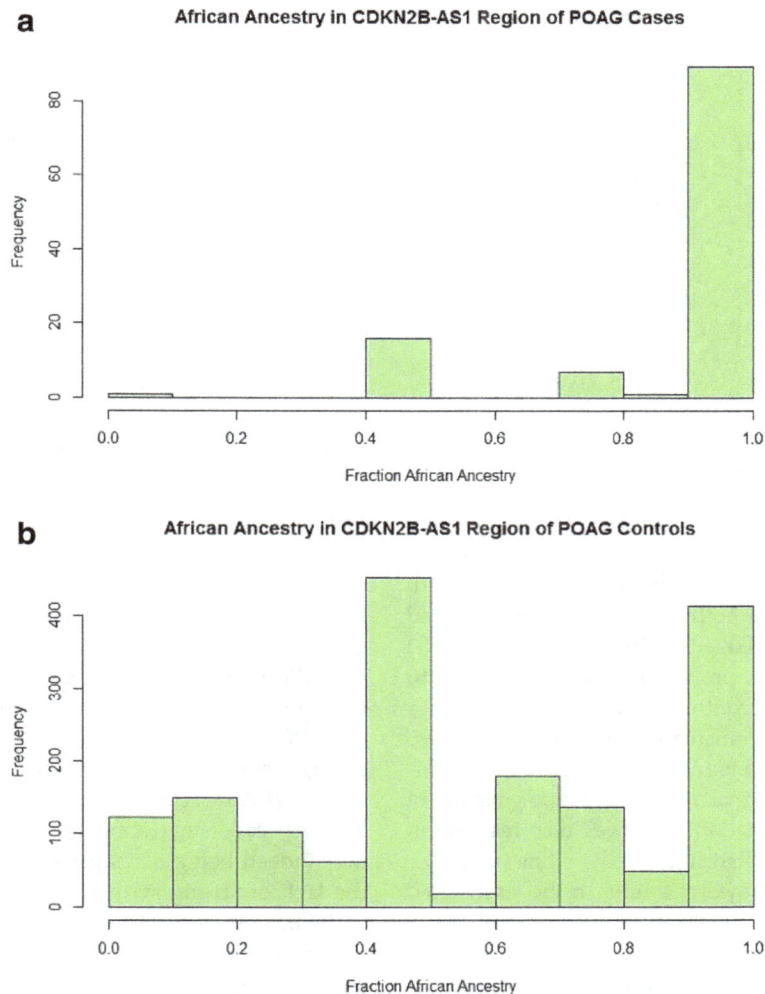

Fig. 1 Distribution of African ancestry at *CDKN2B-AS1* in African American primary open-angle glaucoma cases and controls from EAGLE BioVU. Fraction of African ancestry, estimated by LAMP using genotype data available for *CDKN2B-AS1* from the Illumina Metabochip, is plotted on the x-axis with frequency on the y-axis for primary open-angle glaucoma (POAG) **a** cases ($n = 138$) and **b** controls ($n = 1376$). Plots were graphed in R

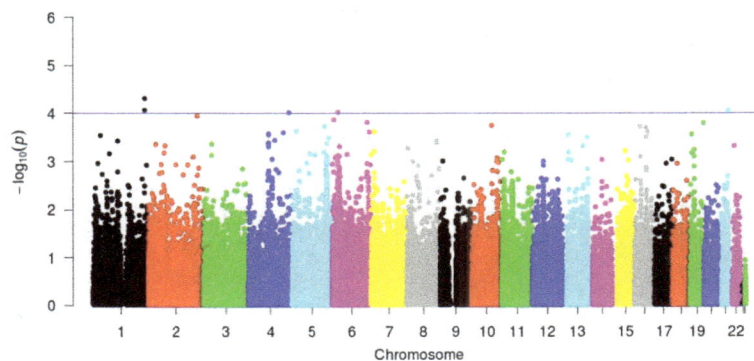

Fig. 2 Manhattan plot of EAGLE BioVU primary open-angle glaucoma Metabochip-wide tests of association in African Americans. Logistic regression assuming an additive genetic model was performed for 138 cases and 1376 controls adjusted by age, sex, principal components, and median diastolic blood pressure. *P*-values [(−log$_{10}$) on the y-axis] for each test of association are plotted by chromosome (x-axis). The blue line depicts a suggestive significance threshold of $p < 5.0 \times 10^{-4}$

Table 2 Ten most significant results for primary open-angle glaucoma Metabochip-wide genetic associations in African Americans

CHR	SNP	Gene	CA	CAF	OR	95% CI	p-value
1	rs4846835	GALNT2	A	0.11	2.37	1.56–3.60	5.00×10^{-5}
1	rs34783939	GALNT2	C	0.15	2.09	1.44–3.02	8.73×10^{-5}
21	rs9982695	C21orf33	A	0.24	2.09	1.44–3.02	8.74×10^{-5}
4	rs3775202	VEGFC	G	0.43	1.92	1.38–2.66	9.70×10^{-5}
2	rs13423742	FN1	C	0.06	3.04	1.73–5.36	1.14×10^{-4}
6	rs7454156	BMP6	G	0.18	2.08	1.42–3.02	1.37×10^{-4}
6	rs9479726	RGS17-OPRM1	A	0.24	0.41	0.25–0.64	1.54×10^{-4}
19	rs1671152	GP6	A	0.32	1.91	1.36–2.68	1.60×10^{-4}
10	rs286489	LOC101929727	A	0.28	1.90	1.35–2.66	1.80×10^{-4}
5	rs4336354	HTR4	G	0.09	2.51	1.54–4.07	1.86×10^{-4}

Logistic regression assuming an additive genetic model was performed for 138 cases and 1376 controls adjusted by age, sex, principal components, and median diastolic blood pressure. For the ten most significant associations, chromosome (CHR), SNP ID (rs number), gene, coded allele (CA), coded allele frequency (CAF), odds ratio (OR), 95% confidence interval (CI), and p-value are given

frequency of 24% in the overall population, with 10.8% of cases and 37.6% of controls being heterozygous carriers.

One SNP (i.e., rs7454156) was consistently associated with POAG at $p < 5.0 \times 10^{-4}$ in both the additive (Table 2) and recessive genetic models (Table 3). This intronic variant (G) in the bone morphogenetic protein 6 (BMP6) was found to be homozygous in 5% of controls and 2.5% of cases. In a mouse model of hemochromatosis, mutations in a BMP6 co-receptor (i.e., HJV) were found to result in an accumulation of iron in mouse retinal tissues and upregulation of BMP6 along with upregulation of VEGF that resulted in subsequent abnormal vascularization of the retina [57].

While certain variants were found to be associated with POAG in both dominant/additive and recessive/additive models, we found that no SNPs were consistently associated with POAG in both dominant and recessive models.

Discussion

Epidemiologic and clinical studies have demonstrated that POAG risk is higher in African-descent populations compared with other populations such as European Americans. To identify genetic variants associated with POAG risk that are specific to African-descent populations or shared across world populations, we identified African American POAG cases and controls in a clinic setting using electronic health records to conduct genetic associations studies in the fine-mapped region of CDKN2B-AS1 and Metabochip-wide [34]. Overall, we found evidence that the percentage of African ancestry at CDKN2B-AS1 was strongly correlated with POAG case status ($p = 2 \times 10^{-6}$). POAG cases on average contained 90% African ancestral alleles at the CDKN2B-AS1 region versus controls which were only 58% African, suggesting that African-specific variation may indeed being driving risk at this locus. Additionally, the lack of strong statistical associations with individual SNPs but an association with gene-based African ancestry suggests that gene x gene or gene x environment interactions may be involved but which will require larger sample sizes to accurately assess the possibility.

Common variants in CDKN2B-AS1 are consistently associated with POAG in European-descent populations [25, 27, 51]. We [34] and others [27, 52, 53] have demonstrated that these same variants are inconsistently associated with POAG in African-descent populations. The lack of association in African-descent populations is likely due to limited power, a consequence of smaller

Table 3 Primary open-angle glaucoma Metabochip-wide genetic associations in African Americans for dominant and recessive models that overlap with the most significant results for the additive genetic model

CHR	SNP	Gene	CA	OR	95% CI	p-value	Genetic model
1	rs4846835	GALNT2	A	2.43	1.56–3.74	6.59×10^{-5}	dominant
1	rs34783939	GALNT2	C	2.24	1.47–3.39	1.6×10^{-4}	dominant
2	rs13423742	FN1	C	2.82	1.63–4.86	2.02×10^{-4}	dominant
6	rs9479726	RGS17-OPRM1	A	0.42	0.26–0.67	2.5×10^{-4}	dominant
19	rs1671152	GP6	A	2.24	1.42–3.53	5.2×10^{-4}	dominant
6	rs7454156	BMP6	G	5.14	2.54–10.37	4.87×10^{-6}	recessive

Logistic regression assuming a dominant genetic model adjusted by age, sex, principal components, and median diastolic blood pressure. Chromosome (CHR), SNP ID (rs number), gene, coded allele (CA), odds ratio (OR), 95% confidence interval (CI), p-value, and assumed genetic model are given

sample sizes and considerably lower allele frequencies compared with studies of European-descent populations. For example, *CDKN2B-AS1* rs2157719 has a minor allele frequency of 3 and 46% in African Americans (ASW) and Europeans (CEU), respectively, in phase 3 of the 1000 Genomes Project. Originally discovered in a European POAG cohort [25], rs2157719 was found to be associated with optic nerve degeneration in glaucoma patients with an odds ratio of 1.45. The present study is powered (80%) to detect associations for common variants (≥15% MAF) with large effect sizes (at least 2.9 odds ratio) at genome-wide significance (5×10^{-8}). The small sample size of this study is underpowered to detect associations for less frequent variants and/or variants with smaller effect sizes. Although we could not generalize these associations in this study sample, we note that this locus is still important in POAG risk as evidenced by the association between African ancestry at this locus and POAG. It is also interesting to note that the *CDKN2B-AS1* rs2157719 allele associated with lower odds of POAG (C/G) is the ancestral allele yet the minor allele in all 1000 Genomes Project populations. The high frequency of the derived allele at rs2157719 may be due to chance, positive selection (and possible antagonistic pleiotropy), or an error in ancestral allele assignment, among other possibilities.

Conclusions

Here, we show a significant association between POAG risk and local African genetic ancestry at *CDKN2B-AS1* ($p = 2 \times 10^{-6}$). While not identifying significant single SNP-POAG associations after adjusting for multiple testing, the results still suggest that *CDKN2B-AS1* is an important locus of POAG risk among African Americans, warranting further investigation to identify genetic variants or epigenetic regulators that may be acting in conjunction with this locus. When gauging the strengths and limitations of this study, perhaps its greatest strength is the expansion of knowledge in African Americans, a population far too often underrepresented in biomedical research [58]. Additional strengths involve the utilization of electronic health records as a cost efficient and data-dense resource for studies. A major limitation of our study is statistical power. Nevertheless, this study is one of only a handful to assess the genetic architecture of POAG in African Americans.

Abbreviations

EAGLE: Epidemiologic Architecture for Genes Linked to Environment; GWAS: Genome-wide association studies; HDL-C: High density lipoprotein cholesterol; IRB: Vanderbilt Institutional Review Board; LAMP: Local Ancestry in admixed Populations; MAF: Minor allele frequency; OR: Odds ratio; PAGE: Population Architecture using Genomics and Epidemiology; PC: Principal components; POAG: Primary open-angle glaucoma; VUMC: Vanderbilt University Medical Center

Funding

This work was supported by National Institutes of Health U01 HG004798 and its ARRA supplements. The cost of publication was funded by Case Western Reserve University' Institute for Computational Biology. NAR was supported by the National Institutes of Health (NIH) Quantitative Ocular Genomics Training Program Pre-doctoral Trainee (1T32EY021453). The dataset (s) used for the analyses described were obtained from Vanderbilt University Medical Center's BioVU which is supported by institutional funding and the National Center for Research Resources, Grant UL1 RR024975–01 (now at the National Center for Advancing Translational Sciences, Grant 2 UL1 TR000445–06).

Authors' contributions

DCC and NAR designed the study. NAR and EFE collected and prepared the data, and NAR and SL analyzed the data. NAR drafted the manuscript. DCC, SL, and EFE were major contributors in revising the manuscript critically for all important intellectual content. All authors gave approval to the final version of the manuscript and agreed to be accountable to all aspects of the work.

Competing interests

The authors declare that they have no competing interests.

Author details

¹Department of Population and Quantitative Health Sciences, Institute for Computational Biology, Case Western Reserve University, 2103 Cornell Road, Wolstein Research Building, Suite 2-527, Cleveland, OH 44106, USA. ²Eastern Virginia Medical School, Norfolk, VA, USA. ³Vanderbilt Institute for Clinical and Translational Research, Vanderbilt University Medical Center, Nashville, TN, USA.

References

1. The Eye Diseases Prevalence Research Group. Causes and prevalence of visual impairment among adults in the United States. Arch Ophthalmol. 2004;122(4):477–85. https://doi.org/10.1001/archopht.122.4.477.
2. Stein JD, Kim DS, Niziol LM, Talwar N, Nan B, Musch DC, et al. Differences in rates of glaucoma among Asian Americans and other racial groups, and among various asian ethnic groups. Ophthalmology. 2011;118(6):1031–7. https://doi.org/10.1016/j.ophtha.2010.10.024. PMC3109193
3. Friedman DS, Wolfs RC, O'Colmain BJ, Klein BE, Taylor HR, West S, et al. Prevalence of open-angle glaucoma among adults in the United States. Arch Ophthalmol. 2004;122(4):532–8. https://doi.org/10.1001/archopht. 122.4.532. PMC2798086
4. Quigley HA, Broman AT. The number of people with glaucoma worldwide in 2010 and 2020. Br J Ophthalmol. 2006;90(3):262–7. https://doi.org/10. 1136/bjo.2005.081224. PMC1856963
5. Ladapo JA, Kymes SM, Ladapo JA, Nwosu VC, Pasquale LR. Projected clinical outcomes of glaucoma screening in African American individuals. Arch Ophthalmol. 2012;130(3):365–72. https://doi.org/10.1001/archopthalmol.2011.1224.
6. Leske M, Connell AS, Wu S, Hyman LG, Schachat AP. Risk factors for open-angle glaucoma: the Barbados eye study. Arch Ophthalmol. 1995;113(7): 918–24. https://doi.org/10.1001/archopht.1995.01100070092031.
7. Pan C-W, Cheung CY, Aung T, Cheung C-M, Zheng Y-F, Wu R-Y, et al. Differential associations of myopia with major age-related eye diseases: the Singapore Indian eye study. Ophthalmology. 2013;120(2):284–91. https://doi. org/10.1016/j.ophtha.2012.07.065.
8. Chandrasekaran S, Cumming RG, Rochtchina E, Mitchell P. Associations between elevated intraocular pressure and Glaucoma, use of Glaucoma medications, and 5-year incident cataract: the Blue Mountains eye study. Ophthalmology. 2006; 113(3):417–24. https://doi.org/10.1016/j.ophtha.2005.10.050.
9. Jiang X, Varma R, Wu S, Torres M, Azen SP, Francis BA, et al. Baseline risk factors that predict the development of open-angle Glaucoma in a population: the Los Angeles Latino eye study. Ophthalmology. 2012;119(11): 2245–53. https://doi.org/10.1016/j.ophtha.2012.05.030. PMC3474872

10. Budde WM. Heredity in primary open-angle glaucoma. Curr Opin Ophthalmol. 2000;11(2):101–6.

11. Tielsch JM, Katz J, Sommer A, Quigley HA, Javitt JC. Family history and risk of primary open angle glaucoma: the Baltimore eye survey. Arch Ophthalmol. 1994;112(1):69–73. https://doi.org/10.1001/archopht.1994.01090130079022.

12. Freeman EE, Roy-Gagnon M-H, Descovich D, Massé H, Lesk MR. The heritability of glaucoma-related traits corneal hysteresis, central corneal thickness, intraocular pressure, and choroidal blood flow pulsatility. PLoS One. 2013;8(1):e55573. https://doi.org/10.1371/journal.pone.0055573. PMC3559508

13. van Koolwijk LME, Despriet DDG, van Duijn CM, Pardo Cortes LM, Vingerling JR, Aulchenko YS, et al. Genetic contributions to Glaucoma: heritability of intraocular pressure, retinal nerve Fiber layer thickness, and optic disc morphology. Invest Ophthalmol Vis Sci. 2007;48(8):3669–76. https://doi.org/10.1167/iovs.06-1519.

14. Charlesworth J, Kramer PL, Dyer T, Diego V, Samples JR, Craig JE, et al. The path to open-angle glaucoma gene discovery: endophenotypic status of intraocular pressure, cup-to-disc ratio, and central corneal thickness. Invest Ophthalmol Vis Sci. 2010;51(7):3509–14. https://doi.org/10.1167/iovs.09-4786. PMC2904007

15. Chang TC, Congdon NG, Wojciechowski R, Muñoz B, Gilbert D, Chen P, et al. Determinants and heritability of intraocular pressure and cup-to-disc ratio in a defined older population. Ophthalmology. 2005;112(7):1186–91. https://doi.org/10.1016/j.ophtha.2005.03.006. PMC3124001

16. Findl O, Rainer G, Dallinger S, Dorner G, Polak K, Kiss B, et al. Assessment of optic disk blood flow in patients with open-angle glaucoma. Am J Ophthalmol. 2000;130(5):589–96. https://doi.org/10.1016/S0002-9394(00)00636-X.

17. Fontana L, Poinoosawmy D, Bunce CV, O'Brien C, Hitchings RA. Pulsatile ocular blood flow investigation in asymmetric normal tension glaucoma and normal subjects. Br J Ophthalmol. 1998;82(7):731–6. https://doi.org/10.1136/bjo.82.7.731. PMC1722652

18. Stone EM, Fingert JH, Alward WLM, Nguyen TD, Polansky JR, Sunden SLF, et al. Identification of a gene that causes primary open angle Glaucoma. Science. 1997;275(5300):668–70. https://doi.org/10.1126/science.275.5300.668.

19. Rezaie T, Child A, Hitchings R, Brice G, Miller L, Coca-Prados M, et al. Adult-onset primary open-angle Glaucoma caused by mutations in Optineurin. Science. 2002;295(5557):1077–9. https://doi.org/10.1126/science.1066901.

20. Monemi S, Spaeth G, DaSilva A, Popinchalk S, Ilitchev E, Liebmann J, et al. Identification of a novel adult-onset primary open-angle glaucoma (POAG) gene on 5q22.1. Hum Mol Genet. 2005;14(6):725–33. https://doi.org/10.1093/hmg/ddi068.

21. Adam MF, Belmouden A, Binisti P, Brézin AP, Valtot F, Béchetoille A, et al. Recurrent mutations in a single exon encoding the evolutionarily conserved Olfactomedin-homology domain of TIGR in familial open-angle Glaucoma. Hum Mol Genet. 1997;6(12):2091–7. https://doi.org/10.1093/hmg/6.12.2091.

22. Suzuki Y, Shirato S, Taniguchi F, Ohara K, Nishimaki K, Ohta S. Mutations in the TIGR gene in familial primary open-angle Glaucoma in Japan. Am J Hum Genet. 1997;61(5):1202–4. https://doi.org/10.1086/301612. PMC1716051

23. Nakano M, Ikeda Y, Tokuda Y, Fuwa M, Omi N, Ueno M, et al. Common variants in CDKN2B-AS1 associated with optic-nerve vulnerability of glaucoma identified by genome-wide association studies in Japanese. PLoS One. 2012;7(3):e33389. https://doi.org/10.1371/journal.pone.0033389. PMC3299784

24. Osman W, Low SK, Takahashi A, Kubo M, Nakamura Y. A genome-wide association study in the Japanese population confirms 9p21 and 14q23 as susceptibility loci for primary open angle glaucoma. Hum Mol Genet. 2012;21(12):2836–42. https://doi.org/10.1093/hmg/dds103.

25. Wiggs JL, Yaspan BL, Hauser MA, Kang JH, Allingham RR, Olson LM, et al. Common variants at 9p21 and 8q22 are associated with increased susceptibility to optic nerve degeneration in Glaucoma. PLoS Genet. 2012;8(4):e1002654. https://doi.org/10.1371/journal.pgen.1002654. PMC3342074

26. Thorleifsson G, Walters GB, Hewitt AW, Masson G, Helgason A, DeWan A, et al. Common variants near CAV1 and CAV2 are associated with primary open-angle glaucoma. Nat Genet. 2010;42(10):906–9. https://doi.org/10.1038/ng.661. PMC3222888

27. Li Z, Allingham RR, Nakano M, Jia L, Chen Y, Ikeda Y, et al. A common variant near TGFBR3 is associated with primary open angle glaucoma. Hum Mol Genet. 2015;24(13):3880–92. https://doi.org/10.1093/hmg/ddv128. PMC4459396

28. Liu W, Liu Y, Challa P, Herndon LW, Wiggs JL, Girkin CA, et al. Low prevalence of myocilin mutatons in an African American population wiht primary open-angle glaucoma. Mol Vision. 2012;18:2241–6. PMC3429360

29. Matise TC, Ambite JL, Buyske S, Carlson CS, Cole SA, Crawford DC, et al. The next PAGE in understanding complex traits: design for the analysis of population architecture using genetics and epidemiology (PAGE) study. Am J Epidemiol. 2011;174(7):849–59. https://doi.org/10.1093/aje/kwr160. PMC3176830

30. Buyske S, Wu Y, Carty CL, Cheng I, Assimes TL, Dumitrescu L, et al. Evaluation of the Metabochip genotyping Array in African Americans and implications for fine mapping of GWAS-identified Loci: the PAGE study. PLoS One. 2012;7(4):e35651. https://doi.org/10.1371/journal.pone.0035651. PMC3335090

31. Roden DM, Pulley JM, Basford MA, Bernard GR, Clayton EW, Balser JR, et al. Development of a large-scale De-identified DNA biobank to enable personalized medicine. Clin Pharmacol Ther. 2008;84(3):362–9. https://doi.org/10.1038/clpt.2008.89. PMC3763939

32. Pulley J, Clayton E, Bernard GR, Roden DM, Masys DR. Principles of Human Subjects Protections Applied in an Opt-Out, De-identified Biobank. Clin Transl Sci. 2010;3(1):42–8. https://doi.org/10.1111/j.1752-8062.2010.00175.x. PMC3075971

33. Crawford DC, Goodloe R, Farber-Eger E, Boston J, Pendergrass SA, Haines JL, et al. Leveraging epidemiologic and clinical collections for genomic studies of complex traits. Hum Hered. 2015;79(3–4):137–46. https://doi.org/10.1159/000381805. PMC4528966

34. Restrepo NA, Farber-Eger E, Goodloe R, Haines JL, Crawford DC. Extracting primary open-angle glaucoma from electronic medical records for genetic association studies. PLoS One. 2015;10(6):e0127817. https://doi.org/10.1371/journal.pone.0127817. PMC4465698

35. Voight BF, Kang HM, Ding J, Palmer CD, Sidore C, Chines PS, et al. The Metabochip, a custom genotyping array for genetic studies of metabolic, cardiovascular, and anthropometric traits. PLoS Genet. 2012;8(8):e1002793. https://doi.org/10.1371/journal.pgen.1002793. PMC3410907

36. Crawford DC, Goodloe R, Brown-Gentry K, Wilson S, Robberson J, Gillani NB, et al. Characterization of the Metabochip in diverse populations from the International HapMap Project in the Epidemiologic Architecture for Genes Linked to Environment (EAGLE) Project. Pac Symp Biocomput. 2013;18:188–99. PMC3584704

37. Price AL, Patterson NJ, Plenge RM, Weinblatt ME, Shadick NA, Reich D. Principal components analysis corrects for stratification in genome-wide association studies. Nat Genet. 2006;38(8):904–9.

38. Patterson N, Price AL, Reich D. Population structure and Eigenanalysis. PLoS Genet. 2006;2(12):e190. https://doi.org/10.1371/journal.pgen.0020190.

39. Purcell S, Neale B, Todd-Brown K, Thomas L, Ferreira MA, Bender D, et al. PLINK: a tool for whole-genome association and population-based linkage analysis. Am J Hum Genet. 2007;81(3):559–75.

40. Johnson AD, Handsaker RE, Pulit S, Nizzari MM, ODonnell CJ, de Bakker PI. SNAP: a web-based tool for identification and annotation of proxy SNPs using HapMap. Bioinformatics. 2008;24(24):2938–9. https://doi.org/10.1093/bioinformatics/btn564. PMC2720775

41. Gauderman WJ. Sample size requirements for association studies of gene-gene interaction. Am J Epidemiol. 2002;155(5):478–84.

42. Baran Y, Pasaniuc B, Sankararaman S, Torgerson DG, Gignoux C, Eng C, et al. Fast and accurate inference of local ancestry in Latino populations. Bioinformatics. 2012;28(10):1359–67. https://doi.org/10.1093/bioinformatics/bts144. PMC3348558

43. R: A language and environment for statistical computing. Vienna, Austria: R Foundation for Statistical Computing; 2013.

44. Raj A, Stephens M, Pritchard JK. fastSTRUCTURE: Variational inference of population structure in large SNP data sets. Genetics. 2014;197(2):573–89. https://doi.org/10.1534/genetics.114.164350. PMC4063916

45. Francis RM. pophelper: an R package and web app to analyse and visualize population structure. Mol Ecol Resour. 2017;17(1):27–32. https://doi.org/10.1111/1755-0998.12509.

46. Parra EJ, Marcini A, Akey J, Martinson J, Batzer MA, Cooper R, et al. Estimating African American admixture proportions by use of population-specific alleles. Am J Hum Genet. 1998;63(6):1839–51. https://doi.org/10.1086/302148. PMC1377655

47. Baharian S, Barakatt M, Gignoux CR, Shringarpure S, Errington J, Blot WJ, et al. The great migration and African-American genomic diversity. PLoS Genet. 2016;12(5):e1006059. https://doi.org/10.1371/journal.pgen.1006059. PMC4883799

48. Willer CJ, Sanna S, Jackson AU, Scuteri A, Bonnycastle LL, Clarke R, et al. Newly identified loci that influence lipid concentrations and risk of coronary artery disease. Nat Genet. 2008;40(2):161–9. https://doi.org/10.1038/ng.76. PMC5206900

49. Kathiresan S, Melander O, Guiducci C, Surti A, Burtt NP, Rieder MJ, et al. Six new loci associated with blood low-density lipoprotein cholesterol, high-density lipoprotein cholesterol or triglycerides in humans. Nat Genet. 2008; 40(2):189–97. https://doi.org/10.1038/ng.75. PMC2682493

50. Beecham GW, Hamilton K, Naj AC, Martin ER, Huentelman M, Myers AJ, et al. Genome-wide association meta-analysis of neuropathologic features of Alzheimer's disease and related dementias. PLoS Genet. 2014;10(9): e1004606. https://doi.org/10.1371/journal.pgen.1004606. PMC4154667

51. Pasquale LR, Loomis SJ, Kang JH, Yaspan BL, Abdrabou W, Budenz DL, et al. CDKN2B-AS1 genotype–glaucoma feature correlations in primary open-angle glaucoma patients from the United States. Am J Ophthalmol. 2013; 155(2):342–53.e5. https://doi.org/10.1016/j.ajo.2012.07.023. PMC3544983

52. Williams SE, Carmichael TR, Allingham RR, Hauser M, Ramsay M. The genetics of POAG in black South Africans: a candidate gene association study. Sci Rep. 2015;5:8378. https://doi.org/10.1038/srep08378. PMC4323640

53. Cao D, Jiao X, Liu X, Hennis A, Leske MC, Nemesure B, et al. CDKN2B polymorphism is associated with primary open-angle glaucoma (POAG) in the Afro-Caribbean population of Barbados, West Indies. PLoS One. 2012; 7(6):e39278. https://doi.org/10.1371/journal.pone.0039278. PMC3384655

54. Jandrot-Perrus M, Busfield S, Lagrue A-H, Xiong X, Debili N, Chickering T, et al. Cloning, characterization, and functional studies of human and mouse glycoprotein VI: a platelet-specific collagen receptor from the immunoglobulin superfamily. Blood. 2000;96(5):1798-807.

55. Lonsdale J, Thomas J, Salvatore M, Phillips R, Lo E, Shad S, et al. The Genotype-Tissue Expression (GTEx) project. Nat Genet. 2013;45(6):580-85.

56. Yu NY-L, Hallström BM, Fagerberg L, Ponten F, Kawaji H, Carninci P, Forrest ARR. The FANTOM Consortium, Yoshihide Hayashizaki, Mathias Uhlén, Carsten O. Daub. Complementing tissue characterization by integrating transcriptome profiling from the Human Protein Atlas and from the FANTOM5 consortium. Nucleic Acids Res. 2015;43(14):6787-98.

57. Arjunan P, Gnanaprakasam JP, Ananth S, Romej MA, Rajalakshmi V-K, Prasad PD, Martin PM, Gurusamy M, Thangaraju M, Bhutia YD, Ganapathy V. Increased Retinal Expression of the Pro-Angiogenic Receptor GPR91 via BMP6 in a Mouse Model of Juvenile Hemochromatosis. Investigative Opthalmology & Visual Science. 2016;57(4):1612.

58. Popejoy AB, Fullerton SM. Genomics is failing on diversity. Nature 2016; 538(7624):161-164

9

Genomic analyses based on pulmonary adenocarcinoma in situ reveal early lung cancer signature

Dan Li[1,2], William Yang[3], Yifan Zhang[2], Jack Y Yang[2], Renchu Guan[1,2], Dong Xu[1,4] and Mary Qu Yang[2*]

From Selected articles from the IEEE BIBM International Conference on Bioinformatics & Biomedicine (BIBM) 2017: medical genomics
Kansas City, MO, USA. 13-16 November 2017

Abstract

Background: Non-small cell lung cancer (NSCLC) represents more than about 80% of the lung cancer. The early stages of NSCLC can be treated with complete resection with a good prognosis. However, most cases are detected at late stage of the disease. The average survival rate of the patients with invasive lung cancer is only about 4%. Adenocarcinoma in situ (AIS) is an intermediate subtype of lung adenocarcinoma that exhibits early stage growth patterns but can develop into invasion.

Methods: In this study, we used RNA-seq data from normal, AIS, and invasive lung cancer tissues to identify a gene module that represents the distinguishing characteristics of AIS as AIS-specific genes. Two differential expression analysis algorithms were employed to identify the AIS-specific genes. Then, the subset of the best performed AIS-specific genes for the early lung cancer prediction were selected by random forest. Finally, the performances of the early lung cancer prediction were assessed using random forest, support vector machine (SVM) and artificial neural networks (ANNs) on four independent early lung cancer datasets including one tumor-educated blood platelets (TEPs) dataset.

Results: Based on the differential expression analysis, 107 AIS-specific genes that consisted of 93 protein-coding genes and 14 long non-coding RNAs (lncRNAs) were identified. The significant functions associated with these genes include angiogenesis and ECM-receptor interaction, which are highly related to cancer development and contribute to the smoking-free lung cancers. Moreover, 12 of the AIS-specific lncRNAs are involved in lung cancer progression by potentially regulating the ECM-receptor interaction pathway. The feature selection by random forest identified 20 of the AIS-specific genes as early stage lung cancer signatures using the dataset obtained from The Cancer Genome Atlas (TCGA) lung adenocarcinoma samples. Of the 20 signatures, two were lncRNAs, BLACAT1 and CTD-2527I21.15 which have been reported to be associated with bladder cancer, colorectal cancer and breast cancer. In blind classification for three independent tissue sample datasets, these signature genes consistently yielded about 98% accuracy for distinguishing early stage lung cancer from normal cases. However, the prediction accuracy for the blood platelets samples was only 64.35% (sensitivity 78.1%, specificity 50.59%, and AUROC 0.747).

(Continued on next page)

---

* Correspondence: mqyang@ualr.edu
[2]MidSouth Bioinformatics Center and Joint Bioinformatics Ph.D. Program of University of Arkansas at Little Rock and Univ. of Arkansas Medical Sciences, 2801 S. Univ. Ave, Little Rock, AR 72204, USA
Full list of author information is available at the end of the article

(Continued from previous page)

Conclusions: The comparison of AIS with normal and invasive tumor revealed diseases-specific genes and offered new insights into the mechanism underlying AIS progression into an invasive tumor. These genes can also serve as the signatures for early diagnosis of lung cancer with high accuracy. The expression profile of gene signatures identified from tissue cancer samples yielded remarkable early cancer prediction for tissues samples, however, relatively lower accuracy for boold platelets samples.

Keywords: Adenocarcinoma in situ, AIS, Lung cancer, Invasive, Early diagnosis, lncRNAs

Background

Lung cancer is one of the most common cancer types and the main cause of cancer-related deaths. About 14% of all new cancers are lung cancers, and about 154,050 deaths from lung cancer are estimated in the United States for 2018 by the American Cancer Society. Non-small cell lung cancer accounts for about 80% of the lung cancer cases and is consist of various subtypes [1]. Generally, most of the deaths caused by lung cancer are in late stages which are due to the distant metastasis and invasion [2]. In contrast, the early stages or non-invasive subtypes of lung cancer can be cured [2].

Lung adenocarcinoma in situ is a subtype of NSCLC and shows non-invasive growth patterns. The 5-year survival rate of AIS is almost 100% with appropriate therapy [3]. However, AIS can develop into an invasive stage of lung cancer that has only approximate 4% patient survival rate [1]. AIS is different from the other lung cancer histologies in that most AIS patients are non-smokers and women [4, 5]. Previous studies of AIS, for purposes of classification and diagnosis, have indicated differences in appearance from these and other types of lung cancer. The studies of AIS at the genetic level have not yet been widely performed, consequenctly, our understanding of the mechanism that causes AIS is limited. On the other hand, AIS cases could be missed diagnosed as pneumonia since sometimes AIS has a varied appearance on CT [6] and generally 62% of the AIS patients do not have symptoms [7]. Similarly, early stage lung cancer often is asymptomatic.

Previous studies have identified gene biomarkers involved in lung cancer progression and development [8], including several critical long non-coding RNAs [2, 9, 10]. More effective and robust molecular biomarkers for early lung cancer diagnosis remained to be uncovered. Currently, studies on AIS progression based on RNA sequencing techniques were performed. Some protein-coding genes and lncRNAs that related to AIS were identified [3] and indicated the evolution of lung cancer from normal to invasive stages. However, large-scale study and comparison of these genes at different disease stage of cancer development are not exploited.

In this study, we first identified the genes that were specifically expressed in AIS tissue samples compared

with normal and invasive cancer cases simultaneously. The differential expression analysis was performed by using two computational methods, the most widely used edgeR [11] and the newly developed Cross-Value Association Analysis (CVAA) [12]. The combined results of these two methods were used for downstream analysis. Only a small group of genes (107) including both protein-coding genes (94) and lncRNAs (13) were found that potentially dominate the AIS and the invasive progression (Additional file 1: Figure S1). Smoking is considered one of the most risk factors that cause lung cancers and about 75% of the lung cancer cases are attributable to tobacco use. The lung cancer in never smokers even considered as different diseases [5]. The AIS-specific genes were significantly enriched of lung cancer related functional annotations such as angiogenesis [13, 14] and the ECM-receptor interaction which is a known pathway contributes the smoke-free lung cancers [15–17]. We further identified 20 early lung cancer signature genes that can be used for distinguishing the early lung cancer cases from normal ones. In particular, we performed an experiment using the random forest method on four independent datasets generated by RNA-seq or microarray techniques and achieved about 98% prediction accuracy for early stage lung cancer in tissue samples but only 64.35% overall accuracy in the blood platelets dataset.

Our results suggested that AIS-specific genes could help us to better understand this uncommon lung cancer subtype. The AIS-specfic genes may also play a critical role in the lung cancer progression. Moreover, the expression profiles of early lung cancer signature genes we identified showed the ability for accurate and robust early cancer prediction.

Results

Comparison of gene expression in AIS and invasive lung cancer

To investigate the genes that dominate the intermediate type of AIS and underlie different phenotypes (normal, AIS and invasive cancer cases), we collected the RNA-seq library (GSE52248) consisted of normal, AIS and invasive cancer samples of six lung cancer patients [3]. The raw RNA-seq data were generated from formalin fixation and paraffin embedding (FFPE) processed tissues. First, the RNA-seq data were processed and the gene expression profile was calculated referring the gene annotation from Ensembl (Methods). Then, the differential expression analysis via edgeR was performed on 16,501 expressed genes consisted of 15,106 protein-coding genes and 1395 lncRNAs. As a result, 1348 significant differentially expressed genes (DEGs) were found between normal and invasive lung cancer samples under the threshold |log2 fold change| > 1 & FDR < 0.05. Based on the same thresholds, 719 DEGs between normal and AIS cases as well as 98 DEGs between AIS and invasive cancer tissues were identified. The gene expression patterns in AIS and invasive cancer tissues demonstrated much more consistency (Additional file 1: Figure S1) despite these two phenotypes was with great differences. Our results indicated that only a small number of genes potentially dominated the evolution of lung cancer from AIS into invasive lung cancer.

Identification of AIS-specific genes

To comprehensively identify the gene set that was specifically expressed in AIS tissue, we applied two differential expression analysis methods, edgeR [11] and CVAA [12], based on the gene expression profiles of paired normal and AIS, AIS and invasive cancer samples. The edgeR is one of the most widely used differential expression (DE) analysis method, while CVAA is a newly developed normalization-free and nonparametric DE analysis method. Unlike the commonly used DE analysis methods, CVAA neither normalizes nor assumes the distribution of the gene expressions. Instead, it reveals the DEGs according to the gene expression comparison and ranking. The DEGs between normal and AIS that, at the same time were differentially expressed in invasive cancer compared with AIS samples were further used as the candidates for AIS-specific genes (Methods). The union set of the DEGs identified by the two methods was collected. As a result, a total of 107 (22 upregulated and 85 downregulated) genes including 93 protein-coding genes and 14 long non-coding RNAs were identified as AIS-specific genes (Methods, Additional file 2: Table S1).

LncRNAs potentially regulate ECM-receptor interaction pathway and involved in lung cancer

We applied the function annotation via David [18] on the 93 protein-coding genes and found a number of enriched functions (Additional file 3: Table S2), including angiogenesis and ECM-receptor interaction which shows the aggressiveness of the tumor and has an important role in metastasis [13, 14]. A previous study of lung cancer [17] indicated that non-smokers also have the risk of the lung cancer. Some well-known cancer-related pathways such as

cell cycle and p53 were enriched of differentially expressed genes in only current smoke patients, whereas ECM-receptor interaction pathway is over-represented in the patients that never smoke and is considered to contribute to smoking-independent lung cancer [17]. Interestingly, it has been found that AIS is more common in women and non-smokers [3] and the disrupted ECM-receptor interaction pathway was also found based on the AIS data in our study. Many ECM proteins are factors that promote the metastatic cascade as they are significantly deregulated during the progression of cancer [16].

The ECM-receptor interaction pathway contains 87 protein-coding genes and three of them (*CD36, SPP1, TNR*) are AIS-specific. We further employed GENIE3 (Gene Network Inference with Ensemble of trees) [19] to predict the regulatory relationships between the 14 AIS-specific lncRNAs and the 87 genes (Methods). As a result, 12 lncRNAs were found to potentially regulate the genes in ECM-receptor interaction pathway (Additional file 4: Figure S2), suggesting their roles in the lung cancer progression. Moreover, the odd ratios of the regulations between the lncRNAs and the ECM-receptor interaction pathway indicated novel lncRNAs, such as FENDRR (OR = 1.53), MEOX2-AIS (OR = 3.22), as regulators interact with this pathway (Methods). Collectively, these results suggested that the AIS-specific genes played critical roles in the progression of AIS and the development of invasive lung cancer.

Early lung cancer signatures identification

AIS is a pre-invasive lung adenocarcinoma lesion. Hence, the AIS-specific genes can potentially serve as gene signatures for early lung cancer detection. We employed random forest for selecting the top genes from the 107 AIS-specific genes that can effectively distinguish normal from early-stage cancer cases (Methods). Using the gene expression profiles of the normal (n = 59) and early-stage (stage I) lung adenocarcinoma cases (n = 286) from TCGA project, random forest reported the importance of each gene by calculating the classification error rate. We found that one gene set composed of 20 genes yielded the lowest error rate (1.16%). Therefore, these 20 genes including two lncRNAs (BLACAT1, CTD-2527I21.15) ranked by the importance scores of random forest were considered to be early lung cancer diagnosis signatures and were used for further validation and analysis (Additional file 5: Table S3). Of the 20 gene signatures, 13 were continually downregulated along with the lung cancer progression from normal to AIS to invasive. In contrast, the expression levels of the other seven genes were significantly increased (Fig. 1) indicating their lung cancer-related functions. Interestingly, all the 20 genes were discovered by CVAA indicating the power of this new method and the necessity of the comprehensively identification of DEGs.

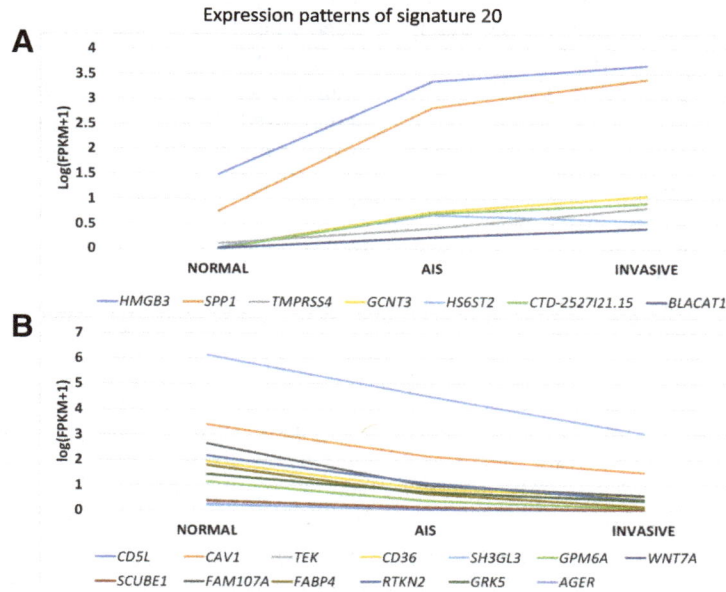

Fig. 1 The gene expression patterns of the 20 early lung cancer signatures. A, seven genes including the two lncRNAs were upregulated along with the lung cancer progression from normal to invasive. B, 13 genes were continually downregulated

Early lung cancer signatures provide insights into early lung cancer diagnosis

A large portion of early-stage NSCLC can be cured [2]. Lung cancer deaths are mainly caused by the distant metastases that drive cancer into late stages [2]. Early diagnosis of lung cancer is critical for patient survival and treatment. The expression patterns of our 20 early lung cancer signatures were distinct between the normal and early stage of the TCGA lung adenocarcinoma samples (Fig. 2) suggesting their potential capability for

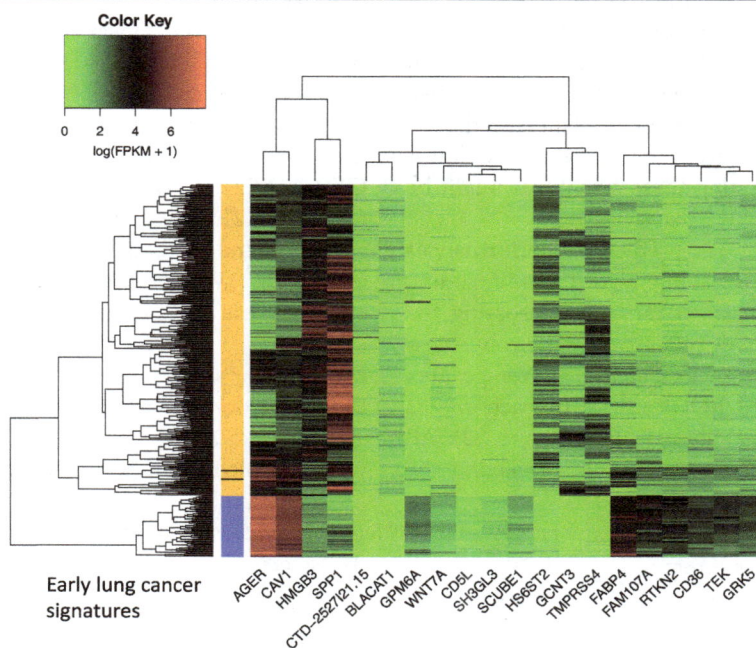

Fig. 2 The expressions of the 20 early lung cancer signatures in TCGA lung adenocarcinoma normal (59, blue) and early (286, gold, stage I) cases

early lung cancer prediction. We next examined the effectiveness of these biomarkers by employing widely used machine learning classification algorithms.

We first applied random forest [20] for detecting the early lung cancer cases (Methods). The gene expression profile of TCGA lung adenocarcinoma dataset consisting of 59 normal and 286 early samples that reported as stage I were downloaded. The expression patterns of the signature genes of this dataset were shown in Fig. 2. The average prediction accuracy of the random forest model was 98.86% (Table 1, Method) based on the expression profiles of these signature genes.

We then collected the second independent early lung cancer dataset: GSE68465 [21] which was generated using the microarray platform (HG-U133A). The dataset consisted of 276 early (stage IA and IB) lung cancer and 19 normal samples. Two lncRNAs (BLACAT1, CTD-2527I21.15) and three protein-coding genes (*SCUBE1, HS6ST2, RTKN2*) of the signatures were not included in this dataset. We achieved 99.51% prediction accuracy, 99.95% sensitivity, and 92.83% specificity in average for this dataset (Table 1). The third dataset (GSE10072) [22] was also microarray platform-based and contained 58 lung cancer and 49 normal cases. The patients were grouped into never, former, and current smokers by their smoking behaviors. Using the expression profile of same genes as the second dataset, we obtained 97.91% accuracy for lung cancer case prediction (sensitivity = 98.05%, specificity = 97.75%).

Blood-based liquid biopsies provide promising non-invasive cancer detection. Blood-based biomarkers have been studied and identified [23]. Based on the age-matched tumor-educated blood platelets (TEPs) early lung cancer samples (GSE89843) [23], we assessed the effectiveness of our 20 gene signatures identified from tissue samples on these TEPs data (Methods). However, the prediction accuracy is relatively lower (64.35%), (Table 1), suggesting these signatures might be tissue-specific.

We further examined the prediction performances using different machine learning algorithms including random forest, SVM [24], and ANNs [25] crossing the four datasets. To comprehensively measure the robustness of our signature genes, we calculated the average area under an ROC curve (AUROC) values of each model for each dataset (Fig. 3, Additional file 6: Figure S3). All the machine learning models succeed in predicting the

early lung cancer tissue samples, excepting the ANNs based model for GSE68465. GSE68465 contained unbalance samples size (19 normal vs. 276 tumor, Methods). In summary, the early lung cancer signature genes we identified showed the robustness and high accuracy for distinguishing normal and early lung cancer cases.

The early lung cancer signature genes were highly lung cancer related

We conducted further literature search and found that majority early lung cancer signature genes we identified were reported to be highly associated with cancer progression, diagnosis, therapy, and patient overall survival. All the 18 protein-coding genes were found to be directly involved in lung cancer development suggested by previous studies (Additional file 5: Table S3). For instance, the protein-coding genes *CD36* [26] and *TMPRSS4* [27] were already identified as potential therapeutic targets of lung cancer, while *TMPRSS4* can induce cancer stem cell-like properties in lung cancer [28]. *HMGB3* and *FABP4* showed their high diagnostic and prognostic value in human NSCLC [29, 30]. *SPP1*, *AGER*, and *RTKN2* regulate the lung cancer-related pathways such as VEGF (vascular endothelial growth factor) signaling pathway and NF-kappaB [31, 32]. The loss of *WNT7A* is a major contributing factor for increased lung cancer tumorigenesis [33]. The expression level of *FAM107A* is decreased in patients with NSCLC [34], whereas the high levels of expression of *HS6ST2* are observed in lung cancer cell lines [35].

The associations of the two lncRNAs and NSCLC are not reported yet. The lncRNA BLACAT1 (Bladder Cancer Associated Transcript 1) was up-regulated in bladder cancer. BLACAT1 also affects cell proliferation, indicates a prognosis of colorectal cancer and is significantly associated with poor overall survival [36]. Our results suggested diagnostic value of BLACAT1 for NSCLC. The other lncRNA CTD-2527I21.15 is a basal-like breast cancer marker. CTD-2527I21.15 locates adjacently to FXYD3 in chromosome 19 and potentially cis-regulates its expression in cancer [37]. Moreover, our results indicated combinatory effect of these genes for early lung cancer diagnosis.

Methods
Data collection and processes
The raw RNA-seq data of the AIS cases (GSE52248) were downloaded. The low-quality reads were trimmed

Table 1 The early lung cancer prediction performances on four different datasets using random forest

Model	Assessment	TCGA	GSE68465	GSE10072	GSE89843 (Blood)
Random Forest	Accuracy	98.68%	99.51%	97.91%	64.35%
	Sensitivity	99.28%	99.95%	98.05%	78.12%
	Specificity	95.68%	92.83%	97.75%	50.59%

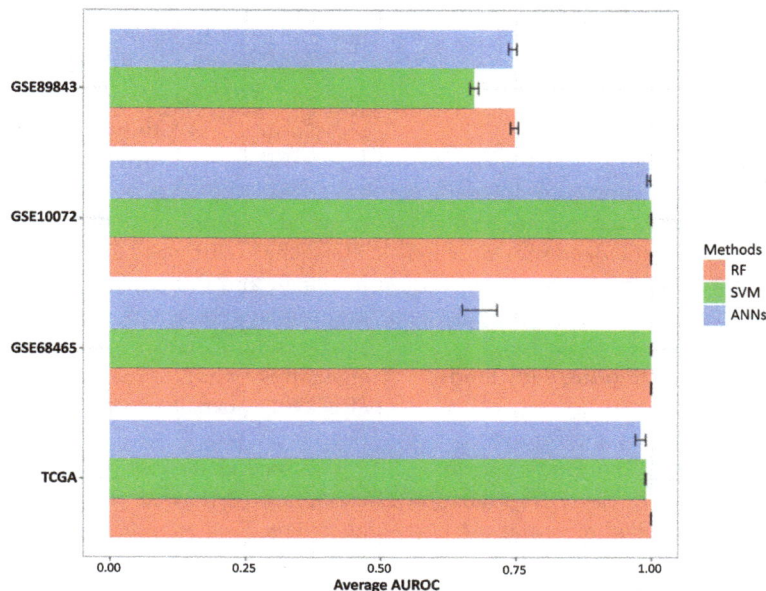

Fig. 3 The performance assessments for early lung cancer prediction using random forest, SVM and artificial neural networks for four lung cancer datasets. The AUROC were calculated based on 100 boostrapping tests.

via Trimmomatic version 0.36 [38]. The human gene annotation of Ensembl was used. We applied STAR (v2.4) [39] followed by Cufflinks (v2.2.1) [40] to calculate the gene expressions. The other four independent lung cancer datasets were TCGA lung adenocarcinoma, GSE68465, and GSE10072 of which the gene expression profiles were available and GSE89843 which was a blood platelets RNA-seq library. The TCGA lung adenocarcinoma dataset was consisted of 596 samples. In this study, only the 59 normal samples and the 286 early lung cancer (stage I) samples were used for the analysis. The dataset GSE68465 was generated by microarray platform HG-U133A and collected from 6 contributing treatment institutions. The patients were around 64 years old on average and 42.3% of the patients were dead in about 4 years after the clinical report. Here, only the gene expression profiles of 19 normal samples and 276 early (stage IA and IB) lung cancer samples were used for the prediction. GSE10072 was also a microarray data and the fresh frozen lung cancer tissue samples were collected from patients with never (20), former (26), and current (28) by smoking behaviors. Additional 49 normal samples were used as control. All the samples were generated by Environment and Genetics in Lung Cancer Etiology (EAGLE). The RNA-seq data of the blood platelets of 53 early locally advanced NSCLC patients were collected from the study of GSE89843 [23]. The other 53 healthy age-matched (range from 48 to 86) samples in the same study were used as normal controls for the prediction. The gene expressions (FPKM) were calculated using the raw RNA-seq reads.

Differentially expressed gene identification

The read counts of the genes were calculated by HTSeq-count (v0.6.1) [41]. Then, the R package edgeR was applied for differential expression analysis between the samples of various types. The threshold $|\log2$ fold change $> 1|$ & FDR < 0.05 was used in our study for defining significantly differentially expressed genes. The R package of the CVAA (version 0.1.0) method was obtained from the author and applied under the default setting [12]. The genes were ranked by CVAA based on the significance of the differential expression. We selected the same number of the top CVAA DEGs and the top edgeR DEGs for the further analysis. The individual sets of AIS-specific genes identified by edgeR and CVAA were combined together.

CVAA is a normalization-free and nonparametric method that identifies DEGs.

Regulation prediction by GENIE3

GEne Network Inference with Ensemble of trees (GENIE3) calculates the regulatory relationships between genes based on the expression patterns [19]. The gene expression profile of normal and early stage of the TCGA lung adenocarcinoma sample was used. The 14 AIS-specific lncRNAs were considered as regulators while all the protein-coding genes were used as potential target genes. All the regulations between lncRNAs and protein-coding genes were ranked by the weight (Additional file 7: Figure S4) and only the regulations over the third quartile of all the weights were considered as confident regulations.

The odd ratios were calculated as:

$$OR = \frac{P_I R_T / P_I R_N}{P_O R_T / P_O R_N}$$

Where $P_I R_T$ represents the number of the target genes of a given lncRNA that in (I) the ECM-receptor interaction pathway (P) whereas $P_I R_N$ represents the non-target genes in the pathway. $P_O R_T$ and $P_O R_N$ in the denominator stand for the number of target and non-target genes outside of (O) the pathway, respectively.

Machine learning models for predicting the early lung cancer

Random forest allows for measuring the importance of the features, which are the genes in our study, for classification. The function of random forest cross-validation for feature selection (rfcv) was applied to reveal the best gene set for the cancer cases prediction. We used the arguments: 5-fold cross-validation, log scale, and 0.9 step which means 10% of the features were removed at each step of testing.

Then we compared classification performances of three machine learning models, random forest, SVM, and ANNs. Random Forest is an ensemble learning method that can be used for classification. The random-Forest package [20] was used with 1000 trees and seed 115 for reproducibility. The e1071 is one widely used R package for performing SVM [24]. The tune function was used for detecting the best parameters of cost and gamma of SVM. The package neuralnet was used for performing the ANNs [25]. Here, we used two hidden layers with 50 and 25 neurons respectively. For each dataset, we randomly selected 2/3 of the samples as training set and the other 1/3 as testing set. Then, the average assessments of the accuracy, sensitivity, specificity, and the area under the receiver operating characteristic curve (AUROC) were calculated by running the experiment 100 times.

Discussions

AIS cases represent the minority of lung cancer cases, however, they provide valuable information about early diagnosis and treatment of the disease. With more attention and the availability of NGS data of AIS cases, we expect more comprehensive analysis for lung cancer can be conducted.

The identification of the differentially expressed genes is critical in cancer studies. Several computational methods for differential expression analysis were developed [11, 12, 40, 42]. Most of these methods are normalized based and assume the distribution of the gene expression profile. On the other hand, the results of these differential expression analysis methods are often not consistent. Here, in addition to apply edgeR, we

employed the newly developed CVAA, a normalization free and nonparametric approach for differential expression analysis. Out of 719 significant DEGs between normal and AIS cases identified by edgeR and CVAA, the overlap rate was about 50% on average (Additional file 8: Figure S5A). Moreover, less than 20% of 98 DEGs between AIS and invasive lung cancer were common genes revealed by both methods (Additional file 8: Figure S5B). Thus, the union set of the AIS-specific genes identified by edgeR and CVAA can provide a more comprehensive and robust gene set as candidate involved in lung cancer progression. Interestingly, the 20 early lung cancer gene signatures, which are the most discriminative genes in classifying normal and early cancer cases, were all identified by CVAA.

The second dataset (GSE68465) is unbalanced, which contained 19 normal samples and 276 lung cancer samples. The prediction performances of the ANNs model was poor compared with random forest and SVM for this data, suggesting performance of ANNs was impacted more by unbalanced dataset. The performance of ANNs on unbalanced data might be improved by optimizing paramters.

Tumor is highly heterogeneous and poses significant challenges in diagnosis and treatment. The gene expression profiles were different between two subtypes of the same tumor or between tissue and liquid sample types from the same patients. Our finding in this study indicted the limitation of the biomarkers that identified from tissue lung cancer samples for predicting the blood-based data.

Conclusions

In this study, we identified the AIS-specific genes that potentially dominate the lung cancer procession from AIS into the invasive tumor. A further analysis of these specific genes in AIS revealed their essential functions and properties in diverse types of lung cancer tissues. We also identified several novel lncRNAs that were involved in lung cancer by interacting with the lung cancer-related pathways. Twenty early lung cancer signature genes were identified. A cross assessment based on diverse machine learning models and independent datasets indicated our signatures were robust for early lung cancer prediction. These signature genes were highly lung cancer-related, and the combined gene group showed the capability to improve the early lung cancer diagnosis with high accuracy.

Additional files

Additional file 1: Figure S1. Gene expression comparison between normal, AIS, and invasion lung cancer cases.

Additional file 2: Table S1. List of the 107 AIS-specific genes.

Additional file 3: Table S2. The functional annotations of the 107 AIS-specific genes.

Additional file 4: Figure S2. The AIS-specific lncRNAs that potentially regulate the target genes in ECM-receptor interaction pathway.

Additional file 5: Table S3. List of the 20 early lung cancer signature genes and their cancer related functions.

Additional file 6: Figure S3. An example ROC curve of three machine learning algorithms on TCGA lung adenocarcinoma dataset. The AUROC values were calculated based on one of the 100 randomly selected training and testing datasets.

Additional file 7: Figure S4. The distribution of the regulatory weights calculated by GENIE3.

Additional file 8: Figure S5. Consistency comparison between the two differential expression analysis methods.

Abbreviations

AIS: Adenocarcinoma in situ; ANNs: Artificial neural networks; AUROC: Average area under an ROC curve; BLACAT1: Bladder Cancer Associated Transcript 1; CVAA: Cross-Value Association Analysis; DE: Differential expression; DEGs: Differentially expressed genes; FFPE: Formalin fixation and paraffin embedding; GENIE3: Gene Network Inference with Ensemble of trees; lncRNA: Long non-coding RNAs; NSCLC: Non-small cell lung cancer; SVM: Support vector machine; TCGA: The Cancer Genome Atlas; TEPs: Tumor-educated blood platelets

Acknowledgements

This research was supported by United States National Institutes of Health (NIH) Academic Research Enhancement Award 1R15GM114739 and National Institute of General Medical Sciences (NIH/NIGMS) 5P20GM103429, United States Food and Drug Administration (FDA) HHSF223201510172C and HHSF223201610111C and Arkansas Science and Technology Authority (ASTA) Basic Science Research 15-B-23 and 15-B-38. However, the information contained herein represents the position of the author(s) and not necessarily that of the NIH and FDA.

Funding

The publication cost of this article was funded by United States National Institutes of Health (NIH) Academic Research Enhancement Award 1R15GM114739.

Authors' contributions

MQY and DX conceived the project, DL and MQY designed the experiments. DL and WY conducted the experiments. DL performed the analysis. YZ, JY and RG participate in discussion. All authors have read and approved final manuscript.

Competing interest

The authors declare that they have no competing interests.

Author details

[1]Key Laboratory of Symbolic Computation and Knowledge Engineering of Ministry of Education, College of Computer Science & Technology, Jilin University, Changchun 130012, China. [2]MidSouth Bioinformatics Center and Joint Bioinformatics Ph.D. Program of University of Arkansas at Little Rock and Univ. of Arkansas Medical Sciences, 2801 S. Univ. Ave, Little Rock, AR 72204, USA. [3]Department of Computer Science, Carnegie Mellon University School of Computer Science, 5000 Forbes Ave, Pittsburgh, PA 15213, USA. [4]Department of Electrical Engineering and Computer Science, Informatics Institute, and Christopher S. Bond Life Sciences Center, University of Missouri, Columbia, MO 65211, USA.

References

1. Travis WD, Brambilla E, Riely GJ. New pathologic classification of lung Cancer: relevance for clinical practice and clinical trials. J Clin Oncol. 2013; 31:992–1001.
2. Ji P, Diederichs S, Wang W, Böing S, Metzger R, Schneider PM, Tidow N, Brandt B, Buerger H, Bulk E, Thomas M. MALAT-1, a novel noncoding RNA, and thymosin β4 predict metastasis and survival in early-stage non-small cell lung cancer. Oncogene. 2003;22(39):8031.
3. Morton ML, Bai X, Merry CR, Linden PA, Khalil AM, Leidner RS, et al. Identification of mRNAs and lincRNAs associated with lung cancer progression using next-generation RNA sequencing from laser micro-dissected archival FFPE tissue specimens. Lung Cancer Amst Neth. 2014;85:31–9.
4. Bracci PM, Sison J, Hansen H, Walsh KM, Quesenberry CP, Raz DJ, et al. Cigarette smoking associated with lung adenocarcinoma in situ in a large case-control study (SFBALCS). J Thorac Oncol. 2012;7:1352–60.
5. Sun S, Schiller JH, Gazdar AF. Lung cancer in never smokers—a different disease. Nature Reviews Cancer. 2007;7(10):778.
6. Patsios D, Roberts HC, Paul NS, Chung T, Herman SJ, Pereira A, et al. Pictorial review of the many faces of bronchioloalveolar cell carcinoma. Br J Radiol. 2007;80:1015–23.
7. Thompson WH. Bronchioloalveolar Carcinoma Masquerading as Pneumonia. Respir Care. 2004;49:1349–53.
8. Zhao Y, Lu H, Yan A, Yang Y, Meng Q, Sun L, Pang H, Li C, Dong X, Cai L. ABCC3 as a marker for multidrug resistance in non-small cell lung cancer. Sci Rep. 2013;3:3120.
9. Clemson CM, Hutchinson JN, Sara SA, Ensminger AW, Fox AH, Chess A, et al. An architectural role for a nuclear non-coding RNA: NEAT1 RNA is essential for the structure of Paraspeckles. Mol Cell. 2009;33:717–26.
10. Jen J, Tang YA, Lu YH, Lin CC, Lai WW, Wang YC. Oct4 transcriptionally regulates the expression of long non-coding RNAs NEAT1 and MALAT1 to promote lung cancer progression. Mol Cancer. 2017;16(1):104.
11. Robinson MD, McCarthy DJ, Smyth GK. edgeR: a Bioconductor package for differential expression analysis of digital gene expression data. Bioinformatics. 2010;26:139–40.
12. Li Q-G, He Y-H, Wu H, Yang C-P, Pu S-Y, Fan S-Q, et al. A normalization-free and nonparametric method sharpens large-scale transcriptome analysis and reveals common gene alteration patterns in cancers. Theranostics. 2017;7: 2888–99.
13. Nishida N, Yano H, Nishida T, Kamura T, Kojiro M. Angiogenesis in Cancer. Vasc Health Risk Manag. 2006;2:213–9.
14. Folkman J. Angiogenesis in cancer, vascular, rheumatoid and other disease. Nat Med. 1995;1(1):27.
15. Zhou W, Yin M, Cui H, Wang N, Zhao L-L, Yuan L-Z, et al. Identification of potential therapeutic target genes and mechanisms in non-small-cell lung carcinoma in non-smoking women based on bioinformatics analysis. Eur Rev Med Pharmacol Sci. 2015;19:3375–84.
16. Venning FA, Wullkopf L, Erler JT. Targeting ECM disrupts cancer progression. Front Oncol. 5:224.
17. Hu Y, Chen G. Pathogenic mechanisms of lung adenocarcinoma in smokers and non-smokers determined by gene expression interrogation. Oncol Lett. 2015;10:1350–70.
18. Huang DW, Sherman BT, Lempicki RA. Systematic and integrative analysis of large gene lists using DAVID bioinformatics resources. Nat Protoc. 2008;4:44–57.
19. Huynh-Thu VA, Irrthum A, Wehenkel L, Geurts P. Inferring Regulatory Networks from Expression Data Using Tree-Based Methods. Isalan M, editor. PLoS ONE. 2010;5:e12776.
20. Liaw A, Wiener M. Classification and regression by randomForest. R news. 2002;2(3):18–22.
21. Director's Challenge Consortium for the Molecular Classification of Lung Adenocarcinoma, Shedden K, JMG T, Enkemann SA, Tsao M-S, Yeatman TJ, et al. Gene expression–based survival prediction in lung adenocarcinoma: a multi-site, blinded validation study. Nat Med. 2008;14:822–7.
22. Landi MT, Dracheva T, Rotunno M, Figueroa JD, Liu H, Dasgupta A, et al. Gene Expression Signature of Cigarette Smoking and Its Role in Lung Adenocarcinoma Development and Survival. Albertson D, editor. PLoS ONE. 2008;3:e1651.
23. Best MG, Sol N, SGJG I 't V, Vancura A, Muller M, Niemeijer A-LN, et al. Swarm Intelligence-Enhanced Detection of Non-Small-Cell Lung Cancer Using Tumor-Educated Platelets. Cancer Cell. 2017;32:238–252.e9.
24. Meyer D, Dimitriadou E, Hornik K, Weingessel A, Leisch F. e1071: misc functions of the department of statistics, probability theory group (formerly: E1071), TU Wien. R package version 1.6–7.

25. Günther F, Fritsch S. neuralnet: Training of neural networks. R J. 2010;2(1):30–8.
26. Pascual G, Avgustinova A, Mejetta S, Martín M, Castellanos A, Attolini CS-O, et al. Targeting metastasis-initiating cells through the fatty acid receptor CD36. Nature. 2017;541:41–5.
27. de Aberasturi AL, Calvo A. TMPRSS4: an emerging potential therapeutic target in cancer. Br J Cancer. 2015;112:4–8.
28. de Aberasturi AL, Redrado M, Villalba M, Larzabal L, Pajares MJ, Garcia J, et al. TMPRSS4 induces cancer stem cell-like properties in lung cancer cells and correlates with ALDH expression in NSCLC patients. Cancer Lett. 2016; 370:165–76.
29. Song N, Liu B, Wu J-L, Zhang R-F, Duan L, He W-S, et al. Prognostic value of HMGB3 expression in patients with non-small cell lung cancer. Tumour Biol. 2013;34:2599–603.
30. Tang Z, Shen Q, Xie H, Zhou X, Li J, Feng J, et al. Elevated expression of FABP3 and FABP4 cooperatively correlates with poor prognosis in non-small cell lung cancer (NSCLC). Oncotarget. 2016;7:46253–62.
31. Lin J, Marquardt G, Mullapudi N, Wang T, Han W, Shi M, et al. Lung Cancer transcriptomes refined with laser capture microdissection. Am J Pathol. 2014;184:2868–84.
32. Psallidas I, Stathopoulos GT, Maniatis NA, Magkouta S, Moschos C, Karabela SP, et al. Secreted phosphoprotein-1 directly provokes vascular leakage to foster malignant pleural effusion. Oncogene. 2013;32:528–35.
33. Bikkavilli RK, Avasarala S, Scoyk MV, Arcaroli J, Brzezinski C, Zhang W, et al. Wnt7a is a novel inducer of β-catenin-independent tumor-suppressive cellular senescence in lung cancer. Oncogene. 2015;34:5317–28.
34. Pastuszak-Lewandoska D, Czarnecka KH, Migdalska-Sęk M, Nawrot E, Domańska D, Kiszałkiewicz J, et al. Decreased FAM107A expression in patients with non-small cell lung Cancer. Adv Exp Med Biol. 2015;852:39–48.
35. HATABE S, KIMURA H, ARAO T, KATO H, HAYASHI H, NAGAI T, et al. Overexpression of heparan sulfate 6-O-sulfotransferase-2 in colorectal cancer. Mol Clin Oncol. 2013;1:845–50.
36. Su J, Zhang E, Han L, Yin D, Liu Z, He X, et al. Long noncoding RNA BLACAT1 indicates a poor prognosis of colorectal cancer and affects cell proliferation by epigenetically silencing of p15. Cell Death Dis. 2017;8:e2665.
37. Bradford JR, Cox A, Bernard P, Camp NJ. Consensus analysis of whole transcriptome profiles from two breast cancer patient cohorts reveals long non-coding RNAs associated with intrinsic subtype and the tumour microenvironment. PloS one. 2016;11(9):e0163238.
38. Bolger AM, Lohse M, Usadel B. Trimmomatic: a flexible trimmer for Illumina sequence data. Bioinformatics. 2014;30:2114–20.
39. Dobin A, Davis CA, Schlesinger F, Drenkow J, Zaleski C, Jha S, et al. STAR: ultrafast universal RNA-seq aligner. Bioinformatics. 2013;29:15–21.
40. Trapnell C, Williams BA, Pertea G, Mortazavi A, Kwan G, van Baren MJ, et al. Transcript assembly and quantification by RNA-Seq reveals unannotated transcripts and isoform switching during cell differentiation. Nat Biotechnol. 2010;28:511–5.
41. Anders S, Pyl PT, Huber W. HTSeq—a Python framework to work with high-throughput sequencing data. Bioinformatics. 2015;31:166–9.
42. Love MI, Huber W, Anders S. Moderated estimation of fold change and dispersion for RNA-seq data with DESeq2. Genome Biol. 2014;15(12):550.

10

Identification of differential gene expression profile from peripheral blood cells of military pilots with hypertension by RNA sequencing analysis

Xing-Cheng Zhao[1][*][†] , Shao-Hua Yang[2†], Yi-Quan Yan[1,3†], Xin Zhang[2], Lin Zhang[1], Bo Jiao[1], Shuai Jiang[1] and Zhi-Bin Yu[1*]

Abstract

Background: Elevated blood pressure is an important risk factor for cardiovascular disease and is also an important factor in global mortality. Military pilots are at high risk of cardiovascular disease because they undergo persistent noise, high mental tension, high altitude hypoxia, high acceleration and high calorie diet. Hypertension is the leading cause of cardiovascular disease in military pilots. In this study, we want to identify key genes from peripheral blood cells of military pilots with hypertension. Identification of these genes may help diagnose and control hypertension and extend flight career for military pilots.

Methods: We use RNA sequencing technology, bioinformatics analysis and Western blotting to identify key genes from peripheral blood cells of military pilots with hypertension.

Results: Our study detected 121 up-regulated genes and 623 down-regulated genes in the peripheral blood mononuclear cells (PBMCs) from hypertensive military pilots. We have also identified 8 important genes (*NME4, PNPLA7, GGT5, PTGS2, IGF1R, NT5C2, ENTPD1* and *PTEN*), a number of gene ontology categories and biological pathways that may be associated with military pilot hypertension.

Conclusions: Our study may provide effective means for the prevention, diagnosis and treatment of hypertension for military pilot and extend their flight career.

Keywords: Hypertension, Military pilots, Peripheral blood cells, RNA sequencing

Background

Elevated blood pressure (BP) is an important risk factor of cardiovascular disease (CVD) and is also an important factor in global mortality, leading to about 9.4 million deaths per year [1]. The morbidity and mortality of CVD are associated with degrees of increased BP. For every increase of 20 mmHg in the systolic BP above 115 mmHg, the incidence of CVD risk will double [2]. In general, the threshold of hypertension is set to systolic pressure of 140 mmHg (150 mmHg for older adults) or diastolic pressure of 90 mmHg based on BP measurement in quiescent condition [3]. One-third American adults over 18 years old of age have hypertension, and 54% of old people (55- to 64-year-olds) have high BP. Among those over 75 years old of age in the United States, nearly 80% have hypertension [4].

Military pilots are at high risk of CVD because they are undergo persistent noise, high mental tension, high altitude hypoxia, high acceleration and high calorie diet [5]. Hypertension is the leading cause of CVD in military pilots. Although hypertension itself will not cause sudden disability in flight, but it is a main risk factor for disability in flight career and it is also one of the major reasons to cause the pilot grounded [6]. Wenzel et al. reported that the incidence of hypertension in Brazilian Air Force is about 22% [7]. Grossman et al. found 2.4%

* Correspondence: xingcheng_zhao@163.com; yuzhib@fmmu.edu.cn
†Xing-Cheng Zhao, Shao-Hua Yang and Yi-Quan Yan contributed equally to this work.
[1]Department of Aerospace Physiology, Fourth Military Medical University, Changle West Road 169#, Xi'an 710032, People's Republic of China
Full list of author information is available at the end of the article

of the pilots had moderate or higher blood pressure in a 7.5-year follow-up study of Israeli Air Force pilots [8]. The hypertension prevalence rate was 9.7% in Chinese Air Force pilots, and the grounded rate of pilots was 21.7% among students in the flight academy because of hypertension or increased blood pressure [9]. Essential hypertension is a disease caused by complex, multifactorial and multigenic changes, and it is the result of both gene regulation and environmental impact [10]. In this study, we use RNA sequencing technology, bioinformatics analysis and Western blotting to identify key genes from peripheral blood cells of military pilots with hypertension. Identification of these genes may help diagnose and control hypertension and extend flight career for military pilots.

Methods

Study subject

For RNA-Seq, six samples of peripheral blood cell from military pilot (3 hypertensives and 3 normotensives) were collected. For quantitative RT-PCR and Western blotting analysis, another 8 samples of peripheral blood cell from fighter pilot (4 hypertensives and 4 normotensives) were collected. All samples collected with the help of doctors from Lintong Aviation Medical Evaluating and Training Center of Air Force, Xi'an, China. The average systolic blood pressure (SBP) of these hypertension pilots was above 160 mmHg and the average diastolic blood pressure (DBP) was above 100 mmHg. The average SBP of these normotensive pilots was below 135 mmHg and the average DBP was below 85 mmHg.

Peripheral blood mononuclear cells (PBMCs) isolation

Five milliliter whole blood collected was transferred to a 15 ml sterile centrifuge tube, 5 ml phosphate buffer saline (PBS) was added to dilute the whole blood. Five milliliter lymphocyte separation medium was added to another 15 ml sterile centrifuge tube. The diluted whole blood was transferred to the lymphocyte separation medium gently to avoid mixing. Then the blood was centrifuged at 2000 rpm for 20 min, room temperature. The white membrane cells of PBMSs were sucked into another sterile 15 ml centrifuge tube. Add 5 ml PBS and centrifuge at 1000 rpm for 10 min. Aspirate supernatant and add 2 ml ACK buffer to the tube, suspend the cells and keep standing for 5 min. Add 5 ml PBS and centrifuge at 1000 rpm for 10 min. Aspirate the supernatant, and the cells were quickly frozen in liquid nitrogen and used for further analysis.

RNA sequencing

RNA sequencing was entrusted to Novel Bioinformatics Co., Ltd., Shanghai, China. Using high-throughput Life technologies Ion Proton Sequencer, the transcript with poly(A)-containing RNA of Human were analyzed.

Quality control

Fast - QC software (http://www.bioinformatics.babraham.ac.uk/projects/fastqc/) was employed to evaluate the overall quality of sequencing data.

Gene expression calculation

The expression of genes is mainly calculated by RPKM (Reads Per Kb per Million reads) method. The formula is: $RPKM = \frac{10^6 C}{NL/10^3}$ RPKM is gene expression, C is the unique number of reads on the gene, and N is the unique number of total reads in the reference gene, and L is the base number of the gene coding region. RPKM method can eliminate the effects of gene length and sequencing on the expression of genes, which can be directly used to compare the gene expression differences between different samples.

Principal component analysis

We applied the PCA analysis based the whole gene expression table and the R script utilizing following package: MASS, evd, rgl and pvclust. Command we used was described as followings:

R script:

dat < – read.table("all.rpkm.exp.txt",sep = "\t", header = T).

colnameall = colnames(dat).

colname = colnames(dat[,2:length(colnameall)]).

dat.pca < –princomp(dat[2:length(colnameall)]).

summary(dat.pca).

plot<–plot3d(dat.pca$loadings[,1],dat.pca$loadings[,2],dat.pca$loadings[,3],type = "s",col. = col.,size = 0.8,xlab = "PC1",ylab = "PC2",zlab = "PC3").

texts3d(dat.pca$loadings[,1],dat.pca$loadings[,2]-0.02,-dat.pca$loadings[,3],texts = colname,font = 5).

GO analysis

The difference of gene analysis based on the database from BP, MF, CC GO annotation in the three dimensions and all GOs were obtained. Each GO significance level was obtained by using the Fisher test (P Value) and so gene enrichment significant difference GOs were screened out [11, 12].

Pathway analysis

The differential expression genes filter out were annotated in KEGG database (http://www.genome.jp/kegg/) for Pathway annotations, and all the Pathway Terms of different genes involved were got. The Pathway of significance level is obtained by using the Fisher test (P Value), and the significant Pathway Term of differential expression gene enrichment was screened out.

Gene-act-network

The construction of gene interaction is to sort out the regulation of all the genes, and through the construction of signal transduction network, we could easily find the vein of gene signal transduction. Based on KEGG database, we could get gene interactions. So, we constructed gene and adjacency matrix using gene interactions [13–17].

Western blotting

PBMCs were isolated as before. Total protein was extracted by using the RIPA reagent (Beyotime, Shanghai, China). The sample protein concentration was tested by measured by BCA Protein Assay reagents (Thermo Scientific, Rockford, IL). After the protein electrophoresis, the samples were transferred to the PVDF membrane, which was then incubated for primary antibodies overnight at 4 °C, and then the membrane was incubated for horseradish peroxidase (HRP)-conjugated secondary antibodies for 2 h at room temperature. The primary antibodies used were as follows: NT5C2 rabbit polyclonal antibody (Proteintech, Wuhan, China), ENTPD1 rabbit polyclonal antibody (Proteintech, Wuhan, China), GGT5 rabbit polyclonal antibody (Proteintech, Wuhan, China), COX2 (PTGS2) rabbit polyclonal antibody (Proteintech, Wuhan, China), PTEN rabbit polyclonal antibody (Proteintech, Wuhan, China), IGF1R rabbit polyclonal antibody (Proteintech, Wuhan, China), rabbit anti-NME4 (Bioss Antibodies, Beijing, China), rabbit anti-PLCG2 (Bioss Antibodies, Beijing, China), rabbit anti-PI3 Kinase p110 delta (PIK3D) (Bioss Antibodies, Beijing, China), anti-PNPLA7 (Santa Cruz Biotechnology, Dallas, TX), anti-β-actin (Santa Cruz Biotechnology, Dallas, TX). The membrane was chemiluminescence using the chemiluminescent reagents (Millipore Corporation, Billerica, MA) and image-forming system Tanon 4200 (Tanon Science & Technology Co., Ltd., Shanghai, China).

Results

Overview of RNA sequencing data

We used Fast-QC online software (http://www.bioinformatics.babraham.ac.uk/projects/fastqc/) to assess the quality of sequencing results (Results were not shown). The results showed that the sequencing data of all samples were qualified. Total raw reads of these six samples were about 12–15 million. GC content of these six samples was about 53%. The average reads mapped to human genome sequence were about $1.28 \pm 0.78 \times 10^7$ reads (96% of the total reads) in the six samples (Additional file 1: Table S1) and about 92% of the total reads ($1.24 \pm 0.74 \times 10^7$ reads) were mapped to human genome sequence uniquely. MapSplice was employed to map the reads. According to the mapping results, about 1×10^7 reads were mapped to the transcript exon, 7×10^6 reads were mapped to CDS, 2×10^6 reads were mapped to intron, 2×10^6 reads were mapped to the UTR regions and the rest reads (about 5% or less) were mapped to intergenic regions, TSS (transcription start site) and TES (transcription end site) (Fig. 1a). We also detected the distribution on chromosomes of these sample mapped reads (Fig. 1b). The results showed that the most reads were aligned to chromosome 1 (about 10% or more) and the least reads were aligned to chromosome Y (less than 0.2%).

Differential gene expression profiles between PBMCs from hypertensives and normotensives military pilots and GO analysis

The six samples were screened for difference gene expression with 3:3. The total number was 26, lower than the minimum standard of data analysis. Two discrete samples (Con4 and Hyp3) were deleted according to results of principal component analysis, and 744 differential genes were acquired. This number was enough for further analysis, so we adopted difference gene expression screened with 2:2.

To characterize the gene expression changes between hypertensives and normotensives military pilots' PBMCs, differentially expressed genes were screened by the following standard: $\text{Log}_2\text{FC} > 0.585$ or $\text{Log}_2\text{FC} < -0.585$, FDR < 0.05 and P value < 0.05. We found 744 differentially expressed genes between hypertensives and normotensives military pilots' PBMCs. Of these genes, 121 genes were up-regulated in hypertensives military pilots' PBMCs and 623 genes were down-regulated. PCA (principal components analysis) cluster analysis was used to compare differential expression of these two groups. The differential gene expression patterns of these samples were showed by gene thermal map (Fig. 2). Gene ontology analysis was used to seek the functions of these differentially expressed genes. The results showed that there were 337 genes belonged to protein binding and 64 genes belonged to ATP binding for molecular function (MF). There were 91 genes belonged to signal transduction and 70 genes belonged to small molecule metabolic process for biological process (BP). As for cellular component (CC), there were 311 genes belonged to membrane and 248 genes belonged to cytoplasm. Results from GO term analyzing showed that inflammatory response, protein binding and phagolysosome were the most significant for BP, MF and CC respectively (Fig. 3).

Pathways analysis of differential expression genes

The differential expression genes were involved in multiple GO, so we constructed functional relation network with significant GO-Term (p-value < 0.05) to reveal relationship between genes clearly based on hierarchical structure of GO (Additional file 2: Figure S1). Of these pathways, protein phosphorylation, toll-like receptor

A

B

Fig. 1 An overview of Reads Distribution and Chromosome Distribution of RNA sequencing. **a** Reads number onto the regions of CDS, exons, intergenic region (InterGenic), introns, transcription end site (TES), transcription start site (TSS), 3'-UTR and 5'-UTR. **b** Distribution of reads on chromosomes

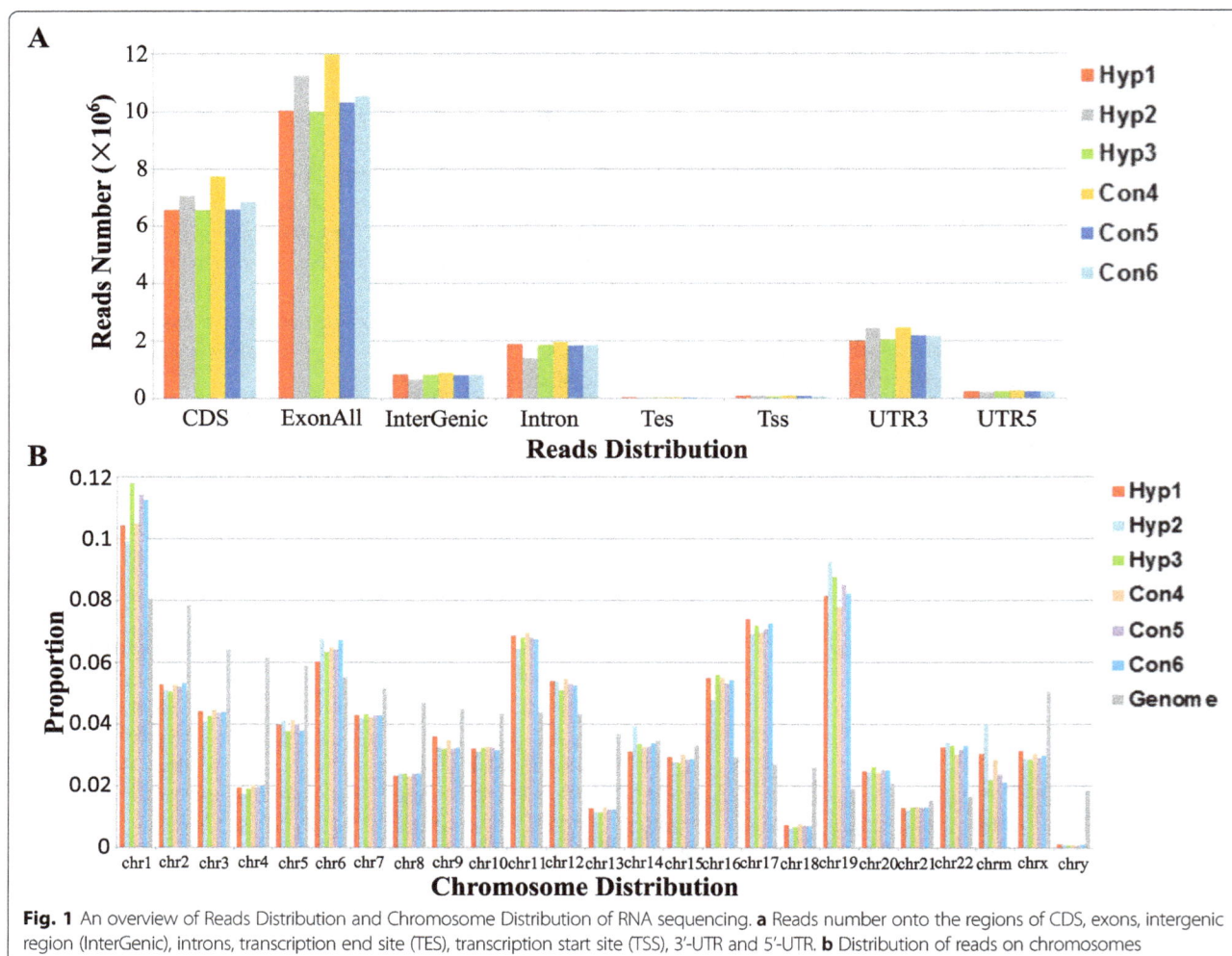

signaling pathway and cell surface receptor signaling pathway were in the core position (Additional file 2: Figure S1). Then, pathway-analysis was carried out to detect significant and important pathways of these differential expression genes. Influenza A and osteoclast differentiation were the most significant (Fig. 4a). Also, the top 20 of pathway enrichment was displayed in Fig. 4b. *P*-Value and gene number was indicated as circle size and color. Next, the pathways interaction network was built to analysis deeply. The analysis results showed that the most important pathways were apoptosis, Jak-STAT signaling pathway, toll-like receptor signaling and cytokine-cytokine receptor interaction (Additional file 3: Figure S2). Because these four pathways are located at the center of the all significant pathways and have the most arrowheads around, these four pathways are likely to be most important in the elevated blood pressure of military pilots. This result suggested that differential expression genes related to apoptosis, Jak-STAT signaling pathway, toll-like receptor signaling and cytokine-cytokine receptor interaction may have important

role in the occurrence and development of elevated blood pressure of military pilots.

Gene act network of differentially expressed genes
Although we got four important pathways related to elevated blood pressure of military pilots, we know that one gene may be involved in multiple signal transduction pathways at the same time. So next, we built gene act network based on the relationships between the differentially expressed genes including expression, binding, inhibition, activation and compound. This analysis method can form the corresponding regulation relationship between gene and gene and is easier to find important related genes under the intervention measures. By analysis the gene act network, we found that *NME4*, *PNPLA7*, *GGT5*, *PTGS2*, *IGF1R*, *PLCG2*, *NT5C2*, *ENTPD1*, *PIK3CD* and *PTEN* these ten genes were located at the center of the all significant genes and have the most arrowheads around (Fig. 5). And also, these ten genes were

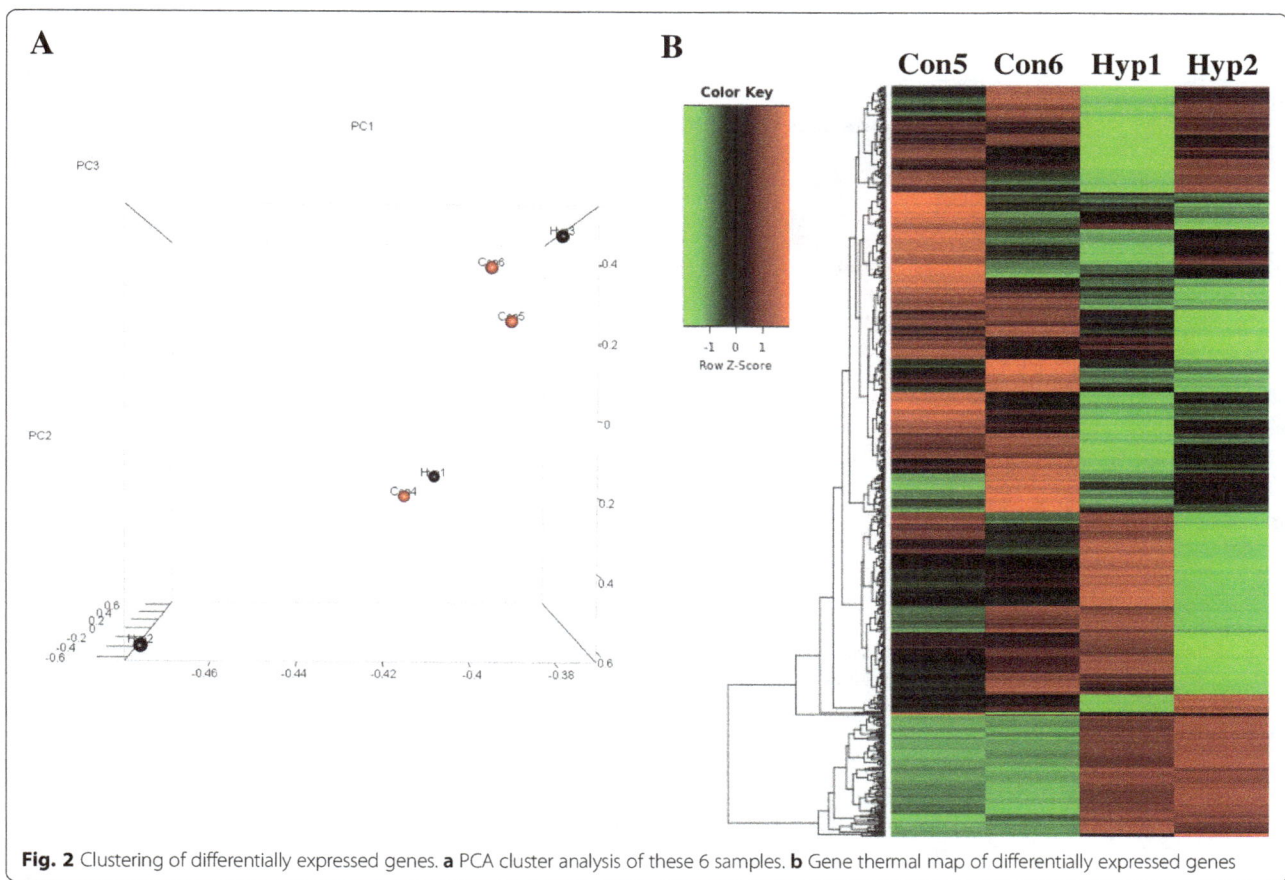

Fig. 2 Clustering of differentially expressed genes. **a** PCA cluster analysis of these 6 samples. **b** Gene thermal map of differentially expressed genes

involved in apoptosis, Jak-STAT signaling pathway, toll-like receptor signaling and cytokine-cytokine receptor interaction signaling pathway previously mentioned. So Next, we will confirm changes of these genes in military pilots' PBMCs of hypertensives and normotensives with Western blotting.

Validation of representative differentially expressed genes by western blotting

The expression of *NME4*, *PNPLA7*, *GGT5*, *PTGS2*, *IGF1R*, *PLCG2*, *NT5C2*, *ENTPD1*, *PIK3CD* and *PTEN* from PBMCs of hypertensive and normotensive military pilots were detected by Western blotting. The results from

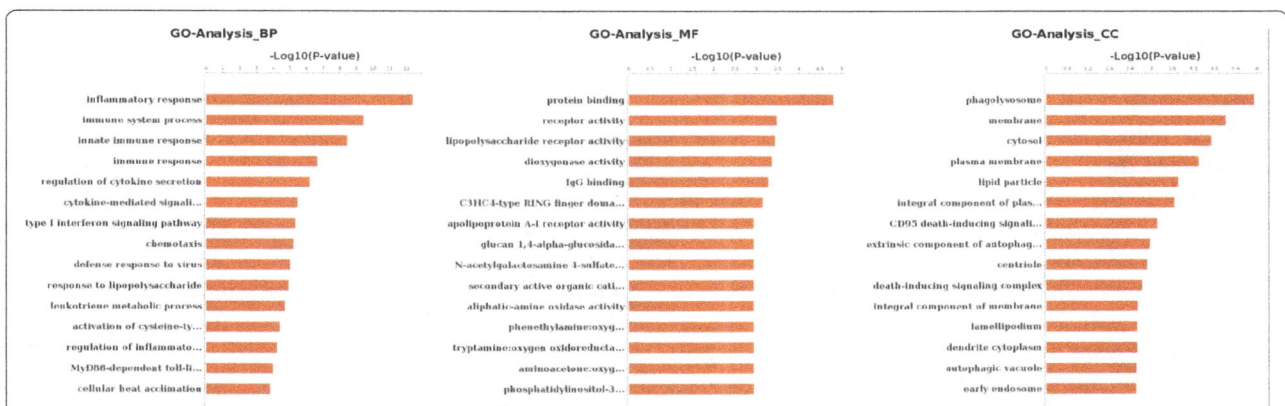

Fig. 3 Gene Ontology (GO) Analysis of differentially expressed genes. GO analysis was annotated from three levels: BP, MF and CC. -Log₁₀(*P*-value) was showed at abscissa axis and GO terms was showed at longitudinal axis. *P* value < 0.05 for all significant GO terms. BP: Biological Process; CC: Cellular Component; MF: Molecular Function

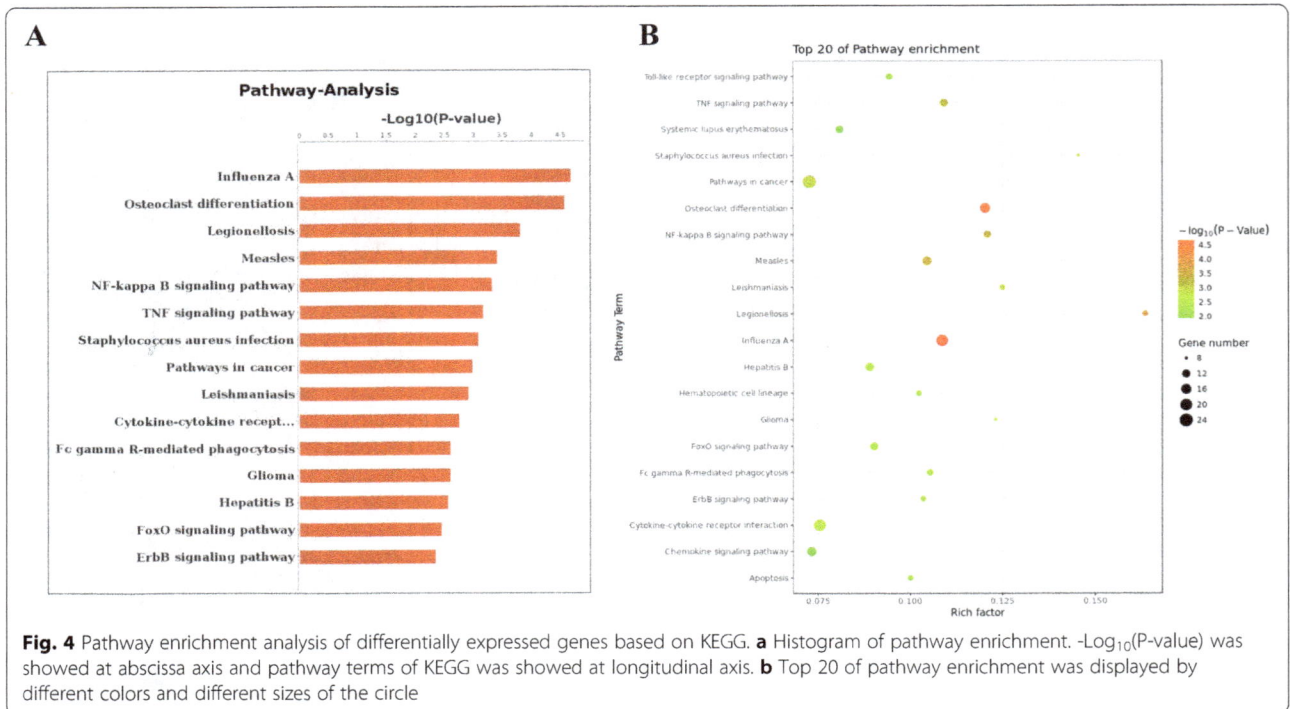

Fig. 4 Pathway enrichment analysis of differentially expressed genes based on KEGG. **a** Histogram of pathway enrichment. -Log$_{10}$(P-value) was showed at abscissa axis and pathway terms of KEGG was showed at longitudinal axis. **b** Top 20 of pathway enrichment was displayed by different colors and different sizes of the circle

Western blotting showed that NME4 and PNPLA7 these two genes were up-regulated significantly and *GGT5*, *PTGS2*, *IGF1R*, *NT5C2*, *ENTPD1* and *PTEN* these six genes were down-regulated significantly in PBMCs of military pilots with hypertension (Fig. 6). Although the expression change of *PLCG2* and *PIK3CD* was not significant between hypertensives and normotensives, there was downward trend in PBMCs of hypertensive military pilots (Fig. 6). The results indicated that the expression change of *NME4*, *PNPLA7*, *GGT5*, *PTGS2*, *IGF1R*, *NT5C2*, *ENTPD1* and *PTEN* could be as sign of elevation of blood pressure for military pilots.

Discussion

Military pilots are in a state of persistent noise, high mental tension, high altitude hypoxia, high acceleration and their high calorie diet, so hypertension is a very common disease in this group. To identify the key genes that related to hypertension of military pilots is very necessary for prevention, diagnosis and treatment of this disorder. In this study, we used RNA sequencing of PBMCs to identify differential gene expression profile between the hypertensive and normotensive military pilots.

Six samples were sequenced and the difference gene expression was compared with 3:3. Because two samples (Con4 and Hyp3) were discrete, so we took them out and adopted different gene expression screened with 2:2. 121 up-regulated genes and 623 down-regulated genes were identified as different expressed genes between

hypertensive and normotensive military pilots. We selected 10 important and significant genes according to results of gene act network analysis. Western blotting was employed to validate the expression change of the 10 genes above. The results showed that expression change of *NME4*, *PNPLA7*, *GGT5*, *PTGS2*, *IGF1R*, *NT5C2*, *ENTPD1* and *PTEN* were consistent with the results of RNA sequencing.

NME4 (also known as *NDPK-D*, *Nm23-H4*) belongs to the *Nm23* family, which includes 10 isoforms (*NME1* to *NME10*) [18]. The classical function of *NME4* as a group I isoform is its NDP kinase activity [19]. *PNPLA7* (also known as *NTE-R1* or *NRE*) is a member of the *PNPLAs* family, and its encoded protein is very conservative in mice, rats and human. *PNPLA7* plays an important role in the hydrolysis of triglycerides, energy metabolism, lipid formation and adipocyte differentiation [20]. Up-regulation of *PNPLA7* indicates elevated blood lipids, which has some correlation with hypertension.

The main expression of *Gamma-glutamyl transferase 5* (*GGT5*) is on the surface of cell membrane, and the role of *GGT5* is to hydrolyze the gamma-glutamyl bond glutathione [21]. There is no phenotypic abnormality in *GGT5* knockout mice under normal conditions. But *GGT5* gene knockout mice were unable to metabolize *LTC4*, resulting in diminished potential of neutrophils infiltrating into the peritoneum. The expression and function of *GGT5* in human are rarely reported [22]. *PTGS2*(also known as *COX-2*) could promote carcinogenesis and

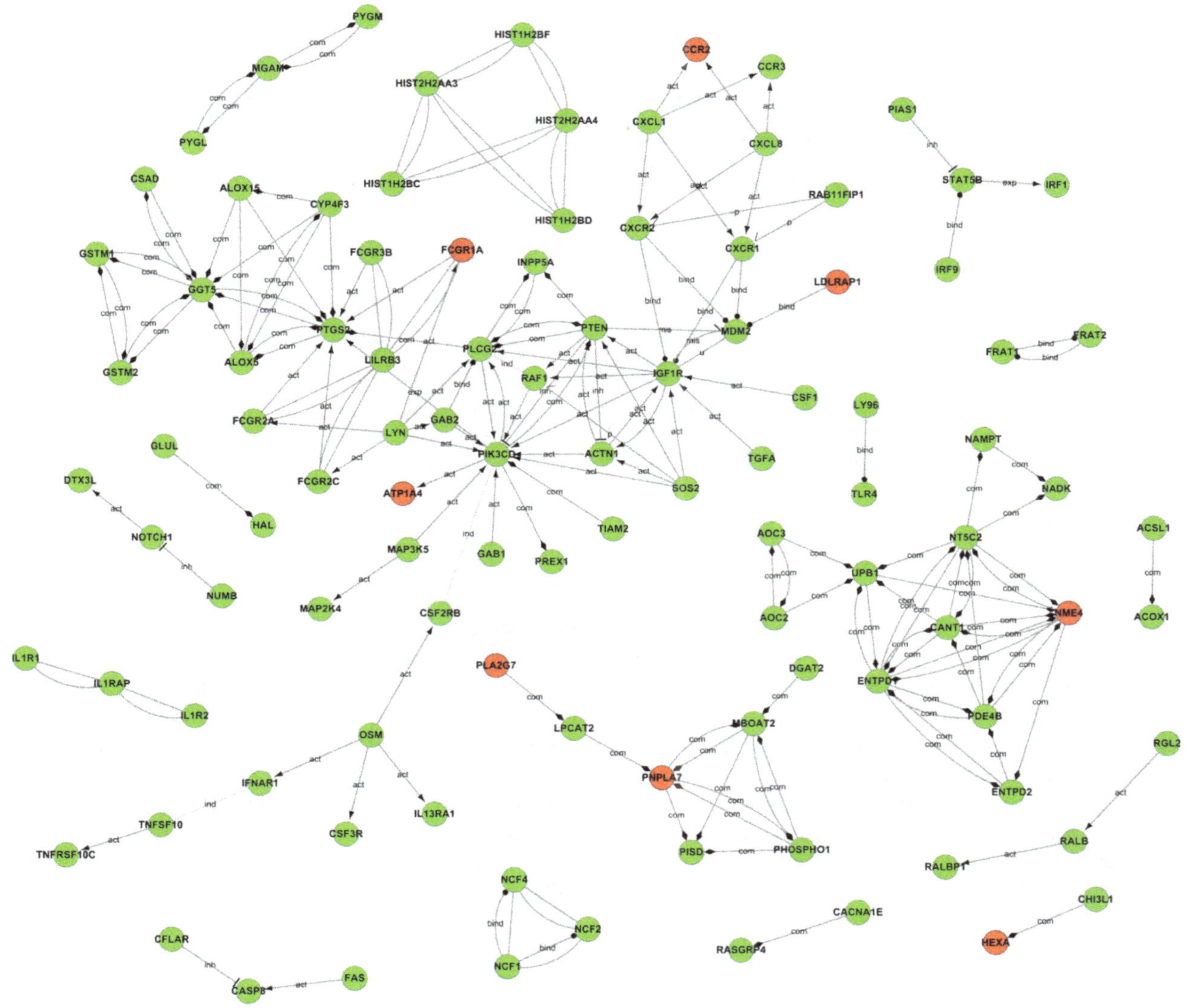

Fig. 5 Gene Act network analysis. Red circles represent up-regulated genes in hypertension group; Green circles represent down-regulated genes in hypertension group, arrows indicate the direction of regulation

metastasis of multiple types of tumors. Expression of *PTGS2* could be dramatically up-regulated by high levels of noise exposure and high altitude hypoxia [23, 24]. Park et al. reported that high fat diet could reduce *PTGS2* expression [25], indicating that expression change of *PTGS2* may be caused by noise exposure, high altitude hypoxia and high fat diet. *IGFR* is a member of the receptor tyrosine family and can form homodimers with insulin receptor (InsR) to identify and bind to the ligand of insulin receptor *IGF1* and *IGF2* [26]. Heterozygous deficiency of *Igf1r* reduced postnatal growth and develop age-dependent insulin resistance. Old-aged *Igf1r*$^{+/-}$ mice had increased adiposity and exhibited increased adipogenesis [27], indicated that reduced expression of *IGF1R* may have a correlation with hypertension. *NT5C2* plays an important role in

purine metabolism. Some papers reported that there were some relationships between somatic mutations of *NT5C2* and T-acute lymphoblastic leukemias (T-ALL) [28, 29]. *ENTPD1* (also known as *CD39*) is a plasma membrane protein and its role is to hydrolyze extracellular ATP and ADP to AMP. Helenius et al. reported that the expression of *ENTPD1* was significantly reduced in small arterial endothelial cells in patients with pulmonary arterial hypertension (PAH). The attenuation function of *ENTPD1* is closely related to vascular dysfunction, suggested that *ENTPD1* may be a novel target for PAH therapy [30]. Their results strongly suggested that down-regulation of *ENTPD1* may be a sign of hypertension, consistent with our results. *PTEN* signaling pathway is one of the most important signaling pathways that regulate

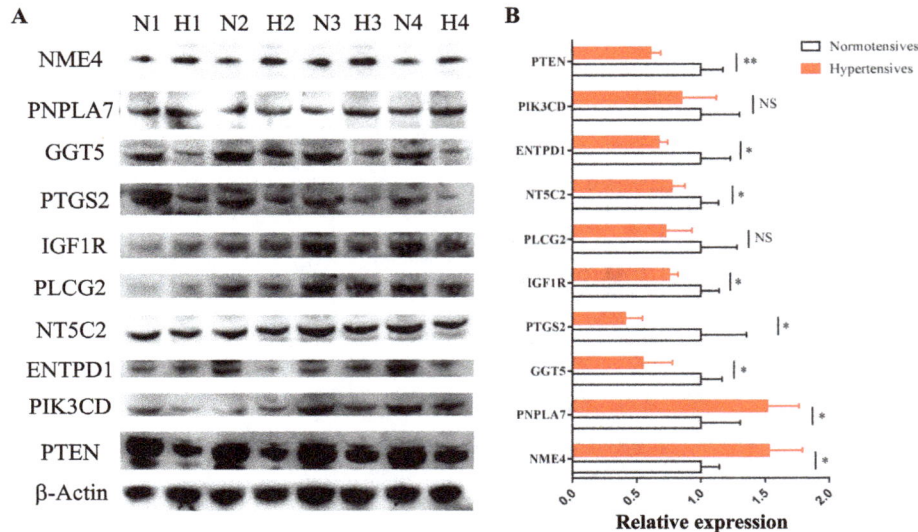

Fig. 6 Western blotting validation of relative expression levels of representative differentially expressed genes. **a** Western blotting of 10 representative differentially expressed genes from 4 hypertensive (H1, H2 H3 and H4) and 4 normotensive (N1, N2, N3, N4) military pilots. **b** Statistics of relative expression of Western blotting. Bars = means ± SD. $^*P < 0.05$, $^{**}P < 0.01$, NS, not significant, $n = 4$

individual development, and participate in the process of cell proliferation, differentiation, aging and apoptosis. Schwerd et al. reported that mutation of *PTEN* led severe macrocephaly and mild intellectual disability in adolescent [31]. Skalska-Sadowska et al. reported that mutations of *PTEN* induced T-ALL [32]. These results suggested that abnormal expression of *PTEN* could lead nervous system abnormalities and hematologic disease, maybe have some relationship with hypertension.

Some of the above eight genes are associated with a high-fat diet, some are associated with noise and high-altitude hypoxia, some may be associated with high mental tension. We hypothesized that the expression change of these genes may affect the level of insulin-like growth factor and small vessel remodeling to induce hypertension under the long-term impact of flight environment. Therefore, we should pay attention to the expression changes of these eight genes in the prevention and control of military pilots' hypertension. Early prevention and early treatment according to the expression change of these eight genes, may extend flight career of military pilots.

At last, we acknowledge that the lack of non-pilot controls is a limitation of the study. The eight differential genes we identified may not be pilots specific. Therefore, our results may lead to some errors in the prevention, diagnosis and treatment of pilot hypertension. But our study still has good guidance for the prevention, diagnosis, and treatment of hypertension in pilots, because the samples used in RNA sequencing and Western blotting experiments in this study are all from military pilots. We will employ non-pilot controls including hypertensives and normotensives to identify differential genes more accurate in the future.

Conclusions

In summary, this study detected gene expression difference in PBMCs between military pilot hypertension and normotensives. We have also identified 8 important genes (*NME4, PNPLA7, GGT5, PTGS2, IGF1R, NT5C2, ENTPD1* and *PTEN*), a few GO categories and biological pathways that may be associated with the military pilot hypertension. Our study may provide effective means for the prevention, diagnosis and treatment hypertension of military pilot, extend their flight career.

Abbreviations
BP: Blood pressure; CC: Cellular component; CDS: Coding sequence; CVD: Cardiovascular disease; DBP: Diastolic blood pressure; FDR: False discovery rate; GO: Gene ontology; HRP: Horseradish peroxidase; MF: Molecular function; PBMCs: Peripheral Blood Mononuclear Cells; PBS: Phosphate buffer saline; PVDF: Polyvinylidene fluoride; RPKM: Reads per Kb per million reads; SBP: Systolic blood pressure; T-ALL: T-acute lymphoblastic leukemias; TES: Transcription end site; TSS: Transcription start site

Acknowledgements
We are indebted to the members of our laboratories at the Department of Aerospace Physiology, Fourth Military Medical University.

Funding
This work was supported by the grant of Youth Training Project of PLA Medical Science and Technology, Funded by the General Logistics Department of PLA, China (Grant No:15QNP066). The cost of some reagents of this study was supported by Natural Science Foundation of Shaanxi, China (Grant No:2016JQ8002; 2012JQ4001) and Natural Science Foundation of China (Grant No:31300979). The publication cost of this article was sponsored by Youth Training Project of PLA Medical Science and Technology, China (Grant No:15QNP066).

Authors' contributions

XCZ and ZBY conceived and designed the study. XCZ, SHY, YQY, LZ, BJ and SJ performed the experiments. SHY and XZ collected the blood sample. YQY, LZ and SJ extracted and quantified protein sample. XCZ, SHY, XZ and BJ did Western blotting and data analysis. XCZ, YQY, LZ and SJ analyzed the sequencing data. XCZ interpreted the data and wrote the paper. ZBY revised the manuscript. All authors read and approved the final manuscript.

Competing interests

The authors declared that they have no competing interests.

Author details

[1]Department of Aerospace Physiology, Fourth Military Medical University, Changle West Road 169#, Xi'an 710032, People's Republic of China. [2]Lintong Aviation Medical Evaluating and Training Center of Air Force, Xi'an 710600, China. [3]Department of Traditional Chinese Medicine, Xijing Hospital, Fourth Military Medical University, Xi'an 710032, China.

References

1. Lim SS, Vos T, Flaxman AD, Danaei G, Shibuya K, Adair-Rohani H, Amann M, Anderson HR, Andrews KG, Aryee M, et al. A comparative risk assessment of burden of disease and injury attributable to 67 risk factors and risk factor clusters in 21 regions, 1990-2010: a systematic analysis for the global burden of disease study 2010. Lancet. 2012;380(9859):2224–60.

2. Lewington S, Clarke R, Qizilbash N, Peto R, Collins R. Age-specific relevance of usual blood pressure to vascular mortality: a meta-analysis of individual data for one million adults in 61 prospective studies. Lancet. 2002;360(9349):1903–13.

3. Weber MA, Schiffrin EL, White WB, Mann S, Lindholm LH, Kenerson JG, Flack JM, Carter BL, Materson BJ, Ram CV, et al. Clinical practice guidelines for the management of hypertension in the community a statement by the American Society of Hypertension and the International Society of Hypertension. J Hypertens. 2014;32(1):3–15.

4. Mozaffarian D, Benjamin EJ, Go AS, Arnett DK, Blaha MJ, Cushman M, Das SR, de Ferranti S, Despres JP, Fullerton HJ, et al. Executive summary: heart disease and stroke statistics–2016 update: a report from the American Heart Association. Circulation. 2016;133(4):447–54.

5. Shamiss A, Meisel S, Rosenthal T. Acute hypertensive response to +Gz acceleration in mildly hypertensive pilots. Aviat Space Environ Med. 1993; 64(8):751–4.

6. McCrary BF, Van Syoc DL. Permanent flying disqualifications of USAF pilots and navigators (1995-1999). Aviat Space Environ Med. 2002;73(11):1117–21.

7. Wenzel D, Souza JM, Souza SB. Prevalence of arterial hypertension in young military personnel and associated factors. Rev Saude Publica. 2009;43(5):789–95.

8. Grossman C, Grossman A, Koren-Morag N, Azaria B, Goldstein L, Grossman E. Interventricular septum thickness predicts future systolic hypertension in young healthy pilots. Hypertens Res. 2008;31(1):15–20.

9. Quan SZ, Ma HY, Luo D, Dong L, Zhou JL, Zhu MC. Dependability research on hypertension and risk factors of cardiovascular disease in pilots. Chin J Clinicians (Electronic Version). 2012;6(4):68–71.

10. Korkor MT, Meng FB, Xing SY, Zhang MC, Guo JR, Zhu XX, Yang P. Microarray analysis of differential gene expression profile in peripheral blood cells of patients with human essential hypertension. Int J Med Sci. 2011;8(2):168–79.

11. The Gene Ontology (GO) project in. Nucleic. Acids Res. 2006;34(Database issue):D322–6.

12. Ashburner M, Ball CA, Blake JA, Botstein D, Butler H, Cherry JM, Davis AP, Dolinski K, Dwight SS, Eppig JT, et al. Gene ontology: tool for the unification of biology. The Gene Ontology Consortium. Nat Genet. 2000;25(1):25–9.

13. Jansen R, Greenbaum D, Gerstein M. Relating whole-genome expression data with protein-protein interactions. Genome Res. 2002;12(1):37–46.

14. Li C, Li H. Network-constrained regularization and variable selection for analysis of genomic data. Bioinformatics. 2008;24(9):1175–82.

15. Wei Z, Li H. A Markov random field model for network-based analysis of genomic data. Bioinformatics. 2007;23(12):1537–44.

16. Zhang JD, Wiemann S. KEGGgraph: a graph approach to KEGG PATHWAY in R and bioconductor. Bioinformatics. 2009;25(11):1470–1.

17. Spirin V, Mirny LA. Protein complexes and functional modules in molecular networks. Proc Natl Acad Sci U S A. 2003;100(21):12123–8.

18. Schlattner U, Tokarska-Schlattner M, Ramirez S, Tyurina YY, Amoscato AA, Mohammadyani D, Huang Z, Jiang J, Yanamala N, Seffouh A, et al. Dual function of mitochondrial Nm23-H4 protein in phosphotransfer and intermembrane lipid transfer: a cardiolipin-dependent switch. J Biol Chem. 2013;288(1):111–21.

19. Schlattner U, Tokarska-Schlattner M, Epand RM, Boissan M, Lacombe ML, Klein-Seetharaman J, Kagan VE. Mitochondrial NM23-H4/NDPK-D: a bifunctional nanoswitch for bioenergetics and lipid signaling. Naunyn Schmiedeberg's Arch Pharmacol. 2015;388(2):271–8.

20. Zhang X, Zhang J, Wang R, Guo S, Zhang H, Ma Y, Liu Q, Chu H, Xu X, Zhang Y, et al. Hypermethylation reduces the expression of PNPLA7 in hepatocellular carcinoma. Oncol Lett. 2016;12(1):670–4.

21. Wickham S, West MB, Cook PF, Hanigan MH. Gamma-glutamyl compounds: substrate specificity of gamma-glutamyl transpeptidase enzymes. Anal Biochem. 2011;414(2):208–14.

22. Hanigan MH, Gillies EM, Wickham S, Wakeham N, Wirsig-Wiechmann CR. Immunolabeling of gamma-glutamyl transferase 5 in normal human tissues reveals that expression and localization differ from gamma-glutamyl transferase 1. Histochem Cell Biol. 2015;143(5):505–15.

23. Faoro V, Fink B, Taudorf S, Dehnert C, Berger MM, Swenson ER, Bailey DM, Bartsch P, Mairbaurl H. Acute in vitro hypoxia and high-altitude (4,559 m) exposure decreases leukocyte oxygen consumption. Am J Physiol Regul Integr Comp Physiol. 2011;300(1):R32–9.

24. Sun Y, Yu J, Lin X, Tang W. Inhibition of cyclooxygenase-2 by NS398 attenuates noise-induced hearing loss in mice. Sci Rep. 2016;6:22573.

25. Park S, Park NY, Valacchi G, Lim Y. Calorie restriction with a high-fat diet effectively attenuated inflammatory response and oxidative stress-related markers in obese tissues of the high diet fed rats. Mediat Inflamm. 2012; 2012:984643.

26. Ii M, Li H, Adachi Y, Yamamoto H, Ohashi H, Taniguchi H, Arimura Y, Carbone DP, Imai K, Shinomura Y. The efficacy of IGF-I receptor monoclonal antibody against human gastrointestinal carcinomas is independent of k-ras mutation status. Clin Cancer Res. 2011;17(15):5048–59.

27. Thakur S, Garg N, Zhang N, Hussey SE, Musi N, Adamo ML. IGF-1 receptor haploinsufficiency leads to age-dependent development of metabolic syndrome. Biochem Biophys Res Commun. 2017;486(4):937–44.

28. Meyer JA, Wang J, Hogan LE, Yang JJ, Dandekar S, Patel JP, Tang Z, Zumbo P, Li S, Zavadil J, et al. Relapse-specific mutations in NT5C2 in childhood acute lymphoblastic leukemia. Nat Genet. 2013;45(3):290–4.

29. Tzoneva G, Perez-Garcia A, Carpenter Z, Khiabanian H, Tosello V, Allegretta M, Paietta E, Racevskis J, Rowe JM, Tallman MS, et al. Activating mutations in the NT5C2 nucleotidase gene drive chemotherapy resistance in relapsed ALL. Nat Med. 2013;19(3):368–71.

30. Helenius MH, Vattulainen S, Orcholski M, Aho J, Komulainen A, Taimen P, Wang L, de Jesus Perez VA, Koskenvuo JW, Alastalo TP. Suppression of endothelial CD39/ENTPD1 is associated with pulmonary vascular remodeling in pulmonary arterial hypertension. Am J Physiol Lung Cell Mol Physiol. 2015;308(10):L1046–57.

31. Schwerd T, Khaled AV, Schurmann M, Chen H, Handel N, Reis A, Gillessen-Kaesbach G, Uhlig HH, Abou Jamra R. A recessive form of extreme macrocephaly and mild intellectual disability complements the spectrum of PTEN hamartoma tumour syndrome. Eur J Hum Genet. 2016;24(6):889–94.

32. Skalska-Sadowska J, Dawidowska M, Szarzynska-Zawadzka B, Jarmuz-Szymczak M, Czerwinska-Rybak J, Machowska L, Derwich K. Translocation t(8;14)(q24;q11) with concurrent PTEN alterations and deletions of STIL/TAL1 and CDKN2A/B in a pediatric case of acute T-lymphoblastic leukemia: a genetic profile associated with adverse prognosis. Pediatr Blood Cancer. 2017;64(4)

11

African ancestry is associated with cluster-based childhood asthma subphenotypes

Lili Ding[1], Dan Li[2], Michael Wathen[3], Mekibib Altaye[1] and Tesfaye B. Mersha[3*]

Abstract

Background: Childhood asthma is a syndrome composed of heterogeneous phenotypes; furthermore, intrinsic biologic variation among racial/ethnic populations suggests possible genetic ancestry variation in childhood asthma. The objective of the study is to identify clinically homogeneous asthma subphenotypes in a diverse sample of asthmatic children and to assess subphenotype-specific genetic ancestry in African-American asthmatic children.

Methods: A total of 1211 asthmatic children including 813 in the Childhood Asthma Management Program and 398 in the Childhood Asthma Research and Education program were studied. Unsupervised cluster analysis on clinical phenotypes was conducted to identify homogeneous subphenotypes. Subphenotype-specific genetic ancestry was estimated for 167 African-American asthmatic children. Genetic ancestry association with subphenotypes/clinical phenotypes were determined.

Results: Three distinct subphenotypes were identified: a moderate atopic dermatitis (AD) group with negative skin prick test (SPT) and preserved lung function; a high AD group with positive SPT and airway hyperresponsiveness; and a low AD group with positive SPT and lower lung function. African ancestry at asthma genome-wide association study (GWAS) SNPs differed between subphenotypes (64, 89, and 94% for the three subphenotypes, respectively) and was inversely correlated with AD; each additional 10% increase in African ancestry was associated with 1.5 fold higher in IgE and 6.3 higher odds of positive SPT (all p-values < 0.0001).

Conclusions: By conducting phenotype-based cluster analysis and assessing subphenotype-specific genetic ancestry, we were able to identify homogeneous subphenotypes for childhood asthma that showed significant variation in genetic ancestry of African-American asthmatic children. This finding demonstrates the utility of these complementary approaches to understand and refine childhood asthma subphenotypes and enable more targeted therapy.

Keywords: Childhood asthma, Cluster analysis, Genetic ancestry, Subphenotypes

Background

Childhood asthma is a heterogeneous chronic airway disease with various clinical phenotypes [1, 2]. Its phenotypic and biologic heterogeneity contributes to the challenges clinicians face in its diagnosis and effective management [3]. It is therefore crucial to clearly define subphenotypes of asthma with homogeneous clinical characteristics in order to search for better asthma management and to develop novel therapeutic strategies. Although a large number of clinical phenotypes are often collected in childhood asthma studies, asthma genetic study has been mostly focused on case-control disease status. Such an endpoint-based analysis ignores the complexity of asthma phenotype [4–6]. In addition, although there is ample evidence for an intrinsic genetic variation among racial/ethnic populations [7, 8] suggesting possible genetic ancestry variation in childhood asthma, most genetic analyses rely on self-reported race thus do not account for the potential contribution of genetic ancestry to disease variation in diverse populations.

An approach to overcome the phenotypic heterogeneity of childhood asthma is to identify homogeneous subgroups by establishing either classical "endotype", based on experts' criteria, or statistical phenotype clustering on asthma clinical phenotypes. The latter has been successfully applied to identify clinically relevant

* Correspondence: tesfaye.mersha@cchmc.org
[3]Division of Asthma Research, Department of Pediatrics, Cincinnati Children's Hospital Medical Center, University of Cincinnati, 3333 Burnet Ave, Cincinnati, OH 45229, USA
Full list of author information is available at the end of the article

subgroups of asthmatics and other airway diseases [9–17]. However, these studies differ in some key elements: variation in phenotyping, analytical approaches used and the patient population under study. These differences limit the comparability of the identified subphenotypes and pose difficulty in applying clustering results to individual patients. Furthermore, little is understood regarding the genetic ancestry of the identified subphenotypes.

The objective of the study is to investigate childhood asthma phenotypic heterogeneity and genetic ancestry variations and their relationships. Specifically, we used childhood asthma data from the NIH controlled database of Genotype and Phenotype (dbGaP) to identify homogeneous subphenotypes, determine clinical phenotypes, estimate subphenotype-specific genetic ancestry, and analyze the relationship between ancestry and subphenotypes using a stepwise approach incorporating cluster analysis, classification tree analysis, and genetic ancestry analyses [9–16, 18, 19]. Our goal is to combine both cluster and genetic ancestry to identify biologically-relevant subphenotypes in childhood asthma.

Methods
Data
The database of Genotypes and Phenotypes (dbGaP) is the repository for both genotype and phenotype data from most NIH-funded GWAS and other whole-genome or exome sequence data. We used baseline data from the SNP Health Association Resource (SHARe) Asthma Resource Project (SHARP) (phs000166.v2.p1), the National Heart, Lung, and Blood Institute's clinical research trials on asthma, specifically, the Childhood Asthma Management Program (CAMP) and the Childhood Asthma Research and Education (CARE) network. The CAMP is a multi-center, randomized, double-masked clinical trial designed to determine the long-term effects of three inhaled treatments for mild to moderate childhood asthma [20]. The CARE data evaluates current and novel therapies and management strategies for children with asthma. Individual level data with asthma diagnosis is available for 1211 subjects through Authorized Access, including 813 in CAMP and 398 in CARE.

An array of phenotypic variables have been harmonized across the CAMP and CARE datasets, including demographics and participant characteristics; intermediate asthma phenotypes such as lung function, skin prick test (SPT), serum total immunoglobulin (IgE), and atopic dermatitis (AD), as well as environmental exposure. See Table 1 for a complete list of variables. We downloaded CAMP and CARE genotype data which were performed using 1 million single nucleotide polymorphisms (SNPs) in the Affymetrix 6.0 chip and stored in the database of dbGaP (accession number

phs000166.v2.p1). Quality control criteria included minor allele frequency ≥ 0.05, Hardy-Weinberg equilibrium ($p \geq 10^{-5}$), $\leq 5\%$ missing rate per person, $\leq 5\%$ missing rate per SNP, families with less than 5% Mendel errors and SNPs with less than 10% Mendel error rate [21].

Hierarchical cluster analysis (HCA)
HCA is a hypothesis free statistical method to group subjects into relatively homogeneous sub-clusters according to similarity quantification based on a set of critical characteristic variables. The grouping is constructed such that the similarity is strong between members of the same cluster and weak between members of different clusters. The baseline phenotypic measures listed in Table 1 were included in the cluster analysis. To reduce collinearity, we examined the variables for absolute correlation (> 0.80). We also assessed missing pattern of the phenotypes and planned to exclude measures with $\geq 10\%$ missingness from the analysis. Blood eosinophils (EOS) and IgE were log transformed.

Since we have mixed types of variables, i.e., continuous and categorical, Gower's distance [22] was used as a similarity index. To avoid inconsistent cluster solutions due to changes in scale of the variables and heavy impact of variables with larger standard deviations, Gower's standardization, based on the range, was applied. HCA was then carried out with Ward's minimum-variance method [23]. Consensus between a pseudo F and a pseudo t^2 statistics [24, 25] was used to select the number of clusters. The number of clusters was also guided by clinical characteristics in addition to statistical considerations.

Descriptive statistics of all variables were obtained and compared across clusters using analysis of variance, Kruskal-Wallis, or Chi-square tests as appropriate. Conditional inference trees [26], a non-parametric class of regression trees that embeds tree structured regression models into a well-defined theory of conditional inference procedures, was used to identify intermediate phenotypes that distinguish the subphenotypes. The cluster analysis was first carried out on the CAMP data and repeated on the CARE data. Replication of the clustering results was examined between the two studies as well as with previously published studies.

Additional analyses were run to investigate if the subphenotypes were associated with clinical outcomes. Two clinical outcomes were examined, number of prednisone bursts (an anti-inflammatory oral steroid medication) since last visit, and number of ER visit or hospitalizations since last visit. Number of prednisone bursts since last visit was modeled as a count variable using Poisson regression with a random subject effect. Number of ER

Table 1 Demographic, clinical phenotypes and environmental exposures of CAMP and CARE study participants

	CAMP (N = 813)	CARE(N = 398)	p-value
Age, Mean (SD), years	8.9 (2.1)	10.6 (2.8)	< 0.0001
Gender, No. (%)			0.8152
Male	500 (61.5)	242 (60.8)	
Female	313 (38.5)	156 (39.2)	
Race, No. (%)			< 0.0001
Caucasian	557 (68.5)	215 (54)	
African American	107 (13.2)	70 (17.6)	
Hispanic	77 (9.5)	78 (19.6)	
Other	72 (8.9)	35 (8.8)	
BMIZ at baseline, Mean (SD)	0.5 (1.0)	0.8 (1.0)	< 0.0001
Age of onset[a], Mean (SD), years	3.0 (2.4)	3.7 (3.3)	< 0.0001
FEV1 PC20 meth[b], Mean (SD), mg/ml	2.0 (2.4)	2.2 (3.1)	0.3602
FEV1 percent predicted[c], Mean (SD)	93.4 (14.1)	97.1 (12.8)	< 0.0001
FVC percent predicted[d], Mean (SD)	103.7 (13.1)	106.7 (12.2)	0.0002
FEV1/FVC ratio[e], Mean (SD)	79.6 (8.3)	80.1 (8.0)	0.2937
Bronchodilator percent change[f], Mean (SD)	10.7 (9.9)	9.4 (8.4)	0.0236
Blood eosinophils, Mean (SD), mm³	485.7 (409.2)	408.8 (319.5)	0.0011
IgE, Mean (SD), ng/ml	1129.8 (2081.9)	330.6 (445.4)	< 0.0001
Average AM peak flow[g], Mean (SD), L/min	250.9 (64.4)	271.1 (92.4)	< 0.0001
Average AM symptoms[h], Mean (SD)	0.61 (0.45)	0.51 (0.40)	< 0.0001
Environmental smoke[i], No. (%)	339 (41.7)	166 (41.7)	0.0256
In utero smoke[j], No. (%)	107 (13.2)	54 (13.6)	0.8060
Atopic dermatitis[k], No. (%)	199 (24.4)	155 (38.9)	< 0.0001
One or more positive SPT[l], No. (%)	716 (88.1)	312 (78.4)	0.0002

[a]Age at first asthma symptoms
[b]The dose of methacholine that is required to decrease FEV1 by 20%
[c]Forced expiratory volume, the maximal amount of air one can forcefully exhale in one second converted to a percentage of normal based on one's height, weight, body composition, and race
[d]Forced vital capacity, the amount of air a person can expire after a maximum inspiration second converted to a percentage of normal based on one's height, weight, body composition, and race
[e]Also called Tiffeneau-Pinelli index, is a calculated ratio used in the diagnosis of obstructive and restrictive lung disease. It represents the proportion of a person's vital capacity that they are able to expire in the first second of expiration
[f]Post bronchodilator percent change from baseline: 100*(POSFEV - PREFEV)/PREFEV
[g]The maximum flow rate generated during a forceful exhalation, starting from full lung inflation; average of daily measurements up to 4 weeks prior to visit with a minimum of 7 days, recorded in daily diary card
[h]Maximum of daily wheezing and coughing then average of daily measurements up to 4 weeks prior to visit with a minimum of 7 days, recorded in daily diary card
[i]Either parent smoked during trial or home exposure to smoke prior to trial enrollment
[j]Mother smoked when pregnant with participant
[k]Child had atopic dermatitis for 2 years and was seen by a doctor for it
[l]One or more skin prick test positive

visit or hospitalizations since last visit was dichotomized (given over 95% of the subjects did not had an ER visit or hospitalization), and modeled using a logistic regression with a random subject effect. Potential covariates included age, sex, race, visit month, time since last visit, treatment, and subphenotypes that were significantly associated with the outcome (adjusted p-value < 0.05). All analyses were run for CAMP and CARE data separately. All the above analyses were conducted in SAS version 9.3 (SAS Institute Inc., Cary, NC, USA) and R [27].

Genetic ancestry analysis

Genetic ancestry was estimated using both genome-wide SNPs and asthma-specific GWAS SNPs for African-American asthmatic individuals in CAMP and CARE. Supervised approach in the ADMIXTURE software program [28] was use to estimated global genetic ancestry, where SNP data of 108 YRI (Yoruba in Ibadan, Nigeria) and 99 CEU (Utah Residents (CEPH) with Northern and Western Ancestry) individuals from the 1000 Genomes Project were included as surrogates for

European and African ancestry. The reference populations and the CAMP/CARE subjects shared 857,127 genetic markers across all autosomes, which reduced to 225,374 SNPs after linkage disequilibrium (LD) pruning with window of 50 (kb), 10 kb window shift and a r2 value of 0.2.

Asthma GWAS SNPs, 157 in total, were retrieved from the GWAS catalog [29] and STRUCTURE software [30] was used to estimate African ancestry proportion at asthma GWAS SNPs. CEU and YRI individuals from the 1000 Genomes Project were used as parental populations.

Correlations between genetic ancestry and the subphenotypes derived by clustering and the discriminate factors of the subphenotypes were examined using the Kruskal-Wallis test, Wilcoxon rank-sum test, Spearman correlation coefficient, or linear regression as appropriate.

Results

Participants from CAMP and CARE were different except in sex, exposure to in utero smoking, PC20, and FEV1/FVC ratio (Table 1). All pairwise Spearman correlation coefficients were less than 0.60, except between FEV1 percent predicted and FVC percent predicted (0.71) and between FEV1/FVC and maximum bronchodilator percent change (− 0.65). No variables had more than 10% of missing values.

HCA identified distinct subphenotypes
Clustering on CAMP cohort identified distinct subphenotypes

Three clusters were identified from CAMP data (Table 2). Members of cluster 1 had a moderate AD rate (15.3%) and all but one had negative SPT (99%). This group also had the lowest age at baseline, age at onset of asthma, bronchodilator percent change, EOS, IgE level, AM peak flow, and AM symptoms, and highest body mass index z-sore (BMIZ), PC20, FEV1 percent predicted, and FEV1/FVC ratio. All these characteristics, but BMIZ and AM symptoms, were statistically different across the clusters at a significant level of 0.05. This is the moderate AD group with negative SPT and preserved lung function.

Members of cluster 2 had a high rate of AD (97.7%) and all had one or more positive SPT. This group also

Table 2 CAMP hierarchical clustering results

	Cluster 1 (N = 98)	Cluster 2 (N = 171)	Cluster 3 (N = 544)	p-value
Age (years)	7.8 (1.9)	8.7 (2.1)	9.2 (2.1)	< 0.0001
Gender No. (%)				0.0675
Male	50 (51.0)	105 (61.4)	345 (63.4)	
Female	48 (49.0)	66 (38.6)	199 (36.6)	
Race No. (%)				0.0153
Caucasian	82 (83.7)	116 (67.8)	359 (66.0)	
African American	9 (9.2)	25 (14.6)	73 (13.4)	
Hispanic	5 (5.1)	12 (7.0)	60 (11.0)	
Other	2 (2.0)	18 (10.5)	52 (9.6)	
BMIZ	0.7 (1.0)	0.6 (1.1)	0.5 (1.0)	0.0929
Age of onset (years)	2.4 (2.2)	2.8 (2.2)	3.2 (2.5)	0.0017
FEV1 PC20 meth (mg/ml)	2.9 (2.8)	1.8 (2.2)	2.0 (2.4)	0.0005
FEV1 percent predicted	96.3 (14.5)	95.0 (14.5)	92.4 (13.9)	0.0117
FVC percent predicted	103.5 (14.3)	104.1 (13.6)	103.6 (12.7)	0.895
FEV1/FVC ratio	82.9 (7.0)	80.6 (8.2)	78.7 (8.3)	< 0.0001
Bronchodilator percent change	7.3 (6.9)	11.4 (10.1)	11.1 (10.1)	0.0012
Blood eosinophils (mm³)	228.9 (197.9)	579.7 (442.4)	504 (408.8)	< 0.0001
IgE (ng/ml)	200.5 (449.1)	1579 (2624.2)	1161 (2022.7)	< 0.0001
Average AM peak flow (L/min)	230.9 (55)	249.8 (67.5)	254.8 (64.4)	0.0040
Average AM symptoms	0.52 (0.40)	0.61 (0.46)	0.63 (0.45)	0.100
Environmental smoke No. (%)	42 (42.9)	60 (35.1)	237 (44.1)	0.1291
In utero smoke No. (%)	19 (19.4)	11 (6.4)	77 (14.2)	0.0046
Atopic dermatitis No. (%)	15 (15.3)	167 (97.7)	17 (3.1)	< 0.0001
Positive SPT No. (%)	1 (1)	171 (100)	544 (100)	< 0.0001

Mean and SD for continuous variables and No. (%) for categorical variables

had the highest EOS and IgE level, and lowest bronchodilator percent change among the 3 clusters. This is the high AD group with positive SPT and airway hyperresponsiveness.

Members of cluster 3 had the highest age at baseline and age onset of asthma and lowest BMIZ. This group had also the lowest FEV1 percent predicted and FEV1/FVC ratio, and highest AM symptoms. Furthermore, members of cluster 3 were mostly AD free and all had one or more positive SPT, moderate EOS and IgE levels, but lower lung function measures and higher AM symptoms compared to the other clusters. This is the low AD group with positive SPT and lower lung function.

Clustering on CARE cohort replicated the subphenotypes identified in CAMP

Three clusters were identified in CARE (Table 3). Members of cluster 1 had a moderate rate of AD (35%) and none of them had a positive SPT. This group also had the lowest bronchodilator percent change, EOS, IgE, AM peak flow, and lowest AM symptoms. All these characteristics, but the last, were statistically different

across the clusters at a significant level of 0.05. This is the moderate AD group with negative SPT and preserved lung function similarity identified in CAMP.

Members of cluster 2 had a high rate of AD (98.4%) and one or more positive SPT (95.3%). This group also had the highest EOS and IgE level among the 3 clusters. This is the high AD asthma group with positive SPT and airway hyperresponsiveness similarly identified in CAMP.

Members of cluster 3 had the highest age at baseline and age onset of asthma, were mostly AD free (3.3%) and all had one or more positive SPT (92.2%), had moderate EOS and IgE levels, but higher AM symptoms compared to the other clusters. This is the low AD group with positive SPT and lower lung function similarly identified in CAMP.

Atopic dermatitis status and SPT distinguished the subphenotypes

Conditional inference trees analysis revealed that, in both CAMP and CARE data, AD and one or more positive SPT were the top two variables that best discriminated the individuals into the subphenotypes (Fig. 1,

Table 3 CARE hierarchical clustering results

	Cluster 1 ($N = 60$)	Cluster 2 ($N = 129$)	Cluster 3 ($N = 209$)	p-value
Age (years)	10.1 (2.4)	10.1 (2.5)	11.0 (3.1)	0.0124
Gender No. (%)				0.1185
Male	30 (50)	77 (59.7)	135 (64.6)	
Female	30 (50)	52 (40.3)	74 (35.4)	
Race No. (%)				0.4519
Caucasian	40 (66.7)	67 (51.9)	108 (51.7)	
African American	8 (13.3)	24 (18.6)	38 (18.2)	
Hispanic	8 (13.3)	24 (18.6)	46 (22.0)	
Other	4 (6.7)	14 (10.9)	17 (8.1)	
BMIZ	0.9 (0.9)	0.8 (1.0)	0.8 (1.0)	0.5920
Age of onset (years)	3.6 (3.5)	3.1 (2.6)	4.1 (3.5)	0.0215
FEV1 PC20 meth (mg/ml)	3.3 (3.3)	1.6 (2.4)	2.3 (3.4)	0.0031
FEV1 percent predicted	97.2 (13.4)	96.3 (13.1)	97.6 (12.5)	0.655
FVC percent predicted	104.7 (10.7)	107.2 (12.5)	106.9 (12.3)	0.378
FEV1/FVC ratio	81.6 (8.5)	79.0 (8.0)	80.4 (7.9)	0.101
Bronchodilator percent change	6.7 (7.4)	9.9 (7.4)	9.8 (9.0)	0.0271
Blood eosinophils (mm³)	245.7 (211.5)	444.4 (322.1)	435.0 (330.2)	< 0.0001
IgE (ng/ml)	63.5 (133.9)	424.5 (537.1)	347.4 (430.1)	< 0.0001
Average AM peak flow (L/min)	255.4 (68.7)	258.6 (81.0)	283.3 (102.3)	0.0209
Average AM symptoms	0.43 (0.32)	0.50 (0.40)	0.53 (0.42)	0.202
Environmental smoke No. (%)	28 (46.7)	62 (48.1)	104 (49.8)	0.8985
In utero smoke No. (%)	1 (1.7)	18 (14.0)	35 (16.9)	0.0121
Atopic dermatitis No. (%)	21 (35)	127 (98.4)	7 (3.3)	< 0.0001
Positive SPT No. (%)	0 (0)	123 (95.3)	189 (92.2)	< 0.0001

Mean and SD for continuous variables and No. (%) for categorical variables

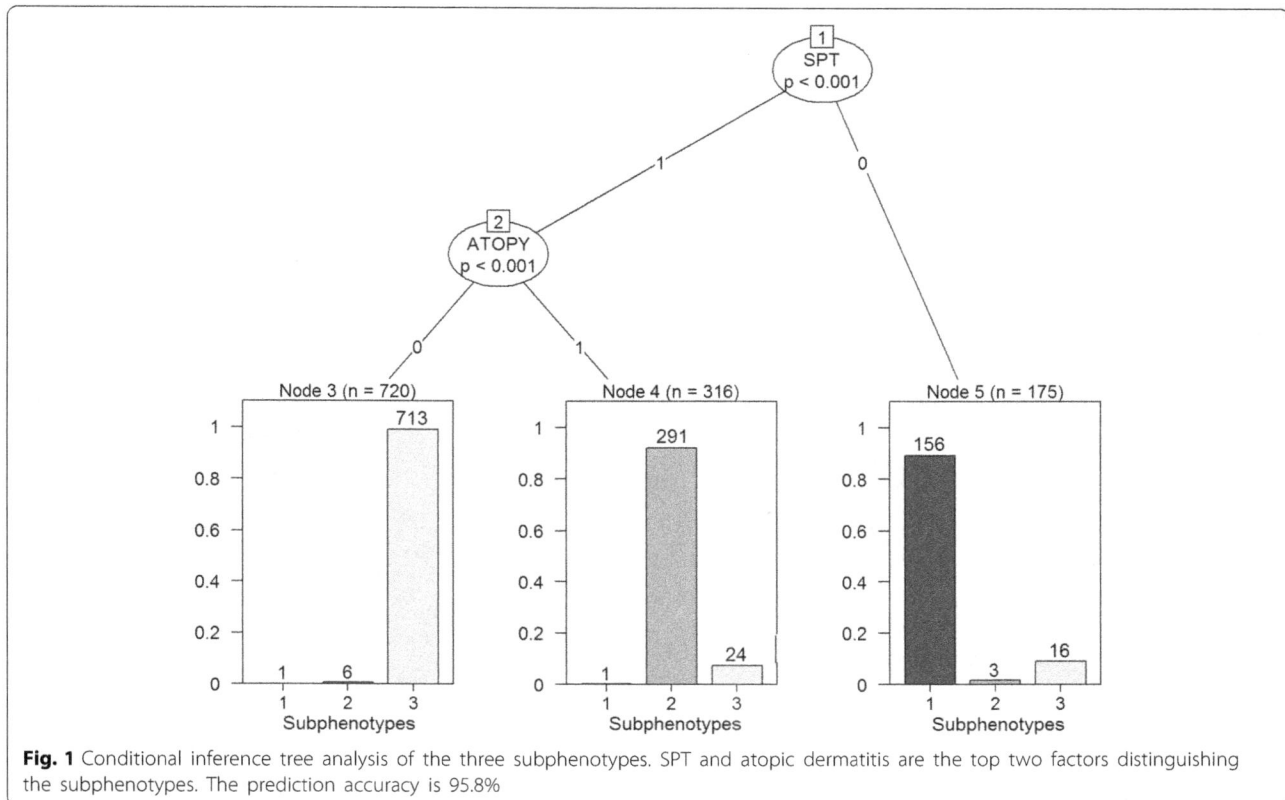

Fig. 1 Conditional inference tree analysis of the three subphenotypes. SPT and atopic dermatitis are the top two factors distinguishing the subphenotypes. The prediction accuracy is 95.8%

prediction accuracy 95.8%). Given the consistent findings across CAMP and CARE data, we combined the two datasets and grouped the three clusters individually identified in CAMP and CARE into three subphenotypes. One subphenotype was the moderate AD group with negative SPT and preserved lung function (subphenotype 1, n = 158), one was the high AD group with positive SPT and airway hyperresponsiveness (subphenotype 2, n = 300), and one was the low AD group with positive SPT and lower lung function (subphenotype 3, n = 753).

Subphenotypes were associated clinical outcomes

Table 4 shows the association between the subphenotypes and clinical outcomes. In CAMP data, the incident rate of prednisone bursts since last visit for subphenotype 2 is 2.63 (1.45, 2.70) times the incident rate for subphenotype 1, and the incident rate of prednisone bursts since last visit for subphenotype 3 is 2.04 (1.56, 2.70) times the incident rate for subphenotype 1. Also in CAMP data, the odds of any ER visit or hospitalizations since last visit for subphenotype 3 is 1.54 (1.01, 2.23) times the odds for subphenotype 1. For CARE data, the odds of any ER visit or hospitalizations since last visit for subphenotype 2 is 0.32 (0.13, 0.98) times the odds for subphenotype 1, and the odds of any ER visit or hospitalizations since last visit for subphenotype 3 is 3.45 (1.47, 7.69) times the odds for subphenotype 2.

Genetic ancestry proportion varied at asthma GWAS SNPs among asthma subphenotypes

The three subphenotypes had 15, 49, and 103 African American individuals, respectively. Global African ancestry proportion varies from 71.2 to 100% with mean 96.6% and standard deviation (SD) 7.2%. Higher global African ancestry was associated with AD (mean ± SD of African origin is 0.96 ± 0.08 for AD free vs. 0.98 ± 0.06 for AD subjects, p-value = 0.0294), but not with other clinical phenotypes. Proportion of African ancestry at asthma GWAS SNPs was correlated with the subphenotypes (mean 64.9, 89.4 and 94.4% for subphenotypes 1, 2, and 3, respectively, p-value < 0.0001, Figs. 2 and 3(a)). The subphenotypes were associated with lung function: FEV1 percent predicted is 96.8 ± 14.1, 95.3 ± 13.9, and 93.9 ± 13.7 (p-value = 0.0083); and FEV1/FVC ratio is 81.9 ± 7.6, 80.5 ± 8.1, and 79.0 ± 8.2 (p-value < 0.0001) for subphenotypes 1, 2, and 3, respectively. Furthermore, African ancestry at asthma GWAS SNPs was inversely associated with AD (median 0.95 with IQR (0.93, 0.95) for AD free vs. 0.92 (0.89, 0.94) for AD subjects, p-value < 0.0001, Fig. 3(b)). Additionally, genetic ancestry at asthma GWAS SNPs was associated with positive SPT with median and interquartile range (IQR) 0.94 (0.92, 0.95) for positive SPT individuals vs. 0.74 with IQR (0.59, 0.78) for negative SPT individuals (p-value < 0.0001, Fig. 3(c)). The odds of one or more positive SPT

Table 4 Association between subphenotypes and number of prednisone bursts and any ER visit or hospitalizations since last visit

Number of prednisone bursts since last visit

CAMP

Predicted number of event			Incident rate ratios		
Subphenotype	Estimate (95% CI)	p-value	Subphenotypes	IRR (95% CI)	p-value
1	0.10 (0.08, 0.13)	< 0.0001	2 vs. 1	2.63 (1.45, 2.70)	< 0.0001
2	0.20 (0.16, 0.24)		3 vs. 1	2.04 (1.56, 2.70)	< 0.0001
3	0.20 (0.18, 0.22)		3 vs. 2	1.02 (0.83, 1.27)	0.8153

CARE

Predicted number of event			Incident rate ratios		
Subphenotype	Estimate (95% CI)	p-value	Subphenotypes	IRR (95% CI)	p-value
1	0.08 (0.05, 0.14)	0.3534	2 vs. 1	0.93 (0.57, 1.54)	0.7880
2	0.08 (0.05, 0.12)		3 vs. 1	1.19 (0.76, 1.89)	0.4420
3	0.10 (0.07, 0.14)		3 vs. 2	1.28 (0.90, 1.82)	0.1666

Any ER visit or hospitalizations since last visit

CAMP

Predicted probability			Odds ratios		
Subphenotype	Estimate (95% CI)	p-value	Subphenotypes	OR (95% CI)	p-value
1	0.03 (0.02, 0.04)	0.1232	2 vs. 1	1.52 (0.95, 2.44)	0.0776
2	0.04 (0.03, 0.05)		3 vs. 1	1.54 (1.01, 2.33)	0.0434
3	0.04 (0.03, 0.04)		3 vs. 2	1.01 (0.75, 1.37)	0.9474

CARE

Predicted probability			Odds ratios		
Subphenotype	Estimate (95% CI)	p-value	Subphenotypes	OR (95% CI)	p-value
1	0.02 (0.01, 0.05)	0.0155	2 vs. 1	0.35 (0.13, 0.98)	0.0458
2	0.01 (0.004, 0.02)		3 vs. 1	1.20 (0.56, 2.63)	0.6296
3	0.03 (0.02, 0.04)		3 vs. 2	3.45 (1.47, 7.69)	0.0039

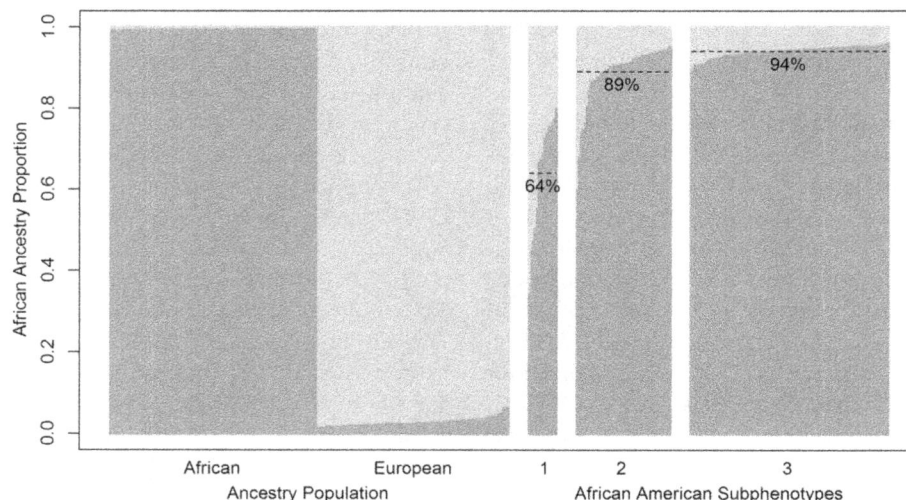

Fig. 2 Population ancestry estimates of African American asthmatic individuals in CAMP and CARE at asthma GWAS SNPs by subphenotypes. Dashed lines indicate average proportions of African ancestry proportion at the asthma GWAS SNPs. Ibadan, Nigeria (YRI) and northern and western European (CEU) from the 1000 Genomes project were used as parental populations

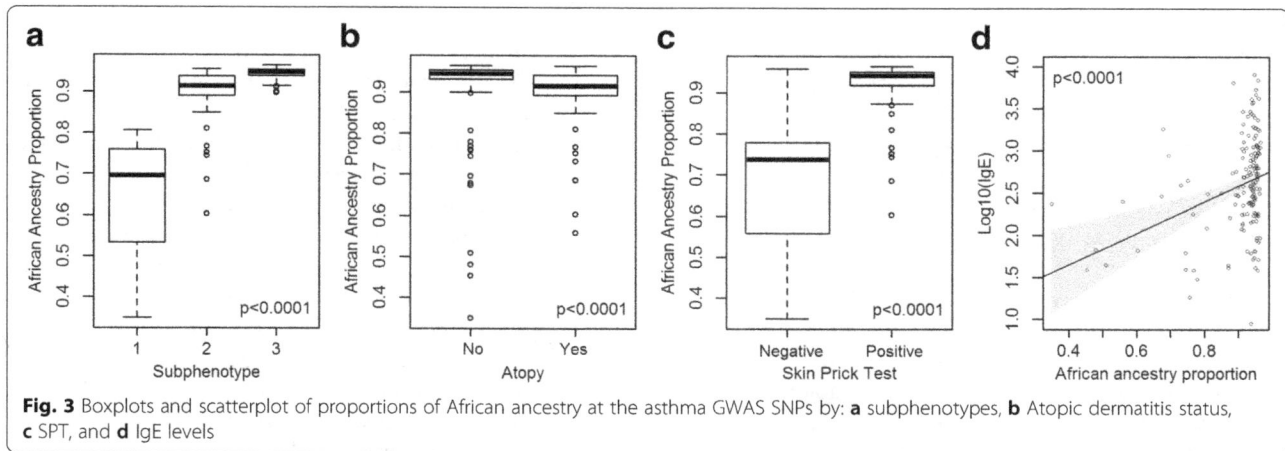

Fig. 3 Boxplots and scatterplot of proportions of African ancestry at the asthma GWAS SNPs by: **a** subphenotypes, **b** Atopic dermatitis status, **c** SPT, and **d** IgE levels

was 6.3 higher (95% confidence interval: (3.4, 13.8), p-value < 0.0001) with each additional 10% of African origin at asthma GWAS SNPs. African origin at asthma GWAS SNPs was also associated with IgE levels (Spearman correlation coefficient = 0.27, p-value = 0.0004) and IgE was 1.5 fold higher with each additional 10% of African origin (Fig. 3(d)).

Discussion

Current clinical practice in childhood asthma treatment tends to use average patient care strategies. Such a "one size fits all" treatment approach faces major challenges when it is becoming clearer that childhood asthma is heterogeneous in pathogenesis. Our unbiased cluster and genetic ancestry analyses pointed toward three distinct phenotypic clusters with differences in clinical characteristics, genetic ancestry, and clinical outcomes, underscoring the clinical and genetic heterogeneity of asthma [10, 13, 17, 31]. Previous studies have also identified clusters with atopic or non-atopic asthma, clusters with preserved or lower lung function, and clusters with mild asthma [13, 14, 32]. It is reassuring that the two independent studies replicated the clustering results and there are similarities with previous clustering-based childhood asthma subphenotypes.

We determined genetic ancestry [33] using genome-wide SNPs and asthma GWAS SNPs for African-American asthmatic individuals in CAMP and CARE data. Our estimate of African global ancestry in asthmatic children is higher than what has been reported in different general populations confirming the higher prevalence of asthma in individuals with higher African ancestry than others. Our results showed that genetic ancestry at asthma GWAS SNPs differed between the childhood asthma subphenotypes and was associated with lung function, SPT, IgE levels, and AD. Previous studies have also showed association between genetic ancestry and asthma prevalence and related clinical phenotypes [34–42]. To our best

knowledge, our study is the first to show the association between genetic ancestry at asthma GWAS SNPs and cluster-based subphenotypes in childhood asthma. Leveraging ancestry and cluster analyses to derive genetic and phenotypic homogeneity subgroups in childhood asthma demonstrates the utility of these approaches to characterize and understand the complexity of asthma towards individual based precision medicine strategies.

This study demonstrates that genetic ancestry at asthma GWAS SNPs is more strongly associated with asthma subgroups sharing similar clinical characteristics compared to broadly defined asthma. The results suggest that validation of genetic studies are more likely to be successful for replication studies carried-out in more homogeneous asthma cohorts (sharing similar clinical characteristics) compared to the multifactorial case-control status. In addition, the results indicate that ancestry-specific genetic loci of asthma are likely to be found by focusing on better defined asthma patients. Furthermore, genetic ancestry analysis in homogeneous asthma subgroups is suitable to refine the biological role of asthma susceptibility variants from GWAS studies in a given phenotype. For example, SNPs at STARD3/PGAP3 are strongly associated with the high atopic dermatitis subgroup suggesting that STARD3/PGAP3 may act on the allergic component of asthma [43]. Another example is that ORMDL3/17q locus is associated with asthma in multiple studies in the European ancestry but not in African ancestry asthmatic individuals [44]. We also investigated associations between asthma GWAS SNPs with the identified subphenotypes in CAMP and CARE data (methods and results in Additional file 1: Table S1). Several significant associations were identified at $p = 0.05$, but none after multiplicity adjustment, possibly due to small sample size and limited statistical power.

Our study had several limitations. First, participants in CAMP and CARE represent studies of childhood asthma, thus the results herein may not be applicable to adulthood asthma. Second, although we identified clinically relevant subphenotypes of childhood asthma using clinical phenotypes [45], the integration of this result with molecular and physiologic phenotyping may help to better understand childhood asthma pathogenesis for possibly more personalized therapeutic strategies. Furthermore, subgroup analyses of asthma may limit sample sizes and impair statistical power. However, given asthma is a highly heterogeneous phenotype, studying homogeneous subgroups of asthma patients not only recovers power limitation, but achieves more statistically significant results. Classifying asthma patients in more homogenous groups may help us to identify new susceptibility or modifying subphenotype-specific genes. Our ability to better define subtypes might help to predict who may respond to treatment vs subjects who may not. Future studies need to elucidate the mechanisms that distinguish each ancestral and clinical clusters to facilitate the development of targeted therapies and providing personalized treatments.

The present study has notable strengths. First, we were able to dissect childhood asthma heterogeneity into subphenotypes using cluster analysis of clinical phenotypes in one study and replicate the findings in an independent study. Second, we were able to show associations between the identified subphenotypes with asthma clinical outcomes. Third, analysis of genetic ancestry at asthma GWAS SNPs in childhood asthma clinical phenotypes provide biologically relevant subphenotype-specific results. Lastly, our study used a more accurate and direct assessment of genetic ancestry instead of self-reported race to determine the relationship between ancestry and childhood asthma subphenotypes and relevant clinical phenotypes. Studies have shown that people with the same self-reported race could have drastically different levels of genetic ancestry, and self-reported race may not be as accurate as direct assessment of genetic ancestry in predicting treatment outcomes [33]. Future studies to identify genetic ancestry-specific variants associated with a specific subphenotype are important as we move towards applying precision medicine paradigm. The finding indicates that African genetic ancestry at asthma GWAS SNPs are differentially associated with the asthma clinical subphenotypes. Unraveling the reasons why individuals with higher African origin at asthma GWAS SNPs had higher IgE level or rate of positive SPT is necessary to determine the potential clinical applications of our findings. In addition, genetic analysis based on more refined phenotypes may increase the statistical power and allow for the detection of population structure-specific phenotype-genotype associations that are undetectable otherwise.

Conclusions

In conclusion, through our systematic clinical phenotype analysis, we identified distinct subphenotypes for childhood asthma using cluster analysis. Further genetic ancestry analysis showed correlations between African ancestry at asthma GWAS SNPs and childhood asthma subphenotypes and related clinical outcomes. Our results demonstrated that cluster analyses on clinical phenotypes followed by ancestry analysis can enhance the understanding of the phenotypic and genetic heterogeneity of childhood asthma. Our approach is distinct from previous efforts in that we developed cluster-based subphenotype and applied genetic ancestry analysis to define subphenotype-ancestry relationships which can be subsequently used as the basis of genetic ancestry based clinical risk prediction. Our findings suggest that defining asthma heterogeneous subgroups on the basis of clinical phenotypes and genetic ancestry proportion is an essential step to understand and refine patient subsets and enable more targeted therapy.

Abbreviations

AD: Atopic dermatitis; BMIZ: Body mass index z-sore; CAMP: the Childhood Asthma Management Program; CARE: the Childhood Asthma Research and Education network; CEU: Utah Residents with Northern and Western Ancestry; dbGaP: The database of Genotypes and Phenotypes; EOS: Blood eosinophils; FEV1: Forced expiratory volume, the maximal amount of air one can forcefully exhale in 1 s converted to a percentage of normal based on one's height, weight, body composition, and race; FVC: Forced vital capacity, the amount of air a person can expire after a maximum inspiration second converted to a percentage of normal based on one's height, weight, body composition, and race; GWAS: Genome-wide association study; HCA: Hierarchical cluster analysis; IgE: Serum total immunoglobulin; IQR: Interquartile range; LD: Linkage disequilibrium; PC20: The dose of methacholine that is required to decrease FEV1 by 20%; SD: Standard deviation; SHARe: The SNP Health Association Resource; SHARP: The SNP Health Association Resource Asthma Resource Project; SNP: Single nucleotide polymorphism; SPT: Skin prick test; YRI: Yoruba in Ibadan, Nigeria

Funding

This work was supported by NIH Grant R01HL132344 and R03HL133713, Health Disparities Award of the Cincinnati Children's Research Foundation, the National Institutes of Health (NIH) Clinical and Translational Science Award (CTSA) program, grant 1UL1TR001425–01, Methods grant from the Center for Clinical and Translational Science and Training, Cincinnati Children's Hospital Medical Center. There is no role of the funding body in the design of the study and collection, analysis, and interpretation of data and in writing the manuscript.

Authors' contributions

LD conceptualized and designed the study, carried out and supervised the analyses, drafted the manuscript, and approved the final manuscript as submitted. DL carried out the initial analyses, reviewed and revised the manuscript, and approved the final manuscript as submitted. MW carried out the analyses, reviewed and revised the manuscript, and approved the final manuscript as submitted. MA supervised data analyses, critically reviewed the manuscript, and approved the final manuscript as submitted. TM conceptualized and designed the study, critically reviewed the manuscript, and approved the final manuscript as submitted.

Competing interests

The authors declare that they have no competing interests.

Author details

[1]Division of Biostatistics and Epidemiology, Department of Pediatrics, Cincinnati Children's Hospital Medical Center, Cincinnati, OH, USA. [2]Alzheimer's Therapeutic Research Institute, Keck School of Medicine, University of Southern California, San Diego, CA, USA. [3]Division of Asthma Research, Department of Pediatrics, Cincinnati Children's Hospital Medical Center, University of Cincinnati, 3333 Burnet Ave, Cincinnati, OH 45229, USA.

References

1. Borish L, Culp JA. Asthma: a syndrome composed of heterogeneous diseases. Ann Allergy Asthma Immunol. 2008;101(1):1–8. quiz -11, 50
2. Siroux V, Garcia-Aymerich J. The investigation of asthma phenotypes. Curr Opin Allergy Clin Immunol. 2011;11(5):393–9.
3. Yeatts K, Sly P, Shore S, Weiss S, Martinez F, Geller A, et al. A brief targeted review of susceptibility factors, environmental exposures, asthma incidence, and recommendations for future asthma incidence research. Environ Health Perspect. 2006;114(4):634–40.
4. Guerra S, Martinez FD. Asthma genetics: from linear to multifactorial approaches. Annu Rev Med. 2008;59:327–41.
5. Lotvall J, Akdis CA, Bacharier LB, Bjermer L, Casale TB, Custovic A, et al. Asthma endotypes: a new approach to classification of disease entities within the asthma syndrome. J Allergy Clin Immun. 2011;127(2):355–60.
6. Manolio TA, Collins FS, Cox NJ, Goldstein DB, Hindorff LA, Hunter DJ, et al. Finding the missing heritability of complex diseases. Nature. 2009;461(7265):747–53.
7. Akinbami LJ, Schoendorf KC, Parker J. US childhood asthma prevalence estimates: the impact of the 1997 National Health Interview Survey redesign. Am J Epidemiol. 2003;158(1):99–104.
8. Gamble C, Talbott E, Youk A, Holguin F, Pitt B, Silveira L, et al. Racial differences in biologic predictors of severe asthma: data from the severe asthma research program. J Allergy Clin Immunol. 2010;126(6):1149–56. e1
9. Green RH, Brightling CE, Bradding P. The reclassification of asthma based on subphenotypes. Curr Opin Allergy Clin Immunol. 2007;7(1):43–50.
10. Haldar P, Pavord ID, Shaw DE, Berry MA, Thomas M, Brightling CE, et al. Cluster analysis and clinical asthma phenotypes. Am J Respir Crit Care Med. 2008;178(3):218–24.
11. Just J, Gouvis-Echraghi R, Rouve S, Wanin S, Moreau D, Annesi-Maesano I. Two novel, severe asthma phenotypes identified during childhood using a clustering approach. Eur Respir J. 2012;40(1):55–60.
12. Kim TB, Jang AS, Kwon HS, Park JS, Chang YS, Cho SH, et al. Identification of asthma clusters in two independent Korean adult asthma cohorts. Eur Respir J. 2013;41(6):1308–14.
13. Moore WC, Meyers DA, Wenzel SE, Teague WG, Li HS, Li XN, et al. Identification of asthma phenotypes using cluster analysis in the severe asthma research program. Am J Respir Crit Care Med. 2010;181(4):315–23.
14. Siroux V, Basagana X, Boudier A, Pin I, Garcia-Aymerich J, Vesin A, et al. Identifying adult asthma phenotypes using a clustering approach. Eur Respir J. 2011;38(2):310–7.
15. Wardlaw AJ, Silverman M, Siva R, Pavord ID, Green R. Multi-dimensional phenotyping: towards a new taxonomy for airway disease. Clin Exp Allergy. 2005;35(10):1254–62.
16. Weatherall M, Travers J, Shirtcliffe PM, Marsh SE, Williams MV, Nowitz MR, et al. Distinct clinical phenotypes of airways disease defined by cluster analysis. Eur Respir J. 2009;34(4):812–8.
17. Amat F, Saint-Pierre P, Bourrat E, Nemni A, Couderc R, Boutmy-Deslandes E, et al. Early-onset atopic dermatitis in children: which are the phenotypes at risk of asthma? Results from the ORCA cohort. PLoS One. 2015;10(6):e0131369.
18. Pillai SG, Tang Y, van den Oord E, Klotsman M, Barnes K, Carlsen K, et al. Factor analysis in the genetics of asthma international network family study identifies five major quantitative asthma phenotypes. Clin Exp Allergy. 2008;38(3):421–9.
19. Weinmayr G, Keller F, Kleiner A, du Prel JB, Garcia-Marcos L, Batllés-Garrido J, et al. Asthma phenotypes identified by latent class analysis in the ISAAC phase II Spain study. Clin Exp Allergy. 2013;43(2):223–32.
20. Cherniack R, Adkinson NF, Strunk R, Szefler S, Tonascia J, Weiss S, et al. The childhood asthma management program (CAMP): design, rationale, and methods. Control Clin Trials. 1999;20(1):91–120.
21. Ding L, Abebe T, Beyene J, Wilke RA, Goldberg A, Woo JG, et al. Rank-based genome-wide analysis reveals the association of ryanodine receptor-2 gene variants with childhood asthma among human populations. Hum Genomics. 2013;7:16.
22. Gower JC. A general coefficient of similarity and some of its properties. Biometrics. 1971;27:857–74.
23. Ward JH Jr. Hierarchical grouping to optimize an objective function. J Am Stat Assoc. 1963;58:236–44.
24. Milligan GW, Cooper MC. An examination of procedures for determining the number of clusters in a data set. Psychometrika. 1985;50(2):159–79.
25. Cooper MC, Milligan GW. The effect of error on determining the number of clusters. Proceedings of the International Workshop on Data Analysis, Decision Support and Expert Knowledge Representation in Marketing and Related Areas of Research; 1988. p. 319–28.
26. Hothorn T, Hornik K, Zeileis A. Unbiased recursive partitioning: a conditional inference framework. J Comput Graph Stat. 2006;15(3):651–74.
27. Team RDC. R: a language and environment for statistical computing. R Foundation for Statistical Computing: Vienaa; 2010.
28. Alexander DH, Novembre J, Lange K. Fast model-based estimation of ancestry in unrelated individuals. Genome Res. 2009;19(9):1655–64.
29. Welter D, MacArthur J, Morales J, Burdett T, Hall P, Junkins H, et al. The NHGRI GWAS catalog, a curated resource of SNP-trait associations. Nucleic Acids Res. 2014;42(Database issue):D1001–6.
30. Pritchard JK, Stephens M, Donnelly P. Inference of population structure using multilocus genotype data. Genetics. 2000;155(2):945–59.
31. Wenzel SE. Asthma phenotypes: the evolution from clinical to molecular approaches. Nat Med. 2012;18(5):716–25.
32. Fitzpatrick AM, Teague WG, Meyers DA, Peters SP, Li XN, Li HS, et al. Heterogeneity of severe asthma in childhood: confirmation by cluster analysis of children in the National Institutes of Health/National Heart, Lung, and Blood Institute severe asthma research program. J Allergy Clin Immun. 2011;127(2):382–U973.
33. Mersha TB, Abebe T. Self-reported race/ethnicity in the age of genomic research: its potential impact on understanding health disparities. Hum Genomics. 2015;9:1.
34. Salam MT, Avoundjian T, Knight WM, Gilliland FD. Genetic ancestry and asthma and rhinitis occurrence in Hispanic children: findings from the Southern California Children's health study. PLoS One. 2015;10(8):e0135384.
35. Rumpel JA, Ahmedani BK, Peterson EL, Wells KE, Yang M, Levin AM, et al. Genetic ancestry and its association with asthma exacerbations among African American subjects with asthma. J Allergy Clin Immunol. 2012;130(6):1302–6.
36. Pino-Yanes M, Thakur N, Gignoux CR, Galanter JM, Roth LA, Eng C, et al. Genetic ancestry influences asthma susceptibility and lung function among Latinos. J Allergy Clin Immunol. 2015;135(1):228–35.
37. Ortega VE, Kumar R. The effect of ancestry and genetic variation on lung function predictions: what is "normal" lung function in diverse human populations? Curr Allergy Asthma Rep. 2015;15(4):516.
38. Vergara C, Murray T, Rafaels N, Lewis R, Campbell M, Foster C, et al. African ancestry is a risk factor for asthma and high Total IgE levels in African admixed populations. Genet Epidemiol. 2013;37(4):393–401.
39. Menezes AM, Wehrmeister FC, Hartwig FP, Perez-Padilla R, Gigante DP, Barros FC, et al. African ancestry, lung function and the effect of genetics. Eur Respir J. 2015;45(6):1582–9.
40. Brehm JM, Acosta-Perez E, Klei L, Roeder K, Barmada MM, Boutaoui N, et al. African ancestry and lung function in Puerto Rican children. J Allergy Clin Immunol. 2012;129(6):1484–90. e6
41. Chen W, Brehm JM, Boutaoui N, Soto-Quiros M, Avila L, Celli BR, et al. Native American ancestry, lung function, and COPD in Costa Ricans. Chest. 2014;145(4):704–10.
42. Kumar R, Seibold MA, Aldrich MC, Williams LK, Reiner AP, Colangelo L, et al. Genetic ancestry in lung-function predictions. N Engl J Med. 2010;363(4):321–30.
43. Moffatt MF, Gut IG, Demenais F, Strachan DP, Bouzigon E, Heath S, et al. A large-scale, consortium-based genomewide association study of asthma. N Engl J Med. 2010;363(13):1211–21.
44. Sleiman PM, Annaiah K, Imielinski M, Bradfield JP, Kim CE, Frackelton EC, et al. ORMDL3 variants associated with asthma susceptibility in north Americans of European ancestry. J Allergy Clin Immunol. 2008;122(6):1225–7.

12

Discovery and disentanglement of aligned residue associations from aligned pattern clusters to reveal subgroup characteristics

Pei-Yuan Zhou, Antonio Sze-To and Andrew K. C. Wong[*]

From Selected articles from the IEEE BIBM International Conference on Bioinformatics & Biomedicine (BIBM) 2017: medical genomics
Kansas City, MO, USA. 13-16 November 2017

Abstract

Background: A protein family has similar and diverse functions locally conserved. An aligned pattern cluster (APC) can reflect the conserved functionality. Discovering aligned residue associations (ARAs) in APCs can reveal subtle inner working characteristics of conserved regions of protein families. However, ARAs corresponding to different functionalities/subgroups/classes could be entangled because of subtle multiple entwined factors.

Methods: To discover and disentangle patterns from mixed-mode datasets, such as APCs when the residues are replaced by their fundamental biochemical properties list, this paper presents a novel method, Extended Aligned Residual Association Discovery and Disentanglement (E-ARADD). E-ARADD discretizes the numerical dataset to transform the mixed-mode dataset into an event-value dataset, constructs an ARA Frequency Matrix and then converts it into an adjusted Statistical Residual (SR) Vector Space (SRV) capturing statistical deviation from randomness. By applying Principal Component (PC) Decomposition on SRV, PCs ranked by their variance are obtained. Finally, the disentangled ARAs are discovered when the projections on a PC is re-projected to a vector space with the same basis vectors of SRV.

Results: Experiments on synthetic, cytochrome c and class A scavenger data have shown that E-ARADD can a) disentangle the entwined ARAs in APCs (with residues or biochemical properties), b) reveal subtle AR clusters relating to classes, subtle subgroups or specific functionalities.

Conclusions: E-ARADD can discover and disentangle ARs and ARAs entangled in functionality and location of protein families to reveal functional subgroups and subgroup characteristics of biological conserved regions. Experimental results on synthetic data provides the proof-of-concept validation on the successful disentanglement that reveals class-associated ARAs with or without class labels as input. Experiments on cytochrome c data proved the efficacy of E-ARADD in handing both types of residue data. Our novel methodology is not only able to discover and disentangle ARs and ARAs in specific statistical/functional (PCs and RSRVs) spaces, but also their locations in the protein family functional domains. The success of E-ARADD shows its great potential to proteomic research, drug discovery and precision and personalized genetic medicine.

Keywords: Pattern discovery, Disentanglement, Aligned residue associations, Aligned pattern clusters, Subgroup characteristics

* Correspondence: akcwong@uwaterloo.ca
Systems Design Engineering, University of Waterloo, Waterloo, ON, Canada

Background

Proteins and their interactions control the biological process of a living organism. Within the same family, proteins have similar functions. Thus, discovering conserved sequence patterns from a family is crucial for revealing domain functionality. However, due to mutations and/or multiple functionality, even these conserved patterns may have substantial differences in species or even functions. Hence, identifying subgroup characteristics are of fundamental importance. We have developed a novel method to obtain knowledge-rich [1] Aligned Pattern Clusters (APC) [2–4] from protein families (Fig. 1(a) and (b)) to represent biological conserved regions. Figures 1(b) and (c) show its pattern space (APC) and data space (APC-D) respectively [2–4]. When a local functional domain is identified, and class labels are given, it is easy to see how the ARs and ARAs are entangled among different classes within the conserved domain (Fig. 1(c)) if the data size is small. We may be able to disentangle their class relation. However, if the size of data is large and more subtle classes or subgroups are present while the class labels are unknown (Fig. 1(d)), the task of ARA disentanglement becomes extreme difficult. To overcome this challenge, a novel algorithm denoted as Aligned Residue Association Discovery and Disentanglement (ARADD) [5], has been developed by us, where ARADD is originated from our recent best-paper-award work [6], by considering the aligned sites in an APC as attributes and residues on a site as attribute values. Hence, we extend AVADD to E-ARADD (Aligned Residue Association Discovery and Disentanglement) to obtain succinct disentangled subgroups of ARAs, revealing more succinct stereo physiochemical knowledge of the conserved regions with or without explicit reliance of class labels. Since this knowledge is not obvious in the data, we refer it as deep knowledge discovered.

It should be noted that to discover knowledge at the physiochemical level, we have to handle mixed-mode data, i.e. data containing both categorical and numerical values. This becomes an interesting challenge since physiochemical properties in Aligned Pattern Clusters [2–4], apart from our early work [7] have not yet been seriously explored. In the following paragraphs, we provided a brief introduction of the related work, ranging from association rule mining to pattern discovery in protein sequences.

Pattern discovery and association rule mining

In the field of data mining, association rule mining [8] is common to mine itemset from relational tables. Algorithms such as Apriori [9] and FP-growth [10] are used to capture associations from relational dataset. However, the above algorithms are extremely sensitive to parameters and thresholds setting, such as probabilistic thresholds, the number of clusters, distance measure and so on. Furthermore, a challenging problem encountered that the discovered patterns may be masked or obscure in the data due to the entanglement of unknown factors in their source environment [5, 6]. Therefore, for the real-world applications in Bioinformatics with noise in the data, it is important to discover patterns in a robust manner to enhance biological comprehension and interpretation.

Protein functional regions represented by aligned pattern clusters

Protein sequence analysis is crucial for identifying and understanding the functional regions, as protein structures are expansive to obtain. Multiple Sequence Alignment (MSA) and Motif Discovery are the two major methods. Given an entire set of protein sequences, MSA [11–13] aligns them globally to identify the conserved regions. However, MSA is limited as it is only suitable

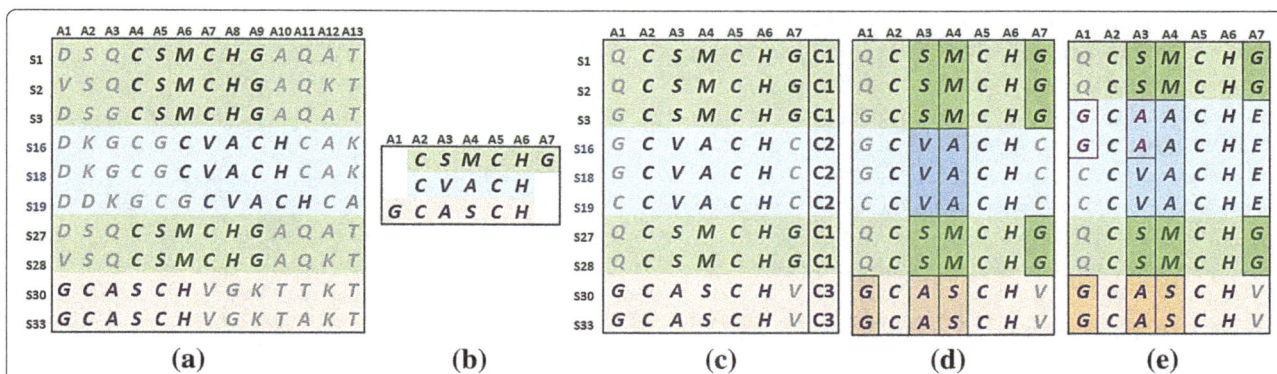

Fig. 1 Pattern and Data Spaces of APC and ARAs. **a** A portion of protein sequence dataset with discovered high order patterns (in bold) [2] with labels on the top row denote the aligned sites, on the first column denote the sequence ID; (**b**) Aligned Pattern Cluster (APC) Pattern Space obtained [3]. **c** APC Data Space (APC-D). C1, C2, C3 represents three classes. **d** An discovered ARA Cluster contains three partitioned subgroups and displayed in green, blue and red shade associate with class C1, C2 and C3 respectively. **e** Entangled ARAs. For example, in S3 S16, the AVAs A1G and A3A in C2 are from C3 entangling with its ARAs A4A and A7E

for globally homologous sequences with a high level of sequence similarity [13]. Different from MSA, Motif Discovery [14, 15] locates and aligns similar subsequences locally to construct a probabilistic model for representing the aligned amino acids. However, motif discovery makes unrealistic assumption that there is independence between residue columns to represent the conserved sequence patterns, where in reality it is clearly not the case [16, 17]. Aligned Pattern Cluster (APC) [2–4] was thus developed to discover sequence patterns directly, and to capture functional conserved residue association in order to identify clusters of aligned patterns from the sequence data. Since APCs conserve both strong statistical sequence associations and homologous sites, it is more knowledge rich [2, 3] to reveal similar yet diverse functional associations in protein families.

Physiochemical properties in aligned pattern clusters

In this study, we extend ARADD [5] to E-ARADD to discover physiochemical subgroup patterns in APCs at the residue (amino acid) level and the deeper level with mixed-mode residue physiochemical property. Hence, the ARPA clusters discovered can directly reveal the physiochemical characteristics of the APCs. We refers them as APPC patterns. In the notations, we insert term "Property" by adding the character "P" into AR, ARA and APC as ARP, ARPA and APPC respectively while the theory and the algorithm are not affected. We thus use them interchangeably except in some specific situation.

Novelty and contributions

The novelty of this study, is the consolidation of our recent work [5] and the extension of our ARADD algorithm [5] into E-ARADD. We introduced into E-ARADD the Aligned Residue Property (ARP), an ordered tuple for five biochemical properties for Aligned Residue Property Association (ARPA) Pattern Discovery and Disentanglement. Additional experimental analyses were conducted to support our proposed algorithms. Besides, we used the Adjusted Statistical Residual instead of standard statistical residual to measure the significance of discovered associations so as to give a more accurate indication of how far the observed count deviates from the expected count to evaluate the statistical significance of ARA/ARPA.

The major contributions of our study are three-folded.

1. We extended the previous ARADD into E-ARADD to handle the mixed-mode physiochemical protein data with chemical properties for direct residue biochemical association interpretation.
2. We showed that sequence patterns could be discovered and disentangled from APCs, even if the patterns were mixed or entangled in functionality and location.

3. We validated that E-ARADD could reveal functional subgroups and subgroup characteristics of APCs and locate their residing domains through the case study on Class A Scavenger Receptor family (SR-A). Understanding subgroup characteristics of conserved regions in proteins could render new knowledge for gene therapy applications [18].

Methods

This study focuses on discovering inherent ARAs/ARPA from APCs; clustering them into subgroups to reveal the functionalities of proteins within conserved functional regions and discover deep knowledge (PC/RSRVs) from APCs. Table 1 gives an abbreviation of terms and Fig. 2 provides a schematic overview of our method.

To show that ARADD can go one level deeper to discover and disentangle ARA at the aligned residue chemical property level, we replace each aligned residue in an APC by its five-tuples of chemical properties referred to as APPC. Given a mixed-mode APC dataset, E-ARADD can accomplish the followings in steps as circled in Fig. 2. In addition, Fig. 3 shows how E-ARADD could be easily shifted from operating modes of APC and APPC via an Interactive GUI to visualize the use of the proposed algorithm.

In the most general setting, an APC/APPC is represented by $\mathbf{R}$. Every tuple in $\mathbf{R}$, denoted as A = $\{A_1, A_2, ...A_N\}$, is described by N amino acid sites or the five chemical properties of the residues (ARP tuples) in the aligned sites.

First, to discover event (residue property) associations, the numerical values of the source data need to be discretized into intervals. Discretization can minimize the impact of noisy data in the data mining process [19]. It also can help smooth data to reduce noise [20], speed up classification process [21] and make classification result more

Table 1 Notations and terminologies

APC	Aligned Pattern Cluster (with categorical amino acid symbols)
APPC	Aligned Property Pattern Cluster (with mixed-mode chemical properties)
AR	Aligned Residue (for amino acid symbols in APC dataset)
ARP	Aligned Residue Property (for mixed-mode chemical properties in APC dataset)
ARA	Aligned Residue Association (Significant co-occurrence of two ARs in APCs)
ARPA	Aligned Residue Property Association (for APPC)
ARA/ARPA FM	ARA/ARPA Frequency Matrix
SR	adjusted Statistical Residual between two ARs/ARPs
SRV	ARA/ARPA adjusted Statistical Residual Vector Space
PCD	Principle Component Decomposition
RSRV	Re-projected SRV

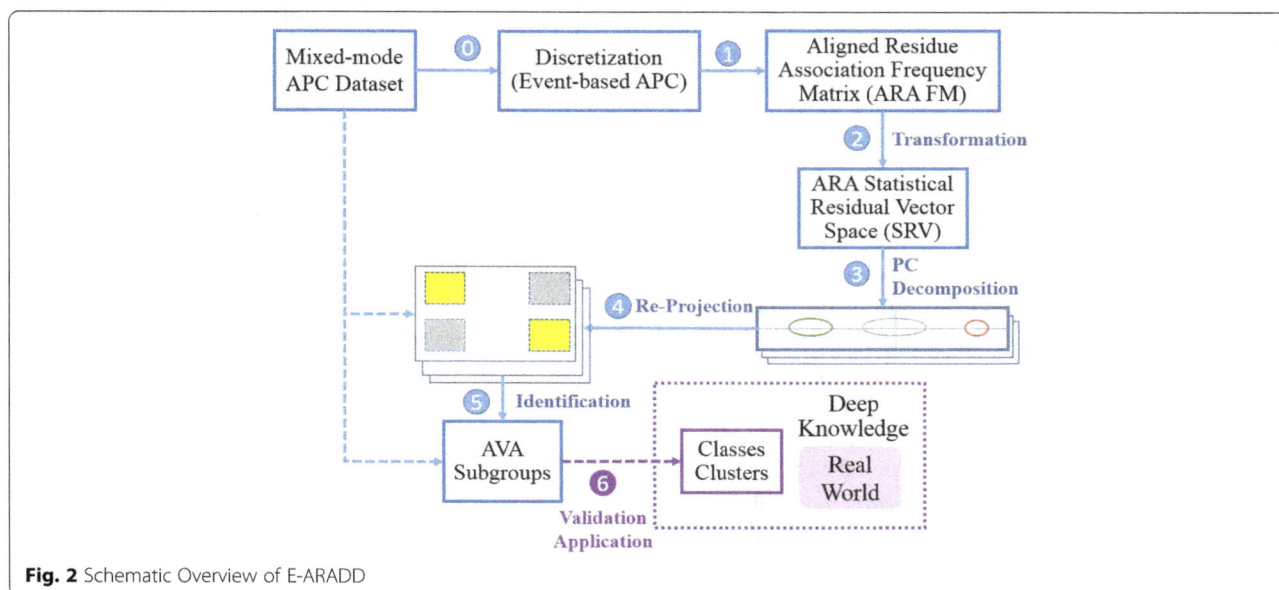

Fig. 2 Schematic Overview of E-ARADD

meaningful and easier-to-understand [22]. Hence, as Fig. 2 shows, in step 0, a mixed-mode APC is first converted to a categorical APC by discretizing all the numerical (ordinal) chemical properties of amino acid into intervals.

Equal Width and Equal Frequency are two simplest discretization methods. However, if uncharacteristic extreme values (outliers) exist in the data set, *Equal Width* can hardly handle this situation [22]. Hence, we transform numerical chemical properties of amino acid into discrete value using *Equal Frequency* [22] algorithm. Besides, we also implemented two other algorithms, class-driven discretization [23], called Optimal Class-Dependent Discretization OCDD, when class labels are given, and equal probability maximizing the entropy [24]

when class labels are not given. As Fig. 3 shows, the original mixed-mode APC can be transformed into a categorical one after selecting a discretization method and pushing the button labeled "Partition".

Therefore, each amino acid site or chemical property A_n can assume a numerical value or a categorical value.

1. For a continuous value, A_n is partitioned into I_n bins by transforming the original numerical values of A_n into interval event values, denoted as $A_n = \{A_n^i | i = 1, 2, \ldots I_n\}$. If the distinct value of numerical A_n is less than three, we treat it as a categorical attribute.
2. For categorical attribute, $A_{n'}$ contains $I_{n'}$ values, we denote it as $A_n = \{A_n^j | j = 1, 2, \ldots I_{n'}\}$.

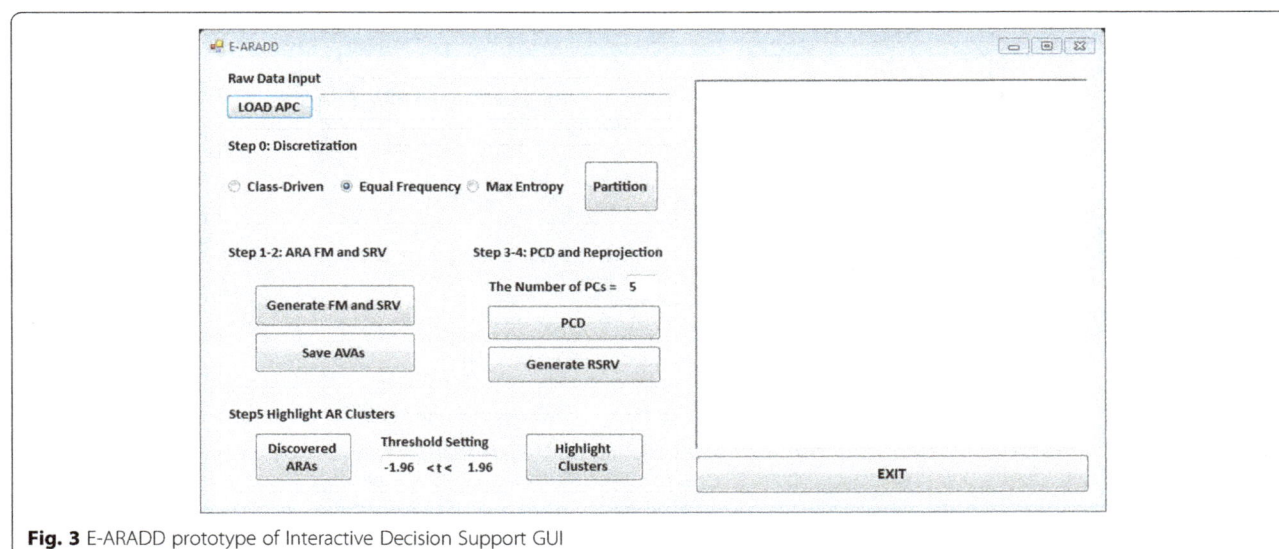

Fig. 3 E-ARADD prototype of Interactive Decision Support GUI

After transforming the mixed-mode dataset into an event-value dataset, all the values of an attribute (A_n) can be denoted as $A_n = \{A_n^1, A_n^2, ... A_n^{I_n}\}$.

Then, we will present the methodology through the algorithmic process with formal definitions and theoretical content as below

1. **Construct ARAFM** In step 1 (Fig. 2) we scan through the APC/APPC to construct an ARAFM/ ARPAFM which is obtained from the frequency counts between two ARs/ARPs, say $FM(A_n^i \leftrightarrow A_{n'}^j)$, where A_n^i denotes the ith value on the nth aligned site/ property in the APC/APPC, and A_n^j denotes the jth value on the n'^{th} aligned site/property in the APC/ APPC ($n \neq n'$). Hence ARAFM/ARPAFM is a $I \times I$ matrix, where $I = \sum_{n=1}^N I_n$ represents the total number of event values of all sites in an APC/APPC.

2. **Obtain SRV.** In order to disentangle the statistical residuals by Principal Component Decomposition (PCD) [25], we first convert the ARAFM/ARPAFM into an adjusted statistical residual (SR) matrix, referred to as a SR Space (SRV), (Step 2 in Fig. 2) by converting each ARA/ARPA frequency in the ARAFM/ARPAFM into an adjusted SR value to account for the deviation of the observed frequency

against the expected frequency if that ARA/ARPA is a random happening.

Formally, ARAFM/ARPAFM is transformed into SRV by converting each ARA frequency into an SR, denoted as $SR(A_n^i \leftrightarrow A_{n'}^j) = SR_{ij} = \frac{o_{ij} - e_{ij}}{\sqrt{e_{ij}}}$. o_{ij} represents the total number of occurrence when $A_n = A_n^i$ and $A_{n'} = A_{n'}^j$; e_{ij} represents the expected value of o_{ij}. SR_{ij} measures whether o_{ij} is significantly deviating from e_{ij} to reveal the statistical significance of an ARA/ARPA. At the confidence level of 95%, the discovered ARA/ ARPA is positive significant or negative significant when its SR > 1.96 or SR < − 1.96; and if the SR is between − 1.96 and 1.96, the ARA/ARPA is considered as irrelevant or random occurrence.

In order to disentangle the statistics in the SR matrix, we treat it as a vector space, denoted as SRV, where each row represents a vector corresponding to an AR (referred to as an AR-vector or just an a-vector) whose coordinates are the SRs of that AR associating with other distinct ARs (of other attributes) represented by the column a-vectors. Then, SRV can be represented as a set of vectors, denoted as, SRV $= <SRV_{A_1^1}, ... SRV_{A_1^{I_1}}, ...$ $SRV_{A_n^i}, ... SRV_{A_N^{I_N}}>$, where $SRV_{A_n^i} = \{SR(A_n^i \leftrightarrow A_1^1), ...$ $SR(A_n^i \leftrightarrow A_1^{I_1}), ... SR(A_n^i \leftrightarrow A_N^{I_N})\}$ and $SR(A_n^i \leftrightarrow A_n^i) = 0$.

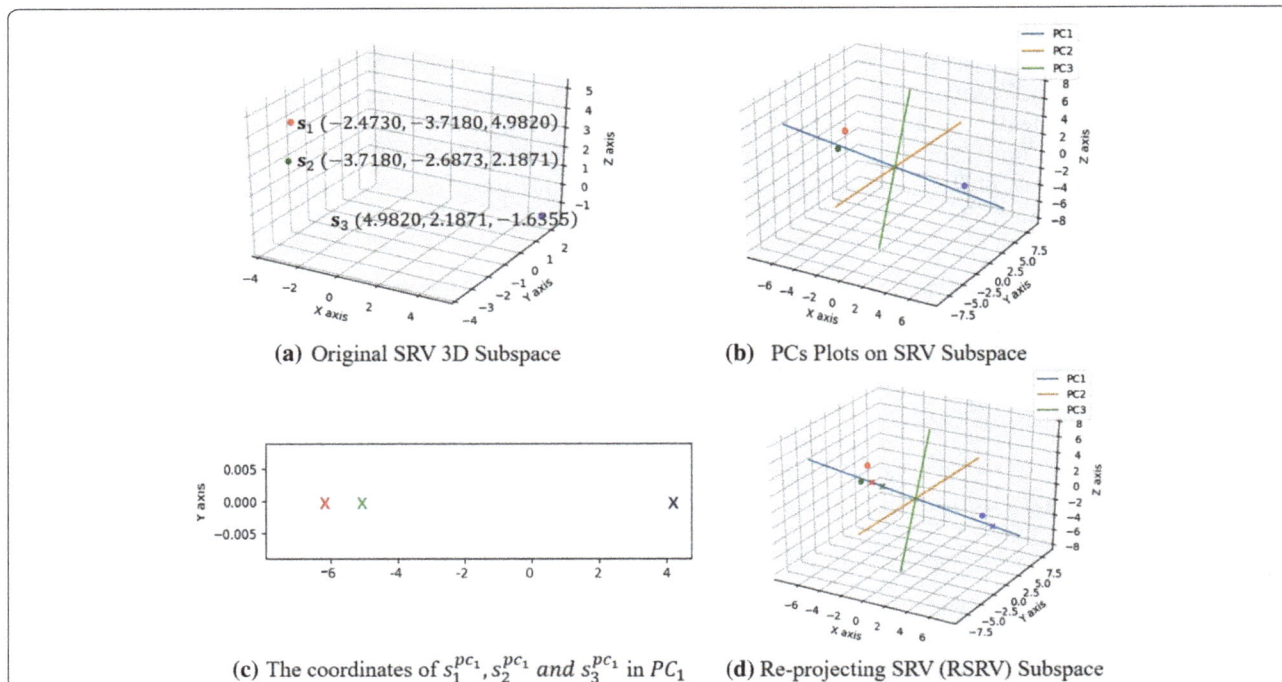

(a) Original SRV 3D Subspace

(b) PCs Plots on SRV Subspace

(c) The coordinates of $s_1^{pc_1}, s_2^{pc_1}$ and $s_3^{pc_1}$ in PC_1

(d) Re-projecting SRV (RSRV) Subspace

Fig. 4 Diagrammatic Illustration of SRV, PC Plots and Their Coordinates in SRV and RSRV Subspaces. **a** Original data space: three a-vectors from the experiment is display in the 3-dimensional SRV Subspace. **b** PCs Plots: a-vectors position after applying PCD on SRV. **c** The coordinates of $s_1^{pc_1}, s_2^{pc_1}$ and $s_3^{pc_1}$ in pc_1: the projection of the transformed a-vectors on the PC (as colored crosses). **d** Re-projecting the Coordinates in PCs: Re-projection of a-vector projections on the PC to RSRV subspace (as crosses on the blue axis). The colored dots are their original position in the SRV subspace

3. **Disentangle the SRV by PCD**. In Step 3, we conduct PCD to disentangle the SRV into PCs ranked according to the descending order of their eigenvalues. In PCD, PCs are a sets k PCs, denoted as $PC = \{PC_1, PC_2, ...PC_k\}$, where PC_n is a set of projections of the a-vectors from SRV on it and denoted as $PC_n = \{PC_n(A_n^i) \mid n = 1, 2, ...N, i = 1, ... I_n\}$, where N represents the total number of all ARs/ARPs and I_n represents the total number of distinct values of A_n. Fig. 4 (a) to (c) give a diagrammatic illustration of applying PCD to the SRV. Considering a matrix, A (i.e. a three-dimensional subspace of SRV) with 3 points as shown in Fig. 4(a) of the original data space. After applying PCD, we obtain eigenvectors and eigenvalues, sorted in descending order according to the magnitude of their eigenvalues. Fig. 4(b) shows the PC axis induced by their projection of the a-vectors that maximize their variance on that PC. Fig. 4(c) shows the coordinates of the projection of the a-vectors on the PC.

4. **Re-project the a-vector projections on each PC**. In step 4, we re-project the projections of the a-vectors on the PC back to an SRV with the same basis vectors of the previous SRV. We refer this new SRV as the Re-projected SRV (denoted as RSRV) with subscript k in $RSRV_k$ corresponding to that in PC_k. $RSRV_k$ is the SRV containing the transformed positions of a-vector on PC_k via $RSRV_k = SRV \cdot PC_k \cdot PC_k^T$.

   Figure 4(d) shows the new positions of the a-vectors representing their projection on the PC to the RSRV. In each RSRV, like SRV, each row represents an a-vector corresponding to an AR with a new set of coordinates accounting the statistical strength SRs of that AR associating with other ARs captured by the PC governed by certain specific underlying factors.

5. **Identify ARAs/ARPAs and AR/ARP Clusters in each PC.** Since each row a-vector in SRV represents an AR or their properties associating with other ARs or properties as its coordinates, the PC transformation will bring out in the PC the highest variance of the a-vectors with high SR coordinate values and display them at the far ends from the center (with zero coordinate value) of the PC. We may not see the reason why an a-vector is significant at the surface, but when viewing it in the RSRV, we would find out that the coordinate(s) of an a-vector of an AR/ARP reflect the statistic strength of its ARAs/ARPAs with another AR(s)/ARP(s) contributing to its high variance on the PC. In general, PCD is sensitive to the relative scaling of the original variables, often masking their distinctiveness. However, by converting the AR(P)AFM into SRV with uniform SR scale and statistical weights, both ARADD and E-ARADD utilize the statistical strength and functional decomposition to reveal more stable, subtle yet significant statistical associations that might be masked in the original frequency space. Hence, in this step, the significant AR(P)As discovered and disentangled are more distinct, stable and specific as manifested in separate RSRVs. Therefore, a cluster of ARs can be generated by AR(P)s that share strong AR(P)As. As Fig. 3 shows the GUI of E-ARADD server, for step 1–2, when pressing the button labeled "Generated FM and SRV" on E-ARADD server, both ARAFM and SRV are constructed for original data. Then, for step 3–4, the set of top PCs and their corresponding RSRVs are generated depending on the values of parameters (i.e. the number of PCs) are assigned in the box. Finally, in step 5, the sub-cluster results are highlighted according to the assigned confidence interval in the box.

Finally, we can validate the output RSRVs and AR(P) clusters when apply E-ARADD in specific application. We summarize the results as below.

1. The significant disentangled AR(P)As. These can be found from the distinct AR(P)s and the AR(P) clusters in the PCs based on their distance from the center (with zero value) of the PCs. When AR(P)As were entangled, the SRV disentanglement to reveal distinct AR(P)s in the PCs is crucial for yielding highly distinct, stable, and specific results as manifested in the RSRVs obtained from both datasets.

2. AR(P)s Sub-clusters. On one hand, the disentangled PCs can reveal significant AR(P)s/AR(P)-Clusters on a one-dimensional space; on the other hand, the SR of the AR(P)As in RSRVs can further reveal the significance of the AR(P)As and the AR(P)-Clusters. The AR(P) subgroups that are obtained in different orthogonal PC spaces may have functional meaning leading to established or new biological interpretation.

Results

In this study, we conducted both experiments on synthetic data and bio-sequence data. We hereby illustrate the experimental results and their analysis in this section.

Synthetic dataset

We first generated a 300×6 matrix with the first column representing class labels and the following 5 representing 5 attributes values AVs (equivalent to aligned residues ARs). First for each entry of an attribute column, we stochastically generated characters from a uniform distribution of the characters via a pseudo random number generator. We

Table 2 Synthetic dataset with embedded entangled patterns

Classes	Attribute Values are Significant Associated with Class Label
C1	A1A, A2C, A3E, (A4 H/G, A5M/N) where A4 and A5 are random patterns
C2	A1A, A2D, A3F, (A4 H/G, A5M/N) where A4 and A5 are random patterns
C3	A1B, A2D, A3E, (A4 H, A5M/N) where A4 and A5 are random patterns

then embedded patterns of three different classes 1, 2 and 3 (C_1, C_2, and C_3) as shown in Table 2. To simplify the notation, from here on we represent an attribute (say A1) assuming a certain value (say A) by A1A.

In Table 2, we can find that the attribute values A1A, A4H, A5N are entangled for class 1 and class 2; attribute values A3E, A4H, A5M and A5N are entangled in class 1 and class 3; and attribute values A2D, A4H, A5M, A5N are entangled in class 2 and class 3.

Figure 5 show the result using adjusted residual as the measurement. In Fig. 5(a), we found that A1A is entangled in class 1 and class 2; A2D is entangled in class 2 and class 3; and A3E is entangled in class 2 and class 3. Later, after the disentanglement, the AVAs results are shown in RSRVs (Fig. 5(b)-(d)). We noted that the class patterns are disentangled. In Fig. 5(b), after disentanglement, RSRV1 captured the disentangled AVA patterns for class 1 and class 2. An interesting characteristic of this association is that they share the same AV in A2 but with different residues D and E. Their AV-vectors are on the opposite side of the same PC. RSRV2 reveals another set of associations between class 2 and class 3. Here they both involve A1 but with different values A and B. This shows that Class 2 has two association patterns, one associated with Class 1 and another associating with Class 3, just as what we implanted. They were disentangled in different PCs and RSRVs. Fig. 5(c) and (d)

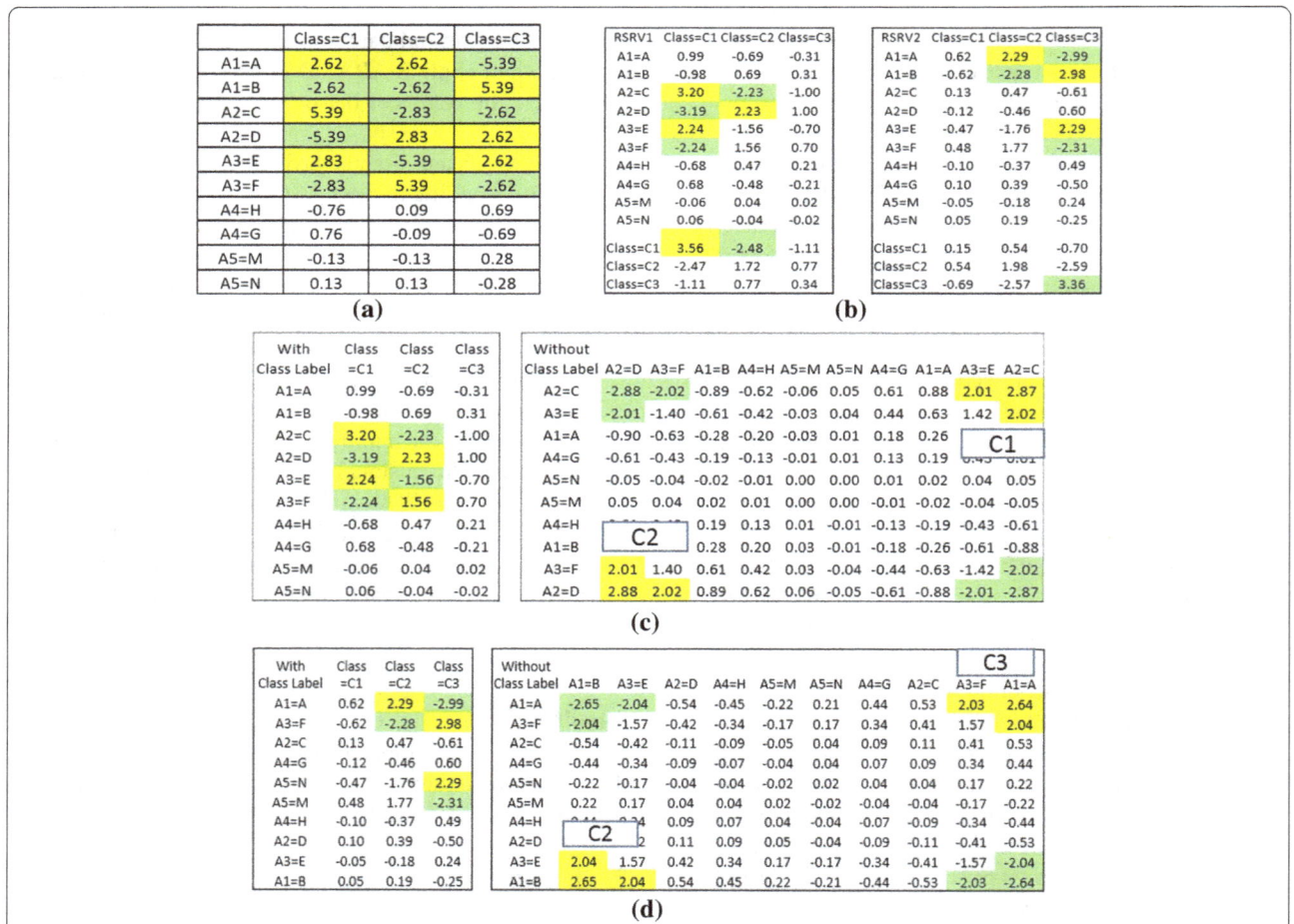

Fig. 5 Pattern entanglement and disentanglement. ARA patterns are shown in significant SR colored in yellow. **a** A1A is entangled in class 1 and class 2; A2D is entangled in class 2 and class 3; and A3E is entangled in class 2 and class 3. **b** AR patterns disentangled in two RSRVs, pattern for classes 1 and 2 in RSRV1 and classes 2 and 3 in RSRV2. Note the different ARAs of class 2 --- one with the same residue site A2 as Class 1 but different ARs (A2C and A2D) while the other with site A1 with different ARs (A1A and A1B) with class 3. **c** and (**d**) show the two different sets of ARs, one associating with classes 1 and 2 and another with classes 2 and 3

SRV	Mammal	Plant	Fungi	Insect
71=L	2.65	2.32	-6.36	1.23
73=E	5.92	-5.44	-2.29	2.04
76=E	4.70	-8.16	1.88	2.19
76=L	-4.45	8.64	-2.77	-2.07
90=A	4.76	-4.31	-3.60	3.95
92=L	-8.69	4.45	3.28	2.37
95=P	-6.21	6.08	-1.05	2.08

(a)

RSRV1	Mammal	Plant	Fungi	Insect
71=L	1.31	-1.37	-0.06	0.08
73=E	5.63	-5.06	-1.15	0.35
76=E	5.50	-4.96	-1.12	0.34
76=L	-5.61	4.55	1.69	-0.35
90=A	4.60	-4.18	-0.89	0.28
92=L	-6.20	5.05	1.83	-0.39
95=P	-5.44	4.40	1.64	-0.34

(b)

RSRV2	Mammal	Plant	Fungi	Insect
71=L	1.64	3.02	-5.13	0.06
73=E	0.13	0.05	-0.20	0.00
76=E	-0.82	-1.81	2.89	-0.03
76=L	1.23	2.21	-3.78	0.04
90=A	0.49	0.75	-1.37	0.02
92=L	-0.44	-1.07	1.66	-0.02
95=P	0.79	1.35	-2.36	0.03

(c)

RSRV3	Mammal	Plant	Fungi	Insect
71=L	-0.59	-0.51	0.15	1.48
73=E	-0.34	-0.39	0.20	0.81
76=E	-0.44	-0.44	0.18	1.09
76=L	0.35	-0.06	0.35	-0.94
90=A	-0.81	-0.62	0.10	2.02
92=L	-0.46	-0.45	0.18	1.44
95=P	-0.51	-0.47	0.17	1.25

(d)

Fig. 6 Discovered ARAs by E-ARADD for Dataset 1 with Amino Acid. (**a**) Entangled ARAs associating with classes in SRV; (**b**) Disentangled ARAs associating with Mammal and Plant in RSRV1; (**c**) Disentangled ARAs associating with Plant and Fungi in RSRV2; (**d**) Disentangled ARAs associating with Insect in RSRV3

unveil all their disentangled patterns as implanted, with or without class labels given --- a robust demonstration of the deep knowledge discovered from the entangled source environment without the explicit reliance of prior knowledge or posteriori fixing.

Bio-sequence dataset (cytochrome c protein family)

For protein study, we used three datasets. Dataset 1 and Dataset 2 are APCs obtained from two distinct localized regions from the dataset in [3] collected from the cytochrome c protein family with taxonomic class labels. In addition, Dataset 3 is the APC obtained from the class A scavenger receptors (SR-A) dataset in our previous paper [26] where we have reported some experimental result. In this paper we just highlight the use of address table in ARADD to track down the

locations of ARAs we discovered and disentangled as detailed in [26].

Dataset 1 is an APC dataset (width: 27) used in [3, 7] that contains 85 samples from four classes: Mammals, Plants, Fungus, and Insects. To compress this dataset, we reduced the number of aligned sites from 27 to 9 by removing the aligned sites with low SR2 value [13].

Dataset 2 is an APC dataset (width:36) used in [3, 7] that contains 147 samples from six classes: Mammals, Birds, Fish, Insects, Metazoas and Plants. Like the dimensionality reduction process in Dataset 1, we reduced the dimensions from 36 to 17.

Dataset 3 is an APC dataset (width: 12) used in [26] converting 95 protein sequences from five classes: Macro, Sra, Scara3, Scara4, Scara5 of class A scavenger receptors (SR-A) originally taken from a dataset with 106 sequences used in [27], one with the highest coverage. All five

SRV	Bird	Fish	Metazoa	Insect	Mammal	Plant
A84 = F	-1.11	-0.96	2.15	6.79	-2.15	-1.93
A79 = N	-0.93	2.94	0.45	3.80	-1.79	-1.60
A80 = Q	-0.44	2.27	2.27	-0.49	-0.85	-0.76
A73 = N	0.82	-2.12	-1.18	-2.74	1.58	1.18
A84 = M	1.63	0.08	-1.69	-2.18	4.16	-3.38
...	...	...	...	...	...	...

(a)

RSRV1	Bird	Fish	Insect	Mammal	Metazoa	Plant
74 = M	-0.78	-0.8	-0.74	-2.19	-0.43	4
75 = A	-1.01	-1.21	-1.03	-2.94	-0.73	5.51
76 = V	-0.96	-1.11	-0.96	-2.77	-0.66	5.16
79 = E	-0.75	-0.77	-0.71	-2.12	-0.4	3.85
84 = Y	-1.01	-1.2	-1.03	-2.94	-0.73	5.5
85 = D	-1.03	-1.23	-1.05	-2.99	-0.75	5.61
88 = L	-1.04	-1.25	-1.06	-3.02	-0.76	5.66
100 = V	-0.86	-0.94	-0.84	-2.44	-0.53	4.5
102 = P	-1.01	-1.21	-1.03	-2.94	-0.73	5.51
104 = L	-0.7	-0.68	-0.65	-1.96	-0.34	3.52
107 = P	-0.87	-0.97	-0.86	-2.5	-0.56	4.63
108 = Q	-0.94	-1.09	-0.95	-2.73	-0.65	5.07

(b)

RSRV3	Bird	Fish	Insect	Mammal	Metazoa	Plant
73 = A	-0.87	1.07	1.91	-2.06	1.88	0.1
84 = F	-0.86	1.06	1.88	-2.04	1.86	0.1
85 = V	-0.9	1.1	1.97	-2.12	1.93	0.09
108 = N	-0.88	1.08	1.94	-2.08	1.9	0.1

(c)

RSRV4	Bird	Fish	Insect	Mammal	Metazoa	Plant
73 = E	0.02	2.42	-2.31	0.41	-1.3	0.46
84 = N	0.02	2.42	-2.31	0.41	-1.3	0.46
88 = Q	0.02	2.42	-2.31	0.41	-1.3	0.46
100 = N	0.02	2.42	-2.31	0.41	-1.3	0.46
108 = R	0.02	2.42	-2.31	0.41	-1.3	0.46

(d)

RSRV5	Bird	Fish	Insect	Mammal	Metazoa	Plant
79 = K	-0.58	0.27	-1.41	-0.36	2.64	0.19
80 = N	-0.58	0.27	-1.41	-0.37	2.65	0.19
107 = Z	-0.55	0.27	-1.3	-0.36	2.47	0.19

(e)

RSRV13	Bird	Fish	Insect	Mammal	Metazoa	Plant
108 = S	0.78	0.11	0.04	-0.65	0.27	0.06
108 = A	0.54	0.13	0.03	-0.57	0.28	0.10

(f)

Fig. 7 Discovered ARAs by E-ARADD for Dataset 2 with Amino Acid. (**a**) Entangled ARAs associating with classes in SRV; (**b-f**) Disentangled ARAs in RSRV1, RSRV3, RSRV4, RSRV5 and RSRV13

subclasses of proteins contain domains: Cytoplasmic, Collagenous, Transmembrane, a-helical and coiled-coil motifs. Macro, Sra, and Scara5 contain the Collagenous domain. Only Sra contains the SRCR domain.

In this paper, we first reported the results when E-ARADD was applied to the two datasets above, using both their APCs and APPCs. Analysis I focuses on evaluating and comparing the entangled ARAs and disentangled ARAs results for APCs composed of amino acid symbols for Dataset 1 and Dataset 2. Analysis II shows how E-ARADD being applied to the mixed-mode APPC for both datasets. Then, in the Discussion Section, we summarized the results of our work on dataset 3 reported in [26], highlighting how ARADD is able to reveal and locate all the significant ARs and ARAs inherent in an APC obtained from the sequence data of SR-A protein family. Since the AR and ARA ID Address Table reported in [26] is a special module of E-ARADD, we will include a brief summary the work in [26] in the discussion of this paper. We will briefly describe how

E-ARADD is able to unveil the crucial functional information, of "what" and "where" of a protein family through the APCs discovered in the data [26].

Analysis I – Cytochrome c APCs in amino acid symbols

In Analysis I, we applied E-ARADD on APCs in amino acid symbols from data of dataset 1 and dataset 2. First, we compared the discovered ARAs obtained in RSRVs by using E-ARADD with those using only the adjusted statistical residual in SRV [28] with the same threshold 1.96. Figures 6 and 7 show the result of dataset 1 and dataset 2 respectively.

Figure 6(a) presents the results when the SRV was used to reveal the ARs associating with classes in dataset 1. From the SRV obtained from the APC, we observed that different species share the same ARs. For example, both Mammal and Plant share A71L. In another word, the ARs are entangled among different classes. However, after the E-ARADD disentanglement, we noted that the

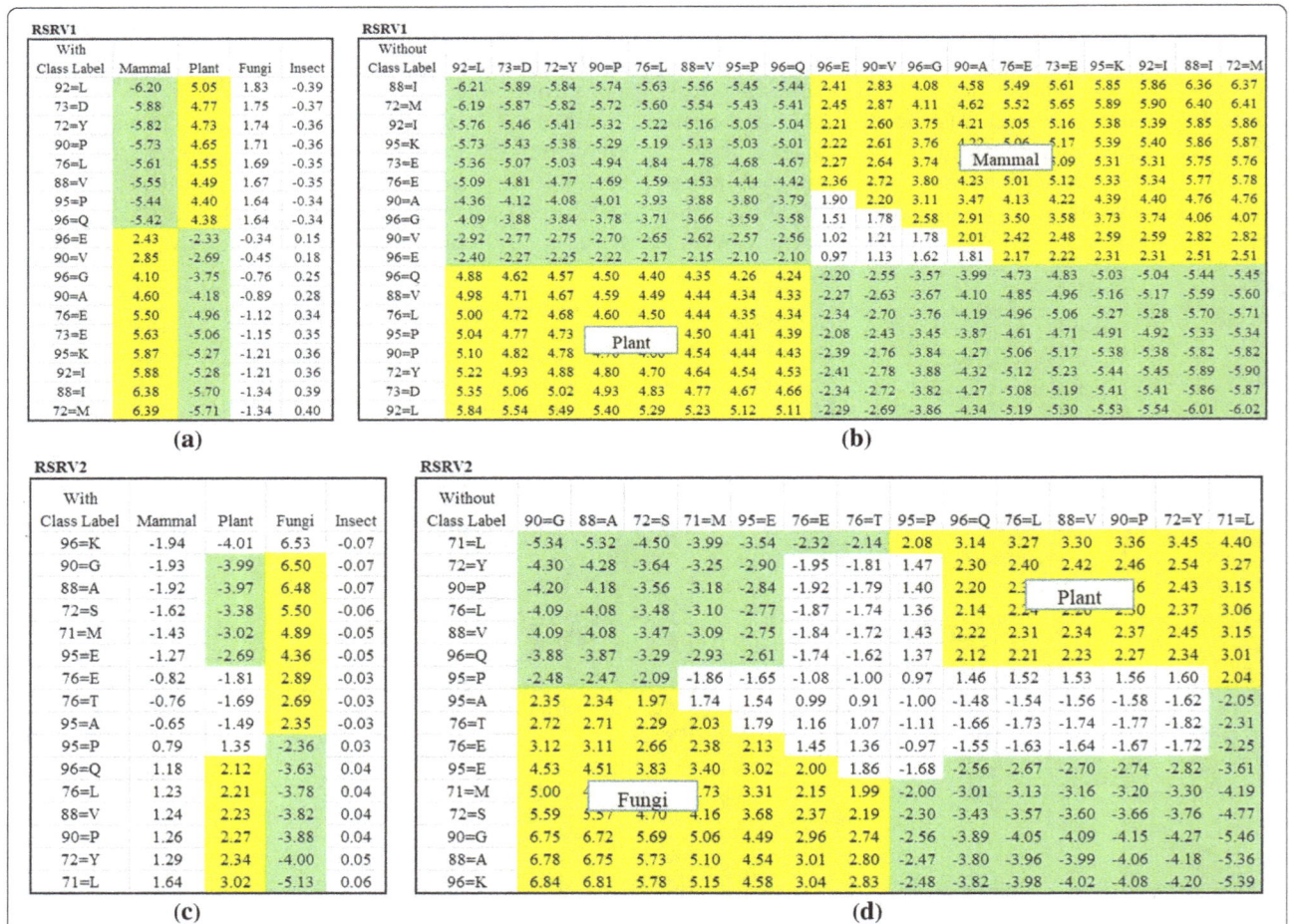

Fig. 8 The Result of AR Clusters captured in PCs and the corresponding ARAs reflected in RSRVs for APC Dataset 1 with amino acid. **a** ARA Clustering Result with Class Label on RSRV1; (**b**) ARA Clustering Result without Class Labels on RSRV1 (**c**) ARA Clustering Result with Class Label on RSRV2; and (**d**) ARA Clustering Result without Class Labels on RSRV2

ARAs associating with class were disentangled as manifested in the RSRVs (Fig. 6b-d). In Fig. 6(b), ARs associating with Mammal were disentangled with those with Plant whereas most of them were quite mixed in the SRV (Fig. 6(a)). For instance, A92L was entangled among Plant, Fungi and Insect in SRV, but associates with Plant but not Mammal in the specific statistic/functional space RSRV1; and with Fungi in RSRV2 and Insect in RSRV3. This indicates that 192 L play different role in three uncorrelated statistic/functional spaces (though the latter could be weak, with SR = 2.02 and 1.44 respectively). We also observed that in RSRV3, only A90A and A92L associating with Insect were picked up. Note that the weak association of A92L with Insect (SR = 1.44) will play a strong role (SR = 5.05) in Plant in RSRV1 and a weaker role (SR = 1.66) in RSRV2. The importance of E-ARADD Disentanglement of ARAs with different classes were clearly revealed in different statistical/functional spaces, RSRV1, RSRV2 and RSRV3, as captured through their corresponding PCs.

Similarly, Fig. 7 shows the discovered ARAs on SRV and RSRVs from the APC in amino acid symbols from dataset 2. Figure 7(a) shows the result in SRV. Here, we observed that "Mammal" stands out with positive SR

associating with A84M while other ARs were entangled with different classes. Note that from the SRV obtained from this APC, Birds and even Plants were irrelevant. We also noted that ARs associating with Metazoa, Insect and Fish were mixed. However, after the disentanglement, the result of RSRVs shown in Fig. 7(b-f) told a different story. In Fig. 7(d) Fish stands out from Insect and Metazoa. In Fig. 7(e) Metazoa separates from Insect and Fish. The ARA with specific classes stood out in different disentangled spaces. More surprising is that the AR missing in the Bird class appeared in PC_{13} and $RSRV_{13}$ with low SR but its ARA values still stand out from the SRs of all the other ARAs. This indicates the capability of ARADD in revealing weak ARAs (rare events) encountered in the imbalanced class problem that has plagued data mining for sometimes [29].

This experimental result shows that, beside discovering and disentangling the ARAs, E-ARADD can discover AR Clusters (ARCs) and significant ARs captured in orthogonal PCs and their corresponding RSRVs. It demonstrated the Explainable AI (XAI) [36] capability without the reliance of explicit a priori knowledge and a posteriori processing.

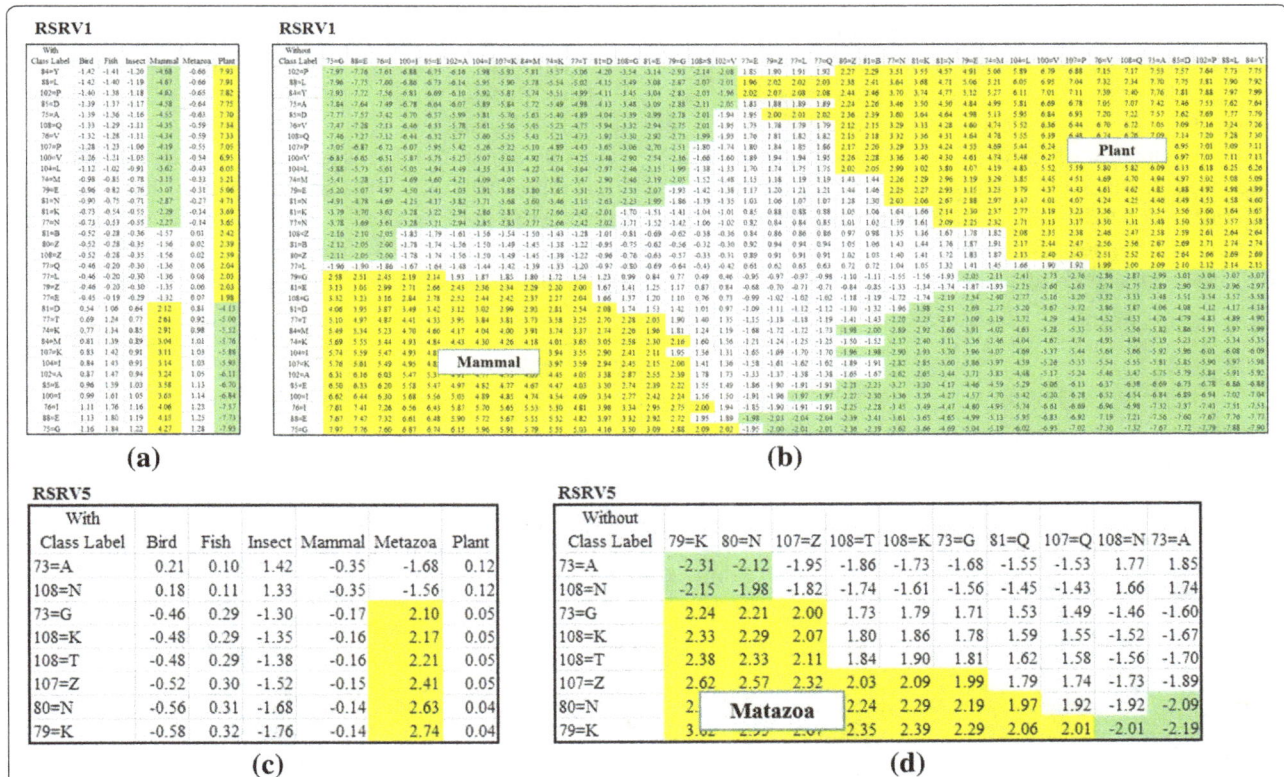

RSRV5 (c) — With Class Label

Class Label	Bird	Fish	Insect	Mammal	Metazoa	Plant
73=A	0.21	0.10	1.42	-0.35	-1.68	0.12
108=N	0.18	0.11	1.33	-0.35	-1.56	0.12
73=G	-0.46	0.29	-1.30	-0.17	2.10	0.05
108=K	-0.48	0.29	-1.35	-0.16	2.17	0.05
108=T	-0.48	0.29	-1.38	-0.16	2.21	0.05
107=Z	-0.52	0.30	-1.52	-0.15	2.41	0.05
80=N	-0.56	0.31	-1.68	-0.14	2.63	0.04
79=K	-0.58	0.32	-1.76	-0.14	2.74	0.04

RSRV5 (d) — Without Class Label

Class Label	79=K	80=N	107=Z	108=T	108=K	73=G	81=Q	107=Q	108=N	73=A
73=A	-2.31	-2.12	-1.95	-1.86	-1.73	-1.68	-1.55	-1.53	1.77	1.85
108=N	-2.15	-1.98	-1.82	-1.74	-1.61	-1.56	-1.45	-1.43	1.66	1.74
73=G	2.24	2.21	2.00	1.73	1.79	1.71	1.53	1.49	-1.46	-1.60
108=K	2.33	2.29	2.07	1.80	1.86	1.78	1.59	1.55	-1.52	-1.67
108=T	2.38	2.33	2.11	1.84	1.90	1.81	1.62	1.58	-1.56	-1.70
107=Z	2.62	2.57	2.32	2.03	2.09	1.99	1.79	1.74	-1.73	-1.89
80=N	2.	Matazoa		2.24	2.29	2.19	1.97	1.92	-1.92	-2.09
79=K	3.			2.35	2.39	2.29	2.06	2.01	-2.01	-2.19

Fig. 9 The Result of AR Clusters captured in PCs and the corresponding ARAs reflected in RSRVs for APC Dataset 2 with amino acid. **a** ARA Clustering Result with Class Label on RSRV1; (**b**) ARA Clustering Result without Class Labels on RSRV1; (**c**) ARA Clustering Result with Class Label on RSRV5; and (**d**) ARA Clustering Result without Class Labels on RSRV5

SRV	Mammal	Plant	Fungi	Insect
721=NonPolar_aromatic	-3.44	-2.41	1.88	6.30
724=[165.19 181.19]	-6.83	5.97	-1.02	3.17
734=[89.09 147.13]	-5.92	5.44	2.29	-2.04
734=[147.13 147.13]	5.92	-5.44	-2.29	2.04
761=Polar	4.45	-8.64	2.77	2.07
762=Acidic	4.70	-8.16	1.88	2.19
904=[89.09 117.15]	3.69	2.66	-8.25	1.72
925=[5.98 5.98]	-8.69	4.45	3.28	2.37
951=Nonpolar	-7.16	5.21	0.27	3.03
952=Neutral	-6.51	4.68	0.30	2.75
953=[-1.6 1.8]	-6.32	4.81	-0.10	2.82
955=[6.3 9.59]	2.06	2.66	-5.19	0.03
963=[-3.5 1.8]	3.69	2.66	-8.25	1.72
964=[0 146.15]	5.04	-3.46	-3.70	2.41
964=[146.15 147.13]	-5.04	3.46	3.70	-2.41

(a)

RSRV1	Mammal	Plant	Fungi	Insect
721=NonPolar_aromatic	0.79	-1.10	0.27	0.04
724=[165.19 181.19]	-4.86	5.84	-0.53	-0.38
734=[89.09 147.13]	-4.87	5.85	-0.53	-0.38
734=[147.13 147.13]	4.70	-5.91	0.82	0.33
761=Polar	5.84	-7.31	0.98	0.41
762=Acidic	5.68	-7.11	0.96	0.40
904=[89.09 117.15]	-1.00	1.10	0.02	-0.09
925=[5.98 5.98]	-4.60	5.51	-0.49	-0.36
951=Nonpolar	-5.09	6.12	-0.56	-0.39
952=Neutral	-4.69	5.64	-0.50	-0.37
953=[-1.6 1.8]	-4.73	5.67	-0.51	-0.37
955=[6.3 9.59]	-1.36	1.54	-0.03	-0.12
963=[-3.5 1.8]	-1.00	1.10	0.02	-0.09
964=[0 146.15]	3.01	-3.83	0.58	0.20
964=[146.15 147.13]	-3.18	3.78	-0.29	-0.25

(b)

RSRV2	Mammal	Plant	Fungi	Insect
721=NonPolar_aromatic	-0.65	-0.30	1.16	-0.14
724=[165.19 181.19]	0.52	0.17	-0.83	0.09
734=[89.09 147.13]	-1.50	-0.64	2.59	-0.30
734=[147.13 147.13]	1.56	0.58	-2.59	0.29
761=Polar	-1.07	-0.47	1.87	-0.22
762=Acidic	-0.49	-0.24	0.88	-0.11
904=[89.09 117.15]	4.29	1.68	-7.22	0.81
925=[5.98 5.98]	-2.27	-0.96	3.91	-0.45
951=Nonpolar	-0.33	-0.18	0.62	-0.08
952=Neutral	-0.24	-0.14	0.46	-0.06
953=[-1.6 1.8]	-0.13	-0.10	0.28	-0.04
955=[6.3 9.59]	3.00	1.16	-5.03	0.56
963=[-3.5 1.8]	4.29	1.68	-7.22	0.81
964=[0 146.15]	2.37	0.91	-3.96	0.44
964=[146.15 147.13]	-2.30	-0.97	3.96	-0.45

(c)

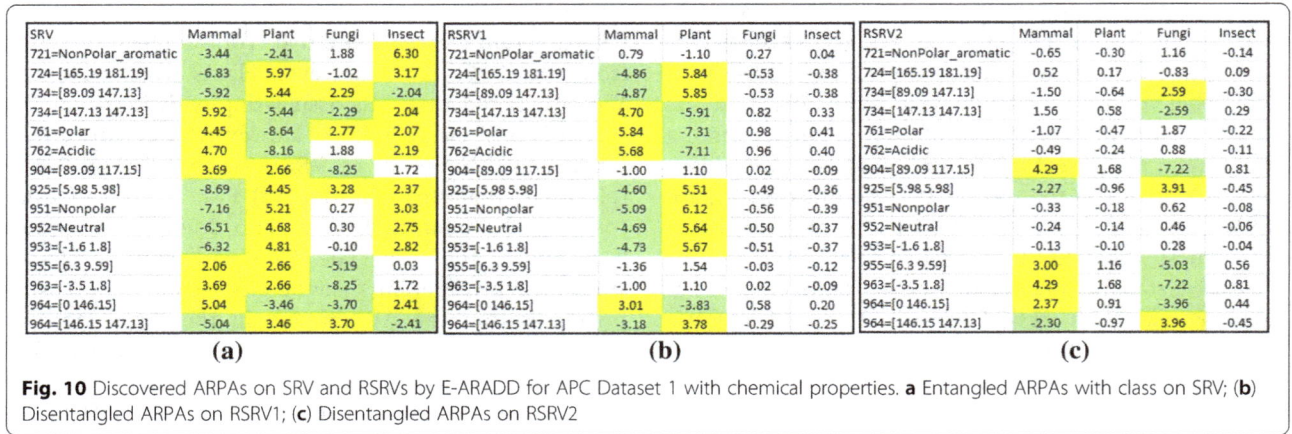

Fig. 10 Discovered ARPAs on SRV and RSRVs by E-ARADD for APC Dataset 1 with chemical properties. **a** Entangled ARPAs with class on SRV; (**b**) Disentangled ARPAs on RSRV1; (**c**) Disentangled ARPAs on RSRV2

To reveal the ARAs obtained for dataset 1 in greater depth, we made a careful comparison of the ARs in the PCs with the ARAs in their corresponding RSRVs to see how the ARAs grouping reflecting the distinctness of the AR sub-clusters in the RSRVs. Fig. 8 shows the AR clusters (yellow cells) that captured on different PCs. In order to show that such functional associations are intrinsic unrelated to class labels, we compared experimental result on APCs with and without class labels. Figure 8 (a-d) showed the AR clusters on the right-handed side and their corresponding RSRV plots obtained from SRV without class labels on the left-handed side. We observed in both that the ARs associating to the class are almost identical. Hence, this further indicates the explainable machine learning capability of E-ARADD in both supervised/unsupervised settings not relying on explicit a priori or a posteriori knowledge. As Figs. 8 and 9 show, in all the experiments, we see little difference in ARA results with or without class labels given.

Analysis II – Cytochrome c APCs in aligned residue property tuples

In Analysis II, the same protein APC datasets in Analysis I were used, but the aligned residues are represented by the five amino acid chemical properties: Side Chain Polarity, Side Chain Acidity / Basicity, Hydropathy Index, Molecular Weight (Da), and Isoelectric Point instead. Thus, we represent an APC in Analysis I by an Aligned Property Pattern Cluster (APPC) and an Aligned Residue (AR) by an Aligned Residue Property Tuple (ARP). Furthermore, instead of using ARAs as our fundamental association from the APC from Dataset 1, we used the Aligned Residue Property Association (ARPA) obtained from APPCs instead.

In this paper, our focus is not to conduct a thorough bio-molecular study of a protein family but rather to explore the performance of E-ARADD on APPCs. That we selected the APCs from cytochrome C based on amino acids and their chemical properties is to examine

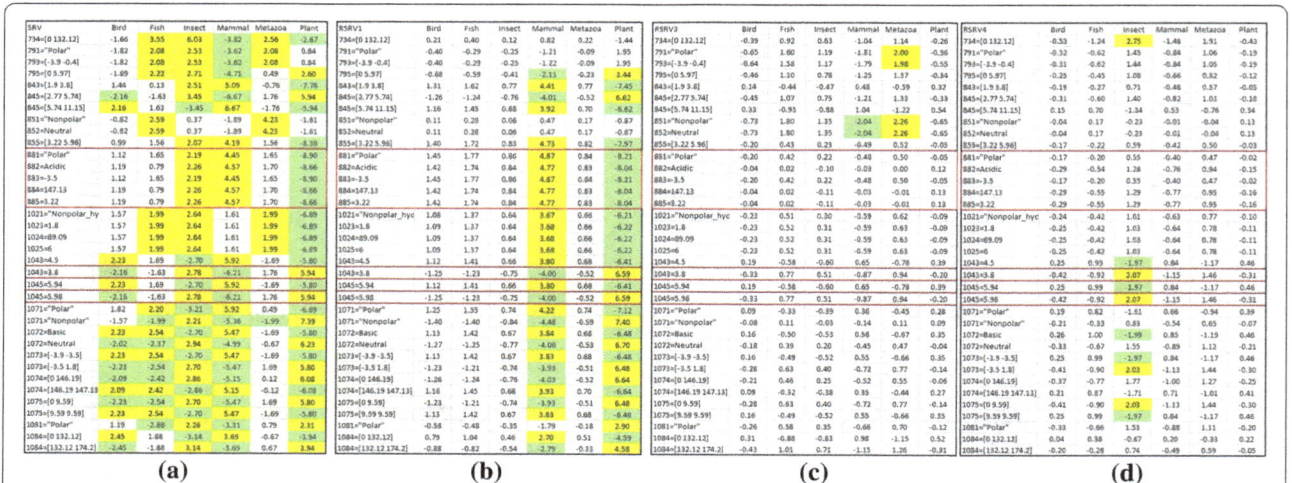

SRV	Bird	Fish	Insect	Mammal	Metazoa	Plant
734=[0 132.12]	-1.66	3.55	6.03	-3.82	2.56	-2.67
791="Polar"	-1.82	2.08	2.53	-3.62	2.08	0.84
793=[-3.9 -0.4]	-1.82	2.08	2.53	-3.62	2.08	0.84
795=[0 5.97]	-1.69	2.22	2.71	-4.71	0.49	2.60
843=[1.9 3.8]	1.44	0.13	2.51	5.09	-0.76	-7.78
845=[2.77 5.74]	-2.16	-1.63	3.45	-6.67	1.76	5.94
845=[5.74 11.15]	2.16	1.63	-3.45	6.67	-1.76	-5.94
851="Nonpolar"	-0.82	2.59	0.37	-1.89	4.23	-1.61
852=Neutral	-0.82	2.59	0.37	-1.89	4.23	-1.61
855=[3.22 5.96]	0.99	1.56	2.07	4.19	1.56	-8.38
881="Polar"	1.12	1.65	2.19	4.45	1.65	-8.90
882=Acidic	1.19	0.79	2.26	4.57	1.70	-8.66
883=-3.5	1.12	1.65	2.19	4.45	1.65	-8.90
884=147.13	1.19	0.79	2.26	4.57	1.70	-8.66
885=3.22	1.19	0.79	2.26	4.57	1.70	-8.66
1021="Nonpolar_hy	1.57	1.99	2.64	1.61	1.99	-6.89
1023=1.8	1.57	1.99	2.64	1.61	1.99	-6.89
1024=89.09	1.57	1.99	2.64	1.61	1.99	-6.89
1025=6	1.57	1.99	2.64	1.61	1.99	-6.89
1043=4.5	2.23	1.69	-2.70	5.92	-1.69	-5.80
1043=3.8	-2.16	-1.63	2.78	-6.21	1.76	5.94
1045=5.94	2.23	1.69	-2.70	5.92	-1.69	-5.80
1045=5.98	-2.16	-1.63	2.78	-6.21	1.76	5.94
1071="Polar"	1.82	2.20	-3.21	5.92	0.49	-6.69
1071="Nonpolar"	-1.57	-1.99	2.21	-5.36	-1.99	7.39
1072=Basic	2.23	2.54	-2.70	5.47	-1.69	-5.80
1072=Neutral	-2.02	-2.37	2.94	-4.99	-0.67	6.23
1073=[-3.9 -3.5]	2.23	2.54	-2.70	5.47	-1.69	-5.80
1073=[-3.5 1.8]	-2.23	-2.54	2.70	-5.47	1.69	5.80
1074=[0 146.19]	-2.09	-2.42	2.86	-5.15	0.12	6.08
1074=[146.19 147.13	2.09	2.42	-2.86	5.15	-0.12	-6.08
1075=[0 9.59]	-2.23	-2.54	2.70	-5.47	1.69	5.80
1075=[9.59 9.59]	2.23	2.54	-2.70	5.47	-1.69	-5.80
1081="Polar"	1.19	-2.88	2.26	-3.31	0.79	2.31
1084=[0 132.12]	2.45	1.88	-3.14	3.69	-0.67	-3.94
1084=[132.12 174.2]	-2.45	-1.88	3.14	-3.69	0.67	3.94

(a)

RSRV1	Bird	Fish	Insect	Mammal	Metazoa	Plant
734=[0 132.12]	0.21	0.40	0.12	0.82	0.22	-1.44
791="Polar"	-0.40	-0.29	-0.25	-1.21	-0.09	1.95
793=[-3.9 -0.4]	-0.40	-0.29	-0.25	-1.22	-0.09	1.95
795=[0 5.97]	-0.68	-0.59	-0.41	-2.11	-0.23	3.44
843=[1.9 3.8]	1.31	1.62	0.77	4.41	0.77	-7.45
845=[2.77 5.74]	-1.26	-1.24	-0.76	-4.01	-0.52	6.62
845=[5.74 11.15]	1.16	1.45	0.68	3.92	0.70	-6.62
851="Nonpolar"	0.11	0.28	0.06	0.47	0.17	-0.87
852=Neutral	0.11	0.28	0.06	0.47	0.17	-0.87
855=[3.22 5.96]	1.40	1.72	0.83	4.73	0.82	-7.97
881="Polar"	1.45	1.77	0.86	4.87	0.84	-8.21
882=Acidic	1.42	1.74	0.84	4.77	0.83	-8.04
883=-3.5	1.45	1.77	0.86	4.87	0.84	-8.21
884=147.13	1.42	1.74	0.84	4.77	0.83	-8.04
885=3.22	1.42	1.74	0.84	4.77	0.83	-8.04
1021="Nonpolar_hyc	1.08	1.37	0.64	3.67	0.66	-6.21
1023=1.8	1.09	1.37	0.64	3.68	0.66	-6.22
1024=89.09	1.09	1.37	0.64	3.68	0.66	-6.22
1025=6	1.09	1.37	0.64	3.68	0.66	-6.22
1043=4.5	1.12	1.41	0.66	3.80	0.68	-6.41
1043=3.8	-1.25	-1.23	-0.75	-4.00	-0.52	6.59
1045=5.94	1.12	1.41	0.66	3.80	0.68	-6.41
1045=5.98	-1.25	-1.23	-0.75	-4.00	-0.52	6.59
1071="Polar"	1.25	1.55	0.74	4.22	0.74	-7.12
1071="Nonpolar"	-1.40	-1.40	-0.84	-4.48	-0.59	7.40
1072=Basic	1.13	1.42	0.67	3.84	0.68	-6.48
1072=Neutral	-1.27	-1.25	-0.77	-4.06	-0.53	6.70
1073=[-3.9 -3.5]	1.13	1.42	0.67	3.83	0.68	-6.48
1073=[-3.5 1.8]	-1.23	-1.21	-0.74	-3.93	-0.51	6.48
1074=[0 146.19]	-1.26	-1.24	-0.76	-4.03	-0.52	6.64
1074=[146.19 147.13]	1.16	1.45	0.68	3.93	0.70	-6.64
1075=[0 9.59]	-1.23	-1.21	-0.74	-3.93	-0.51	6.48
1075=[9.59 9.59]	1.13	1.42	0.67	3.83	0.68	-6.48
1081="Polar"	-0.58	-0.48	-0.35	-1.79	-0.18	2.90
1084=[0 132.12]	0.79	1.04	0.46	2.70	0.51	-4.59
1084=[132.12 174.2]	-0.88	-0.82	-0.54	-2.79	-0.33	4.58

(b)

RSRV3	Bird	Fish	Insect	Mammal	Metazoa	Plant
734=[0 132.12]	-0.39	0.92	0.63	-1.04	1.14	-0.26
791="Polar"	-0.65	1.60	1.19	-1.81	2.00	-0.56
793=[-3.9 -0.4]	-0.64	1.58	1.17	-1.79	1.98	-0.55
795=[0 5.97]	-0.46	1.10	0.78	-1.25	1.37	-0.34
843=[1.9 3.8]	0.14	-0.44	-0.47	0.48	-0.59	0.32
845=[2.77 5.74]	-0.45	1.07	0.75	-1.21	1.33	-0.33
845=[5.74 11.15]	0.33	-0.93	-0.88	1.04	-1.22	0.54
851="Nonpolar"	-0.73	1.80	1.35	-2.04	2.26	-0.65
852=Neutral	-0.73	1.80	1.35	-2.04	2.26	-0.65
855=[3.22 5.96]	-0.20	0.43	0.23	-0.49	0.52	-0.05
881="Polar"	-0.20	0.42	0.22	-0.48	0.50	-0.05
882=Acidic	-0.04	0.02	-0.10	-0.03	0.00	0.12
883=-3.5	-0.20	0.42	0.22	-0.48	0.50	-0.05
884=147.13	-0.04	0.02	-0.11	-0.03	-0.01	0.13
885=3.22	-0.04	0.02	-0.11	-0.03	-0.01	0.13
1021="Nonpolar_hyc	-0.23	0.51	0.30	-0.59	0.62	-0.09
1023=1.8	-0.23	0.52	0.31	-0.59	0.63	-0.09
1024=89.09	-0.23	0.52	0.31	-0.59	0.63	-0.09
1025=6	-0.23	0.52	0.31	-0.59	0.63	-0.09
1043=4.5	0.19	-0.58	-0.60	0.65	-0.78	0.39
1043=3.8	-0.33	0.77	0.51	-0.87	0.94	-0.20
1045=5.94	0.19	-0.58	-0.60	0.65	-0.78	0.39
1045=5.98	-0.33	0.77	0.51	-0.87	0.94	-0.20
1071="Polar"	0.09	-0.33	-0.39	0.36	-0.45	0.28
1071="Nonpolar"	-0.08	0.11	-0.03	-0.14	0.11	0.09
1072=Basic	0.16	-0.50	-0.53	0.56	-0.67	0.35
1072=Neutral	-0.18	0.39	0.20	-0.45	0.47	-0.04
1073=[-3.9 -3.5]	0.16	-0.49	-0.52	0.55	-0.66	0.35
1073=[-3.5 1.8]	-0.28	0.63	0.40	-0.72	0.77	-0.14
1074=[0 146.19]	-0.21	0.46	0.25	-0.52	0.55	-0.06
1074=[146.19 147.13]	0.09	-0.32	-0.38	0.35	-0.44	0.27
1075=[0 9.59]	-0.28	0.63	0.40	-0.72	0.77	-0.14
1075=[9.59 9.59]	0.16	-0.49	-0.52	0.55	-0.66	0.35
1081="Polar"	-0.26	0.58	0.35	-0.66	0.70	-0.12
1084=[0 132.12]	0.31	-0.88	-0.83	0.98	-1.15	0.52
1084=[132.12 174.2]	-0.43	1.01	0.71	-1.15	1.26	-0.31

(c)

RSRV4	Bird	Fish	Insect	Mammal	Metazoa	Plant
734=[0 132.12]	-0.53	-1.24	2.75	-1.48	1.91	-0.43
791="Polar"	-0.32	-0.62	1.45	-0.84	1.06	-0.19
793=[-3.9 -0.4]	-0.31	-0.62	1.44	-0.84	1.05	-0.19
795=[0 5.97]	-0.25	-0.45	1.08	-0.66	0.82	-0.12
843=[1.9 3.8]	-0.19	-0.27	0.71	-0.48	0.57	-0.05
845=[2.77 5.74]	-0.31	-0.60	1.40	-0.82	1.01	-0.18
845=[5.74 11.15]	0.15	0.70	-1.34	0.53	-0.76	0.34
851="Nonpolar"	-0.04	0.17	-0.23	-0.01	-0.04	0.13
852=Neutral	-0.04	0.17	-0.23	-0.01	-0.04	0.13
855=[3.22 5.96]	-0.17	-0.22	0.59	-0.42	0.50	-0.03
881="Polar"	-0.17	-0.20	0.55	-0.40	0.47	-0.02
882=Acidic	-0.29	-0.54	1.28	-0.76	0.94	-0.15
883=-3.5	-0.17	-0.20	0.55	-0.40	0.47	-0.02
884=147.13	-0.29	-0.55	1.29	-0.77	0.95	-0.16
885=3.22	-0.29	-0.55	1.29	-0.77	0.95	-0.16
1021="Nonpolar_hyc	-0.24	-0.42	1.01	-0.63	0.77	-0.10
1023=1.8	-0.25	-0.42	1.03	-0.64	0.78	-0.11
1024=89.09	-0.25	-0.42	1.03	-0.64	0.78	-0.11
1025=6	-0.25	-0.42	1.03	-0.64	0.78	-0.11
1043=4.5	0.25	0.99	-1.97	0.84	-1.17	0.46
1043=3.8	-0.42	-0.92	2.07	-1.15	1.46	-0.31
1045=5.94	0.25	0.99	-1.97	0.84	-1.17	0.46
1045=5.98	-0.42	-0.92	2.07	-1.15	1.46	-0.31
1071="Polar"	0.19	0.82	-1.61	0.66	-0.94	0.39
1071="Nonpolar"	-0.21	-0.33	0.83	-0.54	0.65	-0.07
1072=Basic	0.26	1.00	-1.99	0.85	-1.19	0.46
1072=Neutral	-0.33	-0.67	1.55	-0.89	1.12	-0.21
1073=[-3.9 -3.5]	0.25	0.99	-1.97	0.84	-1.17	0.46
1073=[-3.5 1.8]	-0.41	-0.90	2.03	-1.13	1.44	-0.30
1074=[0 146.19]	-0.37	-0.77	1.77	-1.00	1.27	-0.25
1074=[146.19 147.13]	0.21	0.87	-1.71	0.71	-1.01	0.41
1075=[0 9.59]	-0.41	-0.90	2.03	-1.13	1.44	-0.30
1075=[9.59 9.59]	0.25	0.99	-1.97	0.84	-1.17	0.46
1081="Polar"	-0.33	-0.66	1.53	-0.88	1.11	-0.20
1084=[0 132.12]	0.04	0.38	-0.67	0.20	-0.33	0.22
1084=[132.12 174.2]	-0.20	-0.28	0.74	-0.49	0.59	-0.05

(d)

Fig. 11 Discovered ARAPs on SRV and RSRVs by E-ARADD for APC Dataset 2 with chemical properties. **a** Entangled ARPAs with class on SRV; (**b**) Disentangled ARPAs on RSRV1; (**c**) Disentangled ARPAs on RSRV3. **d** Disentangled ARPAs on RSRV4

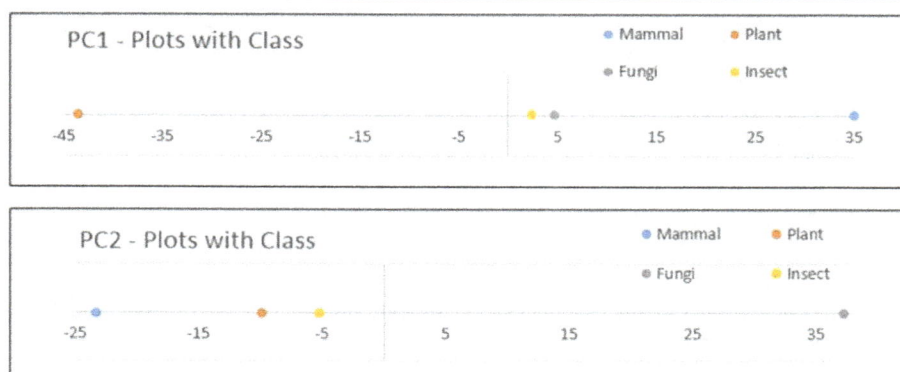

Fig. 12 PC plots results for APPC in dataset 1 with class label

whether ARPAs can be discovered in the disentangled spaces of PCs and RSRVs to reveal the chemical association ARPs at a deeper level. We would also like to find out also whether ARP clusters could be identified to generate ARP subgroups corresponding to taxonomical classes with or without class label provided. Thus, we took the dataset 1 and converted the APC with a width of 9 amino acids into a 9×5 mixed-mode APPC, from which we constructed an SRV. We then applied PCD on the SRV to obtain PCs and RSRVs as we did in Analysis I, ranked them after their eigenvalues. The corresponding set of RSRVs then represent the coordinates of the ARP-vector which were the SRs of each ARPA between ARPs corresponding to the row and column ARP-vectors. Figure 10 shows the disentanglement of the ARPs associating with class labels for dataset 1. The attribute "721 = NonPolar_aromatic" denotes that the aligned 1st chemical property (Side Chain Polarity) of the 72th amino acid in the APPC is "NonPolar_aromatic". Since chemical

properties were used, we observed more disentangled association of the ARP with class labels were obtained in the SRV (Fig. 10(a)). As expected, more succinct disentanglement had also been observed in the RSRVs. In RSRV1 (Fig. 10(b)), we observed succinct disentanglement of ARPAs between Mammal and Plant, and in RSRV2 (Fig. 10(c)), between Mammal and Fungi. Overall, we see that more specific chemical associations between species are discovered in different functional spaces. Such deeper knowledge could help biologists to further their research.

Similarly, Fig. 11 shows the ARPAs with the class labels in disentangled spaces for dataset 2. Figure 11(a) shows the result of ARP Associating with classes in the SRV obtained from the APPC with chemical properties of dataset 2. Note that in SRV, we noted that there are quite a number of ARP entangled with different taxonomical classes. However, after disentanglement, we observed that disentangled ARPs in RSRV1 were distinctly associating Mammal and Plant. Especially for site *1043 = 3.8* (the value of

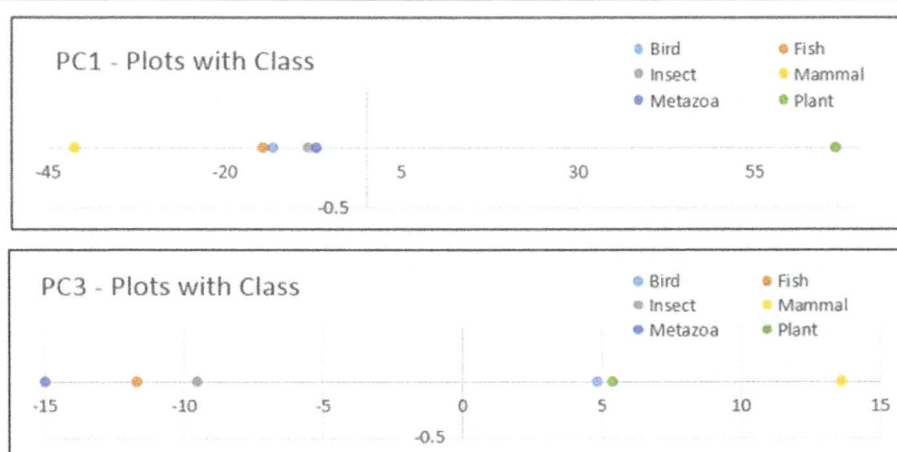

Fig. 13 PC plots results for APPC in dataset 2 with class label

Seq ID \ APC Column Position	Class	1	2	3	4	5	6	7	8	9	10	11	12	Sequence Position
		234	235	236	237	238	239	240	241	242	243	244	245	
68.69, 71-83, 85, 88, 89	scara5	C	R	M	L	G	F	R|H|P	G	V|A	E|K	E|D	V	430-435
70	scara5	C	R	M	L	G	F	R	G	V	E	E	V	393
86	scara5	C	R	M	L	G	Y	R	G	A	T	E	V	347
90 - 102, 104 - 106	sra	C	R	S	L	G	Y	P|R|Q	G	V	Q|L|R|K	A	V	374-390
103	sra	V	A	L	L	G	L	Y	I	L	M	F	G	52

Fig. 14 An Excerpt of Experimental result of AR groups associating with different SR-A classes [28]

the 3th properties of the 104th amino acid), and $1045 = 5.98$, While ARPs of Insect and Plant are entangled in SRV, the ARP of Insect was standing out in RSRV3 and that of Plant was standing out in RSRV1.

We can conclude from the above experimental result that when the class labels are included in APPCs as input, we could disentangle the discovered associations of chemical property relation between ARPs. In addition, we also showed from the PC plots for dataset 1 and 2 how chemical properties of the ARP clusters were associating with class in the PCs as Figs. 12 and 13 show. Since each ARP-cluster consists of a special set of ARPs, biologists could gain significant molecular biological insight for each specific functional space. Such ARP associating with classes were also revealed in other RSRVs.

In summary, from the results of Analysis II, we found that E-ARADD can handle mixed-mode dataset. It can discover the statistically significant ARPAs, though entangled

in the SRV, as well as the ARP Clusters (ARPCs) captured in orthogonal PCs to bring out their separability associating with taxonomical classes.

Discussion

Discovering patterns from biological sequences is of fundamental importance in unraveling the underlying science. It is particularly true in Proteomics, where proteins virtually regulate every biological process of a living organism. A new method has been developed from us to obtain from protein sequences Aligned Pattern Clusters (APCs) [2–4] representing the biological conserved regions. APCs [2–4], comparing with probabilistic methods [1], have captured more complete statistical association of aligned residues. As the column-wise associations are preserved in APCs, contrasting to probabilistic models, e.g. Position Weight Matrix (PWM) [30], we are able to discover the Aligned Residue Associations (ARAs) [5] to

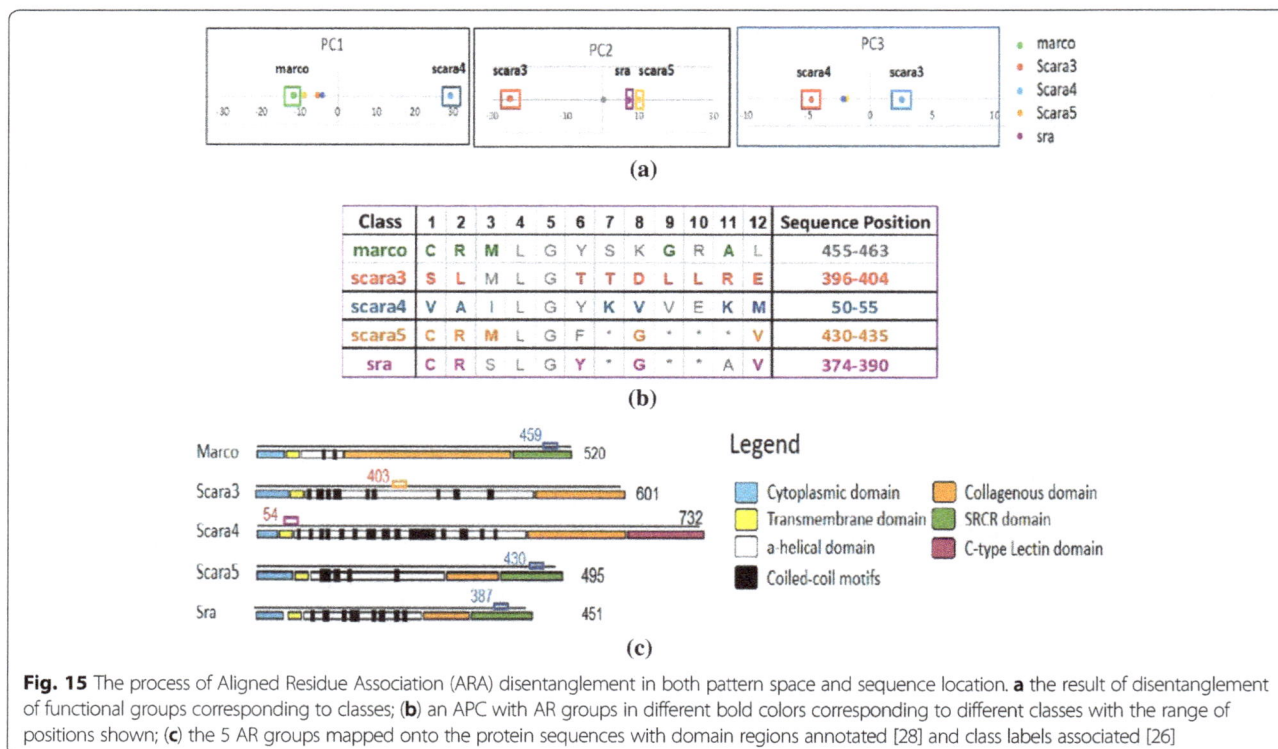

(a)

Class	1	2	3	4	5	6	7	8	9	10	11	12	Sequence Position
marco	C	R	M	L	G	Y	S	K	G	R	A	L	455-463
scara3	S	L	M	L	G	T	T	D	L	L	R	E	396-404
scara4	V	A	I	L	G	Y	K	V	V	E	K	M	50-55
scara5	C	R	M	L	G	F	'	G	'	'	'	V	430-435
sra	C	R	S	L	G	Y	'	G	'	'	A	V	374-390

(b)

(c)

Fig. 15 The process of Aligned Residue Association (ARA) disentanglement in both pattern space and sequence location. **a** the result of disentanglement of functional groups corresponding to classes; (**b**) an APC with AR groups in different bold colors corresponding to different classes with the range of positions shown; (**c**) the 5 AR groups mapped onto the protein sequences with domain regions annotated [28] and class labels associated [26]

reveal subgroup characteristics, in which, these subgroup characteristics, regarding multiple functionalities and/or local stereo physiochemical environments, may have been masked or entangled. We further extended the ARADD algorithm into E-ARADD to handle the mixed-mode biochemical protein data to provide direct biochemical interpretation supported by experimental results.

Experimental results on synthetic data provides the proof-of-concept validation on the successful disentanglement that reveals class-associated ARAs with or without class labels as input, results on cytochrome c and class A scavenger receptors sequence data render scientific validation of our method. In experimental Analysis I, after disentanglement, different ARAs were revealed. They were linked to the species class labels. We validated that the AR results in PCs and ARAS in RSRVs remain essentially the same with or without the inclusion of class labels in the APCs. In experimental Analysis II, we found that different APPAs were associated with different species. The observation, to a certain degree, is consistent to the literature report that certain biological processes of cytochrome c such as oxidization have homologous yet different chemical characterization in different families [31].

Furthermore, in order to show the completeness of the proposed algorithm E-ARADD, we furnish a brief summary of our recent work [26] when ARADD algorithm [5] was applied to a very diverse protein family of class A scavenger receptors (SR-A), dataset 3. In our recent work [26], we showed that ARADD was able not only to discover and disentangle ARs and ARAs in specific PCs and RSRVs, but also their locations in the protein functional domains of SR-A.

Figure 14 demonstrates an excerpt showing the results of only two classes from a figure taken from our recent work [26]. Note that the AR patterns are in bold brown color fonts for Scara5 (CRM****G***V) and in violet color fonts for Sra (CR***Y*G***V). These AR patterns are similar in sequence and thus clustered in the same APC. However, they are in fact in two distant domains. This indicates that not only can ARADD disentangle functional association in an APC, i.e. the pattern space, but also disentangle their sequence locations relating to different family domains [26], e.g. Scara5 and Sra. This provides a strong support to the scientific significance of ARA disentanglement, by revealing the information of "what" and "where" in a protein family.

Figure 15 [26] provides an overview of the discovered results in both pattern and data space. Figure 15(a) from [26] demonstrates that the class labels associating with ARs of their pertaining classes are revealed within their associating clusters in the one-dimensional PC space. As shown in Fig. 14, the AR groups for Scara5 and Sra are close with only a single difference in their significant ARs. Their closeness is also observed in RSRV2 [26].

The two groups differ from other classes significantly. Hence, from the PCs (Fig. 15(a)) and the plots of the significant AR clusters (color rectangular boxes), we have observed both their similarity (i.e. Sra and Scara5 in PC2) and their differences (i.e. scara3 and scara4 in PC3), with statistical backing (the distance of their projection position from the mean in the PCs and their SR magnitude in the RSRVs). From the APC data space as shown by their sequence ID and sequence position in Figs.14(a), 15(b) and (c), we observed that their residing sequence positions and family domain locations of each AR pattern were identified. Surprisingly, they are closely correlated with the domain regions annotated.

Conclusion

In this study, we extend our previous ARADD algorithm [5] into E-ARADD to enable it to handle mixed-mode physiochemical property data, which contains both categorical and numerical values. By applying E-ARADD to the entangled APC obtained from cytochrome c family and class A scavenger receptors, this study has shown that AR clusters (patterns in pattern space), associating with different functional subgroups, regions and domains of the family obtained from an APC, could be succinctly plotted and statistically separated in different PCs and RSRVs as well as in different locations through their sequence ID and sequence position in the protein family data [26].

The most significant finding of this study is that the AR subgroups within the APCs could be found in the disentangled PCs and RSRVS of ARA/ARPA associating with different classes or subgroups, residing in different functional regions or domains of the family. Biologically, entangled ARA/ARPA in the aligned patterns within the conserved regions APC/APPC of class A scavenger receptor, reveal biological functional patterns pertaining to similar or different classes. It is interesting to find that the ARAs/ARPAs within the entangled patterns in APCs of class A scavenger receptor family can be disentangled into subgroups pertaining to different functionality as reflected by the disentangled PCs and RSRVs. This implies that the strong statistical associations of multiple functionalities for different classes/subgroups inherent in the residue associations within the aligned patterns. Hence, in summary, the successful application of ARADD algorithm demonstrates its capability to open a new way for analyzing conserved regions and their distribution, with potential to reveal new knowledge in omics for drug discovery, genetic medicine and gene therapy applications.

Abbreviations
APC: Aligned Pattern Cluster (with categorical amino acid); APPC: Aligned Property Pattern Cluster (with mixed-mode chemical properties); AR: Aligned Residue (for categorical amino acid in APC dataset); ARA: Aligned Residue Association (Significant co-occurrence of two ARs in APC / APC of biochemical properties); ARA/ARPA FM: ARA/ARPA Frequency Matrix; ARP: Aligned Residue Property (for mixed-mode chemical properties in APC dataset);

ARPA: Aligned Residue Property Association (for APPC); PCD: Principle Component Decomposition; RSRV: Re-projected SRV; SR: adjusted Statistical Residual between two ARs/ARPs; SRV: ARA/ARPA adjusted Statistical Residual Vector Space

Acknowledgements
The authors would like to thank Dr. En-Shiun Annie Lee, Lead Research Scientist at VerticalScope Inc., for her valuable input on the experimental data.

Funding
Publication costs were funded by NSERC Discovery Grant (xxxxx 50503–10275 500).

Authors' contributions
PZ and AW directed and designed the study. PZ implemented the algorithm. PZ and AW performed the statistical analyses. AS performed the Bioinformatics analyses. PZ, AS and AW prepared the manuscript. All authors read and approved the final manuscript.

Competing interests
The authors declare that they have no competing interests.

References
1. Durbin R, Eddy S, Krogh A, Mitchison G. Biological sequence analysis: Probabilistic Models of Proteins and Nucleic Acids. Analysis. 1998;356 Available from: https://pdfs.semanticscholar.org/2ed5/d6b35f8971fb9d7434a2683922c3bfcc058e.pdf.
2. Lee E-S, Wong AK. Ranking and compacting binding segments of protein families using aligned pattern clusters. Proteome Sci [Internet]. BioMed Central Ltd; 2013;11:S8. Available from: http://www.proteomesci.com/content/11/S1/S8.
3. Wong AKC, Lee ESA. Aligning and clustering patterns to reveal the protein functionality of sequences. IEEE/ACM Trans Comput Biol Bioinforma. 2014;11:548–60.
4. Sze-To A, Wong AKC. Pattern-Directed Aligned Pattern Clustering. Bioinforma. Biomed. (BIBM), 2017 IEEE Int Conf IEEE; 2017.
5. Zhou P, Sze-Tzo A, Wong AKC. Discovery and disentanglement of protein aligned pattern clusters to reveal subtle functional subgroups, 2017. Kansas: IEEE International Conference on Bioinformatics and Biomedicine (BIBM), MO. 2017; pp. 62–69. http://ieeexplore.ieee.org/stamp/stamp.jsp?tp=&arnumber=8217625&isnumber=8217602.
6. Wong AKC, Zhou P, Sze-To A. Discovering Deep Knowledge from Relational Data by Attribute-Value Association. In: Proceedings of the 13th International Conference on Data Mining (DMIN'17), Las Vegas, NV, USA. 2017. p. 51–57. https://csce.ucmss.com/cr/books/2017/LFS/CSREA2017/DMI8008.pdf.
7. Zhou P, Lee E-SA, Wong AKC. Regrouping of pattern clusters to reveal characteristics of distinct classes and related classes. Proc. - 2013 IEEE Int. Conf. Bioinforma. Biomed. IEEE BIBM 2013. 55–61.
8. Naulaerts S, Meysman P, Bittremieux W, Vu TN, Vanden BW, Goethals B, et al. A primer to frequent itemset mining for bioinformatics. Brief Bioinform. 2015;16:216–31.
9. Agrawal R, Imielinski T, Swami A. Mining Association in Large Databases. Proc 1993 ACM SIGMOD Int Conf Manag data - SIGMOD '93. 1993:207–16.
10. Han J, Pei J, Yin Y, et al. Data Mining and Knowledge Discovery. 2004;8(1): 53–87. https://doi.org/10.1023/B:DAMI.0000005258.31418.83.
11. Edgar RC, Batzoglou S. Multiple sequence alignment. Curr Opin Struct Biol. 2006;16(3):368–73. https://www.sciencedirect.com/science/article/pii/S0959440X06000704?via%3Dihub.
12. Notredame C. Recent evolutions of multiple sequence alignment algorithms. PLoS Comput Biol. 2007;3(8):e123.
13. Thompson JD, Linard B, Lecompte O, Poch O. A comprehensive benchmark study of multiple sequence alignment methods: current challenges and future perspectives. PLoS One. 2011;6.
14. Frith MC, Hansen U, Spouge JL, Weng Z. Finding functional sequence elements by multiple local alignment. Nucleic Acids Res. 2004;32:189–200.
15. Bailey TL, Elkan C. Unsupervised learning of multiple motifs in biopolymers using expectation maximization. Mach Learn. 1995;21:51–80.
16. Altschuh D, Lesk AM, Bloomer AC, Klug A. Correlation of co-ordinated amino acid substitutions with function in viruses related to tobacco mosaic virus. J Mol Biol. 1987;193:693–707.
17. Kass I, Horovitz A. Mapping pathways of allosteric communication in GroEL by analysis of correlated mutations. Proteins Struct Funct Bioinform. 2002; 48(4):611–7.
18. Zani IA, Stephen SL, Mughal NA, Russell D, Homer-Vanniasinkam S, Wheatcroft SB, et al. Scavenger Receptor Structure and Function in Health and Disease. Kalyuzhny AE, ed. Cells. 2015;4(2):178–201. https://doi.org/10.3390/cells4020178.
19. Ma PCH, Chan KCC. Incremental fuzzy mining of gene expression data for gene function prediction. IEEE Trans Biomed Eng. 2011;58:1246–52.
20. Jiawei H, Kamber M, Han J, Kamber M, Pei J. Data Mining: Concepts and Techniques [Internet]. San Fr. CA, itd Morgan Kaufmann. 2012. Available from: http://scholar.google.com/scholar?hl=en&btnG=Search&q=intitle:Data+Mining+Concepts+and+Techniques#1%5Cn, http://scholar.google.com/scholar?hl=en&btnG=Search&q=intitle:Data+mining+concepts+and+techniques%231%5Cn, http://scholar.google.com/scholar?hl=en&btnG=Se.
21. Ramoni M, Sebastiani P, Cohen P. Multivariate clustering by dynamics Marco. Drugs. 2001:1–68.
22. Wong AKC, Wang DCC. Deca: a discrete-valued data clustering algorithm. IEEE Trans Pattern Anal Mach Intell. 1979;PAMI-1(no. 4):342–9.
23. Liu L, Wong AKC, Wang Y. A global optimal algorithm for class-dependent discretization of continuous data. Intell Data Anal. 2004;8:151–70.
24. Wong AK, Wu B, Wu GP, Chan KC. Pattern discovery for large mixed-mode database. Proc 19th ACM Int Conf Inf Knowl Manag. 2010:859–68.
25. Shlens J. A tutorial on principal component analysis. ArXiv. 2014:1–13. https://arxiv.org/pdf/1404.1100.pdf.
26. Zhou P-Y, Lee E-SA, Sze-To A, Wong AKC. Revealing subtle functional subgroups in class a scavenger receptors by pattern discovery and disentanglement of aligned pattern clusters. Proteomes. 2018;6(1):10. https://doi.org/10.3390/proteomes6010010.
27. Lee E-SA, Whelan FJ, Bowdish DME, Wong AKC. Partitioning and correlating subgroup characteristics from aligned pattern clusters. Bioinform. 2016; 32(16):2427–34.
28. Whelan FJ, Meehan CJ, Golding GB, McConkey BJ, E Bowdish DM. The evolution of the class a scavenger receptors. BMC Evol Biol [Internet]. 2012; 12:227. Available from: http://bmcevolbiol.biomedcentral.com/articles/10.1186/1471-2148-12-227.
29. Sun Y, Kamel MS, Andrew KCW, Wang Y. Cost-sensitive boosting for classification of imbalanced data. Pattern Recogn. 2007;40:3358–78.
30. Xia X. Position weight matrix, Gibbs sampler, and the associated significance tests in motif characterization and prediction. Scientifica (Cairo). 2012;2012.
31. Popovic DM, Leontyev IV, Beech DG, Stuchebrukhov AA. Similarity of cytochrome c oxidases in different organisms. Proteins Struct. Funct. Bioinforma. 2010;78:2691–8.

13

Transcriptomic signatures reveal immune dysregulation in human diabetic and idiopathic gastroparesis

Madhusudan Grover[1][*], Simon J. Gibbons[1], Asha A. Nair[2], Cheryl E. Bernard[1], Adeel S. Zubair[1], Seth T. Eisenman[1], Laura A. Wilson[3], Laura Miriel[3], Pankaj J. Pasricha[4], Henry P. Parkman[5], Irene Sarosiek[6], Richard W. McCallum[6], Kenneth L. Koch[7], Thomas L. Abell[8], William J. Snape[9], Braden Kuo[10], Robert J. Shulman[11], Travis J. McKenzie[12], Todd A. Kellogg[12], Michael L. Kendrick[12], James Tonascia[3], Frank A. Hamilton[13], Gianrico Farrugia[1][*]● and the NIDDK Gastroparesis Clinical Research Consortium (GpCRC)

Abstract

Background: Cellular changes described in human gastroparesis have revealed a role for immune dysregulation, however, a mechanistic understanding of human gastroparesis and the signaling pathways involved are still unclear.

Methods: Diabetic gastroparetics, diabetic non-gastroparetic controls, idiopathic gastroparetics and non-diabetic non-gastroparetic controls underwent full-thickness gastric body biopsies. Deep RNA sequencing was performed and pathway analysis of differentially expressed transcripts was done using Ingenuity®. A subset of differentially expressed genes in diabetic gastroparesis was validated in a separate cohort using QT-PCR.

Results: 111 genes were differentially expressed in diabetic gastroparesis and 181 in idiopathic gastroparesis with a $\log_2$fold difference of $| \geq 2 |$ and false detection rate (FDR) < 5%. Top canonical pathways in diabetic gastroparesis included genes involved with macrophages, fibroblasts and endothelial cells in rheumatoid arthritis, osteoarthritis pathway and differential regulation of cytokine production in macrophages and T helper cells by IL-17A and IL-17F. Top canonical pathways in idiopathic gastroparesis included genes involved in granulocyte adhesion and diapedesis, agranulocyte adhesion and diapedesis, and role of macrophages, fibroblasts and endothelial cells in rheumatoid arthritis. Sixty-five differentially expressed genes ($\log_2$fold difference $| \geq 2 |$, FDR < 5%) were common in both diabetic and idiopathic gastroparesis with genes in the top 5 canonical pathways associated with immune signaling. 4/5 highly differentially expressed genes (SGK1, APOLD1, CXCR4, CXCL2, and FOS) in diabetic gastroparesis were validated in a separate cohort of patients using RT-PCR. Immune profile analysis revealed that genes associated with M1 (pro inflammatory) macrophages were enriched in tissues from idiopathic gastroparesis tissues compared to controls ($p < 0.05$).

Conclusions: Diabetic and idiopathic gastroparesis have both unique and overlapping transcriptomic signatures. Innate immune signaling likely plays a central role in pathogenesis of human gastroparesis.

Keywords: Diabetes mellitus, Next generation sequencing, Macrophages, RNA, Signaling

* Correspondence: Grover.madhusudan@mayo.edu;
Farrugia.gianrico@mayo.edu
[1]Enteric NeuroScience Program, Division of Gastroenterology & Hepatology, Mayo Clinic, 200 1st Street SW, Rochester, MN 55905, USA
Full list of author information is available at the end of the article

Background

Diabetic and idiopathic gastroparesis result in significant morbidity and health-care utilization [1]. There is an unmet need for safe and efficacious treatment options [2]. Our mechanistic understanding of gastroparesis has expanded in the last decade; however, actionable therapeutic targets are still missing. We and others have shown that loss of interstitial cells of Cajal (ICC) is a primary cellular injury in animal models and in patients with gastroparesis [3, 4]. In diabetic gastroparesis, this decrease in ICC number correlates with the degree of gastric retention [5]. Ultrastructural studies have allowed us to examine defects in ICC and the broader neuromuscular apparatus [6]. Diabetic gastroparetics had thickened basal lamina around smooth muscles and nerves, whereas, idiopathic gastroparetics had fibrosis, especially around the nerves. This suggests possibility of both overlapping and unique mechanistic aspects for diabetic and idiopathic gastroparesis.

Recent animal studies have provided a paradigm for immune mediated injury of the enteric neuromuscular apparatus, including ICC, to be central in pathogenesis of gastroparesis. In the non-obese diabetic (NOD) mouse model, the proportion of CD206, heme oxygenase-1 (HO1) –positive "M2" macrophages (alternatively activated or anti-inflammatory) increased with development of diabetes. However, the development of delayed gastric emptying was associated with an increase in iNOS expression, a marker for macrophages with a "M1" phenotype (classically activated or pro-inflammatory) [7]. Macrophage-deficient CSF1$^{op/op}$ mice did not develop delayed gastric emptying despite severe diabetes [8]. Decreased CD206$^+$ (M2 macrophages) have also been reported in the gastric antrum of patients with diabetic and idiopathic gastroparesis which correlated with the loss of ICC [9]. Additionally, HO1 expressed in M2 macrophages is directly associated with delayed gastric emptying in diabetic mice and polymorphisms in the HO1 gene (HMOX1) are associated with worse outcomes in human diseases [7].

Despite the advances and insights gained from animal models and human studies, our mechanistic understanding of physiological and clinical changes in human gastroparesis is still limited. The NIDDK Gastroparesis Clinical Research Consortium (GpCRC) collects full thickness gastric tissue from patients with diabetic and idiopathic gastroparesis. We undertook a hypothesis generating approach to attempt to obtain molecular and cellular targets for future mechanistic and therapeutic studies. Our aim was to determine the abundance and relationships between gene transcripts in diabetic and idiopathic gastroparesis by deep sequencing of RNA extracted from the smooth muscle layers including the myenteric plexus of the human gastric body. Secondly, we aimed to identify transcription-based signaling pathways in diabetic and idiopathic gastroparesis.

Methods
Specimens

Full thickness gastric body biopsies were obtained from 7 diabetic gastroparetics, 7 diabetic non-gastroparetic controls, 5 idiopathic gastroparetics and 7 non-diabetic non-gastroparetic controls. Differences between female and male transcriptome are expected and the prevalence of gastroparesis is higher in females. Hence, in this pilot study, only female transcriptome was determined to allow sufficient power for analysis for one sex. The gastroparesis patients were undergoing implantation of a gastric electrical stimulator at the time of tissue procurement, and the controls were undergoing obesity surgery. 37% of gastroparetic patients were obese (BMI > 30 kg/m^2). All patients were > 18 years of age with symptoms of at least 12-weeks duration, delayed gastric emptying on scintigraphy (> 60% retention at 2 h or > 10% retention at 4 h), and no evidence of gastric outlet obstruction. Exclusion criteria included presence of active inflammatory bowel disease, eosinophilic gastroenteritis, neurological conditions, acute liver or renal failure, and history of total or subtotal gastric resection. Tissue collection was done in standardized fashion from the gastric body with established protocols by the participating sites of the GpCRC. As a part of this, the surgeon is required to follow an exact protocol for procuring tissue from a precisely defined location and mark the position on a working sheet. Following this, a member of the research team ensures that the biopsies are promptly preserved in appropriate solutions. The pathology core at Mayo Clinic prepares and ships fixative solutions to all sites. The tissue is shipped as overnight priority to Mayo Clinic and is subsequently processed using standardized procedures. The mucosa was peeled and the muscularis sample was cryopreserved in RNAlater until further use. All gastroparesis patients provided written informed consent for procurement and use of gastric tissue at the clinical sites of GpCRC. All clinical sites of GpCRC had approval from their institutional IRBs. All control tissues were obtained in a de-identified fashion at Mayo Clinic in an IRB-approved protocol. Oral consent was obtained for use of this tissue.

RNA extraction

Total RNA was isolated from the smooth muscle using RNA-Bee (TelTest, Friendswood, TX) and purified for sequencing using the RNeasy Plus Mini Kit (Qiagen, Valencia CA). Samples were tested by the Mayo Gene Expression Core using the Agilent Bioanalyzer and all had a RNA Integrity Numbers (RIN) > 7.0.

RNA sequencing

Samples were sequenced using the Illumina TruSeq v2 library prep kit with 3 samples in each lane using a paired end index read with 51 base reads. RNA-Seq data were analyzed by the Mayo Clinic Division of Biomedical Statistics and Informatics using a comprehensive bioinformatics pipeline, defined MAP-RSeq (version 2.1.1), a streamlined pipeline for processing paired-end RNA sequencing reads with low intervention during the analysis stage [10]. The MAP-RSeq utilized a variety of freely available bioinformatics tools along with in-house developed methods to align, assess and provide multiple genomic features from transcriptomic sequencing data for further downstream analysis.

Differential expression analysis

The data were subjected to principal component analysis (PCA) using the Partek Suite to establish whether the samples in each group had differing expression profiles. Differentially expressed genes were determined using the edgeR package [11]. The criterion for considering a gene transcript to be differentially expressed was having an adjusted probability of significance (adjusted P) less than 0.05 (or false discovery rate, FDR < 5%). Separately, transcripts with a $\log_2$ fold difference of 2 and higher or -2 and lower ($\log_2$FC |2|) were used for creating heat maps and for pathway analysis. We used R packages, edgeR [11] and RNASeqPower [12] to obtain coefficient of variation and perform statistical power analysis. In our cohort, 90% of the expressed genes have a coefficient of variation less than 0.42. Using the formula from RNA-SeqPower, setting the type I error to 0.05 and the power to 80%, 13 samples per group would be needed to observe a 2-fold expression in a gene. Seven subjects per group provide 51% power to detect a 2-fold expression in a gene.

Pathway analysis

Ingenuity pathway analysis (IPA) was used to determine pathways and other associations connecting the differentially expressed transcripts [13].

Immune profile analysis

To determine the immune cell composition of the gastroparesis and control RNA samples, normalized gene counts (reads per kilobase per million mapped reads, RPKM) generated from MAP-RSeq were subset to the LM22 signature gene set from CIBERSORT [14]. The probability values reported by CIBERSORT for M1 and M2 macrophages were assessed for differences between the diabetic and idiopathic gastroparesis groups compared to their controls using a 2-sided non-parametric unpaired t-test. A $p < 0.05$ was considered statistically significant.

RT-PCR for validation

Transcripts that are altered in both diabetic and idiopathic gastroparesis were determined. Subsequently, genes with putative biological significance for gastroparesis were identified and their expression was determined in a separate validation cohort of full thickness gastric body tissue from 6 diabetic gastroparesis subjects and 6 diabetic controls using RT PCR. β-actin was used as the housekeeping gene and delta Ct values were calculated. The following genes were sequenced: SGK, serum/glucocorticoid regulated kinase 1; APOLD1, apolipoprotein L domain containing 1; CXCR4, C-X-C motif chemokine receptor 4; CXCL2, C-X-C motif chemokine ligand 2; and FOS, Fos proto-oncogene.

Results

Patient characteristics

Table 1 highlights the demographic and disease characteristics of diabetic gastroparetics, diabetic non-gastroparetic controls, idiopathic gastroparetics and non-diabetic non-gastroparetic controls. The median age was similar among the 4 groups. The overall gastroparesis cardinal symptom index (GCSI) score and the subtype scores (nausea, fullness and bloating) were similar between diabetic and idiopathic gastroparetics.

Sequencing depth

RNA samples had a minimum RIN value of 7.4 and at least 80 million reads were obtained from each sample (Additional file 1: Table S1). At least 60,000,000 reads mapped to 64,253 identified gene transcripts. The gene annotation used was from Ensembl release 78. The transcript identifiers were obtained from the gene definition file for *Homo sapiens* GRCh38.78, obtained from the Ensembl ftp server (ftp://ftp.ensembl.org/pub/release-78/gtf/homo_sapiens/). Samples were enriched for markers of smooth muscle (ACTG2, ACTB, ACTA2), neurons (UCHL1), glia (S100B) and, to a lesser extent, ICC (Kit, Ano1) indicating that the tissue was enriched for cells from the muscularis propria of the gastric wall. Minimal contamination with RNA derived from the mucosa was detected as indicated by low numbers of reads for genes enriched in the mucosal layers of the GI including trefoil factors (TFF1 and TFF2), gastric lipase (LIPF), gastric intrinsic factor (GIF) and pepsinogens (PGA3 and PGA5). The dataset has been submitted to Gene Expression Omnibus (GSE115601).

Differentially expressed genes in diabetic gastroparesis

Three hundred and seventy-three gene transcripts were differentially expressed (FDR < 5%) among diabetic gastroparetics and diabetic non-gastroparetic controls (Additional file 2: Table S2). 104 of the 373 were upregulated and the remaining genes were downregulated in diabetic gastroparesis. Expression levels in RPKM for one hundred and eleven genes with a $\log_2$fold difference in expression of $|\geq 2|$ as compared to diabetic controls are shown in the heatmap (Fig. 1a). When

Table 1 Demographic and disease characteristics of the gastroparesis patients (diabetic, idiopathic) and controls (diabetic, non-diabetic)

	Diabetic Gastroparesis	Diabetic Control	Idiopathic Gastroparesis	Non-diabetic Control
Age (median, range)	39; 24–59	46; 33–57	40; 26–64	39; 26–48
Diabetes, Type	I: 6; II: 1	–	–	–
% Gastric emptying				
2 h	46.2 (25.6)	–	41.5 (8.7)	–
4 h	36.5 (30)	–	18.7 (11.9)	–
GCSI, overall	3.7 (0.9)	–	3.5 (0.7)	–
Nausea	3.5 (1.5)	–	2.8 (1.7)	–
Fullness	4.2 (0.6)	–	3.5 (0.3)	–
Bloating	3.5 (1.3)	–	4.1 (0.6)	–

diabetic gastroparetics were compared with non-diabetic controls, 568 genes were differentially expressed (Additional file 3: Table S3); 130 of those had a $\log_2$fold difference in expression of $|\geq 2|$.

Genes with $\log_2$fold difference in expression of $|\geq 2|$ ($n = 111$) were analyzed using the Ingenuity pathway analysis. The 3 top canonical pathways were associated with role of macrophages, fibroblasts and endothelial cells in rheumatoid arthritis (p-value 1.12E-07), osteoarthritis pathway (p-value 3.63E-07) and differential regulation of cytokine production in macrophages and T helper cells by IL-17A and IL-17F (p-value 9.74E-07). However, only 3–22% differentially expressed genes in our dataset overlapped with the total genes known to be associated with these pathways in the Ingenuity database. Four genes that were common to at least 2/3 top canonical pathways were CCL2, IL6, IL1RL1 and ADAMTS4, all downregulated in diabetic gastroparesis. Hematological system development and function was the leading physiological function identified linked by 49 of the 130 molecules with quantity of leucocytes as the key annotated function associated with 34 of those molecules (Increased ALOX15 and RORC; Decreased ATF3, CCL2, CCL4, CD69, CDKN1A, CLEC4E, CSF3, CXCL2, CXCR2, CXCR4, DUSP1, DUSP5, EGR1, F3, FOS, FOSB, FPR1, GADD45B, GADD45G, IL1RL1, IL6, IL17R, KLF4, MYC, OSM, RGS1, S100A8, S100A9, SERPINE1, SOCS3, THBS1, and ZFP36). The top biological gene interaction containing the most number of differentially expressed genes in our group was "inflammatory disease, cellular movement, hematological system development and function".

Differentially expressed genes in idiopathic gastroparesis

Seven hundred and twenty-seven gene transcripts were differentially expressed between idiopathic gastroparetics and non-diabetic non-gastroparetic controls (Additional file 4: Table S4). Of those, 73 genes were upregulated in idiopathic gastroparesis and the remaining genes were downregulated. Expression levels in RPKM are shown for one hundred eighty-one genes with at least a $|\geq 2|$ $\log_2$fold difference in

expression as compared to controls are shown in the heatmap (Fig. 1b).

Genes with $\log_2$fold difference ($n = 181$) in expression of $|\geq 2|$ were analyzed using the Ingenuity pathway analysis. This revealed the 3 top canonical pathways with genes associated with granulocyte adhesion and diapedesis (p-value 3.49E-20), agranulocyte adhesion and diapedesis (p-value 2.68E-13), and role of macrophages, fibroblasts and endothelial cells in rheumatoid arthritis (p-value 4.74E-12). All of these genes were downregulated in idiopathic gastroparesis. Five genes that were common to all three top canonical pathways were C5AR1, CCL2, CXCL8, IL1B and SELE. There was 6–12% overlap in genes associated with these functions in these top pathways and the differentially expressed genes in the Ingenuity dataset. A fourth canonical pathway contained 7 of the 18 genes (CCL2, CCL3, CCL4, CSF3, IL6, IL10 and IL1B) that have been associated with differential regulation of cytokine production in macrophages and T helper cells by IL-17A and IL-17F. Immune cell trafficking was the leading physiological function identified linked by 82 of the 181 molecules with leucocyte migration as the key annotated function associated with 71 of those molecules. The top biological gene interaction network containing the most number of differentially expressed genes in our group was "cellular movement, immune cell trafficking, cell-to-cell signaling and interaction".

Differentially expressed genes common to diabetic and idiopathic gastroparesis

Two hundred genes were differentially expressed in both diabetic and idiopathic gastroparesis as compared to their controls (Additional file 5: Table S5). Distribution of common and overlapping genes between the two comparison groups with a $\log_2$fold difference of $|\geq 2|$ is shown in Fig. 2a. Sixty five genes were common to both groups and all of them were downregulated in gastroparesis (Fig. 2b). The top 3 canonical pathways had genes associated with granulocyte adhesion and diapedesis (CCL2, CCL4, CSF3, CXCL2, CXCR2, CXCR4, FPR1, and IL1R1,

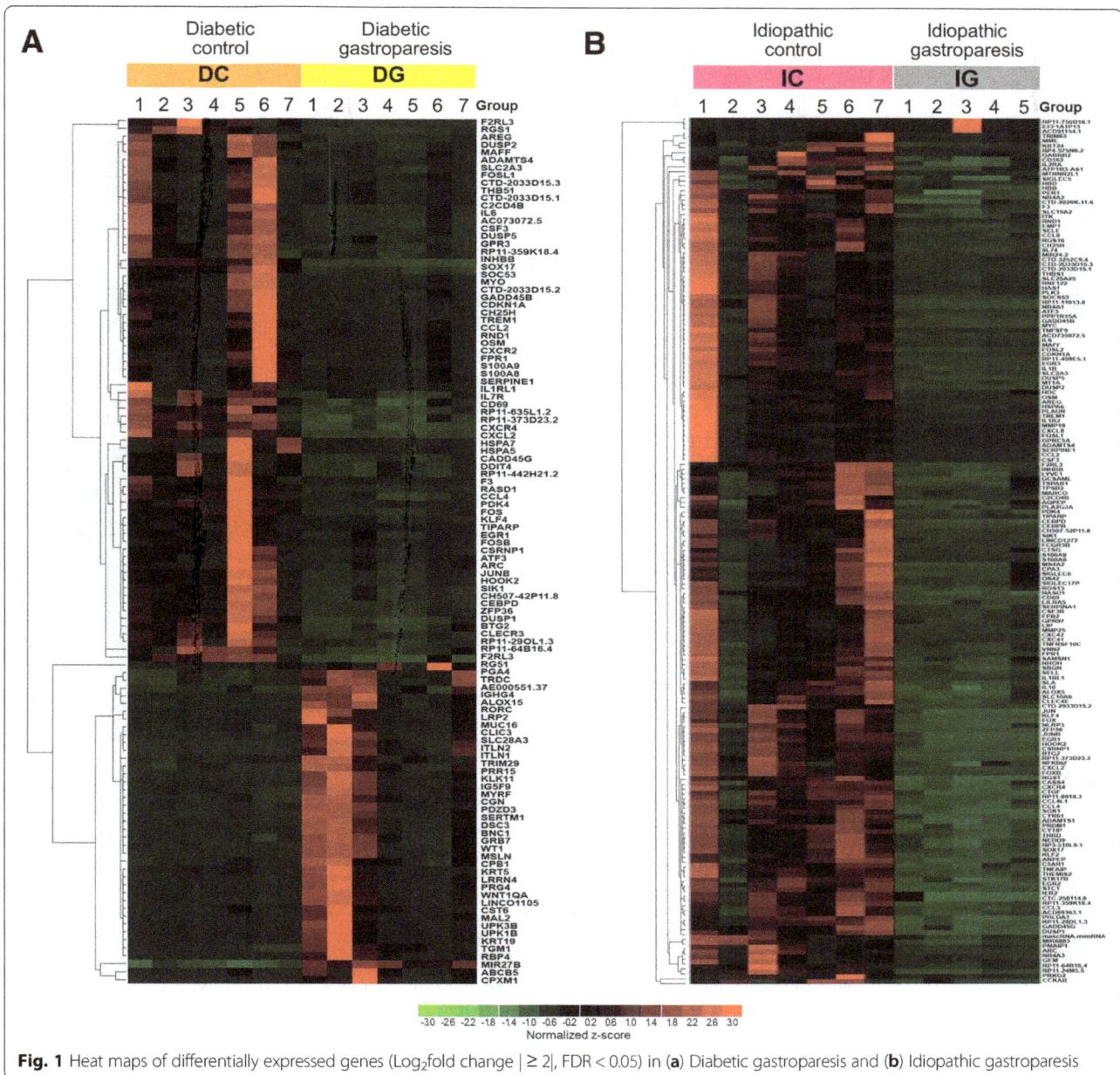

Fig. 1 Heat maps of differentially expressed genes (Log₂fold change | ≥ 2|, FDR < 0.05) in (**a**) Diabetic gastroparesis and (**b**) Idiopathic gastroparesis

$p = 1.74E\text{-}08$), role of macrophages, fibroblasts and endothelial cells in rheumatoid arthritis (ADAMTS4, CCL2, CEBPD, FOS, IL6, IL1R1, MYC, OSM, and SOCS3, $p = 9.13E\text{-}08$), and differential regulation of cytokine production in macrophages and T helper cells by IL-17A and IL-17F (CCL2, CCL4, CSF3 and IL6, $p = 1.15E\text{-}07$) (Fig. 2c). The differential regulation of cytokine production in macrophages and T helper cells by IL-17A and IL-17F had 4 genes overlapping with 18 associated with that pathway (22% overlap). Hematological system development and function (41 genes) and tissue morphology (38 genes) were the two top physiological systems affected with the function "quantity of leucocytes" linking most differentially expressed genes.

RT-PCR validation of common genes

Five highly differentially expressed genes in diabetic gastroparesis were selected for validation studies (SGK1, serum/glucocorticoid regulated kinase 1; APOLD1, apolipoprotein L domain containing 1; CXCR4, C-X-C motif chemokine receptor 4; CXCL2, C-X-C motif chemokine ligand 2; and FOS, Fos proto-oncogene). Four of these were significantly downregulated in diabetic gastroparesis (APOLD1, CXCR4, CXCL2, and FOS) as observed in the RNA seq analysis (Fig. 3). The one gene that was not found to be statistically different on RT-PCR had significant but lower log₂fold changes in expression on RNA seq (SGK1–1.77). The most robust differences were

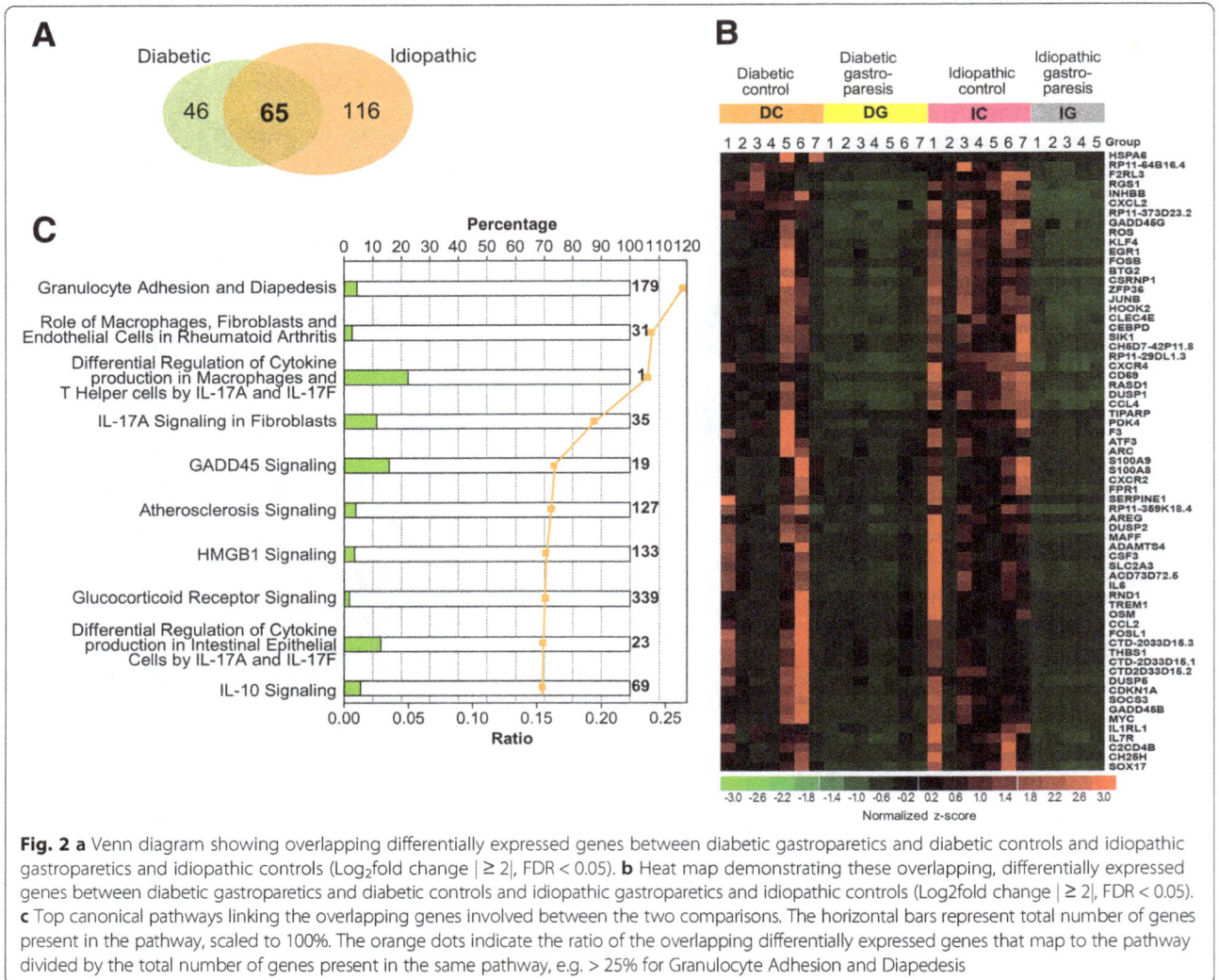

Fig. 2 a Venn diagram showing overlapping differentially expressed genes between diabetic gastroparetics and diabetic controls and idiopathic gastroparetics and idiopathic controls (Log2fold change | ≥ 2|, FDR < 0.05). **b** Heat map demonstrating these overlapping, differentially expressed genes between diabetic gastroparetics and diabetic controls and idiopathic gastroparetics and idiopathic controls (Log2fold change | ≥ 2|, FDR < 0.05). **c** Top canonical pathways linking the overlapping genes involved between the two comparisons. The horizontal bars represent total number of genes present in the pathway, scaled to 100%. The orange dots indicate the ratio of the overlapping differentially expressed genes that map to the pathway divided by the total number of genes present in the same pathway, e.g. > 25% for Granulocyte Adhesion and Diapedesis

seen in APOLD1, apolipoprotein L domain containing 1 ($\Delta\Delta$CT = 3.595, $P < 0.0001$) and FOS, Fos proto-oncogene ($\Delta\Delta$CT = 3.588, P < 0.0001).

Immune profile analysis

The CIBERSORT immune cell analysis revealed no significant differences in enrichment of M1 or M2 macrophage associated genes in the diabetic gastroparesis and diabetic control samples. However, M1 (pro-inflammatory) macrophage associated genes were significantly more highly represented in idiopathic gastroparetic samples than in non-diabetic, non-gastroparetic controls (Mean (SD): 0.04 (0.03) % vs 0.004 (0.007) % M1 associated genes in idiopathic gastroparesis and idiopathic controls respectively, $p = 0.02$). The quantification for percentage of genes associated with these macrophage subtypes in diabetic and idiopathic gastroparesis vs their controls are displayed in Fig. 4.

Discussion

Recent advancements made in molecular understanding of gastroparesis using animal models and human samples have elucidated an important role of the innate immune system [15]. This is likely driven by a shift in polarization of macrophages and associated expression of pro- and anti-inflammatory cytokines. The current proposed central mechanism for gastroparesis includes macrophage driven loss of or functional abnormalities in ICC and other components of the enteric neuromuscular apparatus which can then affect gastric motility.

This study utilizing deep transcriptional sequencing of the human stomach neuromuscular apparatus further provides evidence for innate immune dysregulation as the key feature of both diabetic and idiopathic gastroparesis. More specifically, it highlights that macrophage function and signaling is associated with this disease process. Additionally, this study identifies pathways that are potentially unique to diabetic and idiopathic gastroparesis. Macrophage and T

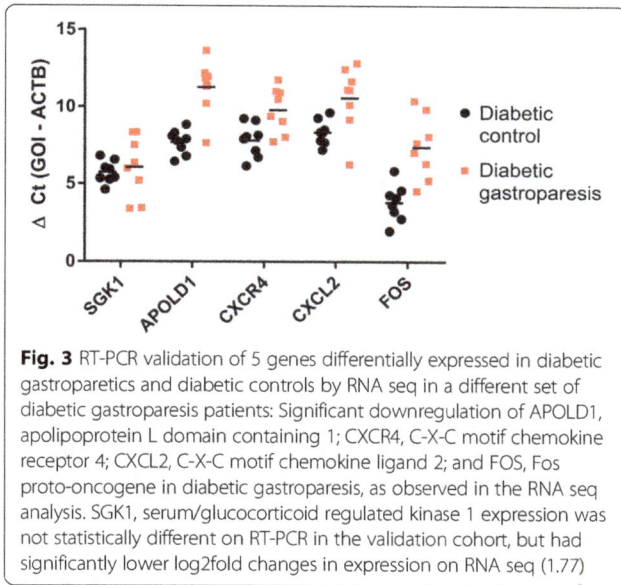

Fig. 3 RT-PCR validation of 5 genes differentially expressed in diabetic gastroparetics and diabetic controls by RNA seq in a different set of diabetic gastroparesis patients: Significant downregulation of APOLD1, apolipoprotein L domain containing 1; CXCR4, C-X-C motif chemokine receptor 4; CXCL2, C-X-C motif chemokine ligand 2; and FOS, Fos proto-oncogene in diabetic gastroparesis, as observed in the RNA seq analysis. SGK1, serum/glucocorticoid regulated kinase 1 expression was not statistically different on RT-PCR in the validation cohort, but had significantly lower log2fold changes in expression on RNA seq (1.77)

helper cell signaling genes were differentially expressed in diabetic gastroparesis, whereas, granulocyte and agranulocyte function genes were associated with pathways involved in idiopathic gastroparesis.

This study builds upon findings from mouse models and in vitro studies. In the NOD mouse model of gastroparesis, animals that retain normal gastric emptying have normal ICC networks and CD206-positive, HO1-positive M2 macrophages (anti-inflammatory spectrum) in the muscularis propria, while animals developing delayed gastric emptying demonstrated damage in ICC networks and express CD206-negative and HO1-negative M1 macrophages (pro-inflammatory spectrum) [7]. Furthermore, the presence of macrophages was found to be essential for development of delayed gastric emptying [8]. Our in vitro work has also provided evidence for M1 macrophage generated TNF-α to be involved in caspase-mediated apoptosis and Kit down regulation in ICC [16]. Finally, human studies have shown a positive correlation between the number of ICC and M2 macrophages in diabetics and diabetic gastroparesis [17]. The loss of ICC has been correlated with impairment in gastric emptying [5].

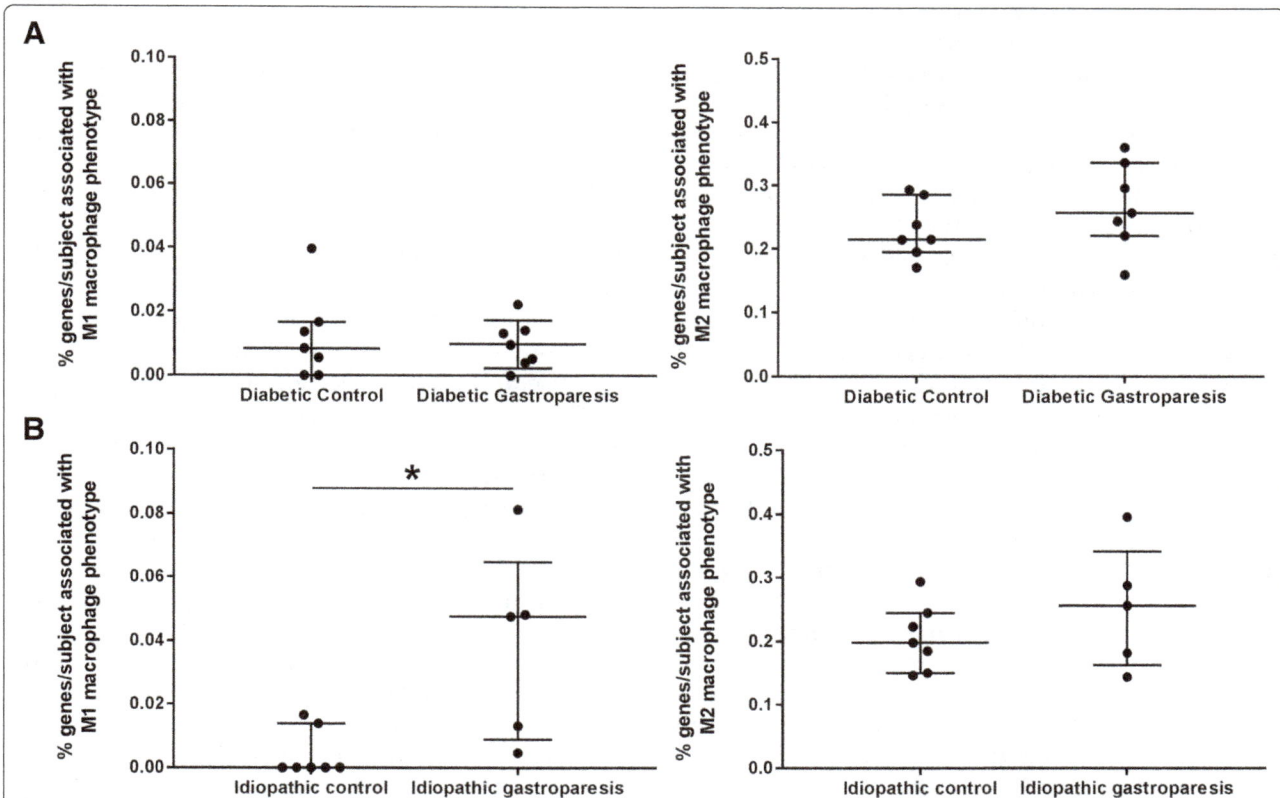

Fig. 4 CIBERSORT analysis displaying distribution of patients with M1 and M2 macrophage associated genes in (**a**) Diabetic controls and diabetic gastroparesis: No differences were seen in % genes/subject associated with M1 or M2 macrophage phenotype (**b**) Idiopathic controls and idiopathic gastroparesis: Significantly greater number of idiopathic gastroparesis patients express % genes associated with an M1 (proinflammatory) macrophage phenotype (Mean (SD): 0.04 (0.03) % vs 0.004 (0.007) % M1 associated genes in idiopathic gastroparesis and idiopathic controls respectively, $p = 0.02$). No differences were seen in % genes/subject associated with M2 macrophage phenotype

A large number of transcripts were found to be significantly altered in both diabetic and idiopathic gastroparesis patients compared to their controls. Four transcripts common to top canonical pathways in diabetic gastroparesis include CCL2 (C-C Motif Chemokine Ligand 2), a monocyte chemoattractant protein coding gene; IL6, pro-inflammatory gene involved in differentiation of B-cells, monocyte and generation of Th17 cells and also involved in improving insulin resistance and susceptibility to diabetes mellitus; IL1RL1 (Interleukin 1 Receptor Like 1), a receptor involved in proinflammatory stimuli and function of T helper cells; and ADAMTS4 (ADAM Metallopeptidase with Thrombospondin Type 1 Motif 4), a protease involved in degradation of cartilage protein aggrecan and extracellular matrix protein brevican. All of these transcripts were downregulated in diabetic gastroparesis. In idiopathic gastroparesis, five transcripts common to all three top canonical pathways include C5AR1 (Complement C5a Receptor 1), receptor for inflammatory peptide C5a involved in both innate and adaptive immune response; CCL2 (C-C Motif Chemokine Ligand 2); CXCL8 (C-X-C Motif Chemokine Ligand 8) chemotactic factor for neutrophils, basophils, and T-cells; IL1B (Interleukin 1 Beta), a macrophage produced cytokine involved in acute B and T cell activation and cyclooxygenase 2 activation; and SELE (Selectin E), a leucocyte cell surface adhesion protein. All of these transcripts were downregulated in gastroparesis. It remains to be further investigated whether these changes have an influence on the protein expression and it should be kept in mind that the majority of differentially expressed genes in our dataset did not overlap with the total genes known to be associated with these pathways in the Ingenuity database suggesting that the specific pathways involved may be different. When transcripts common to diabetic and idiopathic gastroparesis were analyzed, five transcripts associated with IL-17A signaling (CCL2, CEBPD, FOS, IL6 and JUN) were found to be involved. IL-17A is a pro-inflammatory cytokine that regulates NF-kappa B and mitogen-activated protein kinases and can stimulate expression of IL6 and COX-2 [18, 19]. It has been shown to stimulate inflammatory activity in human subepithelial myofibroblasts [20] and involved in and production of nitric oxide in endothelial cells [21].

Of interest is the significant overlap of genes between diabetic and idiopathic gastroparesis that was found in this study. There currently is a healthy and vigorous debate on whether idiopathic gastroparesis belongs more to the functional bowel disorder spectrum of diseases or more to the diabetic gastroparesis spectrum. The findings of this study suggest similarities in pathophysiology between diabetic and idiopathic gastroparesis and presents mechanistic insight into idiopathic gastroparesis as a non-functional disease. Interestingly, almost twice the numbers of transcripts were altered in idiopathic gastroparesis compared

to diabetic gastroparesis when compared with their controls.

The CIBERSORT analysis provided a complementary approach at determining associations between abundance of specific cell type associated genes in specific subjects within the disease groups. This showed a higher abundance of genes indicating presence of M1 (pro-inflammatory spectrum) macrophages in the idiopathic gastroparesis tissues when compared to their controls. This is interesting since in in vitro studies, M1 macrophage derived TNFα was found to cause loss of ICC through reduced Kit expression [16].

Significant challenges exist in the studies of human macrophages due to diversity of macrophage phenotypes and considerable differences between markers for mouse and human macrophages. In mice, mucosal monocytes with lymphocyte antigen 6C (Ly6C) expression differentiate into pro-inflammatory (M1) and inflammatory dendritic cells upon entering the tissue [22]. However, in humans Gr1+, an equivalent of mouse Ly6C is not associated with expression of proinflammatory markers [23]. In lung tissue, TGM2 was found to be a robust marker for the anti-inflammatory macrophage subtype; however, this has not been validated in gastrointestinal tissues [24]. The marker used to study macrophage subtypes depend upon disease, species and sites involved. In general, the dichotomous differentiation of M1 and M2 phenotype is currently discouraged and these phenotypes should be seen in a spectrum. iNOS is expressed robustly in mouse macrophages in inflammation but is repressed epigenetically in human macrophages [25]. Arginase-1 and Ym1 are examples of other proteins that are expressed in mouse but not human M2 macrophages [26]. Therefore, classification of human macrophages continues to be a work in progress. In both mice and human, muscularis macrophages have been identified in close proximity to ICC suggesting a role in their function [27]. A variety of neurotransmitter receptors on macrophages regulate their functional phenotype. Additionally, neurons express receptors for macrophage-derived signaling molecules that alter neuronal activity and survival including bone morphogenetic protein 2 [28] and TNFα [29]. Nitric oxide produced by iNOS in mouse (but not human) macrophages suppresses neuronal [30] and smooth muscle excitability [31]. A recent study of idiopathic gastroparetics revealed decreased expression of PDGFRα and its ligands PDGFA and PDGFB, smooth muscle proteins (MYH11, MYLK1, and PAK1), non-specific macrophage marker (CD68), gene encoding HO1 (HMOX1) and immunosuppressive cytokine TGFβ1 [32]. Functional interactions between macrophages and ICC and other components of neuromuscular apparatus in humans need to be studied.

A limitation of the study is the small sample size. Seven subjects per group provide 51% power to detect a

2-fold expression in a gene, indicating that certain important genes may have been missed. These findings will require validation in a larger cohort of gastroparesis patients. This will also be necessary to determine if there are subsets within gastroparesis with distinct transcriptional profiles based on symptoms, gastric emptying delay or overlap with other diagnoses. Secondly, all controls were obese, whereas, only 37% of gastroparesis patients were obese. Since obesity is also a proinflammatory state, this could have confounded the results of the analysis. However, in our previous study no differences in global immune cell population (CD45 immunoreactive cells) were seen between obese and non-obese subjects [3]. Third, the databases used for Ingenuity pathway analysis are enriched in transcripts associated with immune and cancer biology. This may skew pathways analyses towards those biological functions. Another observation from the current study is lack of evidence of pathways linking transcripts for neuromuscular function which synchronizes with our findings at protein level, where nerve and neuronal changes were seen in only a subset of patients with gastroparesis. Although, this may be due to limitations of the Ingenuity platform, another possibility includes that cumulative transcriptional expression in a complex biological sample containing multiple cell types may mask changes seen in gene expression in specific cell-types.

Conclusions

This study is the first to determine whole transcriptomic changes in deeper neuromuscular apparatus in gastroparesis (or any gastrointestinal motility disorder). Several important observations are made. First, diabetic and idiopathic gastroparesis have both unique and overlapping changes in the transcriptome. However, immune signaling predominates the pathways linking most of the differentially expressed transcripts. Second, most patients with idiopathic gastroparesis differentially expressed transcripts compared to controls that have been associated with pro-inflammatory (M1) macrophage phenotype. Third, transcriptomics provides reliable targets for future mechanistic work considering the validation of selected genes achieved in a separate set of diabetic gastroparesis patients. These findings make a case for targeting innate immune system for development of future treatment approaches to gastroparesis but the molecular targets identified will need further investigations in animal models to determine the optimal timing of intervention aimed at preventing or reversing damage to the gastric function.

Abbreviations

GI: Gastrointestinal tract; HO1: Heme oxygenase 1; ICC: Interstitial cells of Cajal; IL10: Interleukin 10; IL6: Interleukin 6; iNOS: Inducible NOS; NOD: Non-obese diabetic; op/op: Osteopetrotic mouse; TNFα: Tumor necrosis factor-α

Acknowledgements

The authors also acknowledge Dr. Jose Serrano MD, PhD, Project Officer, NIDDK. Dr. Linda Nguyen, MD (Stanford University), and Dr. William Hasler, MD (University of Michigan) as past members of the GpCRC. The authors wish to thank Ms. Kristy Zodrow for administrative assistance.

Funding

The Gastroparesis Clinical Research Consortium (GpCRC) is supported by the National Institute of Diabetes and Digestive and Kidney Diseases (NIDDK) (grants U01DK073975, U01DK074007, U01DK073974, U01DK074008). Additionally, Dr. Grover is supported by K23 DK103911.

Authors' contributions

MG study concept and design; acquisition of data; analysis and interpretation of data; drafting of the manuscript; critical revision of the manuscript; statistical analysis; study supervision. SJG study concept and design; acquisition of data; analysis and interpretation of data; critical revision of the manuscript; statistical analysis; study supervision. AN analysis and interpretation of data; critical revision of the manuscript; statistical analysis. CEB analysis and interpretation of data; critical revision of the manuscript. ASZ analysis and interpretation of data; critical revision of the manuscript. SE acquisition of data; critical revision of the manuscript. LW acquisition of data; critical revision of the manuscript. LM acquisition of data; critical revision of the manuscript. PJP acquisition of data; critical revision of the manuscript. HPP acquisition of data; tissue procurement; critical revision of the manuscript. IS acquisition of data; tissue procurement; critical revision of the manuscript. RM acquisition of data; tissue procurement; critical revision of the manuscript. KK acquisition of data; critical revision of the manuscript. TLA acquisition of data; tissue procurement; critical revision of the manuscript. WS acquisition of data; tissue procurement; critical revision of the manuscript. BK critical revision of the manuscript. RS critical revision of the manuscript. TJM tissue procurement; critical revision of the manuscript. TAK tissue procurement; critical revision of the manuscript. MJK tissue procurement; critical revision of the manuscript. JT acquisition of data; analysis and interpretation of data; critical revision of the manuscript. FAH critical revision of the manuscript; study supervision. GF study concept and design; acquisition of data; analysis and interpretation of data; critical revision of the manuscript; study supervision. All authors have read and approved the manuscript.

Competing interests

The authors declare that they have no competing interests.

Author details

[1]Enteric NeuroScience Program, Division of Gastroenterology & Hepatology, Mayo Clinic, 200 1st Street SW, Rochester, MN 55905, USA. [2]Biomedical Statistics and Informatics, Mayo Clinic, Rochester, MN, USA. [3]Johns Hopkins University Bloomberg School of Public Health, Johns Hopkins University, Baltimore, MD, USA. [4]Johns Hopkins University School of Medicine, Baltimore, MD, USA. [5]Temple University, Philadelphia, PA, USA. [6]Texas Tech University, El Paso, TX, USA. [7]Wake Forest University, Winston-Salem, NC, USA. [8]University of Louisville, Louisville, KY, USA. [9]California Pacific Medical Center, San Francisco, CA, USA. [10]Massachusetts General Hospital, Boston, MA, USA. [11]Baylor College of Medicine, Houston, TX, USA. [12]Department of Surgery, Mayo Clinic, Rochester, MN, USA. [13]National Institute of Diabetes and Digestive and Kidney Diseases, Bethesda, MD, USA.

References

1. Wang YR, Fisher RS, Parkman HP. Gastroparesis-related hospitalizations in the United States: trends, characteristics, and outcomes, 1995-2004. Am J Gastroenterol. 2008;103(2):313–22.
2. Pasricha PJ, Camilleri M, Hasler WL, Parkman HP. White Paper AGA: Gastroparesis: clinical and regulatory insights for clinical trials. Clin Gastroenterol Hepatol. 2017;15(8):1184–90.

3.   Grover M, Farrugia G, Lurken MS, Bernard CE, Faussone-Pellegrini MS, Smyrk TC, et al. Cellular changes in diabetic and idiopathic gastroparesis. Gastroenterology. 2011;140(5):1575–85. e1578

4.   Ordog T, Takayama I, Cheung WK, Ward SM, Sanders KM. Remodeling of networks of interstitial cells of Cajal in a murine model of diabetic gastroparesis. Diabetes. 2000;49(10):1731–9.

5.   Grover M, Bernard CE, Pasricha PJ, Lurken MS, Faussone-Pellegrini MS, Smyrk TC, et al. Clinical-histological associations in gastroparesis: results from the gastroparesis clinical research consortium. Neurogastroenterol Motil. 2012;24(6):531–9. e249

6.   Faussone-Pellegrini MS, Grover M, Pasricha PJ, Bernard CE, Lurken MS, Smyrk TC, et al. Ultrastructural differences between diabetic and idiopathic gastroparesis. J Cell Mol Med. 2012;16(7):1573–81.

7.   Choi KM, Kashyap PC, Dutta N, Stoltz GJ, Ordog T, Shea Donohue T, et al. CD206-positive M2 macrophages that express heme oxygenase-1 protect against diabetic gastroparesis in mice. Gastroenterology. 2010;138(7):2399–409. 2409 e2391

8.   Cipriani G, Gibbons SJ, Verhulst PJ, Choi KM, Eisenman ST, Hein SS, et al. Diabetic Csf1(op/op) mice lacking macrophages are protected against the development of delayed gastric emptying. Cell Mol Gastroenterol Hepatol. 2016;2(1):40–7.

9.   Grover M, Bernard CE, Pasricha PJ, Parkman HP, Gibbons SJ, Tonascia J, et al. Diabetic and idiopathic gastroparesis is associated with loss of CD206-positive macrophages in the gastric antrum. Neurogastroenterol Motil. 2017;29(6). https://doi.org/10.1111/nmo.13018. Epub 2017 Jan 9.

10. Kalari KR, Nair AA, Bhavsar JD, O'Brien DR, Davila JI, Bockol MA, et al. MAP-RSeq: Mayo analysis pipeline for RNA sequencing. BMC Bioinformatics. 2014;15:224.

11. Robinson MD, McCarthy DJ, Smyth GK. edgeR: a Bioconductor package for differential expression analysis of digital gene expression data. Bioinformatics. 2010;26(1):139–40.

12. Hart SN, Therneau TM, Zhang Y, Poland GA, Kocher JP. Calculating sample size estimates for RNA sequencing data. J Comput Biol. 2013;20(12):970–8.

13. Kramer A, Green J, Pollard J Jr, Tugendreich S. Causal analysis approaches in ingenuity pathway analysis. Bioinformatics. 2014;30(4):523–30.

14. Newman AM, Liu CL, Green MR, Gentles AJ, Feng W, Xu Y, et al. Robust enumeration of cell subsets from tissue expression profiles. Nat Methods. 2015;12(5):453–7.

15. Cipriani G, Gibbons SJ, Kashyap PC, Farrugia G. Intrinsic gastrointestinal macrophages: their phenotype and role in gastrointestinal motility. Cell Mol Gastroenterol Hepatol. 2016;2(2):120–30. e121

16. Eisenman ST, Gibbons SJ, Verhulst PJ, Cipriani G, Saur D, Farrugia G. Tumor necrosis factor alpha derived from classically activated "M1" macrophages reduces interstitial cell of Cajal numbers. Neurogastroenterol Motil. 2017;29(4). https://doi.org/10.1111/nmo.12984. Epub 2016 Oct 25.

17. Bernard CE, Gibbons SJ, Mann IS, Froschauer L, Parkman HP, Harbison S, et al. Association of low numbers of CD206-positive cells with loss of ICC in the gastric body of patients with diabetic gastroparesis. Neurogastroenterol Motil. 2014;26(9):1275–84.

18. Hata K, Andoh A, Shimada M, Fujino S, Bamba S, Araki Y, et al. IL-17 stimulates inflammatory responses via NF-kappaB and MAP kinase pathways in human colonic myofibroblasts. Am J Physiol Gastrointest Liver Physiol. 2002;282(6):G1035–44.

19. Zhang Z, Andoh A, Inatomi O, Bamba S, Takayanagi A, Shimizu N, et al. Interleukin-17 and lipopolysaccharides synergistically induce cyclooxygenase-2 expression in human intestinal myofibroblasts. J Gastroenterol Hepatol. 2005;20(4):619–27.

20. Yagi Y, Andoh A, Inatomi O, Tsujikawa T, Fujiyama Y. Inflammatory responses induced by interleukin-17 family members in human colonic subepithelial myofibroblasts. J Gastroenterol. 2007;42(9):746–53.

21. Miljkovic D, Cvetkovic I, Vuckovic O, Stosic-Grujicic S, Mostarica Stojkovic M, Trajkovic V. The role of interleukin-17 in inducible nitric oxide synthase-mediated nitric oxide production in endothelial cells. Cell Mol Life Sci. 2003;60(3):518–25.

22. Bain CC, Scott CL, Uronen-Hansson H, Gudjonsson S, Jansson O, Grip O, et al. Resident and pro-inflammatory macrophages in the colon represent alternative context-dependent fates of the same Ly6Chi monocyte precursors. Mucosal Immunol. 2013;6(3):498–510.

23. Auffray C, Sieweke MH, Geissmann F. Blood monocytes: development, heterogeneity, and relationship with dendritic cells. Annu Rev Immunol. 2009;27:669–92.

24. Martinez FO, Helming L, Milde R, Varin A, Melgert BN, Draijer C, et al. Genetic programs expressed in resting and IL-4 alternatively activated mouse and human macrophages: similarities and differences. Blood. 2013;121(9):e57–69.

25. Gross TJ, Kremens K, Powers LS, Brink B, Knutson T, Domann FE, et al. Epigenetic silencing of the human NOS2 gene: rethinking the role of nitric oxide in human macrophage inflammatory responses. J Immunol. 2014;192(5):2326–38.

26. Raes G, Van den Bergh R, De Baetselier P, Ghassabeh GH, Scotton C, Locati M, et al. Arginase-1 and Ym1 are markers for murine, but not human, alternatively activated myeloid cells. J Immunol. 2005;174(11):6561. author reply 6561-6562

27. Mikkelsen HB. Interstitial cells of Cajal, macrophages and mast cells in the gut musculature: morphology, distribution, spatial and possible functional interactions. J Cell Mol Med. 2010;14(4):818–32.

28. Muller PA, Koscso B, Rajani GM, Stevanovic K, Berres ML, Hashimoto D, et al. Crosstalk between muscularis macrophages and enteric neurons regulates gastrointestinal motility. Cell. 2014;158(2):300–13.

29. Coquenlorge S, Duchalais E, Chevalier J, Cossais F, Rolli-Derkinderen M, Neunlist M. Modulation of lipopolysaccharide-induced neuronal response by activation of the enteric nervous system. J Neuroinflammation. 2014;11:202.

30. Green CL, Ho W, Sharkey KA, McKay DM. Dextran sodium sulfate-induced colitis reveals nicotinic modulation of ion transport via iNOS-derived NO. Am J Physiol Gastrointest Liver Physiol. 2004;287(3):G706–14.

31. Hori M, Kita M, Torihashi S, Miyamoto S, Won KJ, Sato K, et al. Upregulation of iNOS by COX-2 in muscularis resident macrophage of rat intestine stimulated with LPS. Am J Physiol Gastrointest Liver Physiol. 2001;280(5):G930–8.

32. Herring BP, Hoggatt AM, Gupta A, Griffith S, Nakeeb A, Choi JN et al. Idiopathic gastroparesis is associated with specific transcriptional changes in the gastric muscularis externa. Neurogastroenterol Motil. 2017; 2017 Oct 20. doi: https://doi.org/10.1111/nmo.13230. [Epub ahead of print].

14

Calculating the statistical significance of rare variants causal for Mendelian and complex disorders

Aliz R. Rao[1]* (iD) and Stanley F. Nelson[1,2,3]

Abstract

Background: With the expanding use of next-gen sequencing (NGS) to diagnose the thousands of rare Mendelian genetic diseases, it is critical to be able to interpret individual DNA variation. To calculate the significance of finding a rare protein-altering variant in a given gene, one must know the frequency of seeing a variant in the general population that is at least as damaging as the variant in question.

Methods: We developed a general method to better interpret the likelihood that a rare variant is disease causing if observed in a given gene or genic region mapping to a described protein domain, using genome-wide information from a large control sample. Based on data from 2504 individuals in the 1000 Genomes Project dataset, we calculated the number of individuals who have a rare variant in a given gene for numerous filtering threshold scenarios, which may be used for calculating the significance of an observed rare variant being causal for disease. Additionally, we calculated mutational burden data on the number of individuals with rare variants in genic regions mapping to protein domains.

Results: We describe methods to use the mutational burden data for calculating the significance of observing rare variants in a given proportion of sequenced individuals. We present SORVA, an implementation of these methods as a web tool, and we demonstrate application to 20 relevant but diverse next-gen sequencing studies. Specifically, we calculate the statistical significance of findings involving multi-family studies with rare Mendelian disease and a large-scale study of a complex disorder, autism spectrum disorder. If we use the frequency counts to rank genes based on intolerance for variation, the ranking correlates well with pLI scores derived from the Exome Aggregation Consortium (ExAC) dataset ($\rho = 0.515$), with the benefit that the scores are directly interpretable.

Conclusions: We have presented a strategy that is useful for vetting candidate genes from NGS studies and allows researchers to calculate the significance of seeing a variant in a given gene or protein domain. This approach is an important step towards developing a quantitative, statistics-based approach for presenting clinical findings.

Keywords: SORVA, Intolerance, Genes, Protein domains, Mutational burden, Significance, Pathogenic

Background

Whole-exome sequencing has enabled the identification of causal genes responsible for causing hundreds of rare, Mendelian disorders in just a few years; however, there remain hundreds, if not thousands, more to be uncovered. The genetic basis has been determined for 4803 of the rare diseases [1], whereas the number of disease phenotypes with a known or suspected Mendelian basis lies close to 6419 based on data in Online Mendelian Inheritance in Man (OMIM) [1]. Next-gen sequencing (NGS) studies are certain to uncover many disease-phenotype relationships in the near future, but for cases involving rare diseases with limited sample sizes, determining causality between phenotypes and novel genes, and distinguishing true pathogenic variants from rare benign variants remains a challenge. Often disease causality of a given rare variant is only clear when additional affected individuals with similar rare variants in the same gene are identified, which can take years

* Correspondence: aliz.rao@ucla.edu
[1]Department of Human Genetics, University of California, Los Angeles, California, Los Angeles, USA
Full list of author information is available at the end of the article

to occur due to the rarity of these disorders. Thus, improvements in determining disease causality or likely pathogenicity would greatly enhance efforts to prioritize genes and gene variants for further molecular analysis, even if only a single affected individual was identified.

Variants identified through broad based NGS technologies are typically classified as pathogenic, likely pathogenic, variant of uncertain significance (VUS) or likely benign according to multiple criteria, largely based on prior knowledge about the specific variant. Novel variants are evaluated individually and placed into discrete categories if they meet complex combinations of criteria, which include thresholds for allele frequency, segregation, number of affected unrelated individuals, and known functional relevance [2, 3]. For example, a variant would be deemed pathogenic if the allele frequency threshold falls below a given threshold and the variant segregates with a disorder in at least two unrelated affected families, or if other criteria are met. In brief, variants are evaluated individually based on variant-specific annotations.

An additional source of information that would aid in variant prioritization would be a gene-specific annotation describing mutational burden in the overall population. To illustrate, consider a gene that has very few functional variants in the general population, and several unrelated patients were found to carry distinct protein-altering, rare missense or potential loss-of-function (LOF) variants in the given gene and within a highly conserved protein domain. Under a model for a rare Mendelian disorder caused by highly penetrant variants, we assume that common variants cannot be considered causal, and rare variants in genes intolerant of mutations are deemed highly suspicious of being causal for disease even if no other information is known about the variants. Therefore, knowing the population-wide mutational burden of a given gene for rare variants would be informative.

While there are gene-ranking methods based on other parameters [4], recently several gene-level ranking systems have emerged based on measures for intolerance to mutations in the general population. The Residual Variation Intolerance Score (RVIS) generates a score based on the frequencies of observed common functional coding variants compared to the total number of observed variants in the same gene or protein domain [5, 6]. A second ranking system, in addition to these parameters, also incorporates the frequency at which genes are found to be affected by rare, likely functional variants, and their findings suggest that disease associations to genes which frequently contain variants, termed as FLAGS, should be evaluated with extra caution [7]. Next, the Exome Aggregation Consortium (ExAC) dataset provides missense Z scores that describe the degree to which a gene is depleted of missense and LOF variants compared to expected values. They base expected values on the

frequency of synonymous variants, and provides pLI scores that describe probabilities of a gene being LOF intolerant [8, 9]. Of these two metrics, pLI is less correlated with coding sequence length and outperforms the Z score as an intolerance metric [8]. Another method, EvoTol, combines genic intolerance with evolutionary conservation of whole protein sequences or their constituent protein domains to prioritize disease-causing genes, and extends the RVIS method by leveraging the information on protein sequence evolution to identify genes where the number of mutations that are likely to be damaging based on evolutionary protein information is higher than expected [10]. Although these methods may be useful in ranking genes and prioritizing variants in order to highlight those in genes that frequently contain variants, neither results in a score that is directly interpretable in order to calculate statistics about NGS findings and determine the significance of seeing a variant in a given number of affected individuals.

One tool that calculates a P-value of finding a true association through clinical exome sequencing, RD-Match [11], allows researchers to calculate the probability of finding phenotypically similar individuals who share variants in a gene through systems such as Matchmaker Exchange. The tool incorporates the probability of an individual having a rare, nonsynonymous variant in a gene by taking the sum of the allele frequencies of all rare (MAF < 0.1%) nonsynonymous variants annotated in ExAC [8]. With higher MAF thresholds and large population sizes, this is problematic because an individual may have multiple variants in a gene that frequently contains rare variation, causing one to overestimate the fraction of the population carrying rare variants in the gene, hence the fixed, low MAF threshold. Furthermore, this tool is applicable to studies in which the affected individuals are selected based on phenotype as well as the prior knowledge that they share rare variants in a given gene. Finally, RD-Match does not allow researchers to customize variant filtering thresholds according to the disease model with regards to minor allele frequency or predicted consequence such as LOF or missense variant.

Another method that calculates the significance of NGS findings, the Transmission And De novo Association test (TADA), is a Bayesian model that combines data from de novo mutations, inherited variants in families, and variants in cases and controls in a population [12]. This method has been used to identify risk-conferring genes in whole-exome sequencing studies of autism spectrum disorders and neurodevelopmental delay [13–15]. While TADA analysis has proven to be a critical first step in the development of quantitative methods to assess risk genes, it is restricted to integrating trio and case-control data and is unable to leverage information from larger pedigrees, and whether siblings or distantly related individuals share the variants observed in the proband. Also, it does not incorporate any information from large reference datasets, and therefore, it cannot be used for calculating the *P*-value of findings in smaller studies.

Here we describe a method, named SORVA for Significance Of Rare VAriants, for ranking genes based on mutational burden. In addition to incorporating information from variant allele frequencies, we use population-derived data to precompute an unbiased, easily interpretable score, which allows one to calculate the significance of observed and novel rare variants and their potential for being causal of disease. One may then answer the question: what is the probability of observing missense variants in three out of ten unrelated affected individuals, for example, given that only one in a thousand individuals in the general population carry a missense variant in the gene? Essentially, a model can be constructed to estimate the probability of drawing *n* unrelated families with similar biallelic genotypes by chance from the general population [16]. Conversely, if one has a large list of variants of unknown significance, the significance level may be useful in prioritizing variants within the same category of pathogenicity, and in improving the interpretation of variants in studies of Mendelian genetic disorders.

Results

For calculating the significance of seeing variants within a gene when sequencing multiple individuals affected for a rare, presumably Mendelian disorder, we first calculated the frequency of observing a variant in each gene in an individual within the population by using a large control dataset and collapsing variants in each gene. Calculations are based on data from 2504 individuals in the 1000 Genomes Project phase 3 dataset, which includes targeted exome sequencing data (mean depth = 65.7×) from individuals from five "superpopulations" (European, African, East Asian, South Asian, and ad-mixed American) [17]. We repeated the analysis for variants filtered according to various minor allele frequency and protein consequence thresholds that researchers may use when filtering variants. First, we filtered out common variants that met various minor allele frequency (MAF) thresholds used in the literature and others: 5, 1, 0.5, 0.1 and 0.05%. We then filtered rare variants according to two scenarios before collapsing variants across genes: 1) we included all protein-altering variants, i.e. those that cause a nonsynonymous change in the protein transcript or have a potential loss-of-function (LOF) consequence, and 2) we filtered for LOF variants only, i.e. splice site, stop codon gain and frameshift variants.

Below, we present general findings in population and molecular genetics that can be gleaned from the dataset, and illustrate how the dataset can be used in multiple studies, as a control group to vet candidate genes and variants.

Population differences

Of 18,877 genes that are in the union of the Ensembl and RefSeq gene sets, most genes contained heterozygous or homozygous missense variants in individuals in all populations; only 2.3% contain no rare variants (MAF < 5%), and 1.0% of genes have an identified variant in only a single population. Lowering our MAF threshold does not decrease the number of genes much. Although, filtering variants to include only LOF variants reduces the number of genes containing variants in the dataset to 9641, or 51.1% of genes in the dataset. (Fig. 1) These results demonstrate that choosing the correct MAF threshold is not nearly as important as identifying the correct protein consequence threshold to use when filtering variants. For instance, including all missense variants when LOF variants are generally causal for a given disease would reduce power to detect the gene associated with the disease.

The number of individuals who carried a heterozygous or homozygous variant in a given gene was generally higher in the African population compared to other populations (Fig. 2a), which is expected given that African individuals are observed to have up to three times as many low-frequency variants as those of European or East Asian origin [17], which reflects ancestral bottlenecks in non-African populations [18]. Conversely, regarding genes for which the number of individuals with a rare variant in the gene differed between populations, the genes having the greatest difference between populations tended to diverge most in the African population. (Fig. 2b) Genes whose mutational burden diverges most between populations are significantly enriched for a large number of biological functional terms, including glycoprotein, olfactory transduction and sensory perception, cell adhesion, various repeats, basement membrane and extracellular matrix part, cadherin, microtubule motor activity, immunoglobulin and EGF-like domain. It is important to note differences between populations, because, in many cases, researchers would be advised to use control populations similar to their study population. However, if a gene is associated with a severe, childhood-onset disorder in one population, it is likely to be associated with disease in other populations, as well, and knowledge that a gene frequently contains variation in African populations would be useful in prioritizing candidate genes even if one is studying variation in another population. In this case, such information would point towards reduced likelihood for disease association.

Properties of known disease genes

To determine whether calculating the frequency of individuals who have a rare variant in a given gene in the general population may be helpful in determining which genes are more likely to cause disease, we compared the

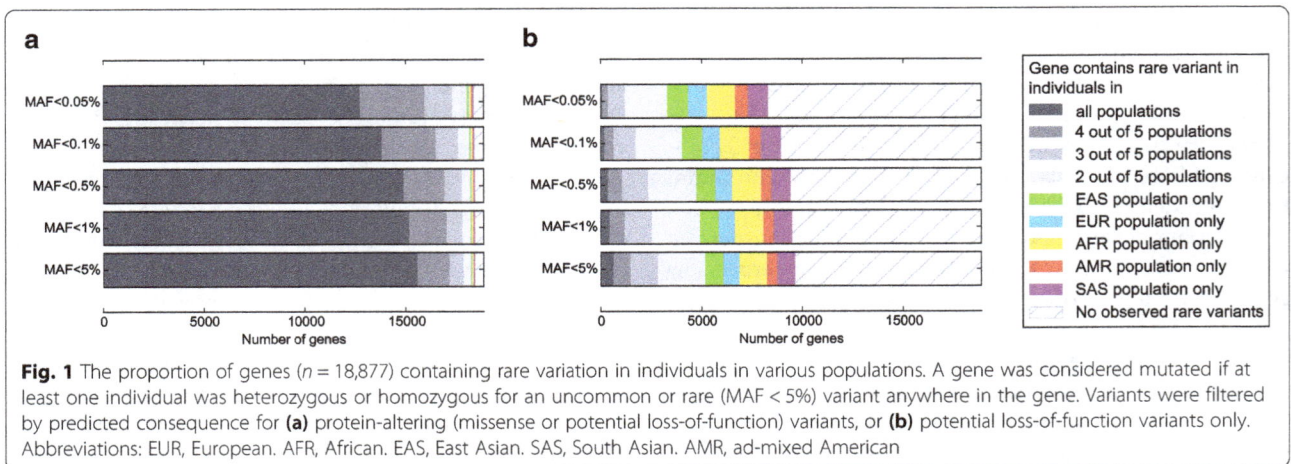

Fig. 1 The proportion of genes (*n* = 18,877) containing rare variation in individuals in various populations. A gene was considered mutated if at least one individual was heterozygous or homozygous for an uncommon or rare (MAF < 5%) variant anywhere in the gene. Variants were filtered by predicted consequence for **(a)** protein-altering (missense or potential loss-of-function) variants, or **(b)** potential loss-of-function variants only. Abbreviations: EUR, European. AFR, African. EAS, East Asian. SAS, South Asian. AMR, ad-mixed American

counts between multiple categories of genes: a) "essential" genes, defined as genes essential for cell survival in human cell lines, b) genes in which variants are known to cause autosomal dominant disorders, c) genes in which variants are known to cause autosomal recessive disorders, d) genes in which variants are known to cause X-linked disorders, and e) all other genes. As expected, fewer individuals carry rare, protein-altering or LOF variants in genes known to cause Mendelian disorders compared to other genes, and genes associated with X-linked disorders tend to be least tolerant of mutations (Fig. 3; Additional file 1). Although frequency counts overlapped between gene categories for every variant filtering

threshold, clusters were most differentiated when plotting the proportion of individuals who are heterozygous for rare LOF variants in a gene. Furthermore, the differentiation between clusters increased as the MAF threshold became more stringent, as the datasets became enriched for deleterious variants that can only subsist at a low allele frequency in a population due to selective pressure. (Additional file 1).

Previous research suggests that 2.0% of adults of European ancestry and 1.1% of adults of African ancestry can be expected to have actionable highly penetrant pathogenic (including novel expected pathogenic) or likely pathogenic single-nucleotide variants (SNVs) in 112

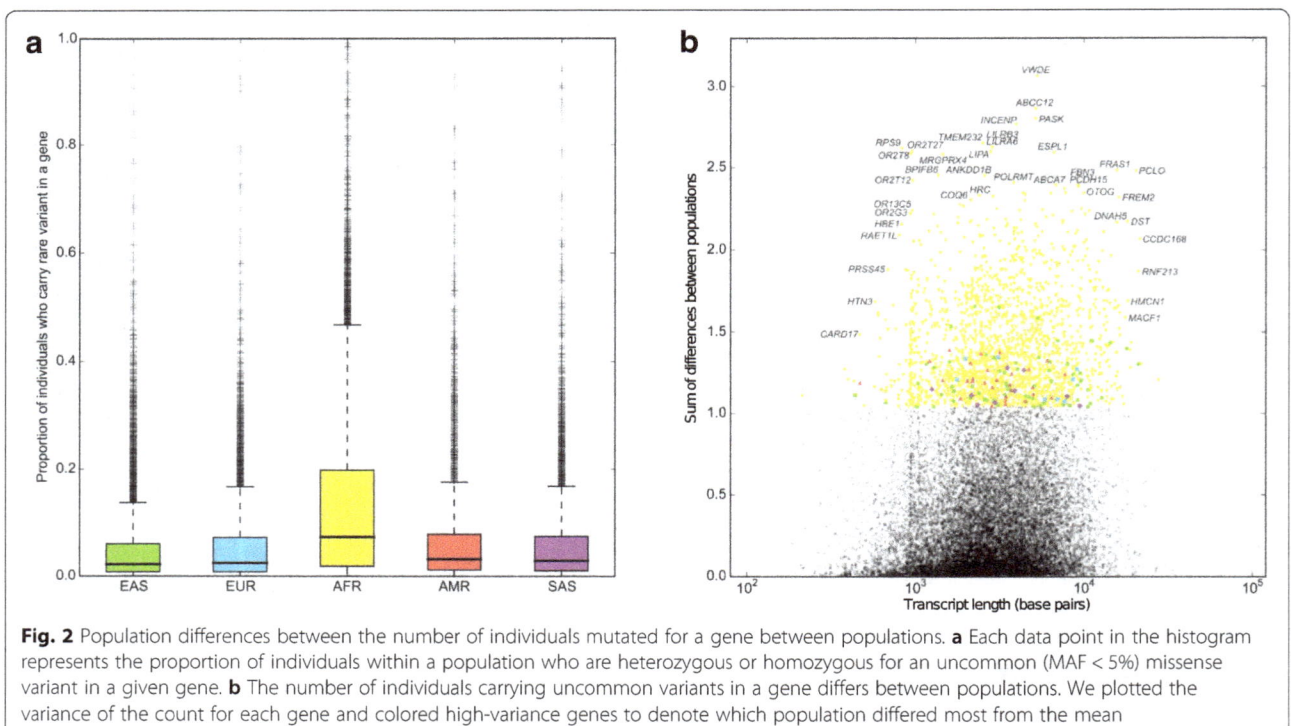

Fig. 2 Population differences between the number of individuals mutated for a gene between populations. **a** Each data point in the histogram represents the proportion of individuals within a population who are heterozygous or homozygous for an uncommon (MAF < 5%) missense variant in a given gene. **b** The number of individuals carrying uncommon variants in a gene differs between populations. We plotted the variance of the count for each gene and colored high-variance genes to denote which population differed most from the mean

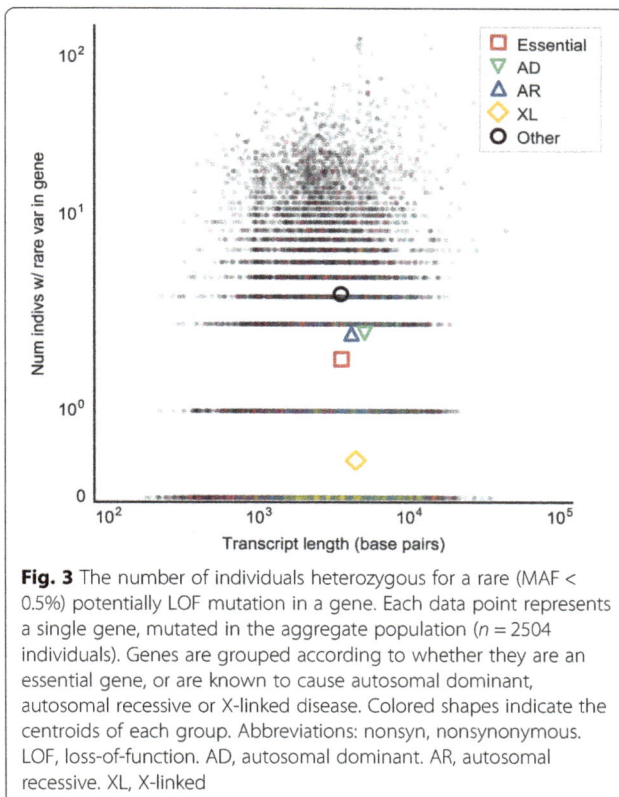

Fig. 3 The number of individuals heterozygous for a rare (MAF < 0.5%) potentially LOF mutation in a gene. Each data point represents a single gene, mutated in the aggregate population (n = 2504 individuals). Genes are grouped according to whether they are an essential gene, or are known to cause autosomal dominant, autosomal recessive or X-linked disease. Colored shapes indicate the centroids of each group. Abbreviations: nonsyn, nonsynonymous. LOF, loss-of-function. AD, autosomal dominant. AR, autosomal recessive. XL, X-linked

medically actionable genes [2]. If we look for rare variants in 1000 Genomes Project individuals—benign as well as pathogenic variants—, we find that a larger proportion of 1000 Genomes Project individuals—5.8% of European individuals and 3.3% of African individuals—are heterozygous or homozygous for extremely rare (MAF < 0.0005) LOF variants in these 112 genes, highlighting the large number of benign variants that are found in the population at low allele frequencies and should be filtered out by manual curation.

Depletion of variants in regions mapping to specific protein domains

It has been suggested previously that collapsing variants by protein domain could lead to improved gene-based intolerance scoring systems, as certain regions of the gene could be much more constrained than others [5]. We incorporated data for 322,772 protein domains from Interpro [19] and calculated the average number of individuals who have a variant in any given type of protein domain (Additional file 2), after filtering for rare (MAF < 0.5%), heterozygous LOF variants. Protein domains that are highly constrained, well covered during exome sequencing and rarely contain variants despite their large size include the Family A G protein-coupled receptor-like protein domain (Superfamily: SSF81321), which is found in 660 genes and has a mean length of 965 base pairs; none of the 2504

individuals carry rare variants in the region mapping to this protein domain. Other highly constrained protein domains that occur throughout the human genome include Glutamic acid-rich region profile (PfScan: PS50313), Proline-rich region profile (PfScan:PS50099), Immunoglobulin (Superfamily: SSF48726), and Cysteine-rich region profile (PfScan: PS50311). (Additional file 2) If an NGS study finds that affected individuals have rare variants in variation intolerant protein domains such as those listed, the variants would become highly suspicious of being causal.

We also calculated whether specific genes contain protein domains that are significantly depleted of variation, given the frequency of variants in the gene overall. Filtering out protein domains in genes with no variants and those with missing information reduced the dataset to 67,138 protein domains in 7004 genes. 77 protein domains in 26 genes were significantly depleted of variation compared to the rest of the gene. Specifically, the number of rare (MAF < 0.5%), heterozygous LOF variants per individual in a protein domain were significantly lower than expected after correcting for multiple testing by the number of genes. (Fig. 4) Functional enrichment analysis in DAVID revealed that the most significant biological functions in the gene list were related to tubulin-tyrosine ligase activity ($P = 0.015$), and G-protein coupled receptor, rhodopsin-like superfamily ($P = 0.05$). Depletion values for all protein domains may be found in Additional file 3. Information about whether a protein domain is significantly depleted of variation despite being in a gene with frequently observed variation may be useful in distinguishing between pathogenic and benign rare variants within genes containing regions under different degrees of evolutionary constraint.

Significance of findings in multi-family studies of rare genetic disorders

Below, we present methods for multiple study designs to calculate the significance of observing a given variant in a given gene. In the simplest case, a study involving a single family, calculating the P-value is relatively simple. Consider a case of a severe, pediatric-onset Mendelian disorder, in which both parents and the affected child are sequenced to identify the causal variant. If only de novo variants are identified within a putative gene, one can easily estimate the probability of at least one de novo mutation occurring in a gene by random chance; one could multiply the per-base mutation rate by the length of the gene transcript and make adjustments to account for CpG content related variation in mutation rates (Additional file 4).

In studies that identify both de novo and inherited variants in more complex family structures, calculating the significance of a variant is more complex. First, we generalize the equation for calculating the significance of observing a de novo mutation in a gene for studies involving multiple families. If multiple families

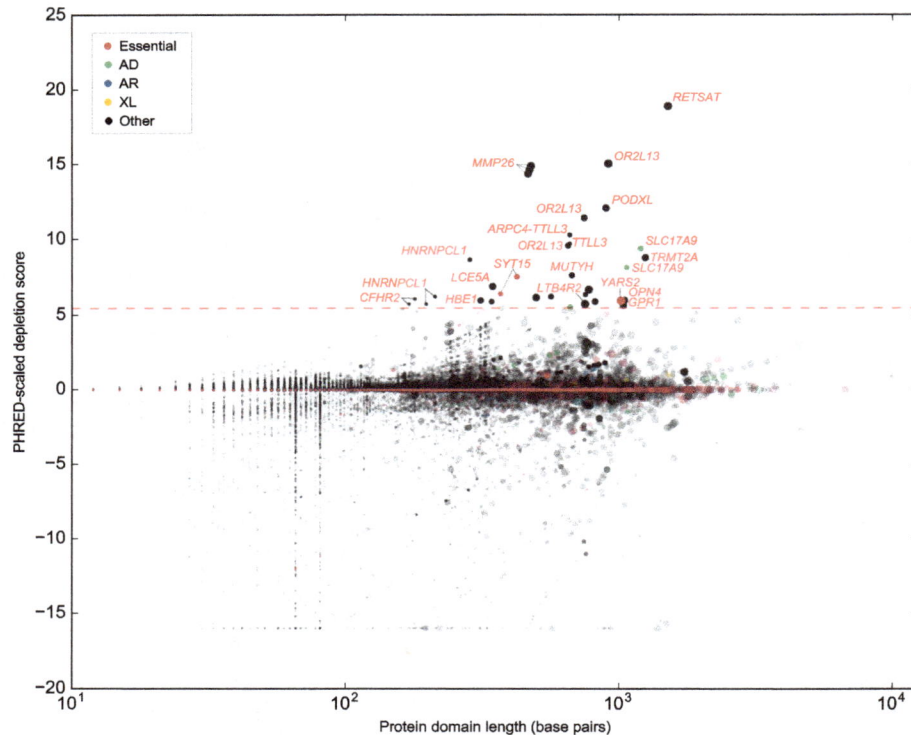

Fig. 4 Depletion of rare, heterozygous LOF variants in regions mapping to protein domains. We plotted scaled protein domain depletion scores for each domain mapping within a gene; high scaled scores indicate that a protein domain is depleted of rare (MAF < 0.5%) mutations compared to the rest of the gene. Darkened points above the red dashed line represent protein domains that are significantly depleted of mutations after correcting for the number of genes remaining after filtering. Larger points indicate protein domains with a greater length in proportion to the transcript length. Points are colored if the protein domain is within a gene that is an essential human gene or is causal for a Mendelian disorder. Abbreviations: AD, autosomal dominant. AR, autosomal recessive. XL, X-linked

sequenced, the *P*-value of observing independent de novo events in the same gene in *s* out of *n* individuals is

$$P = 1 - BinomCDF(s-1, n, l_{tx}dc)$$

where l_{tx} is the length of the transcript in nucleotide bases and *d* is the mean rate of de novo single-nucleotide variants (SNVs) arising per nucleotide per generation, *c* is the fraction of de novo events that meet our protein consequence threshold—2.85% if we consider only splice site altering or nonsense events, and 70.64% if we consider all protein-altering events, i.e. missense or LOF variants [20]—, and BinomCDF denotes the binomial cumulative distribution function. Consider the following example.

Clinical exome sequencing in four independent families identified de novo nonsense mutations in the gene *KAT6A* in all probands displaying significant developmental delay, microcephaly, and dysmorphism [21]. De novo nonsense mutations arising in this gene in all four individuals is highly unlikely by chance ($P = 2.66 \times 10^{-12}$), and the statistical findings would support *KAT6A* as highly suspicious

for causing the disorder. Further experiments and the identification of multiple other affected individuals by a separate study [22] confirmed this result.

If inherited variants are also observed in a gene, calculating the statistical significance of findings requires incorporating information about the number of individuals who carry a variant in the particular gene in the general population. The frequencies of the number of individuals who contain rare variants in a given gene or protein domain for various filtering thresholds may be queried through our online database called SORVA (https://sorva.genome.ucla.edu). (Additional file 5) Researchers can select the variant filtering thresholds identical to those used in hard filtering variants in a given study. Minor allele frequency thresholds range from 5%, useful for studies involving more common, complex disorders where less stringent filtering criteria are used, to 0.05% for studies involving extremely rare disorders. For genes that are rarely mutated, based on the expected number of individuals who carry a variant in the gene or protein domain in question, one can also calculate the significance of seeing the observed number of singletons (variants observed in a single independent individual), doubletons (variants observed in two individuals within a single family) or more complex cases as follows.

Let f_{hom} be the fraction of individuals in the general population with a homozygous variant in a gene or protein domain. Then, the P-value of seeing k individuals with a homozygous variant, out of n total unrelated affecteds is

$$P_{k,n} = 1 - BinomCDF(k-1, n, f_{hom})$$

where BinomCDF denotes the binomial cumulative distribution function.

If we sequence multiple individuals within a family, we can calculate the P-value of observing a given number of individuals with a variant in a gene under the following assumptions: 1) the gene rarely contains variants in the population, i.e. f_{hom} and f_{het} are small, and in this case, $f_{hom} \approx f_{het}$; and 2) the shared alleles within a family are shared identical-by-descent (IBD).

If we sequence full siblings, the P-value of seeing k sib pairs who share homozygous variants in a given gene, out of n total sib pairs is

$$P_{k,n} = 1 - BinomCDF(k-1, n, \yen f_{hom})$$

Another common scenario when sequencing individuals to determine the cause of an autosomal recessive disorder is to sequence distantly related affecteds in a pedigree with consanguineous marriages. In this case, the probability P that two sequenced individuals will share a homozygous can be calculated based on the pedigree structure and the corresponding path diagram, and the P-value becomes

$$P_{k,n} = 1 - BinomCDF\left(k-1, n, f_{het}(\tfrac{1}{2})^{E-1}\right)$$

where E is the number of independent edges in the paths connecting the two sequenced individuals through a single common ancestor. (Additional file 4).

If the affected individuals are heterozygous for the putative variants, the P-value is.

$$P_{k,n,r} = 1 - BinomCDF(k-1, n, rf_{both})$$

where r is the coefficient of relationship [23] or the fraction of the genome shared between affected family members, and f_{both} is the probability of an individual having either a heterozygous or homozygous variant in the gene of interest.

If multiple families and unrelated individuals had been sequenced with different degrees of relatedness, the P-value can be obtained by assuming that the control population is a pool of families with similar pedigree structures, calculating the probabilities of observing a combination of results that is at least as extreme as

the current observation, and taking the sum of these probabilities.

To illustrate, consider that we have sequenced independent cases and sib pairs with a rare, autosomal dominant Mendelian disorder, and we observed that k of n independent cases (singletons) and j of m sib pairs (doubletons) have heterozygous variants in a given gene. We can calculate the probability $P_{n,m,k,j}$ of observing exactly this number of successes based on the proportion of independent cases versus sib pairs and knowledge of the fraction of individuals heterozygous for rare variants in a given gene, f_{het}. As an example, assume that we have sequenced two unrelated cases and four sib pairs concordant for disease status. After variant filtering, we note that three sib pairs and one unrelated case carry rare variants in the same gene. Then, we calculate the probability of observing any of the more extreme possible outcomes: observing 2 singletons and 3 sib pairs, 2 singletons and 4 sib pairs, or 2 singletons and 4 sib pairs who have heterozygous variants in the given gene. Then,

$$P = P_{2,4,1,3} + P_{2,4,2,3} + P_{2,4,2,4} + P_{2,4,1,4}$$

The formula for calculating $P_{n,m,k,j}$ can be found in Methods, and detailed derivations of this and other equations can be found in Additional file 4. The a priori probability p, i.e. values for f_{het}, f_{hom}, and f_{both} for any given gene, can be queried from the SORVA dataset online, and standalone computer software for obtaining p and calculating P-values based on the methods described herein is also available on our website.

Significance of findings in large-scale studies of complex disorders

In complex disorders where most of the genes contributing to risk remain unknown, our dataset may be used to provide additional evidence supporting novel gene findings and provides a simple method to calculate the significance of observing variants in a given gene in a large-scale study. As an example, several large-scale whole-exome sequencing (WES) studies have been carried out to-date in trios and quads to elucidate causal genes underlying autism spectrum disorders (ASD) [24–29]. However, genes identified as containing de novo variants rarely overlap between studies, raising the question of how many genes are truly causal and how likely genes are to be identified as associated with autism by chance in these studies as well as others. We assessed the number of individuals carrying rare (MAF < 0.1%), heterozygous LOF variants in 1145 genes cumulatively associated with ASD by more than a dozen studies, meta-analyses and reviews [14, 27, 30–47]. There was no significant difference between the distribution of values and that of all genes, and assuming that truly causal

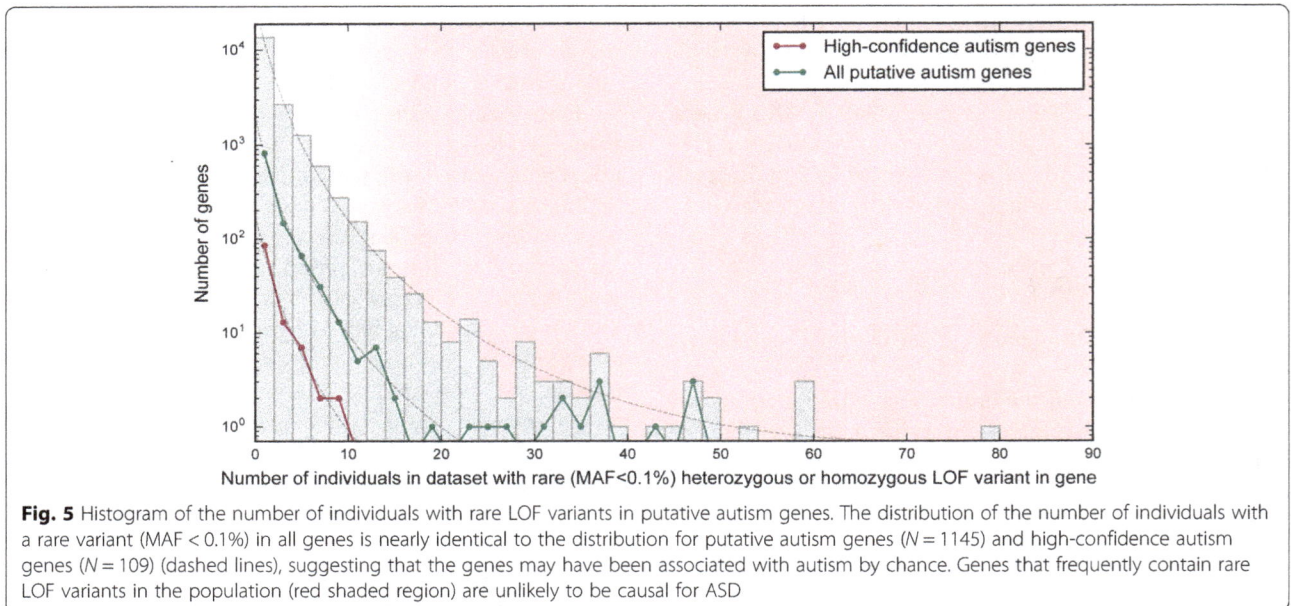

Fig. 5 Histogram of the number of individuals with rare LOF variants in putative autism genes. The distribution of the number of individuals with a rare variant (MAF < 0.1%) in all genes is nearly identical to the distribution for putative autism genes ($N = 1145$) and high-confidence autism genes ($N = 109$) (dashed lines), suggesting that the genes may have been associated with autism by chance. Genes that frequently contain rare LOF variants in the population (red shaded region) are unlikely to be causal for ASD

genes are more intolerant of rare LOF variants, our findings support the hypothesis that many genes could have been randomly associated with the disorder (Fig. 5, Additional file 6). Furthermore, there are 19 putative autism genes in which >0.5% of individuals carry rare, LOF variants. These genes are likely to be false positives, because no single gene contributes to a large proportion of autism cases. Our results highlight the need to perform statistical validation of findings involving genes associated with complex disorders.

Appropriately, several WES studies on ASD calculate the significance of their findings. For example, Sanders et al. demonstrate in a study which identifies de novo coding mutations in 928 individuals that finding two independent de novo mutations in a single gene is highly unlikely by chance, and this occurring is viewed as evidence for association between ASD and the gene *SCN2A* (sodium channel, voltage-gated, type II, α subunit) [28]. Neale et al. also consider the probability of seeing two independent de novo mutations in a single gene when evaluating their findings [25]. Iossifov et al. (2012) demonstrates that disrupted genes are significantly enriched for FRMP-associated function; however, they also highlight several individual non-FRMP-associated genes based on their plausibility to cause an ASD phenotype but make no attempt at applying statistics when considering these. In fact, de novo mutations in genes may have arisen in these genes by chance [24].

To validate our methods, we validated findings by O'Roak et al. (2012) [26], who reported de novo variants as well as inherited LOF variants in ASD cases. In a targeted sequencing study of 44 candidate genes in 2446 ASD probands, the authors found that six individual genes

(*CHD8, GRIN2B, DYRK1A, PTEN, TBR1,* and *TBL1XR1*) had evidence of mutation burden for de novo variants, for which they calculated the *P*-value using simulations. Applying our methods, we find that more cases carry de novo variants than expected by chance in 6 out of the 6 genes. (Table 1). Furthermore, one additional gene, *ADNP*, was found to be significant using our method when only considering de novo variation in the cohort. One advantage to our method is that it allows one to incorporate information about inherited variants, and by doing so, 3 additional genes are found to contain more variation than expected by chance. For genes that rarely contain LOF variation in the population, observing more than one inherited variant in the cohort is unlikely to happen by chance, and the *P*-value decreases. To summarize, our methods approximate *P*-values obtained using more complex and computationally intensive methods such as simulations, with the advantage that it can incorporate information about both inherited and de novo variation, and the fact that it incorporates precomputed population level data makes our methods easy to apply to calculating the statistical significance of observing rare variants in a given gene.

Applications in predictive genomics

If a genetic disease is associated with the presence of variants in a given gene, information about the variants in the gene in affected individuals and in population controls can be used to more accurately assess the probability that a person will develop a disease given their genotype.

Consider a randomly chosen person from the general population who is undergoing prenatal genetic testing. Define A as the event that their child will be born with a

Table 1 Validation of mutational burden findings in autism genes

Gene	Number of indivs with variant			P	$P_{including\ inh\ vars}$
	LOF / de novo	Nonsyn / de novo	Inh / LOF		
ADCY5	0	2	1	0.723	0.446
ADNP	2	0	1	1.1×10^{-3}	1.7×10^{-3}
CHD8	8	1	0	1.7×10^{-21}	1.7×10^{-21}
DYRK1A	3	0	1	5.9×10^{-6}	1.1×10^{-5}
GRIN2B	3	1	0	8.2×10^{-5}	8.2×10^{-5}
LAMC3	0	2	4	0.550	**0.022**
PTEN	1	2	1	8.2×10^{-3}	9.2×10^{-3}
SBF1	0	2	1	0.833	0.502
SETD2	1	1	2	0.078	**0.0110**
SGSM3	0	2	2	0.086	**0.0471**
TBL1XR1	1	1	0	**0.0167**	**0.0167**
TBR1	2	1	0	3.4×10^{-5}	3.4×10^{-5}
UBE3C	0	2	1	0.432	0.291

In a targeted sequencing study of 44 candidate autism genes in 2446 individuals [26], 12 genes contained both recurring de novo variants and inherited LOF variants in multiple individuals, or had evidence of excess mutation burden of de novo variants. Gene names that are in bold were statistically significant in the original study. P-values calculated using our methods validate findings by O'Roak et al. [27] for all 6 of these genes, and one additional gene. If we also consider inherited LOF variants, 3 additional genes are statistically significant using our methods. Inherited nonsynonymous variants were not reported in the original study, hence the P-value is conservative. Abbreviations: *nonsyn* nonsynonymous variant or single amino acid deletion, *LOF* loss-of-function variant, *Inh* inherited

disease, and B as the event that the child carries a rare, LOF variant in a given gene associated with the disease. For many heterogeneic Mendelian disorders, studies of large cohorts provide information regarding the relative contribution of individual causative genes and the genotype–phenotype correlations, giving us the conditional probability $P(B|A)$. The term $P(A)$ can be defined as the disease incidence, and the value of $P(B)$, or the proportion of individuals carrying a rare, LOF variant in the gene, can be queried from our dataset. Then, according to Bayes' theorem

$$P(A|B) = \frac{P(B|A) \times P(A)}{P(B)}$$

we can calculate that the probability that the child will have the disorder. The following example illustrates such an application.

Consider that prenatal testing identified that a fetus is compound heterozygous for novel variants in the gene *POMGNT1*, which suggests a possible phenotype of congenital muscular dystrophy (CMD). It is known that 53% of patients with CMD have homozygous or compound heterozygous variants in one of six known CMD genes, 10% have homozygous or compound heterozygous variants in *POMGNT1*, and the incidence of CMD is estimated to be 1:21,500 [48, 49]. Since most mutations observed in affected individuals are novel and are not found in healthy population controls, we will assume a low MAF threshold of 0.1% for variant filtering. At this threshold, 2 out of 2504

individuals (0.08%) in our dataset have a rare protein-altering variant in the gene *POMGNT1*, therefore $P(B) = 0.0008$, and we calculate that the positive predictive value (PPV), the probability that the child will have the disease given a positive test result, is roughly 1.0%. Using this method, sensitivity, the probability $P(B|A)$, is quite low (10%); whereas specificity is high (1-P(B) = 99.9%). If we aggregate data for all known CMD genes, we can increase sensitivity to 53% with a negligible decrease in specificity, due to the fact that the other CMD genes contains very few, in any variants in our dataset. This example highlights that sensitivity greatly depends on the proportion of cases that can be explained by variants in a given set of genes. This type of analysis thus has implications for interpretation of broad NGS-based prenatal testing and can be extrapolated as well to preconception testing and risk to potential children.

It is important to note that the extreme numbers involved—the very low prevalence of a disorder and in many cases, the fact that no individual on the 1000 Genomes Project dataset had been observed with variants in a gene, i.e. the lack of previous false-positive results—make it difficult to compute the PPV. A previous study suggests that the latter "zero numerator" problem can be solved using a Bayesian approach that incorporates a prior distribution describing the initial uncertainty about the false-positive rate [50]. Alternatively, the number of rare LOF variants observed in a gene has been published as part of the ExAC and GnomAD datasets, which contain information about 60,706 and 123,136 individuals, respectively [8]. Although only nonsense or splice site variants were included in the LOF classification, and they only include values for a single MAF threshold of 0.1%, the number can be used a rough estimate for f. Furthermore, if even the count obtained from GnomAD is zero, we can assume that f is less than 1/123136, or 3/123136 if we are being conservative.

To summarize, for monogenic disorders and disorders where there exist detailed phenotype-genotype correlation data, our dataset will provide the denominator in the equation to calculate the probability that an individual with a rare variant in a known disease gene will have a rare genetic disorder. As further research uncovers novel gene-disease associations, and as we increase the size of the public dataset from which $P(B)$ values can be calculated, we can update expected false-positive rates and calculating PPVs will

become increasingly accurate. As illustrated, our methods will be be useful for applications in predictive genomics, including prenatal testing and testing for late-onset genetic disorders.

Comparison to other gene ranking methods

We applied our method to calculate the significance of several previous studies' findings [51–77]. In all except one study where the Mendelian disorder was found to be caused by inherited disease variants ($N = 20$) [51–68, 76, 77], findings were confirmed to be significant using our methods, and in 11 out of 20 studies, P-values were highly significant ($P < 0.0001$). (Table 2, Additional file 7) In many studies, initial exome sequencing in a limited number of individuals is followed by sequencing of only

Table 2 Statistical significance of variants found to be causal in selected previous studies

Inheritance	Gene	Individuals sequenced	Indivs w/ var in gene	Variant consequence	Zygosity filter	MAF threshold[b]	f^a	P-val	Approximate # of genes targeted	Corrected P-value
AR	ISPD	1 full-sibling doubleton and 5 unrelated affecteds	all	LOF	CHet/Hom	Exclusion	0	4.16E-008	7200	3.00E-004
AD	CDKN1C	1 third-cousin doubleton and 4 unrelated affecteds	all	nonsyn	Het	Exclusion	0.0044	5.24E-015	2500	1.31E-011
AD	MLL2	10 unrelated affecteds	7 / 10[c]	LOF	Het	Exclusion	0.0020	1.51E-017	20,000	3.02E-013
complex	PBRM1	7 unrelated affecteds	4 / 7[d]	LOF	Hom	none stated	0	5.56E-014	20,000	1.11E-009
complex	WDR62	2 affecteds in consanguineous family%	all	LOF	Hom	Exclusion	0	9.75E-008	20,000	1.95E-003
AR	C5orf42	6 unrelated affecteds	all[d]	nonsyn	Het	0.1%	0.0779	2.23E-007	20,000	4.46E-003
AR	C5orf42	2 affecteds in consanguineous family	all	nonsyn	Hom	none stated	0	4.88E-008	20,000	9.75E-004
complex	AP4E1	6 affecteds in a single, large family	all	nonsyn	Het	1%	0.0459	1.44E-003	530	0.76
AR	ANTXR1	2 unrelated affecteds from consanguineous families	all	nonsyn	Hom	0.1%	0	3.04E-013	144	4.38E-011
AR	ITGB6	2 unrelated affecteds	all	nonsyn	CHet/Hom	none stated	0.0012	1.44E-006	20,000	2.87E-002
AR	CSPP1	1 proband sequenced in region of homozygosity	all	LOF	Hom	1%	0	2.00E-004	40	7.99E-003
AR	GMPPB	3 unrelated affecteds and 3 sibs in consanguineous family sequenced in single candidate gene	all[d]	nonsyn	CHet/Hom	1%	0.0032	2.15E-014	1	2.15E-014
AR	DHODH	1 full-sibling doubleton and 2 unrelated affecteds	all	nonsyn	CHet/Hom	Exclusion	0.0004	1.35E-007	20,000	2.69E-003
AR	SCN5A	Gene screened in 10 affecteds from 7 families	5 / 10	nonsyn	CHet/Hom	none stated	0.0012	9.25E-010	1	9.25E-010
AD	MAX	3 unrelated affecteds	all	nonsyn	Het	Exclusion	0.0064	2.61E-007	20,000	5.22E-003
AR	GPSM2	1 proband sequenced in region of homozygosity	all	LOF	Hom	Exclusion	0.0000	2.00E-004	66	1.32E-002
AR	TBC1D24	15 unrelated affecteds	6 / 15	nonsyn	CHet/Hom	1.00%	0.0004	2.02E-017	20,000	4.05E-013
AR	PGM3	3 unrelated affecteds	all	nonsyn	CHet/Hom	0.3%	0.0004	6.37E-011	20,000	1.27E-006

Applying our methods to previous NGS findings, in which researchers filtered variants using various criteria, would have statistically validated findings in silico. See Additional file 7 for more details. [a]The parameter f denotes the proportion of individuals in the 1000 Genomes Project dataset who have a rare variant at least as severe as the identified variants. [b]We used a threshold of MAF < 0.1% for studies with no specific MAF threshold. A MAF threshold labeled exclusion refers to studies where variants were not filtered for a given threshold and variants were excluded based on their presence in public databases such as dbSNP. [c]Follow-up Sanger sequencing identified mutations in 2 out of 3 exome-negative cases. [d]Follow-up sequencing of the given gene identified further mutations in multiple additional cases. Abbreviations: *MAF* minor allele frequency, *AD* autosomal dominant, *AR* autosomal recessive, *XL* X-linked, *nonsyn* nonsynonymous variant, *LOF* loss-of-function variant, *Het* heterozygous, *Hom* homozygous, *CHet/Hom* compound heterozygous or homozygous

the putative causal gene in a large number of individuals. In one such study, the *P*-value resulting from the initial exome sequencing is significant enough to suggest causality, and the follow-up sequencing essentially serves to establish the proportion of cases in which the phenotype is attributed to variants in the gene [61]. In others studies, however, the initial sequencing merely identifies potential candidate genes, and follow-up sequencing is required to achieve genome-wide significance [58, 59, 62, 76, 77]. In these cases, the second round of sequencing is not corrected for multiple testing, because only a single gene is interpreted during follow-up sequencing. (Additional file 7).

The rankings of frequencies at which a gene contains rare, deleterious variants is comparable to previously published gene ranking methods for prioritizing variants. The list of genes sorted and ranked according to the number of individuals carrying rare (MAF < 0.5%) heterozygous, loss-of-function variants correlates well with genes ranked based on pLI scores, which describe the probability that a gene is intolerant of LOF variation ($\rho = 0.515$) [8, 9]. These scores were derived from the ExAC dataset consisting of exome sequencing data from 60,706 individuals. The order in which ExAC pLI score ranks genes correlates more closely with SORVA rankings than rankings based on EvoTol [10] ($\rho = 0.400$), RVIS [5] ($\rho = -0.157$) and FLAGS [7] ($\rho = 0.278$) methods.

We compare methods in their ability to prioritize disease-causing genes from the Online Mendelian Inheritance in Man (OMIM) database [1]. pLI scores, EvoTol, and RVIS outperform SORVA for known autosomal dominant disease genes, however all methods perform similarly for autosomal recessive genes, and SORVA outperforms EvoTol, RVIS, and FLAGS for genes known to cause X-linked disorders. (See Additional file 8 for receiver operating characteristic (ROC) curves.)

Discussion

We demonstrate the utility of using mutational burden data to aid in prioritizing variants in silico and quantifying the significance of seeing a variant within a gene. We have shown this using examples from previous studies encompassing multiple NGS study designs and disease inheritance models. Other metrics such as gene constraint pLI scores and EvoTol rankings [9, 10] are appropriate for prioritizing genes by their likelihood of causing genetic disorders, but our methods will calculate the statistical significance of findings based on the constellation of families and individuals that variants are seen in, independent of how genes were prioritized initially.

Although there was some variation between the frequency of individuals with a rare variant in a given gene between populations, and selecting a comparable population to a study would be ideal when calculating variant significance, this restriction is not necessary. To illustrate, if individuals in the African population frequently carry LOF variants in a gene but this does not hold true for another population that more closely matches the study population, one may nevertheless consider the gene to be less likely to cause a rare Mendelian disorder.

A limitation of this method of ranking genes is that genes are prioritized on the basis of their likelihood of being involved in disease in general rather than in the specific disease of interest [4]. On the other hand, this can be viewed as a benefit in the sense that results are unbiased and do not depend on previously existing annotations, which would bias rankings to prefer known and well-studied genes. This bias is a known issue in the interpretation of clinical variants [78]. To illustrate, Bell et al. discovered that an unexpected proportion (27%) of literature-annotated disease variants in recessive disease-causing genes were incorrect [79], and Piton et al. estimated that 25% of X-linked intellectual disability genes are incorrect or require further review based on allele frequency estimates that have become more accurate with the availability of large-scale sequencing datasets [80]. Disease genes that are incorrectly annotated as disease-causing may explain the lack of difference between the average number of individuals carrying variants in genes causal for autosomal dominant and autosomal recessive genes. One would expect decreased counts for autosomal dominant disease genes due to stronger purifying selection among deleterious variants that arise in these genes, where a single variant may be sufficient to cause disease [81]. Another possibility is that the sample size may be too small to include a sufficient number of individuals who are carriers for rare, deleterious variants in recessive disease genes.

Future improvements to our methods would include increasing the amount of genetic information from unaffected individuals. Our results suggest that for most applications, low MAF thresholds should be used to achieve power to detect genes associated with disease; however, at thresholds of MAF < 0.0005, most genes will lack any data; e.g. there will be no individuals observed who are carriers of LOF variants. The SORVA dataset is useful in its current state with data from a relatively small number of individuals, but increasing the population size by several orders of magnitude will increase the utility of the application. The recently approved Precision Medicine Initiative will fund sequencing and data collection from 1 million or more Americans and make the data accessible to qualified researchers, and the methods described in this manuscript could be applied to this larger dataset and contribute towards the aim of this initiative to generate knowledge applicable to the whole range of health and disease [82].

Additional improvements would include incorporating additional information regarding specific categories of variants, such as the degree to which stop codon gain (also known as nonsense) variants in a gene are constrained to the end of the gene. Knowing whether an essential gene is highly intolerant of nonsense mutations in only certain regions of the gene would allow one to lower the priority of nonsense variants in regions tolerant of mutations when evaluating variants in silico. For example, Li et al. exclude stop-gain variants occurring in the terminal gene exon and those that do not affect all transcripts of a gene when evaluating deleterious LOF mutations in a large cohort of individuals [83]. The limitation to providing individual-level mutational burden counts at such a high level of granularity is that researchers will be restricted to following the same methods of filtering and annotating variants. This would be problematic because, by default, many commonly-used software pipelines do not annotate variants with the information about the proportion of transcript truncated [84–89]. Selecting variant filtering thresholds in SORVA that are identical to those used in one's study is essential in having comparable data with which to calculate variant significance. For this reason, we also did not filter missense variants based on annotations from commonly tools such as SIFT [90], PolyPhen-2 [91], and CADD [92], which provide an interpretation of mutation impacts.

Conclusions

Our methods provide a score for prioritizing variants within a gene that is unbiased and directly interpretable. Restricted by the sample size of our dataset, we provide limited population-level data, and adding more data will greatly improve the utility of our method. However, even in its current state, SORVA is useful for vetting candidate genes from NGS studies and allows researchers to calculate the significance of seeing a variant in a given gene or protein domain, which is an important step towards developing a quantitative, statistics-based approach for presenting clinical findings.

Methods

Datasets

Genomic data and allele frequencies for calculating a priori probabilities of observing a variant within a gene were obtained from the 1000 Genomes Project (phase 3 variant set) [17]. This variant set contains 2504 individuals from 26 populations in Africa (AFR), East Asia (EAS), Europe (EUR), South Asia (SAS), and the Americas (AMR).

Bioinformatics pipeline

Genomic annotations were assigned to each variation using *SNP & Variation Suite (SVS)* v8.1 [84] with the following parameters: gene set Ensembl release 75 [93], human genome version GRCh37.p13. Variants were filtered for coding mutations that result in a change in the amino acid sequence (e.g. missense, nonsense and frameshift mutations), or mutations that reside within a splice site junction (intronic distance of 2 base pairs). Biallelic data was recoded based on an additive model to correct for MAF of variants on the X chromosome for male samples, using a script in SVS. Variants were then filtered for minor allele frequency thresholds of MAF < 5%, < 1%, < 0.5%, < 0.1% and < 0.05%, based on allelic frequency within the dataset. For each filtered list of variants, we collapsed variants by gene and performed the following two scenarios: 1) an individual was counted as having a rare variant in a gene if the variant mapped to any transcript of a gene; 2) we counted the number of variants in a given gene per individual, i.e. if an individual carried two rare mutations within a gene, they were counted twice. In a separate analysis, we collapsed variants by protein domains obtained from Interpro [19] using the Ensembl API [86]. Finally, we repeated each analysis using a subset of the 1000 Genomes Project data grouped according to superpopulation. Variant collapsing methods were performed using a custom Python script run by SVS, and an individual was counted as having a rare variant in a gene if the variant mapped to any transcript of a gene.

In addition to replicating the analysis for gene versus protein domain, for each population, and for each MAF threshold, we also repeated the calculations for multiple categories of predicted variant consequence on the protein transcript. The two categories were 1) nonsynonymous variants or those predicted to be more severe by Ensembl [93], briefly nonsynonymous or LOF variants, and 2) potential LOF variants (includes splice site, protein truncation stop codon gain mutations, and frameshift indels).

Comparison of disease gene categories

To determine whether our results show concordance with studies identifying essential genes critical for the survival of a human, we compared the number of individuals with rare, deleterious mutations between gene lists containing essential human genes, those known to cause Mendelian diseases, and control genes, defined as genes not included in either category. We considered genes to be essential human genes if they were determined as such in at least one of the following two studies. The first essential human gene set is defined as 'core' essential genes that are required for fitness of cells from both the HAP1 and KBM7 cell lines, determined through extensive mutagenesis in near-haploid human cells ($N = 1734$) [94]. The second essential human gene set consists of genes essential to four screened cell lines,

KBM7, K562, Raji and Jiyoye, determined using the CRISPR system. From the latter set, we selected genes with an adjusted P-value CRISPR score < 0.4025 for each cell line ($N = 1878$) [95].

To identify genes known to cause Mendelian disease, we parsed data from Online Mendelian Inheritance in Man (OMIM) [1] and identified phenotype descriptions with known molecular basis. We parsed the genotype description field for the gene name and the following phrases: 'caused by heterozygous/homozygous mutation', 'autosomal recessive', 'autosomal dominant', 'X-linked', 'on chromosome X', and categorized genes as autosomal recessive (AR) ($N = 655$), autosomal dominant (AD) ($N = 785$), and X-linked (XL) ($N = 126$) accordingly.

Comparison of gene ranking methods

Genic mutational intolerance scores were obtained from four previous studies and included the Residual Variation Intolerance Score (RVIS) [5], scores from Shyr et al. 2014 (FLAGS) [7], pLI scores based on the ExAC dataset [8, 9], and EvoTol scores [10]. We considered 15,266 genes that were found in all four datasets, as well as ours, and ranked genes based on scores obtained using each method. Spearman's rho test [96, 97] was used to measure the size and statistical significance of the association between the rankings obtained from ExAC and those obtained by RVIS, FLAGS and SORVA methods. This test measures the strength and direction of association between two ranked variables.

In order to assess the performances of all five methods when prioritizing putative disease genes and plot receiver operating characteristic (ROC) curves, we used the sets of OMIM genes described earlier. We filtered the OMIM gene sets to overlap the 15,266 genes that were scored by all five methods. Genes were ranked according to each metric and a count of the number of disease-causing genes that would be found at each percentile are reported. In order to show the baseline prediction, the result of randomly assigning a percentile to each gene is also shown. SORVA genes were ranked according to the number of 1000 Genomes Project individuals who were heterozygous or homozygous for rare (MAF < 0.005) LOF variants in a given gene, and ties between genes were resolved based on the number or individuals who have rare (MAF < 0.005) LOF or missense variants in a gene, and finally less rare (MAF < 0.05) LOF or missense variants.

Calculating depletion of variants in protein domains

We performed two analyses: first, we calculated whether protein domains in a gene were depleted of variation compared to the rest of the gene, and second, we calculated whether there were any types of protein domains

that were depleted of variation in general across the entire genome.

First, for each protein domain mapping within a gene, we calculated whether domains were depleted of variation compared to the rest of the gene. Depletion was calculated as: (number of variants per individual in protein domain / number of variants per individual in gene × length of protein domain / length of transcript). A value of 1 is expected by chance, and a small value indicates protein domains most intolerant towards mutations. We then calculated the P-value of obtaining such a depletion score using the binomial cumulative density function, under the assumption that each site is equally likely to be mutated. This P-value is then "PHRED-scaled" by expressing the rank in order of magnitude terms rather than the precise rank itself. High scaled scores indicate that a protein domain is depleted of rare (MAF < 0.5%) mutations compared to the rest of the gene, hence protein domains with high scores tend to be enriched for highly mutated genes. We filtered out genes with no observed mutations and protein domains that span more than 50% of the length of the transcript, resulting in 7828 genes remaining.

Next, we calculated whether there were any types of protein domains that were depleted of variation in general across the entire genome. We weighted each gene with instances of the protein domain equally. In other words, if a gene had multiple instances of a protein domain, we first calculated the mean number of heterozygous rare (MAF < =0.5%) LOF variants observed (in the entire dataset of 2504 individuals) in either protein domain within the gene. Next, we calculated the mean and variance of the means for each gene.

To determine whether a protein domain was well covered by sequencing, we calculated the mean coverage of an instance of a protein domain in the 1000 Genomes Project sample HG00096 [17]. We calculated depth of coverage from phase 3 exome alignment data using GATK and custom code, which is available at https://github.com/alizrrao/DepthOfCoveragePerInterval.

Combining P-values when calculating significance of observing given variants in sequenced families

Let's assume that we sequenced individuals in families with multiple family structures, e.g. we have sequenced independent cases and sib pairs with a rare, autosomal dominant Mendelian disorder, and we observed that k of n independent cases (singletons) and j of m sib pairs (doubletons) have heterozygous variants in a given gene. In the control population, the fraction of unrelated individuals heterozygous for a variant in the gene is $f_{het} \approx f_{both} = r_0 f_{both}$ for $f_{het} < < 1$ where the relationship coefficient is $r_0 = 1$, and the fraction of sib pairs who share heterozygous variants in the gene is $r_1 f_{both}$ where the relationship coefficient is $r_1 = \frac{1}{2}$. Weighting these by the fraction of unrelated individuals and sib pairs, the total fraction of "familial units" that do not have or share the variant is

$$F = 1 - \frac{n}{n+m} r_0 f_{both} - \frac{m}{n+m} r_1 f_{both}$$

which equals the probability of a failure in any given trial. The probability $P_{n,m,k,j}$ of having $n+m$ trials and observing exactly k singleton successes and j doubleton successes is equal to:

$$P_{n,m,k,j} = P(X = n + m - k - j) \times P(Y = k)$$

where X is a binomial random variable with $n+m$ trials and probability of success equal to F, and Y is a binomial random variable with $k+j$ trials and probability of success equal to

$$\frac{r_0 n}{r_0 n + r_1 m}$$

Finally, to calculate the P-value for observing k of n independent cases and j of m sib pairs who have heterozygous variants in a given gene, we calculate the probability $P_{n,m,k,j}$ of observing exactly k singleton successes and j doubleton successes or any combination of outcomes that is less likely, and sum these values.

$$P\text{-}value = \sum_{a=0}^{n} \sum_{b=0}^{m} P_{n,m,a,b} [P_{n,m,a,b} \le P_{n,m,k,j}]$$

The P-value can be derived in a similar manner for various experimental designs, where multiple families with different pedigree structures are sequenced to identify heterozygous variants shared by affected cases or, in case of an autosomal recessive disorder, homozygous or potential compound heterozygous variants. Additional details can be found in Additional file 4: Supplementary Methods.

Additional files

Additional file 1: Number of individuals carrying a rare variant in a gene under various filtering thresholds. Each data point represents a single gene which contains a variant in the aggregate population ($n = 2504$ individuals). Calculations were repeated using multiple variant filtering thresholds to determine the scenario that most differentiates between essential genes, those known to cause autosomal dominant, autosomal recessive or X-linked disease, and other genes. We varied filters for type of variant ('LOF or missense' or 'LOF only'), zygosity (Het or Hom) and MAF threshold. Colored shapes indicate the centroids of each group of genes. Abbreviations: LOF, loss-of-function; nonsyn, nonsynonymous or LOF; het, heterozygous; hom, homozygous; ess, essential; AD, autosomal dominant; AR, autosomal recessive; XL, X-linked.

Additional file 2: Mean number of individuals mutated for different types of protein domains. We calculated the mean number of individuals (out of 2504 individuals) who carried mutations in a given type of protein domains, averaging per gene.

Additional file 3: Variant depletion scores for all protein domain in every gene. For each instance of a protein domain in a gene, we calculated variant depletion scores to identify regions within a gene that may be under differing degrees of evolutionary constraint.

Additional file 4: Supplementary methods. Includes derivation of equations and math used for calculating the significance of finding rare variants in a given gene.

Additional file 5: Screenshot of an example query run on SORVA. Users can select variant filtering thresholds such as population, MAF cutoff, zygosity and whether to consider only LOF variants or missense variants, as well. Output includes the number of individuals who carry a rare variant in the gene and in any protein domain that maps to the gene.

Additional file 6: List of candidate autism genes. Genes listed were used to produce Fig. 5.

Additional file 7: Calculating P-values for findings from previous whole-exome or targeted sequencing studies. The parameter f denotes the proportion of individuals in the 1000 Genomes Project dataset who have a rare variant at least as severe as the identified variants. A MAF threshold labeled exclusion refers to studies that did not filter by a given threshold and excluded variants based on their presence in public databases such as dbSNP; in such cases, results were calculated using a MAF threshold of 0.1%. Abbreviations: MAF, minor allele frequency; AD, autosomal dominant; AR, autosomal recessive; XL, X-linked; nonsyn, nonsynonymous variant; LOF, loss-of-function variant; Het, heterozygous; Hom, homozygous; CHet/Hom, compound heterozygous or homozygous.

Additional file 8: ROC curves for the selection of known disease-causing genes from gene rankings. Comparison between gene ranking metrics from SORVA, FLAGS, ExAC pLI score, RVIS, and EvoTol using the OMIM database, showing the cumulative percentage plots for the residual scores for three OMIM gene lists. The OMIM gene categories are **(a)** autosomal dominant disease causing ($N = 681$), **(b)** autosomal recessive disease causing ($N = 556$), and **(c)** X-linked disease causing ($N = 118$). SORVA were based on the number of 1000 Genomes Project individuals who were heterozygous or homozygous for rare (MAF < 0.005) LOF variants in a given gene. Dashed lines indicate control. Abbreviations: ROC, Receiver Operating Characteristic; AUC, area under the curve, LOF, loss-of-function.

Abbreviations

ASD: Autism spectrum disorder; BinomCDF: Binomial cumulative distribution function; CMD: Congenital muscular dystrophy; ExAC: Exome aggregation consortium; IBD: Identical-by-descent; LOF: Loss-of-function; MAF: Minor allele frequency; NGS: Next-generation sequencing; OMIM: Online mendelian inheritance in man; PPV: Positive predictive value; RVIS: Residual variation intolerance score; SNV: Single nucleotide variant; SORVA: Significance Of Rare VAriants; TADA: Transmission and de novo association test; VUS: Variant of uncertain significance; WES: Whole-exome sequencing

Acknowledgements

Funding to ARR was provided by National Institutes of Health (NIH) Training Grant No. T32HG002536. We thank Dr. Janet Sinsheimer for providing statistical advice. We thank the NIH/National Center for Advancing Translational Science (NCATS) (UCLA CTSI Grant Number UL1TR000124) for their support. The funders had no role in study design, data collection and analysis, decision to publish, or preparation of the manuscript.

Authors' contributions

ARR and SFN designed analyses. ARR analyzed data and created the software. ARR and SFN wrote the manuscript. All authors have read and approved the manuscript.

Competing interests

The authors declare that they have no competing interests.

Author details

[1]Department of Human Genetics, University of California, Los Angeles, California, Los Angeles, USA. [2]Department of Psychiatry and Biobehavioral Sciences at the David Geffen School of Medicine, University of California, Los Angeles, California, Los Angeles, USA. [3]Department of Pathology and Laboratory Medicine, University of California, Los Angeles, California, Los Angeles, USA.

References

1. Online Mendelian Inheritance in Man, OMIM®. McKusick-Nathans Institute of Genetic Medicine. Baltimore: Johns Hopkins University; 2015. http://omim.org/
2. Amendola LM, Dorschner MO, Robertson PD, Salama JS, Hart R, Shirts BH, et al. Actionable exomic incidental findings in 6503 participants: challenges of variant classification. Genome Res. 2015;25:305–15.
3. Dorschner MO, Amendola LM, Turner EH, Robertson PD, Shirts BH, Gallego CJ, et al. Actionable, pathogenic incidental findings in 1,000 participants' exomes. Am J Hum Genet. 2013;93:631–40.
4. Gill N, Singh S, Aseri TC. Computational disease gene prioritization: an appraisal. J Comput Biol J Comput Mol Cell Biol. 2014;21:456–65.
5. Petrovski S, Wang Q, Heinzen EL, Allen AS, Goldstein DB. Genic intolerance to functional variation and the interpretation of personal genomes. PLoS Genet. 2013;9:e1003709.
6. Gussow AB, Petrovski S, Wang Q, Allen AS, Goldstein DB. The intolerance to functional genetic variation of protein domains predicts the localization of pathogenic mutations within genes. Genome Biol. 2016;17:9.
7. Shyr C, Tarailo-Graovac M, Gottlieb M, Lee JJ, van KC, Wasserman WW. FLAGS, frequently mutated genes in public exomes. BMC Med Genet. 2014;7:64.
8. Lek M, Karczewski KJ, Minikel EV, Samocha KE, Banks E, Fennell T, et al. Analysis of protein-coding genetic variation in 60,706 humans. Nature. 2016; 536:285–91.
9. Samocha KE, Robinson EB, Sanders SJ, Stevens C, Sabo A, McGrath LM, et al. A framework for the interpretation of de novo mutation in human disease. Nat Genet. 2014;46:944–50.
10. Rackham OJL, Shihab HA, Johnson MR, Petretto E. EvoTol: a protein-sequence based evolutionary intolerance framework for disease-gene prioritization. Nucleic Acids Res. 2015;43:e33.
11. Akle S, Chun S, Jordan DM, Cassa CA. Mitigating false-positive associations in rare disease gene discovery. Hum Mutat. 2015;36:998–1003.
12. He X, Sanders SJ, Liu L, De Rubeis S, Lim ET, Sutcliffe JS, et al. Integrated model of De novo and inherited genetic variants yields greater power to identify risk genes. PLoS Genet. 2013;9:e1003671.
13. Sanders SJ, He X, Willsey AJ, Ercan-Sencicek AG, Samocha KE, Cicek AE, et al. Insights into autism Spectrum disorder genomic architecture and biology from 71 risk loci. Neuron. 2015;87:1215–33.
14. De Rubeis S, He X, Goldberg AP, Poultney CS, Samocha K, Ercument Cicek A, et al. Synaptic, transcriptional and chromatin genes disrupted in autism. Nature. 2014;515:209–15.
15. Berko ER, Cho MT, Eng C, Shao Y, Sweetser DA, Waxler J, et al. De novo missense variants in HECW2 are associated with neurodevelopmental delay and hypotonia. J Med Genet. 2017;54:84–6.
16. Akawi N, McRae J, Ansari M, Balasubramanian M, Blyth M, Brady AF, et al. Discovery of four recessive developmental disorders using probabilistic genotype and phenotype matching among 4,125 families. Nat Genet. 2015;47:1363–9.
17. The 1000 Genomes Project Consortium. An integrated map of genetic variation from 1,092 human genomes. Nature. 2012;491:56–65.
18. Marth G, Schuler G, Yeh R, Davenport R, Agarwala R, Church D, et al. Sequence variations in the public human genome data reflect a bottlenecked population history. Proc Natl Acad Sci. 2003;100:376–81.
19. Mitchell A, Chang H-Y, Daugherty L, Fraser M, Hunter S, Lopez R, et al. The InterPro protein families database: the classification resource after 15 years. Nucleic Acids Res. 2015;43:D213–21.
20. Kryukov GV, Pennacchio LA, Sunyaev SR. Most rare missense alleles are deleterious in humans: implications for complex disease and association studies. Am J Hum Genet. 2007;80:727–39.
21. Arboleda VA, Lee H, Dorrani N, Zadeh N, Willis M, Macmurdo CF, et al. De novo nonsense mutations in KAT6A, a lysine acetyl-transferase gene, cause a syndrome including microcephaly and global developmental delay. Am J Hum Genet. 2015;96:498–506.
22. Tham E, Lindstrand A, Santani A, Malmgren H, Nesbitt A, Dubbs HA, et al. Dominant mutations in KAT6A cause intellectual disability with recognizable syndromic features. Am J Hum Genet. 2015;96:507–13.
23. Wright S. Coefficients of inbreeding and relationship. Am Nat. 1922;56:330–8.
24. Iossifov I, Ronemus M, Levy D, Wang Z, Hakker I, Rosenbaum J, et al. De novo gene disruptions in children on the autistic spectrum. Neuron. 2012; 74:285–99.
25. Neale BM, Kou Y, Liu L, Ma'ayan A, Samocha KE, Sabo A, et al. Patterns and rates of exonic de novo mutations in autism spectrum disorders. Nature. 2012;485:242–5.
26. O'Roak BJ, Vives L, Girirajan S, Karakoc E, Krumm N, Coe BP, et al. Sporadic autism exomes reveal a highly interconnected protein network of de novo mutations. Nature. 2012;485:246–50.
27. O'Roak BJ, Vives L, Fu W, Egertson JD, Stanaway IB, Phelps IG, et al. Multiplex targeted sequencing identifies recurrently mutated genes in autism spectrum disorders. Science. 2012;338:1619–22.
28. Sanders SJ, Murtha MT, Gupta AR, Murdoch JD, Raubeson MJ, Willsey AJ, et al. De novo mutations revealed by whole-exome sequencing are strongly associated with autism. Nature. 2012;485:237–41.
29. Yuen RKC, Thiruvahindrapuram B, Merico D, Walker S, Tammimies K, Hoang N, et al. Whole-genome sequencing of quartet families with autism spectrum disorder. Nat Med. 2015;21:185–91.
30. Betancur C. Etiological heterogeneity in autism spectrum disorders: more than 100 genetic and genomic disorders and still counting. Brain Res. 2011; 1380:42–77.
31. Yu TW, Chahrour MH, Coulter ME, Jiralerspong S, Okamura-Ikeda K, Ataman B, et al. Using whole-exome sequencing to identify inherited causes of autism. Neuron. 2013;77:259–73.
32. Davis LK, Gamazon ER, Kistner-Griffin E, Badner JA, Liu C, Cook EH, et al. Loci nominally associated with autism from genome-wide analysis show enrichment of brain expression quantitative trait loci but not lymphoblastoid cell line expression quantitative trait loci. Mol Autism. 2012;3:3.
33. Li X, Zou H, Brown WT. Genes associated with autism spectrum disorder. Brain Res Bull. 2012;88:543–52.
34. Vorstman J a. S, Staal WG, van Daalen E, van Engeland H, Hochstenbach PFR, Franke L. Identification of novel autism candidate regions through analysis of reported cytogenetic abnormalities associated with autism. Mol Psychiatry. 2005;11:18–28.
35. Novarino G, El-Fishawy P, Kayserili H, Meguid NA, Scott EM, Schroth J, et al. Mutations in BCKD-kinase lead to a potentially treatable form of autism with epilepsy. Science. 2012;338:394–7.
36. Vieland VJ, Hallmayer J, Huang Y, Pagnamenta AT, Pinto D, Khan H, et al. Novel method for combined linkage and genome-wide association analysis finds evidence of distinct genetic architecture for two subtypes of autism. J Neurodev Disord. 2011;3:113–23.
37. Kou Y, Betancur C, Xu H, Buxbaum JD, Ma'ayan A. Network- and attribute-based classifiers can prioritize genes and pathways for autism spectrum disorders and intellectual disability. Am J Med Genet C Semin Med Genet. 2012;160C:130–42.
38. Toma C, Torrico B, Hervás A, Valdés-Mas R, Tristán-Noguero A, Padillo V, et al. Exome sequencing in multiplex autism families suggests a major role for heterozygous truncating mutations. Mol Psychiatry. 2014;19:784–90.
39. Koshimizu E, Miyatake S, Okamoto N, Nakashima M, Tsurusaki Y, Miyake N, et al. Performance comparison of bench-top next generation sequencers using microdroplet PCR-based enrichment for targeted sequencing in patients with autism spectrum disorder. PLoS One. 2013;8:e74167.
40. Liu L, Lei J, Sanders SJ, Willsey AJ, Kou Y, Cicek AE, et al. DAWN: a framework to identify autism genes and subnetworks using gene expression and genetics. Mol Autism. 2014;5:22.
41. Kumar RA, Christian SL. Genetics of autism spectrum disorders. Curr Neurol Neurosci Rep. 2009;9:188–97.
42. Lee MS, Kim YJ, Kim EJ, Lee MJ. Overlap of autism spectrum disorder and glucose transporter 1 deficiency syndrome associated with a heterozygous deletion in the 1p34.2 region. J Neurol Sci. 2015;356:212–4.
43. Michaelson JJ, Shi Y, Gujral M, Zheng H, Malhotra D, Jin X, et al. Whole-genome sequencing in autism identifies hot spots for de novo germline mutation. Cell. 2012;151:1431–42.
44. Butler MG, Rafi SK, Manzardo AM. High-resolution chromosome ideogram representation of currently recognized genes for autism spectrum disorders. Int J Mol Sci. 2015;16:6464–95.
45. Miles JH. Autism spectrum disorders—a genetics review. Genet Med. 2011;13:278–94.
46. Jeste SS, Geschwind DH. Disentangling the heterogeneity of autism spectrum disorder through genetic findings. Nat Rev Neurol. 2014;10:74–81.
47. Turner TN, Sharma K, Oh EC, Liu YP, Collins RL, Sosa MX, et al. Loss of δ-catenin function in severe autism. Nature. 2015;520:51–6.
48. Mercuri E, Messina S, Bruno C, Mora M, Pegoraro E, Comi GP, et al. Congenital muscular dystrophies with defective glycosylation of dystroglycan a population study. Neurology. 2009;72:1802–9.
49. Sparks S, Quijano-Roy S, Harper A, Rutkowski A, Gordon E, Hoffman EP, et al. Congenital muscular dystrophy overview. In: Pagon RA, Adam MP, Ardinger HH, Wallace SE, Amemiya A, Bean LJ, et al., editors. GeneReviews(®). Seattle: University of Washington; 1993. http://www.ncbi.nlm.nih.gov/books/NBK1291/. Accessed 3 May 2016.

50. Smith JE, Winkler RL, Fryback DG. The first positive: computing positive predictive value at the extremes. Ann Intern Med. 2000;132:804–9.

51. Willer T, Lee H, Lommel M, Yoshida-Moriguchi T, de Bernabe DBV, Venzke D, et al. ISPD loss-of-function mutations disrupt dystroglycan O-mannosylation and cause Walker-Warburg syndrome. Nat Genet. 2012;44:575–80.

52. Arboleda VA, Lee H, Parnaik R, Fleming A, Banerjee A, Ferraz-de-Souza B, et al. Mutations in the PCNA-binding domain of CDKN1C cause IMAGe syndrome. Nat Genet. 2012;44:788–92.

53. Ng SB, Bigham AW, Buckingham KJ, Hannibal MC, McMillin MJ, Gildersleeve HI, et al. Exome sequencing identifies MLL2 mutations as a cause of kabuki syndrome. Nat Genet. 2010;42:790–3.

54. Varela I, Tarpey P, Raine K, Huang D, Ong CK, Stephens P, et al. Exome sequencing identifies frequent mutation of the SWI/SNF complex gene PBRM1 in renal carcinoma. Nature. 2011;469:539–42.

55. Bilgüvar K, Öztürk AK, Louvi A, Kwan KY, Choi M, Tatlı B, et al. Whole-exome sequencing identifies recessive WDR62 mutations in severe brain malformations. Nature. 2010;467:207–10.

56. Lopez E, Thauvin-Robinet C, Reversade B, Khartoufi NE, Devisme L, Holder M, et al. C5orf42 is the major gene responsible for OFD syndrome type VI. Hum Genet. 2013;133:367–77.

57. Bayram Y, Aydin H, Gambin T, Akdemir ZC, Atik MM, Karaca E, et al. Exome sequencing identifies a homozygous C5orf42 variant in a Turkish kindred with oral-facial-digital syndrome type VI. Am J Med Genet A. 2015;167:2132–7.

58. Raza MH, Mattera R, Morell R, Sainz E, Rahn R, Gutierrez J, et al. Association between rare variants in AP4E1, a component of intracellular trafficking, and persistent stuttering. Am J Hum Genet. 2015;97:715–25.

59. Stránecký V, Hoischen A, Hartmannová H, Zaki MS, Chaudhary A, Zudaire E, et al. Mutations in ANTXR1 cause GAPO syndrome. Am J Hum Genet. 2013; 92:792–9.

60. Wang S-K, Choi M, Richardson AS, Reid BM, Lin BP, Wang SJ, et al. ITGB6 loss-of-function mutations cause autosomal recessive amelogenesis imperfecta. Hum Mol Genet. 2014;23:2157–63.

61. Tuz K, Bachmann-Gagescu R, O'Day DR, Hua K, Isabella CR, Phelps IG, et al. Mutations in CSPP1 cause primary cilia abnormalities and Joubert syndrome with or without Jeune asphyxiating thoracic dystrophy. Am J Hum Genet. 2014;94:62–72.

62. Belaya K, Cruz PMR, Liu WW, Maxwell S, McGowan S, Farrugia ME, et al. Mutations in GMPPB cause congenital myasthenic syndrome and bridge myasthenic disorders with dystroglycanopathies. Brain. 2015;138:2493–504.

63. Ng SB, Buckingham KJ, Lee C, Bigham AW, Tabor HK, Dent KM, et al. Exome sequencing identifies the cause of a mendelian disorder. Nat Genet. 2010;42:30–5.

64. Benson DW, Wang DW, Dyment M, Knilans TK, Fish FA, Strieper MJ, et al. Congenital sick sinus syndrome caused by recessive mutations in the cardiac sodium channel gene (SCN5A). J Clin Invest. 2003;112:1019–28.

65. Comino-Méndez I, Gracia-Aznárez FJ, Schiavi F, Landa I, Leandro-García LJ, Letón R, et al. Exome sequencing identifies MAX mutations as a cause of hereditary pheochromocytoma. Nat Genet. 2011;43:663–7.

66. Walsh T, Shahin H, Elkan-Miller T, Lee MK, Thornton AM, Roeb W, et al. Whole exome sequencing and homozygosity mapping identify mutation in the cell polarity protein GPSM2 as the cause of nonsyndromic hearing loss DFNB82. Am J Hum Genet. 2010;87:90–4.

67. Campeau PM, Kasperaviciute D, Lu JT, Burrage LC, Kim C, Hori M, et al. The genetic basis of DOORS syndrome: an exome-sequencing study. Lancet Neurol. 2014;13:44–58.

68. Stray-Pedersen A, Backe PH, Sorte HS, Mørkrid L, Chokshi NY, Erichsen HC, et al. PGM3 mutations cause a congenital disorder of glycosylation with severe immunodeficiency and skeletal dysplasia. Am J Hum Genet. 2014;95:96–107.

69. Lee H, Lin MA, Kornblum HI, Papazian DM, Nelson SF. Exome sequencing identifies de novo gain of function missense mutation in KCND2 in identical twins with autism and seizures that slows potassium channel inactivation. Hum Mol Genet. 2014;23:3481–9.

70. Baasch A-L, Hüning I, Gilissen C, Klepper J, Veltman JA, Gillessen-Kaesbach G, et al. Exome sequencing identifies a de novo SCN2A mutation in a patient with intractable seizures, severe intellectual disability, optic atrophy, muscular hypotonia, and brain abnormalities. Epilepsia. 2014;55:e25–9.

71. Dyment DA, Smith AC, Alcantara D, Schwartzentruber JA, Basel-Vanagaite L, Curry CJ, et al. Mutations in PIK3R1 cause SHORT syndrome. Am J Hum Genet. 2013;93:158–66.

72. Lee H, Graham JM, Rimoin DL, Lachman RS, Krejci P, Tompson SW, et al. Exome sequencing identifies PDE4D mutations in acrodysostosis. Am J Hum Genet. 2012;90:746–51.

73. Deardorff MA, Kaur M, Yaeger D, Rampuria A, Korolev S, Pie J, et al. Mutations in cohesin complex members SMC3 and SMC1A cause a mild variant of Cornelia de Lange syndrome with predominant mental retardation. Am J Hum Genet. 2007;80:485–94.

74. Deardorff MA, Bando M, Nakato R, Watrin E, Itoh T, Minamino M, et al. HDAC8 mutations in Cornelia de Lange syndrome affect the cohesin acetylation cycle. Nature. 2012;489:313–7.

75. Vulto-van Silfhout AT, Rajamanickam S, Jensik PJ, Vergult S, de Rocker N, Newhall KJ, et al. Mutations affecting the SAND domain of DEAF1 cause intellectual disability with severe speech impairment and behavioral problems. Am J Hum Genet. 2014;94:649–61.

76. Chudasama KK, Winnay J, Johansson S, Claudi T, König R, Haldorsen I, et al. SHORT syndrome with partial lipodystrophy due to impaired phosphatidylinositol 3 kinase signaling. Am J Hum Genet. 2013;93:150–7.

77. Chen Y-Z, Matsushita MM, Robertson P, Rieder M, Girirajan S, Antonacci F, et al. Autosomal dominant familial dyskinesia and facial myokymia: single exome sequencing identifies a mutation in adenylyl cyclase 5. Arch Neurol. 2012;69:630–5.

78. Wang J, Shen Y. When a "disease-causing mutation" is not a pathogenic variant. Clin Chem. 2014;60:711–3.

79. Bell CJ, Dinwiddie DL, Miller NA, Hateley SL, Ganusova EE, Mudge J, et al. Carrier testing for severe childhood recessive diseases by next-generation sequencing. Sci Transl Med. 2011;3:65ra4.

80. Piton A, Redin C, Mandel J-L. XLID-causing mutations and associated genes challenged in light of data from large-scale human exome sequencing. Am J Hum Genet. 2013;93:368–83.

81. Blekhman R, Man O, Herrmann L, Boyko AR, Indap A, Kosiol C, et al. Natural selection on genes that underlie human disease susceptibility. Curr Biol. 2008;18:883–9.

82. Collins FS, Varmus H. A new initiative on precision medicine. N Engl J Med. 2015;372:793–5.

83. Li AH, Morrison AC, Kovar C, Cupples LA, Brody JA, Polfus LM, et al. Analysis of loss-of-function variants and 20 risk factor phenotypes in 8,554 individuals identifies loci influencing chronic disease. Nat Genet. 2015;47:640–2.

84. SNP & Variation Suite ™ (Version 8.1). Bozeman, MT: Golden Helix, Inc.; Available from http://www.goldenhelix.com. http://www.goldenhelix.com.

85. Wang K, Li M, Hakonarson H. ANNOVAR: functional annotation of genetic variants from high-throughput sequencing data. Nucleic Acids Res. 2010;38:e164.

86. McLaren W, Pritchard B, Rios D, Chen Y, Flicek P, Cunningham F. Deriving the consequences of genomic variants with the Ensembl API and SNP effect predictor. Bioinformatics. 2010;26:2069–70.

87. Lucas FAS, Wang G, Scheet P, Peng B. Integrated annotation and analysis of genetic variants from next-generation sequencing studies with variant tools. Bioinformatics. 2012;28:421–2.

88. Yandell M, Huff C, Hu H, Singleton M, Moore B, Xing J, et al. A probabilistic disease-gene finder for personal genomes. Genome Res. 2011;21:1529–42.

89. Habegger L, Balasubramanian S, Chen DZ, Khurana E, Sboner A, Harmanci A, et al. VAT: a computational framework to functionally annotate variants in personal genomes within a cloud-computing environment. Bioinformatics. 2012;28:2267–9.

90. Kumar P, Henikoff S, Ng PC. Predicting the effects of coding non-synonymous variants on protein function using the SIFT algorithm. Nat Protoc. 2009;4:1073–81.

91. Adzhubei IA, Schmidt S, Peshkin L, Ramensky VE, Gerasimova A, Bork P, et al. A method and server for predicting damaging missense mutations. Nat Methods. 2010;7:248–9.

92. Kircher M, Witten DM, Jain P, O'Roak BJ, Cooper GM, Shendure J. A general framework for estimating the relative pathogenicity of human genetic variants. Nat Genet. 2014;46:310–5.

93. Cunningham F, Amode MR, Barrell D, Beal K, Billis K, Brent S, et al. Ensembl 2015. Nucleic Acids Res. 2015;43:D662–9.

94. Blomen VA, Májek P, Jae LT, Bigenzahn JW, Nieuwenhuis J, Staring J, et al. Gene essentiality and synthetic lethality in haploid human cells. Science. 2015;350:1092–6.

15

Mitochondrial DNA 7908–8816 region mutations in maternally inherited essential hypertensive subjects in China

Ye Zhu[1,2], Xiang Gu[1,2*] and Chao Xu[3]

Abstract

Background: Nuclear genes or family-based mitochondrial screening have been the focus of genetic studies into essential hypertension. Studies into the role of mitochondria in sporadic Chinese hypertensives are lacking. The objective of the study was to explore the relationship between mitochondrial DNA (mtDNA) variations and the development of maternally inherited essential hypertension (MIEH) in China.

Methods: Yangzhou residents who were outpatients or in-patients at the Department of Cardiology in Northern Jiangsu People's Hospital (Jiangsu, China) from June 2009 to June 2015 were recruited in a 1:1 case control study of 600 gender-matched Chinese MIEH subjects and controls. Genomic DNA was isolated from whole blood cells. The most likely sites for hypertension were screened using oligodeoxynucleotides at positions 7908–8816, purified and subsequently analyzed by direct sequencing according to the revised consensus Cambridge sequence. The frequency, density, type and conservative evolution of mtDNA variations were comprehensively analyzed.

Results: We found a statistical difference between the two groups for body mass index, waist circumference, abdominal circumference, triglyceride, low-density lipoprotein cholesterol, fasting blood glucose, uric acid, creatinine and blood urea nitrogen ($P < 0.05$). More amino-acid changes and RNA variants were found in MIEH subjects than the controls ($P < 0.01$). The detection system simultaneously identified 40 different heteroplasmic or homoplasmic mutations in 4 genes: COXII, tRNA^{Lys}, ATP8 and ATP 6. The mtDNA variations were mainly distributed in regions of ATP6 binding sites, and the site of highest mutation frequency was m. 8414C > T. Three changes in single bases (C8414T in ATP8, A8701G in ATP6 and G8584A in ATP6) were significantly different in the MIEH patients and the controls ($P < 0.001$). The m.8273_8281del mutation was identified from 59 MIEH patients.

Conclusions: Our results indicate that novel mtDNA mutations may be involved in the pathological process of MIEH, and mitochondrial genetic characteristics were identified in MIEH individuals.

Keywords: Mitochondria, DNA, Mutation, Essential hypertension, Maternal inheritance

Background

Essential hypertension (EH) is a common chronic disease which is becoming an urgent public health issue worldwide, accounting for 9.4 million deaths each year [1]. EH is characterized by an elevation in arterial pressure and is a major risk factor for many common causes of morbidity and mortality including myocardial infarction, congestive heart failure, stroke and kidney failure in many segments of the population [2]. EH results from the interaction between environmental and inherited risk factors, which can be caused by single-gene or multifactorial conditions.

A family history of hypertension means that individuals are more likely to suffer hypertension [3, 4]. Maternally inherited essential hypertension (MIEH) is EH that shows a pattern of maternal inheritance and is occasionally observed in the clinic [5]. mtDNA can lead to mitochondrial diseases that are exclusively transmitted from the mother. mtDNA mutations have been identified in

---

* Correspondence: guxiang@yzu.edu.cn
[1]Clinical Medical College, Yangzhou University, Yangzhou 225001, Jiangsu, China
[2]Department of Cardiology, Northern Jiangsu People's Hospital, Yangzhou 225001, Jiangsu, China
Full list of author information is available at the end of the article

some pathogenic diseases such as myoclonic epilepsy, lactic acidosis, mitochondrial myopathy, encephalopathy, stroke-like episodes, and ragged-red fibers or maternally inherited diabetes [6]. Accordingly, mutations in mtDNA have also been reported in MIEH [7].

Mitochondria have an inefficient DNA repair and protection system in comparison to that of nuclear DNA [8]. All the homoplasmic mtDNA mutations that have been identified as being related to MIEH have caused functional disorders. The m.4435A > G mutation that is located immediately at the 3'end of the anticodon. This location corresponds to position 37 of tRNAMet affecting codon recognition, structural formation, and stabilization of functional tRNAs [9]. The m.4263A > G mutation reduces the efficiency of the tRNAIle precursor 5'-end cleavage that is catalyzed by RNase P because it is located at the processing site for the tRNAIle 5'-end precursor [10]. The result of these mutations is abnormal mitochondrial respiration that causes oxidative stress, this uncouples the oxidative pathways for ATP synthesis, and leads to cellular energetic processes failing [11].

To date, the roles of somatic mtDNA mutations in MIEH are still poorly understood. The development of blood pressure and this increases with many factors that include the mtDNA mutation/background, nuclear genes and environmental factors [12]. There is some suggestion that gene variations are associated with hypertension; but different results have been seen in different populations [13]. The mitochondrial genome accounts for ~ 5% of the heritability of blood pressure and these increases to ~ 35% for hypertensive pedigrees [14, 15]. With improved genetic analysis techniques, in particular genome-wide association studies, genes can now be identified that are likely to contribute to the development of hypertension within populations [16]. However, most genetic mutations have been identified in the nuclear genome [17]; only a few studies have focused on the investigation of the mitochondrial genome in the development of hypertension in populations. Therefore, it is obvious that understanding mtDNA sequence alteration involvement in MIEH may improve understanding of the genetic basis and pathogenesis of MIEH.

MtDNA mutations mainly distributed in the 7908–8816 region as described previously [18]. In this study, to understand more about the molecular mechanism underlying MIEH, we undertook screening of study in the mtDNA 7908–8816 region in hypertensive and normotensive subjects in a systematic and extensive manner. We explored inherited and clinical evidence to observe the relationship between the mitochondrial genome and MIEH. We decided to focus upon a Chinese Han population, as the morbidity of EH in Chinese adults is nearly 11.8% [19] but there is a limited amount of study on this racial group.

Methods

Subjects

This was a case control study of 300 unrelated patients with MIEH and 300 healthy control subjects. The MIEH participants were selected according to the following inclusion criteria: (1) outpatients or in-patients underwent a regular medical check-up at the Department of Cardiology in Northern Jiangsu People's Hospital from June 2009 to June 2015; (2) more than 18 years old; (3) with a diagnosis of primary hypertension; (4) not receiving antihypertensive medication; (5) diagnosed with MIEH according to the maternal transmission of EH within generations, which was transmitted by the mother or her relatives and not by the father. Patients were excluded if they were diagnosed with: (1) secondary hypertension (for example renal arterial sterosis, hyperaldosteronism, aortic coarctation, and pheochromocytoma); (2) congenital heart diseases; and (3) presence of organic valve diseases.

Three hundred gender-matched healthy subjects were also selected as the control group. Controls were healthy Yangzhou residents who accepted annual examination in the physical examination center of Northern Jiangsu People's Hospital from June 2009 to June 2015. They were chosen randomly from the daily appointment list and were gender matched with the MIEH group. The inclusion criteria for the control subjects were: (1) no personal or family history of hypertension, and (2) a systolic blood pressure (SBP) of < 130 mmHg and a diastolic blood pressure (DBP) of< 85 mmHg. The occurrence of hypertension in one or both biologic parents was considered to be a positive family history of essential hypertension. All study participants were interviewed and then evaluated to identify both personal and medical histories of clinical abnormalities.

Verbal Informed consent, medical history, clinical evaluations and genetic analysis were obtained from all participants involved in the study. The reason for receiving verbal consent is that genetic analysis is used for diagnosis, not for treatment. There was no harm to the patients. The protocol was conducted in accordance with the Helsinki declaration and approved by the ethics committee of the Northern Jiangsu People's Hospital.

Data collection

Height and weight were both measured when the subjects had fasted overnight and were wearing only underwear. Body mass index (BMI) was calculated as weight in kilograms divided by height in squared meters (kg/m^2). Blood pressure was measured by an experienced physician using a mercury column sphygmomanometer according to the World Health Organization (WHO) standardized criteria [20]. The physician was blinded to the study information of the subjects. Systolic and diastolic blood pressure were indicated by the first and fifth Korotkoff sounds, respectively. Three systolic and diastolic blood pressure readings were taken and the mean was used as the blood pressure measurement. The hypertension was defined according to the 2010 Chinese guidelines for the management of hypertension [21]: under the condition of no antihypertensive drugs treatment, the systolic blood pressure is higher than 140 mmHg and/or diastolic blood pressure is higher than 90 mmHg measured three times on different days. After 12-h fast, 4 ml venous blood were drawn from the antecubital vein for the measurement of fasting blood glucose (FBG), total cholesterol (TC), low-density lipoprotein cholesterol (LDL), triglycerides (TG), uric acid (UA), creatinine (CR) and blood urea nitrogen (BUN) by an automatic biochemistry analyzer (Hitach 7600DDP, Japan), using Roche biochemical reaction kits.

Mitochondrial DNA analysis

Genomic DNA was extracted from peripheral blood using standard protocols [22]. DNA was isolated using Promega Wizard Genomic DNA Purification Kit (Madison, WI, USA). Locations considered the main areas for cardiovascular disease as described previously [12] were screened using oligodeoxynucleotides at 7908-8816 bp. Polymerase chain reaction (PCR) was carried out to amplify mitochondrial tRNA^{Lys} gene using the following primers: forward: 5′-ACGAGTACACCGACTACGG C-3′ and reverse: 5′- TGGGTGGTTGGTGTAAATG A-3′. PCR was performed in 30 μl of the reaction mixture, containing 5.2 μl of PCR Master Mix (Qiagen; Hilden, Germany), 2.5 μl of each primer, 1 μl DNA sample, and 18.8 μl of water. The cycling program for PCR consisted of one cycle of 95 °C for 5 min and then 35 - cycles of 95 °C for 30 s, 54 °C for 30 s and 72 °C for 60 s with a full extension cycle of 72 °C for 10 min in a 9700 Thermocycler (Perkin-Elmer Applied Biosystems, Norwalk, USA). Each fragment was purified and subsequently analyzed by direct sequencing with ABI 3730 Sequence Analysis software (Applied Biosystems, Inc., Foster City, CA, USA) using the BigDye Terminator v1.1 kit (ABI Company, Carlsbad, CA, USA), and SeqWeb program GAP(GCG) was used for analysis referring to the updated consensus Cambridge sequence [23]. Pathogenic variants were identified from MitoMap (http://www.mitomap.org/) [24].

Statistical analysis

Statistical analysis was performed using R and SPSS software (version 16.0; SPSS Inc., Chicago, IL, USA). For comparison of the MIEH group and control group, continuous variables were first tested for normal distribution by Kolmogorov-Smirnov test and then presented in terms of mean ± standard deviation (SD). Discrete variables in the groups were expressed as frequency. Student's t test

and Fisher's exact t test were used to identify the associations between potential continuous and discrete factors and MIEH respectively. A multiple testing adjusted P-value of < 0.05 was considered as statistically significant.

Results

Clinical evaluation of baseline characteristics

The general data of study participants is summarized in Table 1. In this study, no significant differences were found in age, gender, or total cholesterol between the two groups. There was a statistical difference for BMI, waist circumference (WC), abdominal circumference (AC), TG, LDL, FBG, UA, CR and BUN ($P < 0.05$) between the two groups.

mtDNA analysis

Data comparing the frequency of mtDNA variants in the 300 balanced cases and controls are presented in Table 2. The distribution of the number of observed mutations in mtDNA 7908~ 8816 bp for all the participants is shown in Fig. 1. As shown in Table 3, we found a total of 40 mutation sites in the 300 MIEH subjects from the mutation analysis (Additional file 1). The mutations were mainly distributed in the regions of the ATP6 binding site, and the site of highest mutation frequency was m. 8414C > T (Fig. 2).

Table 1 Comparison of baseline clinical data between the MIEH and control groups

Subjects	MIEH group	Control group	p-value
Gender(M/F)	300(148/152)	300(145/155)	0.870
Age at test(years)	66.85 ± 7.24	65.37 ± 6.76	0.01*
Age at onset (years)	47.46 ± 6.8	NA	
SBP(mmHg)	148.5 ± 19.8	145.6 ± 18.6	0.065
DBP(mmHg)	94.8 ± 8.9	88.4 ± 12.5	< 0.001*
BMI(kg/m^2)	25.89 ± 2.61	23.55 ± 3.04	< 0.001*
WC (cm)	87.30 ± 10.78	78.08 ± 8.72	< 0.001*
AC (cm)	89.51 ± 10.15	80.98 ± 7.89	< 0.001*
Alcohol, n (%)	72(24)	30(10)	< 0.001*
Current Smoking, n	66(22)	39(13)	0.005*
TG(mmol/L)	1.87 ± 1.22	1.38 ± 0.81	< 0.001*
TC(mmol/L)	4.59 ± 1.90	4.29 ± 1.18	0.021*
LDL(mmol/L)	2.64 ± 1.02	2.03 ± 1.35	< 0.001*
FBG (mmol/L)	5.18 ± 2.19	4.35 ± 0.84	< 0.001*
UA(umol/L)	367.00 ± 127.27	320.38 ± 78.91	< 0.001*
Cr(ummol/L)	103.36 ± 33.71	86.38 ± 30.71	< 0.001*
BUN(mmol/L)	5.75 ± 2.04	4.87 ± 1.78	< 0.001*

Abbreviations: *F* female, *M* male, *SBP* Systolic blood pressure, *DBP* Diastolic blood pressure, *BMI* Body mass index, *WC* waist circumference, *AC* abdomen circumference, *TG* triglyceride, *TC* total cholesterol, *LDL* low-density lipoprotein cholesterol, *FBG* fasting blood glucose, *UA* uric acid, *Cr* creatinine, *BUN* blood urea nitrogen
*: A P value < 0.05 was marked by a star

Table 2 Distribution of mtDNA sequence analyses at positions 7908–8816

Gene	Position	Length	Control group (n(%))	MIEH group (n(%))	Fisher's exact P value
COXII	7908–8269	684	7(2.3%)	28(9.3%)	< 0.001
tRNA^{Lys}	8295–8364	70	0	4(1.3%)	0.124
ATP8	8366–8572	207	11(3.7%)	90(30%)	< 0.001
ATP6	8527–8816	290	14(4.7%)	115(38%)	< 0.001

These results all showed that the MIEH group had more mtDNA variations in frequency and density than the control group. Three SNPs were significantly ($P < 0.001$) different between the MIEH and the control groups: C8414T (leucine to phenylalanine, belongs to haplogroup D) in ATP8 gene, A8701G in ATP6 gene (threonine to alanine, belongs haplogroup M), and G8584A in ATP6 gene (alanine to threonine) (Figs. 3 and 4).

Forty different heteroplasmic or homoplasmic mutations were simultaneously identifed in 4 genes: COXII, tRNA^{Lys}, ATP8 and ATP 6 gene. We found a total of 38 homoplasmic mutations in 182 MIEH subjects. Two heteroplasmic mutations of m.8563A > T and m.8031C > A were found in 2 MIEH subjects. The MIEH subjects harbored more variants ($P < 0.01$) than the controls with respect to the amino-acid changes and coding sequence variants. Among the MIEH individuals, an intriguing observation was that there were m.8273_8281del mutations in 59 MIEH group patients (Fig. 5). These observations suggested a positive correlation between mtDNA mutation and MIEH.

Discussion

This study aimed to investigate mtDNA 7908–8816 region mutations in a Chinese population of patients with MIEH. The results showed that the patients in the MIEH group harbored more mtDNA variants than the control group. We simultaneously identified 40 different heteroplasmic or homoplasmic mutations in 4 genes: COXII, tRNA^{Lys}, ATP8 and ATP6. As previously reported, most pathogenic mtDNA mutations are in tRNAs [25]. Mutations in protein-encoding genes are frequently associated with ATPase dysfunction [26]. Failure in tRNA metabolism will lead to the deficiency of mitochondrial protein synthesis [27]. Defects in mitochondrial translation consequently result in a respiratory phenotype and a decrease in ATP production, may reduce the production of ROS, and subsequently have the potential role to affect the course of hypertension [28]. The mtDNA variations were mainly distributed in regions of ATP6 binding sites, and the site of highest mutation frequency was m.8414C > T. Three single base pair changes were significantly different between the MIEH and control groups, namely C8414T in ATP8, and A8701G and G8584A in ATP6. It is becoming established that mitochondrial damage and dysfunction are important factors in cardiovascular disease [29]. To our best knowledge, this is one of the first large-scale population-based systematic screens for mitochondrial mutations and their effects on MIEH in the Chinese population. Systematic study of the relationship between disease and mtDNA mutation is important to assist with

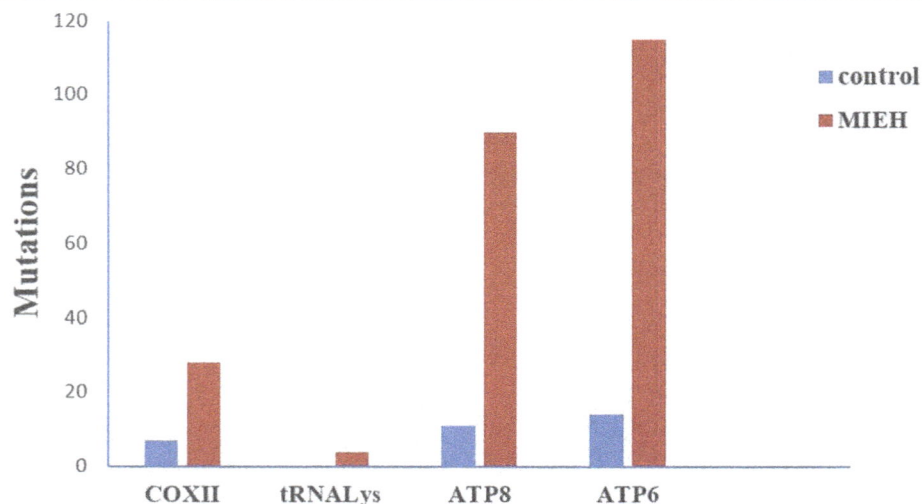

Fig. 1 Distribution histogram of the mtDNA sequences in 7908~ 8816

Table 3 Mutation sites of mtDNA in MIEH individuals and controls

Site of mutation	Gene	Replacement	Number of mutations(n) (MIEH)	(Controls)	Fisher's exact P value	Conservation (H/B/M/X)[a]	Previously reported[b]	Change of Amino acid
8020	COXII	G to A	1	0	1	G/T/C/G	Yes	non-synonymous variant
8027	COXII	G to A	4	2	0.686	G/C/C/A	Yes	non-synonymous variant
8078	COXII	G to A	2	1	1	G/G/A/C	Yes	non-synonymous variant
8149	COXII	A to G	3	1	0.624	A/A/C/T	Yes	non-synonymous variant
8152	COXII	G to A	2	0	0.499	G/A/C/C	Yes	non-synonymous variant
8176	COXII	T to C	2	0	0.499	T/A/C/T	Yes	non-synonymous variant
8200	COXII	T to C	5	1	0.216	T/T/T/C	Yes	non-synonymous variant
8251	COXII	G to A	6	1	0.123	G/T/T/T	Yes	non-synonymous variant
8269	COXII	G to A	2	1	1	G/A/A/C	Yes	non-synonymous variant
8348	tRNA[Lys]	A to G	2	0	0.499	A/T/T/G	Yes	non-synonymous variant
8380	ATP8	T to C	1	0	1	T/T/C/C	No	non-synonymous variant
8392	ATP8	G to A	2	0	0.499	G/A/T/T	Yes	non-synonymous variant
8414	ATP8	C to T	60	7	9.883e-13	C/T/A/T	Yes	non-synonymous variant
8440	ATP8	A to G	1	0	1	A/C/C/T	Yes	non-synonymous variant
8452	ATP8	A to G	1	0	1	A/A/G/T	No	non-synonymous variant
8459	ATP8	A to G	4	1	0.373	A/T/C/G	No	non-synonymous variant
8467	ATP8	C to T	2	0	0.499	C/A/T/T	No	non-synonymous variant
8470	ATP8	A to G	2	0	0.499	A/C/A/T	Yes	non-synonymous variant
8473	ATP8	T to C	4	1	0.373	T/A/A/C	Yes	non-synonymous variant
8557	ATP8	G to A	1	0	1	G/C/G/T	Yes	non-synonymous variant
8563	ATP8	A to G	4	1	0.373	A/T/G/C	Yes	non-synonymous variant
8563	ATP8	A to T	1	0	1	A/T/G/C	No	non-synonymous variant
8584	ATP6	G to A	46	5	5.188e-10	G/T/C/A	Yes	non-synonymous variant
8593	ATP6	A to G	1	0	1	A/C/C/A	No	non-synonymous variant
8654	ATP6	T to C	1	0	1	T/A/A/G	Yes	non-synonymous variant
8656	ATP6	A to G	3	1	0.624	A/G/C/T	No	non-synonymous variant
8684	ATP6	C to T	9	2	0.063	C/G/T/T	Yes	non-synonymous variant
8701	ATP6	A to G	49	6	3.445e-10	A/A/T/A	Yes	non-synonymous variant
8723	ATP6	G to A	1	0	1	G/A/A/T	No	non-synonymous variant
8190	COXII	C to T	1	0	1	C/T/A/A	No	synonymous variant
8343	tRNA[Lys]	A to G	2	0	0.499	A/T/A/C	Yes	synonymous variant
8403	ATP8	T to C	1	0	1	T/A/G/C	No	synonymous variant
8409	ATP8	C to T	3	1	0.624	C/T/A/T	No	synonymous variant
8448	ATP8	T to C	2	0	0.499	T/A/C/G	Yes	synonymous variant
8503	ATP8	T to C	1	0	1	T/T/T/T	Yes	synonymous variant
8604	ATP6	T to C	1	0	1	T/C/A/A	Yes	synonymous variant
8614	ATP6	T to C	1	0	1	T/T/A/T	Yes	synonymous variant
8643	ATP6	C to T	1	0	1	C/C/C/T	No	synonymous variant
8745	ATP6	A to G	1	0	1	A/A/C/G	No	synonymous variant
8749	ATP6	T to C	1	0	1	T/A/T/T	Yes	synonymous variant

[a]H/B/M/X means human/bovine/mouse/xenopus
[b]See http//www.mitomap.org and http://www.genpat.uu.se/mtDB/. Previously reported means the variant was ever reported in a database

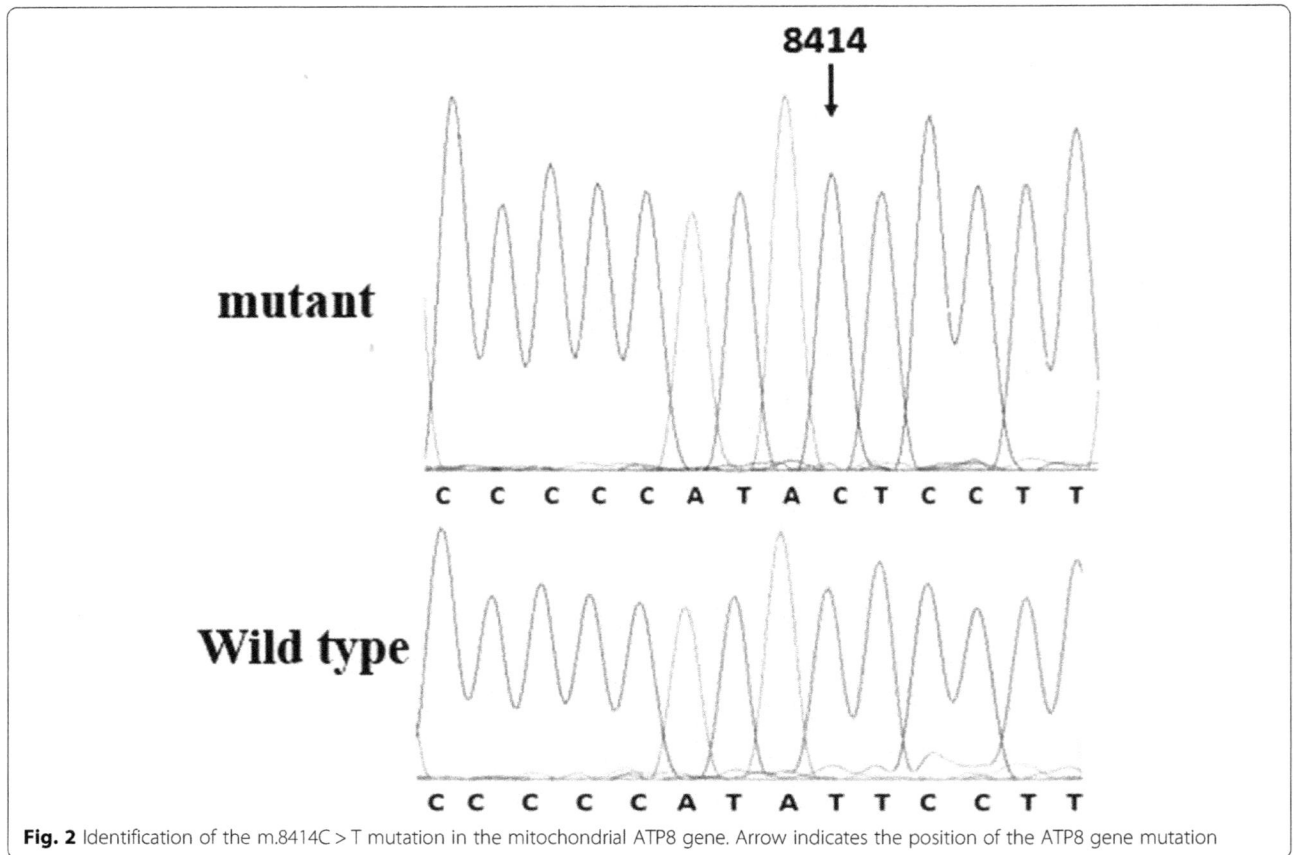

Fig. 2 Identification of the m.8414C > T mutation in the mitochondrial ATP8 gene. Arrow indicates the position of the ATP8 gene mutation

our understanding of the mechanism of the mutation and its relationship to disease, but is also able to improve diagnosis, prevention and treatment of EH.

Blood glucose, blood lipids, creatinine, urea nitrogen and other biochemical abnormalities are all very closely related to the chance of developing primary hypertension [30]. In order to clarify whether mtDNA affects the biochemical indicators of the MIEH individuals, we compared and analyzed the biochemical abnormalities of the MIEH and normal individuals. Clinical examination and evaluation of all available members in this study suggested that MIEH subjects presented significantly higher values than those of non-maternal members in BMI, WC, AC, TG, LDL, FBG, UA, CR and BUN. In our study, participants with MIEH were overweight or obese compared to participants with normal blood pressure. A normal body weight (BMI 18.5–24.9 kg/m^2) should be maintained for prevention and management of hypertension [31]. The occurrence and development of MIEH, can involve these factors or these factors might occur as a result of the development of MIEH, which leads to the damage or deterioration of the target organ.

Many studies, including the analysis of maternally transmitted hypertension in a large Han Chinese pedigree, have acknowledged the role of inherited mtDNA

mutations in familial MIEH [32, 33]. Here, we undertook mutational analysis of the mitochondrial DNA 7908–8816 region using PCR amplification and then sequence analysis of the PCR fragments. The present experiment showed that there were more mtDNA variations in frequency and density in the MIEH patients than those who were normotensives (NT). Among these mutations, ATP6 is a hotspot for pathogenic mutations associated with MIEH. The occurrence of mtDNA mutations in these genetically unrelated subjects affected by MIEH suggests that mutations may participate in key functional development processes of EH. There are hundreds of mitochondria and thousands of mtDNAs in a mammalian cell and the close proximity of mtDNA within mitochondria with ROS generation sites means that mtDNA is vulnerable to a high level of mutation without an efficient DNA protection and repair system [18].

Mutations of mtDNA may lead to disease, and the significant determinant of their clinical outcomes are likely to correlate with the amount of mutated mtDNA [34]. Some MIEH patients in the study were part of one family branch. Among the MIEH individuals, there was a high mutation frequency and density in mtDNA m.8584G > A and m.8701A > G mutations. Specifically, an amino acid change at the m.8414C > T in the ATP8

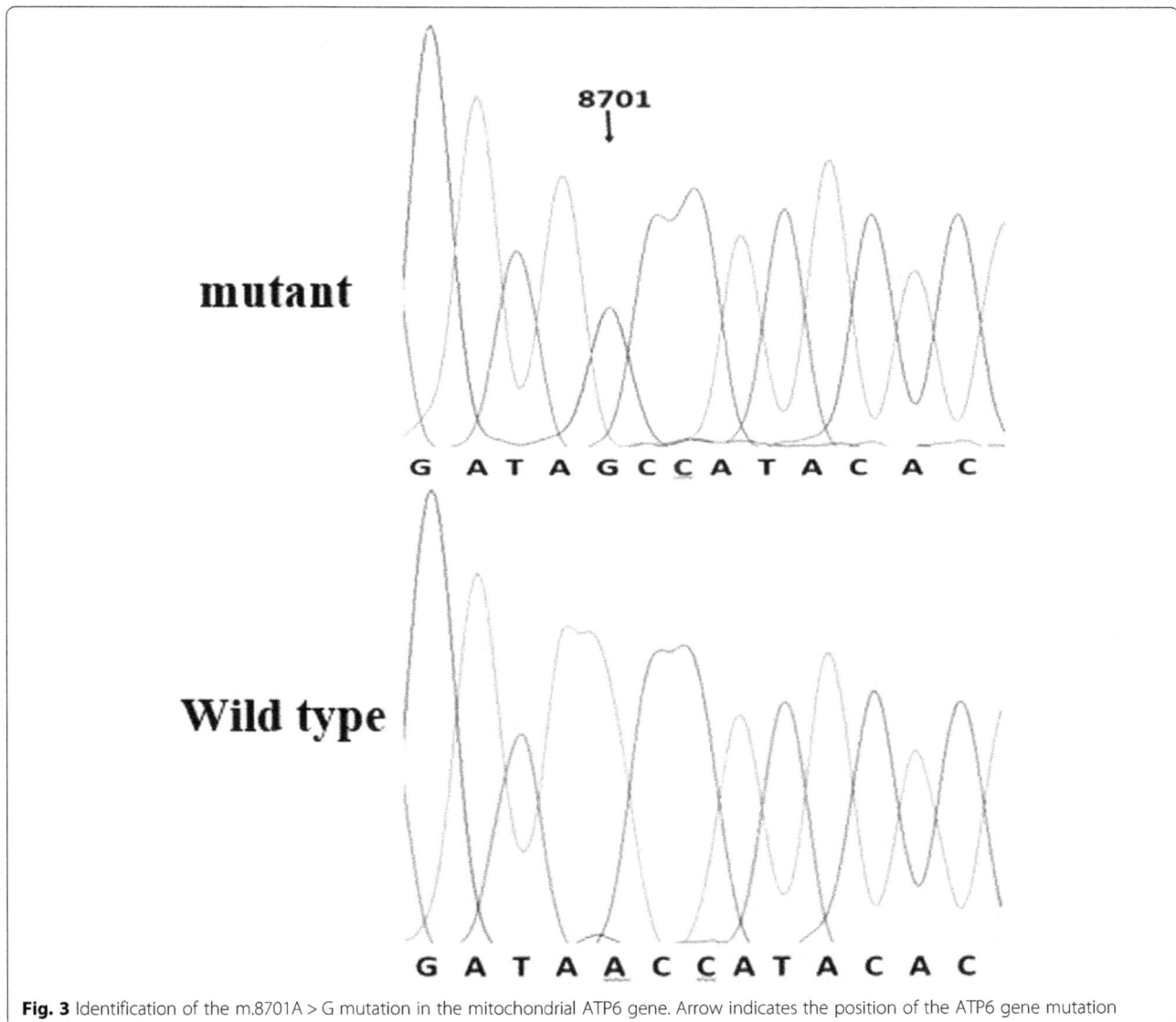

Fig. 3 Identification of the m.8701A > G mutation in the mitochondrial ATP6 gene. Arrow indicates the position of the ATP6 gene mutation

gene (leucine to phenylalanine) shows that mtDNA variants may be able to affect the development of hypertension in China [35]. Ancestral variants of mtDNA define population-specific mtDNA lineages or haplogroups. These were first used to trace the origins of different races and allow reconstruction of the migration of humans throughout our ancient history [36]. MtDNA lineages have been shown recently to be more prone to certain disease symptoms, including type-2 diabetes, obesity and atherothrombotic cerebral infarction. Haplogroups can also protect against myocardial infarction and increase lifespan.

MtDNA mutations, including point mutations, deletions, and duplications that affect transcription and translation of mtDNA are implicated in most mitochondrial diseases [37]. Our intriguing observation is that

there was a m.8273_8281del mutation in 59 MIEH patients. This 9-bp deletion polymorphism is a phylogenetic marker of studies into evolution trends and population migration [38]. Because of its location, this polymorphism could change either downstream or upstream gene expression. Some crucial structural components of the respiratory chain, such as ATP8, ATP6 are located in the downstream of 9-bp deletion polymorphism [39]. This could affect important respiratory chain structural components, including ATP8 and ATP6 that are located downstream of this polymorphism. If these genes are abnormally expressed they could change oxidative phosphorylation and influence oxidative stress levels [40].

Compared to MIEH patients without mtDNA mutations, the onset time of hypertension for patients with

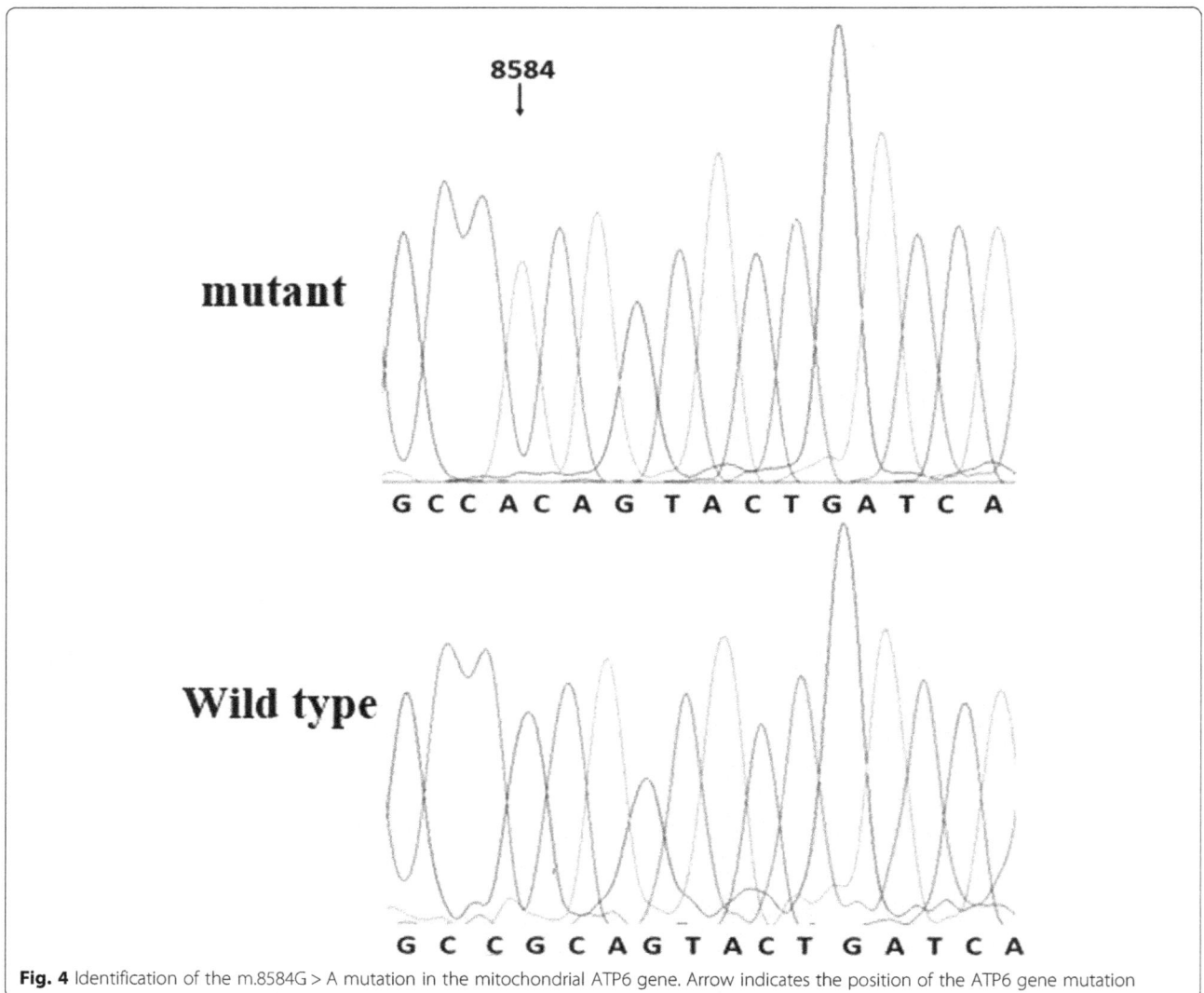

Fig. 4 Identification of the m.8584G > A mutation in the mitochondrial ATP6 gene. Arrow indicates the position of the ATP6 gene mutation

mtDNA mutations was significantly ahead of schedule. This is comparable to the onset time for other Chinese patients with maternally transmitted hypertension [41]. Individuals carrying mtDNA mutations develop hypertension stimulated by environmental factors more easily. Impaired mitochondrial function may contribute increased blood pressure characteristic of aging. Heteroplasmy of mtDNA is strongly associated with hypertension, with the EH mother carrying the gene mutation, and the children with the same mutation more likely to suffer from hypertension. Regarding amino-acid changes and RNAs variants the MIEH subjects harbored more variants than the controls. A possible reason for mtDNA defects pathogenesis in hypertension is that it decreases energy production, increases ROS production, resulting in oxidative stress, disrupting signal transduction, and leading to cardiovascular and renal damage, ultimately initiating hypertension [42, 43]. In consist with previous report [44], mtSNPs may affect the development of hypertension in sporadic Chinese hypertensive subjects. Some specific mtSNP within mitochondria may have potential effect in Chinese hypertensives because of their function. How mitochondrial mtSNPs and/or haplogroups interact synergistically needs to be investigated in further studies. This study was the first step in investigating the role of mitochondria in Chinese hypertensives.

This study has some limitations. One was the small sample size and the single center nature of the study. The conclusions would have been strengthened if the more people had been enrolled. We were not able to control for genetic principal components, which is typically essential in any genomic analysis. Additional limitation was that we were not including people treated with antihypertensives, etc. this would have eliminated quite a large number of people from the analysis.

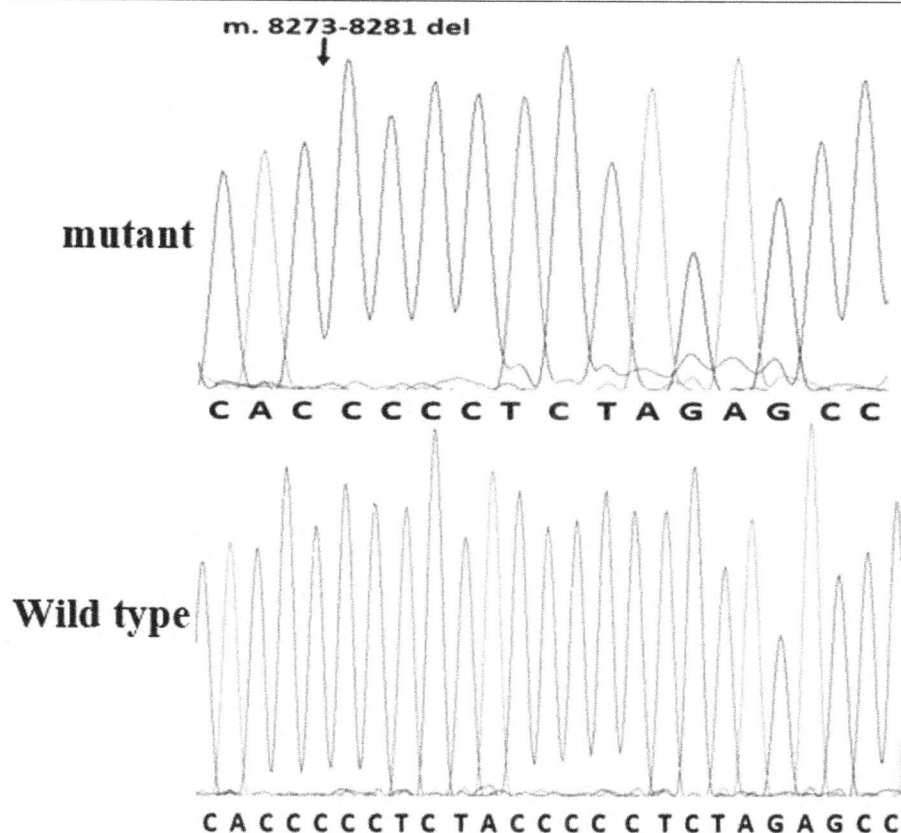

Fig. 5 Identification of the m.8273_8281del mutations. Arrow indicates the position of the deletion mutation

Conclusions

In conclusion, our data convincingly demonstrated the possibility of mitochondrial mutations being involved in the pathological process of MIEH. We also identified mitochondrial genetic characteristics in MIEH individuals. Our findings may be generalizable to other China and Asian populations with a similar lifestyle. The investigation of the role of mitochondrial dysfunction in MIEH provides critical implications on the understanding and treatment of this disorder. The present research serves as a solid foundation for further study on the association between MIEH and mitochondrial dysfunction, and the cause and effect relationship in this population.

Abbreviations
AC: Abdominal circumference; BMI: Body mass index; DBP: Diastolic blood pressure; EH: Essential hypertension; MIEH: Maternally inherited essential hypertension; MtDNA: Mitochondrial DNA; SBP: Systolic blood pressure; WC: Waist circumference

Acknowledgements
We are grateful to Dr. Lei Sun, Dr. Yi Zhang, Dr. Zhengyu Bao and Dr. Jianhua Shen for their valuable advice. We thank the editor and the reviewers whose comments/suggestions helped improve and clarify this manuscript.

Funding
The design and collection of data of the study was supported by Jiangsu Province Outstanding Medical Talented Leader (JS2006038). The analysis, interpretation of data and in writing the manuscript was supported by Science and Technology Department of Jiangsu Province (No. BL2013022).

Authors' contributions
YZ and XG carried out the studies, participated in collecting data, and drafted the manuscript. YZ and CX performed the statistical analysis and participated in its design. CX helped to draft the manuscript. All authors read and approved the final manuscript.

Competing interests
The authors declare that they have no competing interests.

Author details
[1]Clinical Medical College, Yangzhou University, Yangzhou 225001, Jiangsu, China. [2]Department of Cardiology, Northern Jiangsu People's Hospital, Yangzhou 225001, Jiangsu, China. [3]Department of Biostatistics and Epidemiology, University of Oklahoma Health Science Center, Oklahoma City, OK 73134, USA.

References

1. Marian AJ. Mitochondrial genetics and human systemic hypertension. Circ Res. 2011;108(7):784–6.
2. Chen BL, Zhang YZ, Luo JQ, Zhang W. Clinical use of azelnidipine in the treatment of hypertension in Chinese patients. Ther Clin Risk Manag. 2015; 11:309–18.
3. Nemati R, Lu J, Ramachandran V, Etemad A, Heidari M, Yahya MJ, et al. Association between the C34T polymorphism of the AMPD1 gene and essential hypertension in Malaysian patients. Genet Mol Res. 2016;15(2):1–11.
4. Guo H, Zhuang XY, Zhang AM, Zhang W, Yuan Y, Guo L, et al. Presence of mutation m.14484T>C in a Chinese family with maternally inherited essential hypertension but no expression of LHON. Biochim Biophys Acta. 2012;1822(10):1535–43.
5. Qiu Q, Li R, Jiang P, Xue L, Lu Y, Song Y, et al. Mitochondrial tRNA mutations are associated with maternally inherited hypertension in two Han Chinese pedigrees. Hum Mutat. 2012;33(8):1285–93.
6. Schapira AH. Mitochondrial disease. Lancet. 2006;368(9529):70–82.
7. Chen H, Zheng J, Xue L, Meng Y, Wang Y, Zheng B, et al. The 12S rRNA A1555G mutation in the mitochondrial haplogroup D5a is responsible for maternally inherited hypertension and hearing loss in two Chinese pedigrees. Eur J Hum Genet. 2012;20(6):607–12.
8. Liu P, Demple B. DNA repair in mammalian mitochondria: much more than we thought? Environ Mol Mutagen. 2010;51(5):417–26.
9. Lu Z, Chen H, Meng Y, Wang Y, Xue L, Zhi S, et al. The tRNAMet 4435A>G mutation in the mitochondrial haplogroup G2a1 is responsible for maternally inherited hypertension in a Chinese pedigree. Eur J Hum Genet. 2011;19(11):1181–6.
10. Wang S, Li R, Fettermann A, Li Z, Qian Y, Liu Y, et al. Maternally inherited essential hypertension is associated with the novel 4263A>G mutation in the mitochondrial tRNAIle gene in a large Han Chinese family. Circ Res. 2011;108(7):862–70.
11. Muftuoglu M, Mori MP, de Souza-Pinto NC. Formation and repair of oxidative damage in the mitochondrial DNA. Mitochondrion. 2014;17:164–81.
12. Liu Y, Li Y, Gao J, Zhu C, Lan Y, Yang J, et al. Molecular characterization of a Chinese family carrying a novel C4329A mutation in mitochondrial tRNAIle and tRNAGln genes. BMC Med Genet. 2014;15:84.
13. Jia Z, Wang X, Qin Y, Xue L, Jiang P, Meng Y, et al. Coronary heart disease is associated with a mutation in mitochondrial tRNA. Hum Mol Genet. 2013; 22(20):4064–73.
14. Schon EA, DiMauro S, Hirano M. Human mitochondrial DNA: roles of inherited and somatic mutations. Nat Rev Genet. 2012;13(12):878–90.
15. Liu C, Yang Q, Hwang SJ, Sun F, Johnson AD, Shirihai OS, et al. Association of genetic variation in the mitochondrial genome with blood pressure and metabolic traits. Hypertension. 2012;60(4):949–56.
16. Padmanabhan S, Melander O, Johnson T, Di Blasio AM, Lee WK, Gentilini D, et al. Genome-wide association study of blood pressure extremes identifies variant near UMOD associated with hypertension. PLoS Genet. 2010;6(10): e1001177.
17. Assie G, Letouze E, Fassnacht M, Jouinot A, Luscap W, Barreau O, et al. Integrated genomic characterization of adrenocortical carcinoma. 2014; 46(6):607–12.
18. Zhu HY, Wang SW, Martin LJ, Liu L, Li YH, Chen R, et al. The role of mitochondrial genome in essential hypertension in a Chinese Han population. Eur J Hum Genet. 2009;17(11):1501–6.
19. Teng L, Zheng J, Leng J, Ding Y. Clinical and molecular characterization of a Han Chinese family with high penetrance of essential hypertension. Mitochondrial DNA. 2012;23(6):461–5.
20. Chalmers J, MacMahon S, Mancia G, Whitworth J, Beilin L, Hansson L, et al. World Health Organization-International Society of Hypertension Guidelines for the management of hypertension. Guidelines sub-committee of the World Health Organization. Clin Exp Hypertens. 1999;21(5–6):1009–60.
21. Liu LS. Chinese guidelines for the management of hypertension. Zhonghua Xin Xue Guan Bing Za Zhi 2011. 2010;39(7):579–615.
22. Zhu HY, Wang SW, Liu L, Li YH, Chen R, Wang L, et al. A mitochondrial mutation A4401G is involved in the pathogenesis of left ventricular hypertrophy in Chinese hypertensives. Eur J Hum Genet. 2009;17(2):172–8.
23. Gomez-Carballa A, Cerezo M, Balboa E, Heredia C, Castro-Feijoo L, Rica I, et al. Evolutionary analyses of entire genomes do not support the association of mtDNA mutations with Ras/MAPK pathway syndromes. PLoS One. 2011; 6(4):e18348.

24. Ingman M, Gyllensten U. mtDB: human mitochondrial genome database, a resource for population genetics and medical sciences. Nucleic Acids Res. 2006;34(Database issue):D749–51.
25. Jesina P, Tesarova M, Fornuskova D, Vojtiskova A, Pecina P, Kaplanova V, et al. Diminished synthesis of subunit a (ATP6) and altered function of ATP synthase and cytochrome c oxidase due to the mtDNA 2 bp microdeletion of TA at positions 9205 and 9206. Biochem J. 2004;383(Pt. 3):561–71.
26. Liu Y, Zhu Q, Zhu C, Wang X, Yang J, Yin T, et al. Systematic analysis of the clinical and biochemical characteristics of maternally inherited hypertension in Chinese Han families associated with mitochondrial. BMC Med Genet. 2014;7:73.
27. Zheng P, Li S, Liu C, Zha Z, Wei X, Yuan Y. Mitochondrial tRNA(ala) C5601T mutation may modulate the clinical expression of tRNA(met) A4435G mutation in a Han Chinese family with hypertension. Clin Exp Hypertens. 2018;40(6):595–600.
28. Li H, Geng J, Yu H, Tang X, Yang X, Xue L. Mitochondrial tRNA(Thr) 15909A>G mutation associated with hypertension in a Chinese Han pedigree. Biochem Biophys Res Commun. 2018;495(1):574–81.
29. Samuels DC, Li C, Li B, Song Z, Torstenson E, Boyd Clay H, et al. Recurrent tissue-specific mtDNA mutations are common in humans. PLoS Genet. 2013;9(11):e1003929.
30. Lu Y, Xiao T, Zhang F, Chen Y, Liu Y, Li Y, et al. Effect of mitochondrial tRNA(Lys) mutation on the clinical and biochemical characteristics of Chinese essential hypertensive subjects. Biochem Biophys Res Commun. 2014;454(4):500–4.
31. Chobanian AV, Bakris GL, Black HR, Cushman WC, Green LA, Izzo JL Jr, et al. Seventh report of the joint National Committee on prevention, detection, evaluation, and treatment of high blood pressure. Hypertension. 2003;42(6): 1206–52.
32. Akhmedov AT, Marin-Garcia J. Mitochondrial DNA maintenance: an appraisal. Mol Cell Biochem. 2015;409(1–2):283–305.
33. Chen X, Zhang Y, Xu B, Cai Z, Wang L, Tian J, et al. The mitochondrial calcium uniporter is involved in mitochondrial calcium cycle dysfunction: underlying mechanism of hypertension associated with mitochondrial tRNA(Ile) A4263G mutation. Int J Biochem Cell Biol. 2016;78:307–14.
34. Shimizu A, Mito T, Hayashi C, Ogasawara E, Koba R, Negishi I, et al. Transmitochondrial mice as models for primary prevention of diseases caused by mutation in the tRNA(Lys) gene. Proc Natl Acad Sci U S A. 2014;111(8):3104–9.
35. Mohanty K, Dada R, Dada T. Neurodegenerative eye disorders: role of mitochondrial dynamics and genomics. Asia Pac J Ophthalmol (Phila). 2016;5(4):293–9.
36. Kytovuori L, Lipponen J, Rusanen H, Komulainen T, Martikainen MH, Majamaa K. A novel mutation m.8561C>G in MT-ATP6/8 causing a mitochondrial syndrome with ataxia, peripheral neuropathy, diabetes mellitus, and hypergonadotropic hypogonadism. J Neurol. 2016;263(11):2188–95.
37. Shen L, Fang H, Chen T, He J, Zhang M, Wei X, et al. Evaluating mitochondrial DNA in cancer occurrence and development. Ann N Y Acad Sci. 2010;1201:26–33.
38. Yao YG, Watkins WS, Zhang YP. Evolutionary history of the mtDNA 9-bp deletion in Chinese populations and its relevance to the peopling of east and Southeast Asia. Hum Genet. 2000;107(5):504–12.
39. Kleidon J, Plesofsky N, Brambl R. Transcripts and transcript-binding proteins in mitochondria of Neurospora crassa. Mitochondrion. 2003;2(5):345–60.
40. Komandur S, Venkatasubramanian S, Alluri RV, Rao P, Rao P, Hasan Q. Mitochondrial insertion-deletion polymorphism: role in disease pathology. Genet Test Mol Biomarkers. 2011;15(5):361–4.
41. Aure K, Dubourg O, Jardel C, Clarysse L, Sternberg D, Fournier E, et al. Episodic weakness due to mitochondrial DNA MT-ATP6/8 mutations. Neurology. 2013;81(21):1810–8.
42. Moskalev AA, Aliper AM, Smit-McBride Z, Buzdin A, Zhavoronkov A. Genetics and epigenetics of aging and longevity. Cell Cycle. 2014;13(7):1063–77.
43. Nazarewicz RR, Dikalov SI. Mitochondrial ROS in the prohypertensive immune response. Am J Physiol Regul Integr Comp Physiol. 2013;305(2):R98–100.
44. Chen J, Zhao X, Wang H, Chen Y, Wang W, Zhou W, et al. Common variants in TGFBR2 and miR-518 genes are associated with hypertension in the Chinese population. Am J Hypertens. 2014;27(10):1268–76.

16

Association of *NOS1* gene polymorphisms with cerebral palsy in a Han Chinese population: a case-control study

Ting Yu[1†] (iD), Lei Xia[2†], Dan Bi[2], Yangong Wang[1], Qing Shang[3], Dengna Zhu[2], Juan Song[2], Yong Wang[2], Xiaoyang Wang[2,4], Changlian Zhu[2,5*] and Qinghe Xing[1,6*]

Abstract

Background: Cerebral palsy (CP) is the leading cause of motor disability in children; however, its pathogenesis is unknown in most cases. Growing evidence suggests that Nitric oxide synthase 1 (NOS1) is involved in neural development and neurologic diseases. The purpose of this study was to determine whether genetic variants of *NOS1* contribute to CP susceptibility in a Han Chinese population.

Methods: A case-control study involving 652 CP patients and 636 healthy controls was conducted. Six SNPs in the *NOS1* gene (rs3782219, rs6490121, rs2293054, rs10774909, rs3741475, and rs2682826) were selected, and the MassARRAY typing technique was applied for genotyping. Data analysis was conducted using SHEsis online software, and multiple test corrections were performed using SNPSpD online software.

Results: There were no significant differences in genotype and allele frequencies between patients and controls for the SNPs except rs6490121, which deviated from Hardy-Weinberg equilibrium and was excluded from further analyses. Subgroup analysis revealed differences in genotype frequencies between the CP with neonatal encephalopathy group (CP + NE) and control group for rs10774909, rs3741475, and rs2682826 (after SNPSpD correction, $p = 0.004$, 0.012, and 0.002, respectively). The T allele of *NOS1* SNP rs3782219 was negatively associated with spastic quadriplegia (OR = 0.742, 95% CI = 0.600–0.918, after SNPSpD correction, $p = 0.023$). There were no differences in allele or genotype frequencies between CP subgroups and controls for the other genetic polymorphisms.

Conclusions: *NOS1* is associated with CP + NE and spastic quadriplegia, suggesting that NOS1 is likely involved in the pathogenesis of CP and that it is a potential therapeutic target for treatment of cerebral injury.

Keywords: Cerebral palsy, Nitric oxide synthase 1, Single nucleotide polymorphism, Association analysis

Background

Cerebral palsy (CP), the most common cause of motor disability in childhood, is a group of permanent movement and posture disorders attributed to non-progressive abnormalities in the immature brain. Patients with CP often exhibit secondary musculoskeletal problems, epilepsy, and disturbances of sensation, perception, cognition, communication, and behavior [1]. Epidemiologic studies indicate that the incidence of CP is approximately 2–3 per 1000 live births. Despite remarkable advances in obstetric and neonatal care, the overall prevalence of CP has changed little over the past several decades [2]. CP is a lifelong neurologic motor disorder and has a substantial impact on health care and social services costs, family welfare, and patient quality of life [3, 4]. Although known risk factors include prematurity, asphyxia, infection and inflammation, the causes of CP are unknown in most individuals [5, 6]. The pathogenesis and mechanism of CP have been studied and debated for more than 100 years, but the exact pathogenesis remains unclear. Many children with cerebral palsy do not have any known risk factor. Recently, families, twins, population-based, CNV and

---
* Correspondence: zhuc@zzu.edu.cn; xingqinghe@hotmail.com
[†]Ting Yu and Lei Xia contributed equally to this work.
[2]Henan Key Laboratory of Child Brain Injury, Third Affiliated Hospital of Zhengzhou University, Kangfuqian Street 7, Zhengzhou 450052, China
[1]Children's Hospital and Institutes of Biomedical Sciences, Fudan University, Wanyuan Road 399, Minhang District, Shanghai 201102, China
Full list of author information is available at the end of the article

gene-association studies have strongly and directly suggested that genetic factors contribute to the etiology of CP [7–10].

CP is a complex disease. It is highly heterogeneous with regard to phenotype and etiology, and the different subtypes of CP might result from different causal pathways. Some cases may be caused by a single mutation in a single gene, but many may be caused by complex interactions of multiple genetic loci and environmental factors. However, the causes of CP are unknown in most individuals. An increasing association studies have explored the interactions between the susceptibility to CP and SNPs of candidate genes, including those involved in the inflammatory system and the coagulation cascade such as coagulation factor II/V/VII, lymphotoxin-alpha, tumor necrosis factor, IL-6, and IL-8, to determine whether they contribute to the causal pathway of CP [11–14].

Nitric oxide (NO) acts as a pleiotropic gaseous messenger molecule, and it is dynamically controlled during normal development and brain injuries. NO is synthesized from L-arginine by nitric oxide synthase enzymes (NOSs), of which there are three isozyme forms: neuronal NOS (nNOS, NOS1), inducible NOS (iNOS), and endothelial NOS (eNOS) [15]. The *NOS1* gene is the major isoform and is widely expressed throughout the brain, accounting for approximately 90% of NO in the CNS [16]. NO produced from NOS1 is involved in neurogenesis, neuronal differentiation and development [17, 18], and neuroprotection and neuropathology [19]. NO appears to play a critical role in hypoxia-ischemia (HI) brain injury which is a well-known risk factor for CP [20]. During hypoxic insults, excessive NO, which is produced by NOS1 in the cerebral tissue, produces toxic effects leading to neuronal death through several different mechanisms, such as the N -methyl- D –aspartic acid (NMDA) pathway. NMDA play a role in the pathology of multiple neurodegenerative diseases, such as Alzheimer's, Parkinson's and Multiple Sclerosis [21]. Recent studies have revealed that *NOS1* variants are associated with disorders such as Alzheimer's disease [22], schizophrenia [23], and Parkinson's disease [24]. The association of NOS1 with different diseases suggests a pleiotropic role of NOS1 in many physiological processes and a potentially shared pathomechanism.

Genetic and pharmacological studies have also provided valuable insights into the pathophysiology of NOS1. In a neonatal animal model of hypoxia-ischemia (HI), *NOS1* knockout mice were less vulnerable to HI-induced histopathological brain damage than their wild-type counterparts [25]. Selective inhibitors of NOS1, which reduce the NO concentration, were shown to dramatically improve the survival rate of fetal rabbits and ameliorate the symptoms of CP [26]. These results strongly suggest that NOS1

might be involved in the pathogenesis of CP. Although biological plausability for the involvement of NO in the pathogenesis of cerebral palsy is not clear. To our knowledge, no study has reported an association between the *NOS1* gene and CP. Therefore, we performed a comprehensive association study on polymorphisms of the *NOS1* gene and the risk of different subtypes of CP.

Methods

Study population

This was a case-control study based on a Chinese Han population. The study cohort included 652 CP patients and 636 healthy participants who were recruited from the centers for CP rehabilitation and Child Healthcare Departments in the Third Affiliated Hospital of Zhengzhou University, Zhengzhou Children's Hospital and the First Affiliated Hospital of Henan Traditional Chinese Medical College. The CP group consisted of 198 female (30.4%) and 454 male (69.6%) patients ranging in age from 8 to 116 months. The control group was selected from healthy individuals who came to the facility for routine examinations and did not have neurologic conditions or predefined medical conditions; this group was comprised of 214 female (33.2%) and 422 male (66.8%) individuals ranging in age from 8 to 106 months. The diagnosis of CP was made by child neurologists, based on either a clinical examination or medical records and followed the guidelines proposed by the "Surveillance of CP in Europe" network [27]. Written informed consent was obtained from the parents or guardians on behalf of the infant participants. The study was approved by the Ethics Committee of Zhengzhou University.

The database of medical records contains information on the subtypes of CP, such as spastic; CP risk factors, such as preterm and birth asphyxia; symptoms concomitant with CP, such as mental retardation (MR); neonatal complications, such as periventricular leukomalacia (PVL) and hypoxic-ischemic encephalopathy (HIE); maternal factors, such as premature rupture of membrane (PROM); and neonatal encephalopathy (NE) (Table 1). The evaluation standards were consistent with those in our previous published study [13]. NE is a clinical syndrome of disordered neurological function, which includes not only HIE but also intracranial hemorrhage, hypoglycemia, severe hyperbilirubinemia, various metabolic disorders, neurodegenerative disorders, and intracranial infection, among other disorders [28].

SNP selection and genotyping

Altogether, six SNPs (rs3782219, rs6490121, rs2293054, rs10774909, rs3741475, and rs2682826) of the *NOS1* gene with minor allele frequencies in the Chinese Han population greater than 0.1 were selected from the

Table 1 Clinical characteristics of all participants

Characteristic	CP cases (n = 652)	Controls (n = 636)
Sex (male:female)	454:198	422:214
Preterm (< 37 weeks)	37	9
< 2500 g	30	2
BIRTH Asphyxia	187	11
TYPE OF CP		
Spastic CP	438	–
CP with spastic tetraplegia	238	–
COMPLICATION		
CP with PVL	54	–
CP with HIE	91	–
CP with MR	248	–
CP with NE	261	–
MATERNAL FACTORS		
PROM	62	24
TPL	50	27
PIH	22	5

CP cerebral palsy, PVL periventricular leukomalacia, HIE hypoxic-ischemic encephalopathy, MR mental retardation, NE neonatal encephalopathy, PROM premature rupture of membrane, TPL threatened premature labor, PIH pregnancyinduced hypertensio

dbSNP database (www.ncbi.nlm.nih.gov/SNP) and the phase II genotyping data of the HapMap project (http://www.1000genomes.org/). rs2293052 (exon 13) and rs3741475 (exon 22) were synonymous mutation, rs2682826 is located in 3'UTR, while the other three SNPs are located in intron: rs3782219 (intron 1), rs6490121 (intron 10), 10,774,909 (intron 20). Exception for rs10774909, the rest 5 SNPs were reported in published literature online, which were associated with disorders, such as Schizophrenia, Alzheimer's disease, Parkinson's disease.

Genomic DNA was extracted from whole blood of CP patients and controls, using the AxyPrep Blood Genomic DNA Miniprep Kit (Axygen Biosciences, Union City, CA, USA) according to a standard protocol. Probes and primers were designed using the SEQUENOM online tools (https:// http://www.seque-nom.com), and the sequences are available upon request. After the amplification of polymorphism-spanning fragments by multiplex polymerase chain reaction (PCR), the selected SNPs were genotyped using the MassARRAY system (Sequenom, Inc., San Diego, CA) following the manufacturer's directions (http://www.sequenom.com). SpectroTYPER software (Seque-nom, Inc.) was used to automatically perform genotype calling with a set of digital filters optimized for the mass spectra of oligonucleotides. The individual who analyzed the genotype results was blinded to the clinical data.

Statistical analysis

Hardy-Weinberg equilibrium testing was performed to analyze the allele and genotype frequencies, using the SHEsis online software platform (http://analysis.-bio-x.cn/). Linkage disequilibrium was measured using standardized D', and the discrepancies in allele and geno-type frequencies at single loci between patients and con-trols were compared using a Monte Carlo simulation strategy. The number of observations for each haplotype were compared by $\chi 2$ tests. All reported p values are two-tailed, and statistical significance was set at $p < 0.05$. The relative risk was approximated by the estimate of odds ratio (OR), and for each OR, a 95% confidence interval (CI) was computed. All statistical analyses were performed using the Statistical Package for the Social Sciences (SPSS version 19.0) and GraphPad Prism 6.0 software package (version 6.0 for Windows, GraphPad, La Jolla, CA, USA). For all comparisons, multiple testing for each individual SNP was corrected using the SNPSpD program (http://gump.qimr.edu.au/general/daleN/matSpD/), which is based on the linkage disequi-librium. Multiple testing for each haplotype was cor-rected by the Bonferroni correction. Statistical efficacy was evaluated with G.power 3.1 software.

Results
Overall analysis

Power analysis showed that the current sample size had > 85% power for testing a significant association ($\alpha < 0.05$) when an effect size index of 0.1 was used. The genotypic distribution of the selected SNPs, except for rs6490121 ($p = 0.0338$), did not deviate from Hardy-Wein-berg equilibrium ($p > 0.05$) among the control population (Table 2). Therefore, rs6490121 was excluded from further tests. For the other five SNPs, the genotype frequencies of rs2682826 ($p = 0.046$) were different between all CP pa-tients and the controls, but the differences disappeared after SNPSpD correction (Table 2). There were no signifi-cant differences in the allele and genotype frequencies of rs3782219, rs6490121, rs3741475, rs10774909, and rs2293054 between CP cases and controls.

The SNP pairs rs3741475/rs2682826, rs3741475/rs10774909, and rs10774909/rs2682826 exhibited strong linkage disequilibrium (LD) (D' > 0.9) (Additional file 1: Table S1). Haplotype analysis is a powerful strategy for resolving the controversy regarding association studies based on individual polymorphisms and determining whether the SNPs would have greater predictive value when analyzed together. We analyzed only the common haplotypes comprised of rs10774909, rs3741475, and rs2682826 (those with frequency < 0.01 were excluded from the analysis), but no statistically significant dif-ference was found between all patients and controls (data not shown).

Table 2 Allele and genotype frequencies of SNPs in CP patients and controls

Group	Allele frequency		P	OR (95% CI)	Genotype frequency		P	Hardy-Weinberg equilibrium test
rs3782219	C	T			C/C	T/T		
Case	764 (0.586)	540 (0.414)	0.242	0.910	216 (0.331)	104 (0.160)	0.354	0.936
Control	774 (0.608)	498 (0.392)		(0.778~ 1.066)	235 (0.369)	97 (0.153)	0.939	
rs6490121	A	G			A/A	GG		
Case	831(0.637)	473(0.363)	0.888	0.989	268(0.411)	89(0.137)	0.585	0.0470
Control	814(0.640)	458(0.360)		(0.842~ 1.1609)	272 (0.428)	94 (0.148)	0.047	
rs2293054	A	G			A/A	G/G		
Case	270 (0.207)	1034 (0.793)	0.607	1.052	29 (0.044)	411 (0.630)	0.877	0.204
Control	253 (0.199)	1019 (0.801)		(0.868~ 1.274)	26 (0.041)	409 (0.643)	0.204	
rs10774909	C	G			C/C	G/G		
Case	887 (0.680)	417 (0.320)	0.958	1.004463	293 (0.449)	58 (0.089)	0.496	0.107
Control	864 (0.679)	408 (0.321)		(0.8512~ 1.185)	294 (0.462)	66 (0.104)	0.107	
rs3741475	A	G			A/A	G/G		
Case	335 (0.257)	969 (0.743)	0.519	0.944	35 (0.054)	352 (0.540)	0.094	0.918
Control	341 (0.268)	931 (0.732)		(0.792~ 1.125)	52 (0.082)	347 (0.546)	0.918	
rs2682826	A	G			A/A	G/G		
Case	335 (0.257)	969 (0.743)	0.709	0.967	34 (0.052)	351 (0.538)	0.046	0.835
Control	335 (0.263)	937 (0.737)		(0.811~ 1.153)	52 (0.082)	353 (0.555)	0.835	

Subgroup analysis

CP is highly heterogeneous with regard to clinical presentation, etiology, and pathogenesis. Subgroup analysis was performed to evaluate the potential relationship between genotypes and clinical features such as sex, gestational age, CP subtype, and neonatal complications (Tables 3, 4 and 5). The results of the subgroup analysis indicated significant differences in the allele or genotype frequencies in these CP subgroups, including male sex, birth asphyxia, spastic type, spastic tetraplegia, and NE. However, the associations of rs3741475 and rs2682826 with male CP, rs10774909 with CP + birth asphyxia, and rs2682826 with spastic CP disappeared after adjusting for multiple tests, using the program

Table 3 Allele and genotype frequencies of SNPs in CP patients with spastic tetraplegia and controls

Group	Allele frequency		P	OR (95% CI)	Genotype frequency			P
rs3782219	C	T			C/C	C/T	T/T	
Case	255 (0.536)	221 (0.464)	0.006[a]	0.742	63 (0.265)	129 (0.542)	46 (0.193)	0.013
Control	774 (0.608)	498 (0.392)		(0.600~ 0.918)	235 (0.369)	304 (0.478)	97 (0.153)	
rs2293054	A	G			A/A	A/G	G/G	
Case	110 (0.231)	366 (0.769)	0.140	1.211	16 (0.067)	78 (0.328)	144 (0.605)	0.226
Control	253 (0.199)	1019 (0.801)		(0.939~ 1.560)	26 (0.041)	201 (0.316)	409 (0.643)	
rs10774909	C	G			C/C	C/G	G/G	
Case	328 (0.689)	148 (0.311)	0.695	1.047	106 (0.445)	116 (0.487)	16 (0.067)	0.159
Control	864 (0.679)	408 (0.321)		(0.834~ 1.313)	294 (0.462)	276 (0.434)	66 (0.104)	
rs3741475	A	G			A/A	A/G	G/G	
Case	108 (0.227)	368 (0.773)	0.079	0.801	8 (0.034)	92 (0.387)	138 (0.580)	0.043
Control	341 (0.268)	931 (0.732)		(0.625~ 1.027)	52 (0.082)	237 (0.373)	347 (0.546)	
rs2682826	A	G			A/A	A/G	G/G	
Case	109 (0.229)	367 (0.771)	0.142	0.831	8 (0.034)	93 (0.391)	137 (0.576)	0.042
Control	335 (0.263)	937 (0.737)		(0.649~ 1.064)	52 (0.082)	231 (0.363)	353 (0.555)	

[a] After the SNPSpD correction, $p = 0.023$

Table 4 Haplotype analysis between patients with spastic tetraplegia and controls

Haplotype	case(frequency)	control(frequency)	P-value	OR(95% CI)
C G G	323.66 (0.680)	852.26 (0.670)	0.745	1.039 [0.826~ 1.306]
G A A	103.66 (0.218)	324.60 (0.255)	0.099	0.809 [0.629~ 1.041]
G G G	42.34 (0.089)	74.71 (0.059)	0.025*	1.561 [1.054~ 2.312]
Global result			0.034	

Abbreviations: *OR* odds ratio, *CI* confidence interval
Loci chosen for haplotype analysis: rs10774909, rs229305, rs2682826
Haplotype frequency < 0.01 in both control & case has been dropped
*After Bonferroni correction, p = 0.075

SNPSpD. There were no differences in allele or genotype frequencies in the other CP subgroups classified according to gestational age, birth weight, or fetal growth restriction (data not shown).

Notably, the T allele of *NOS1* SNP rs3782219 was negatively associated with spastic quadriplegia (OR = 0.742, 95% CI = 0.600–0.918, after SNPSpD correction, p value = 0.023) (Table 3). The genotype frequencies of rs3782219 (p = 0.013), rs3741475 (p = 0.043), and rs2682826 (p = 0.042) also showed differences between spastic tetraplegia (n = 238) and controls, but the differences disappeared after SNPSpD correction. The haplotype analysis for rs10774909, rs3741475, and rs2682826 revealed a global P-value of 0.034 (Table 4). The haplotype "GGG" was found to be significantly associated with spastic tetraplegia (OR = 1.561, 95% CI = 1.054~ 2.312, p = 0.025), but the differences

disappeared after Bonferroni correction (p = 0.075). There were significant differences in genotype between CP patients with NE (n = 261) and controls at rs10774909, rs3741475, and rs2682826 (p = 0.005, 0.015, and 0.003, respectively, after SNPSpD correction) (Table 5). The haplotype analysis of the three SNPs did not indicate significant differences between CP patients with NE and control subjects (data not shown).

Discussion

The present study is the first to link a genetic variant with NOS1 gene to CP. We conducted a case-control study that included 652 CP patients and 636 healthy controls. Given that the sample size was sufficient for an appropriate statistical analysis, the likelihood of a type II error appears to be considerably low. Our result has shown that there was no significant association between *NOS1* and susceptibility to CP.

CP cases are highly heterogeneous with regard to both etiology and clinical phenotype, and different clinical phenotypes may have different pathogenesis [29]. Genetic factors might be associated with certain sub-types of CP [30]. According to the stratified analysis of factors such as sex, gestational age, birth weight, risk factors, clinical classification, complications and others. The T allele of *NOS1* SNP rs3782219 was negatively associated with spastic quadriplegia, and the genotype frequencies of rs10774909, rs37841475, and rs2682826 were significantly associated with CP + NE. Both spastic tetraplegia and CP + NE are serious forms of CP, suggesting that NOS1 likely plays a more important role in the pathogenesis of severe CP.

Table 5 Allele and genotype frequencies of SNPs in CP patients with neonatal encephalopathy and controls

Group	Allele frequency		P	OR (95% CI)	Genotype frequency			P
rs3782219	C	T			C/C	C/T	T/T	
Case	300 (0.575)	222 (0.425)	0.185	0.869	82 (0.314)	136 (0.521)	43 (0.165)	0.289
Control	774 (0.608)	498 (0.392)		(0.707~ 1.069)	235 (0.369)	304 (0.478)	97 (0.153)	
rs2293054	A	G			A/A	A/G	G/G	
Case	122 (0.234)	400 (0.766)	0.100	1.228	15 (0.057)	92 (0.352)	154 (0.590)	0.256
Control	253 (0.199)	1019 (0.801)		(0.961~ 1.560)	26 (0.041)	201 (0.316)	409 (0.643)	
rs10774909	C	G			C/C	C/G	G/G	
Case	343 (0.657)	179 (0.343)	0.364	0.905	98 (0.375)	147 (0.563)	16 (0.061)	**0.001**[a]
Control	864 (0.679)	408 (0.321)		(0.729~ 1.123)	294 (0.462)	276 (0.434)	66 (0.104)	
rs3741475	A	G			A/A	A/G	G/G	
Case	145 (0.278)	377 (0.722)	0.675	1.050	10 (0.038)	125 (0.479)	126 (0.483)	**0.003**[b]
Control	341 (0.268)	931 (0.732)		(0.836~ 1.319)	52 (0.082)	237 (0.373)	347 (0.546)	
rs2682826	A	G			A/A	A/G	G/G	
Case	145 (0.278)	377 (0.722)	0.531	1.076	9 (0.034)	127 (0.487)	125 (0.479)	**0.0005**[c]
Control	335 (0.263)	937 (0.737)		(0.856~ 1.352)	52 (0.082)	231 (0.363)	353 (0.555)	

[a]After the SNPSpD correction, p = 0.004; [b]After the SNPSpD correction, p = 0.012; [c]After the SNPSpD correction, p = 0.002

The etiology and pathogenesis of NE are not clear, and the known risk factors include HIE, intracranial hemorrhage, hypoglycemia, severe hyperbilirubinemia, a variety of metabolic disorders, neurodegenerative diseases, and intracranial infection [31]. Those also were risk factors for CP. In addition, NOS1 inhibitors can effectively reduce the degree of an ischemic brain injury. In view of the important role of NO in ischemic brain injuries, the association of the NOS1 gene with CP + NE also indirectly suggests that hypoxic brain damage may play an important role in the pathogenesis of CP.

NO is a highly diffusible gas that easily penetrates biological membranes and participates in a variety of important biological processes in the brain, such as immune responses, the release and delivery of neurotransmitters [32–34]. During intrauterine or hypoxic insults, excessive NO is produced by NOS1 in the cerebral tissue. Abnormal levels of NO have negative effects on the developing fetal brain through a wide range of mechanisms, such as glutamate and N-methyl-D-aspartate receptor (NMDAR) activation, resulting in excitotoxicity, oxidative stress, and inflammatory responses [35, 36]. It has been postulated that NMDA receptors play an essential role in the pathogenesis of CP [37, 38]. NMDA receptors are essential for excitatory synaptic transmission in the CNS. During in the process of hypoxic injury, excessive NO trigger the activity of NMDA receptors, leading to intracellular calcium ion influx, lipid peroxidation and free radical production. Those processes ultimately results in neuronal cell injury and irreversible brain damage. NMDA receptors were highly expressed in oligodendrocytes where glutamate toxicity could damage the myelin sheath that implies a role in synaptic stability and neuronal activity [39, 40].

The human NOS1 gene is composed of 29 exons and 28 introns and maps to 12q24, which spans more than a 160 kb genomic region [41]. Moreover, its expression patterns are associated with the promoter-exon1 region [42]. Associations of NOS1 with various diseases have been reported, such as schizophrenia, Parkinson's disease, suicide, achalasia, multiple sclerosis, ischemic stroke, and hypertension. In previous studies found that the T allele of rs2293054 was associated with lower NIHSS scores and with NIHSS scores of ischemic stroke patients in different inherited model [43]. But in our result, rs2293054 showed no relationship with CP. To our knowledge only several studies are to investigate the relationship of rs3782219 SNP and rs3741475 with clinical diseases, it showed no relationship with disorders. However, we found the T allele of NOS1 SNP rs3782219 was negatively associated with spastic quadriplegia. The genotype frequencies of rs3741475 was significantly associated with CP + NE. Therefore, the T-allele of the rs3782219 and genotype of rs3741475 may contribute to the pathogenesis of clinical phenotypes in CP patients.

The synonymous SNP (rs2682826) located in the 3'-UTR of exon 29 of the NOS1 gene was selected as the tag SNP for one of the most frequent haplotypes. The SNP rs2682826 is located close to several miRNA-binding sites in the gene's 3'-UTR, and it likely affects the stability and translational efficiency of mRNA [43–45]. Some polymorphisms in NOS1 gene can directly affect the expression of mRNA, which change the levels of NO [46, 47]. While the majority of SNPs located in intron region do not affect the amino acid sequence, but they may be indirectly involved in the regulation of NOS1 expression or might be in linkage disequilibrium with a functional site. Rujescu et al. (2008) reported that the CGG haplotype which consists of 3 SNPs of NOS1 gene including rs2682826 SNP was significantly associated with suicide attempts [48]. The genotype frequencies of rs107749909, rs37841475, and rs2682826 were significantly associated with CP + NE, respectively. But the haplotype consisted of three highly linkage SNPs was no significantly associated with CP + NE. Future association studies with more systemic SNPs selection are thought to be needed to clarify the involvement of NOS1 in CP.

The etiology and pathogenesis of CP are complex. Regarding the genetic mechanism, CP may exhibit different genetic patterns, and the disease is polygenic in most CP cases. Although genome-wide association studies (GWASs) have been successful in identifying many cerebral disorder-associated loci, no GWAS on CP has been performed, and most of the CP-related genes have not been identified. Because of the complicated genetic architecture of CP, multiple genes might be involved in the etiology of CP, and the effect size of each individual risk allele is likely to be small. Moreover, the factors underlying inter-individual variations in the susceptibility to CP may also include demographic, clinical, and environmental variables. Our results need to be validated or replicated in other, larger population samples.

Conclusions

There was no significant association between NOS1 gene polymorphisms and CP at the total level, but NOS1 was associated with spastic tetraplegia and CP + NE, suggesting that NOS1 may play a more important role in the pathogenesis of severe forms of CP. However, we only assessed five SNPs of the NOS1 gene, and it is necessary to explore more NOS1 gene variants. It is important to note that a comprehensive evaluation of the NOS1 gene and CP requires a large sample for which sample independence can be validated and functional evidence is available. Furthermore, functional studies on the impact of these polymorphisms on gene expression in CP populations might help to define new therapeutic perspectives for CP.

Abbreviations

CI: Confidence interval; CP: Cerebral palsy; HWE: Hardy-weinberg equilibrium; MAF: Minor allele frequency; NE: Neonatal encephalopathy; NOS1: Nitric oxide synthase 1; OR: Odds ratio; SNP: Single nucleotide polymorphism

Acknowledgements

We thank all participants involved in this study and all authors.

Funding

This work was supported by the Shanghai Municipal Commission of Science and Technology Program (14DJ1400101), the Fourth Round of Shanghai Three-year Action Plan on Public Health Discipline and Talent Program: Women and Children's Health (No. 15GWZK0401), the National Natural Science Foundation of China (grants 31611130035,31371274, U1604165), VINNMER–Marie Curie international qualification (VINNOVA, 2015–04780), the Swedish Medical Research Council (VR 2015–06276), Swedish governmental grants to researchers in the public health service (ALFGBG-429271) and the 973 Projects (2011CB710801). The funding sponsors had no role in the design of the study, collection, analysis and interpretation of data and in writing the manuscript.

Authors' contributions

QX and CZ conceived and designed the study. LX, QS, DZ, JS, YW and XW recruited subjects and sorted out clinical information. YW and DB performed all of the laboratory work. TY performed all data and statistical analysis. YT drafted the manuscript. All authors have read and approved the final manuscript.

Competing interests

The authors declare that they have no competing interests.

Author details

[1]Children's Hospital and Institutes of Biomedical Sciences, Fudan University, Wanyuan Road 399, Minhang District, Shanghai 201102, China. [2]Henan Key Laboratory of Child Brain Injury, Third Affiliated Hospital of Zhengzhou University, Kangfuqian Street 7, Zhengzhou 450052, China. [3]Department of Pediatrics, Zhengzhou Children's Hospital, Zhengzhou 450053, China. [4]Perinatal Center, Institute of Neuroscience and Physiology, University of Gothenburg, Gothenburg 40530, Sweden. [5]Center for Brain Repair and Rehabilitation, Department of Clinical Neuroscience, Sahlgrenska Academy, University of Gothenburg, Gothenburg 40530, Sweden. [6]Shanghai Center for Women and Children's Health, Shanghai 200062, China.

References

1. Bax M, Goldstein M, Rosenbaum P, Leviton A, Paneth N, Dan B, Jacobsson B, Damiano D. Proposed definition and classification of cerebral palsy, April 2005. Dev Med Child Neurol. 2005;47(8):571–6.

2. Colver A, Fairhurst C, Pharoah PO. Cerebral palsy. Lancet. 2014;383(9924):1240–9.

3. Tosi LL, Maher N, Moore DW, Goldstein M, Aisen ML. Adults with cerebral palsy: a workshop to define the challenges of treating and preventing secondary musculoskeletal and neuromuscular complications in this rapidly growing population. Dev Med Child Neurol. 2009;51(Suppl 4):2–11.

4. Weichselbraun A, Gindl S, Scharl A. Enriching semantic knowledge bases for opinion mining in big data applications. Knowl Based Syst. 2014;69:78–85.

5. Badawi N, Keogh JM. Causal pathways in cerebral palsy. J Paediatr Child Health. 2013;49(1):5–8.

6. Wu YW, Xing G, Fuentes-Afflick E, Danielson B, Smith LH, Gilbert WM. Racial, ethnic, and socioeconomic disparities in the prevalence of cerebral palsy. Pediatrics. 2011;127(3):e674–81.

7. Rajab A, Yoo SY, Abdulgalil A, Kathiri S, Ahmed R, Mochida GH, Bodell A, Barkovich AJ, Walsh CA. An autosomal recessive form of spastic cerebral palsy (CP) with microcephaly and mental retardation. Am J Med Genet A. 2006;140(14):1504–10.

8. Garne E, Dolk H, Krageloh-Mann I, Holst RS, Cans C. Cerebral palsy and congenital malformations. Eur J Paediatr Neurol. 2008;12(2):82–8.

9. Oskoui M, Gazzellone MJ, Thiruvahindrapuram B, Zarrei M, Andersen J, Wei J, Wang Z, Wintle RF, Marshall CR, Cohn RD, et al. Clinically relevant copy number variations detected in cerebral palsy. Nat Commun. 2015;6:7949.

10. Segel R, Ben-Pazi H, Zeligson S, Fatal-Valevski A, Aran A, Gross-Tsur V, Schneebaum-Sender N, Shmueli D, Lev D, Perlberg S, et al. Copy number variations in cryptogenic cerebral palsy. Neurology. 2015;84(16):1660–8.

11. O'Callaghan ME, Maclennan AH, Gibson CS, McMichael GL, Haan EA, Broadbent JL, Goldwater PN, Painter JN, Montgomery GW, Dekker GA. Fetal and maternal candidate single nucleotide polymorphism associations with cerebral palsy: a case-control study. Pediatrics. 2012;129(2):e414–23.

12. Nelson KB, Dambrosia JM, Iovannisci DM, Cheng S, Grether JK, Lammer E. Genetic polymorphisms and cerebral palsy in very preterm infants. Pediatr Res. 2005;57(4):494–9.

13. Bi D, Chen M, Zhang X, Wang H, Xia L, Shang Q, Li T, Zhu D, Blomgren K, He L, et al. The association between sex-related interleukin-6 gene polymorphisms and the risk for cerebral palsy. J Neuroinflammation. 2014;11:100.

14. Hou R, Ren X, Wang J, Guan X. TNF-alpha and MTHFR polymorphisms associated with cerebral palsy in Chinese infants. Mol Neurobiol. 2016; 53(10):6653–8.

15. Alderton WK, Cooper CE, Knowles RG. Nitric oxide synthases: structure, function and inhibition. Biochem J. 2001;357(Pt 3):593–615.

16. Khaldi A, Chiueh CC, Bullock MR, Woodward JJ. The significance of nitric oxide production in the brain after injury. Ann N Y Acad Sci. 2002;962:53–9.

17. Contestabile A, Ciani E. Role of nitric oxide in the regulation of neuronal proliferation, survival and differentiation. Neurochem Int. 2004;45(6):903–14.

18. Estrada C, Murillo-Carretero M. Nitric oxide and adult neurogenesis in health and disease. Neuroscientist. 2005;11(4):294–307.

19. Contestabile A, Monti B, Contestabile A, Ciani E. Brain nitric oxide and its dual role in neurodegeneration/neuroprotection: understanding molecular mechanisms to devise drug approaches. Curr Med Chem. 2003;10(20):2147–74.

20. Derrick M, Drobyshevsky A, Ji X, Chen L, Yang Y, Ji H, Silverman RB, Tan S. Hypoxia–ischemia causes persistent movement deficits in a perinatal rabbit model of cerebral palsy: assessed by a new swim test. Int J Dev Neurosci. 2009;27(6):549–57.

21. Ma MW, Wang J, Zhang Q, Wang R, Dhandapani KM, Vadlamudi RK, Brann DW. NADPH oxidase in brain injury and neurodegenerative disorders. Mol Neurodegener. 2017;12(1):7.

22. Reif A, Grunblatt E, Herterich S, Wichart I, Rainer MK, Jungwirth S, Danielczyk W, Deckert J, Tragl KH, Riederer P, et al. Association of a functional NOS1 promoter repeat with Alzheimer's disease in the VITA cohort. J Alzheimers Dis. 2011;23(2):327–33.

23. Shinkai T, Ohmori O, Hori H, Nakamura J. Allelic association of the neuronal nitric oxide synthase (NOS1) gene with schizophrenia. Mol Psychiatry. 2002; 7(6):560–3.

24. Hancock DB, Martin ER, Vance JM, Scott WK. Nitric oxide synthase genes and their interactions with environmental factors in Parkinson's disease. Neurogenetics. 2008;9(4):249–62.

25. Ferriero DM, Holtzman DM, Black SM, Sheldon RA. Neonatal mice lacking neuronal nitric oxide synthase are less vulnerable to hypoxic-ischemic injury. Neurobiol Dis. 1996;3(1):64–71.

26. Ji H, Tan S, Igarashi J, Li H, Derrick M, Martasek P, Roman LJ, Vasquez-Vivar J, Poulos TL, Silverman RB. Selective neuronal nitric oxide synthase inhibitors and the prevention of cerebral palsy. Ann Neurol. 2009;65(2):209–17.

27. Sellier E, Surman G, Himmelmann K, Andersen G, Colver A, Krageloh-Mann I, De-la-Cruz J, Cans C. Trends in prevalence of cerebral palsy in children born with a birthweight of 2,500 g or over in Europe from 1980 to 1998. Eur J Epidemiol. 2010;25(9):635–42.

28. Shang Q, Zhou C, Liu D, Li W, Chen M, Xu Y, Wang F, Bi D, Zhang X, Zhao X, et al. Association Between Osteopontin Gene Polymorphisms and Cerebral Palsy in a Chinese Population. Neuromolecular Med. 2016;18(2): 232–8.

29. Chang MC, Jang SH, Yoe SS, Lee E, Kim S, Lee DG, Son SM. Diffusion tensor imaging demonstrated radiologic differences between diplegic and quadriplegic cerebral palsy. Neurosci Lett. 2012;512(1):53–8.

30. Nelson KB. Causative factors in cerebral palsy. Clin Obstet Gynecol. 2008; 51(4):749–62.

31. Battin M, Sadler L, Masson V, Farquhar C. Neonatal encephalopathy in New Zealand: Demographics and clinical outcome. J Paediatr Child Health. 2016; 52(6):632–6.

32. Tan S, Zhou F, Nielsen VG, Wang Z, Gladson CL, Parks DA. Sustained hypoxia-ischemia results in reactive nitrogen and oxygen species production and injury in the premature fetal rabbit brain. J Neuropathol Exp Neurol. 1998;57(6):544–53.

33. Tan S, Zhou F, Nielsen VG, Wang Z, Gladson CL, Parks DA. Increased injury following intermittent fetal hypoxia-reoxygenation is associated with increased free radical production in fetal rabbit brain. J Neuropathol Exp Neurol. 1999;58(9):972–81.

34. Baig MS, Zaichick SV, Mao M, de Abreu AL, Bakhshi FR, Hart PC, Saqib U, Deng J, Chatterjee S, Block ML, et al. NOS1-derived nitric oxide promotes NF-kappaB transcriptional activity through inhibition of suppressor of cytokine signaling-1. J Exp Med. 2015;212(10):1725–38.

35. Costantine MM, Clark EA, Lai Y, Rouse DJ, Spong CY, Mercer BM, Sorokin Y, Thorp JJ, Ramin SM, Malone FD, et al. Association of polymorphisms in neuroprotection and oxidative stress genes and neurodevelopmental outcomes after preterm birth. Obstet Gynecol. 2012;120(3):542–50.

36. Buhimschi CS, Baumbusch MA, Dulay AT, Oliver EA, Lee S, Zhao G, Bhandari V, Ehrenkranz RA, Weiner CP, Madri JA, et al. Characterization of RAGE, HMGB1, and S100beta in inflammation-induced preterm birth and fetal tissue injury. Am J Pathol. 2009;175(3):958–75.

37. Wallin C, Puka-Sundvall M, Hagberg H, Weber SG, Sandberg M. Alterations in glutathione and amino acid concentrations after hypoxia-ischemia in the immature rat brain. Brain Res Dev Brain Res. 2000;125(1-2):51–60.

38. Costantine MM, Drever N. Antenatal exposure to magnesium sulfate and neuroprotection in preterm infants. Obstet Gynecol Clin North Am. 2011; 38(2):351–66.

39. Mayer ML. Glutamate receptors at atomic resolution. Nature. 2006;440(7083): 456–62.

40. Karadottir R, Cavelier P, Bergersen LH, Attwell D. NMDA receptors are expressed in oligodendrocytes and activated in ischaemia. Nature. 2005; 438(7071):1162–6.

41. Hall AV, Antoniou H, Wang Y, Cheung AH, Arbus AM, Olson SL, Lu WC, Kau CL, Marsden PA. Structural organization of the human neuronal nitric oxide synthase gene (NOS1). J Biol Chem. 1994;269(52):33082–90.

42. Bros M, Boissel JP, Godtel-Armbrust U, Forstermann U. Transcription of human neuronal nitric oxide synthase mRNAs derived from different first exons is partly controlled by exon 1-specific promoter sequences. Genomics. 2006;87(4):463–73.

43. Yoo SD, Park JS, Yun DH, Kim HS, Kim SK, Kim DH, Chon J, Je G, Kim YS, Chung JH, et al. Polymorphism of nitric oxide synthase 1 affects the clinical phenotypes of ischemic stroke in Korean population. Ann Rehabil Med. 2016;40(1):102–10.

44. Mignone F, Gissi C, Liuni S, Pesole G. Untranslated regions of mRNAs. Genome Biol. 2002;3(3):S4.

45. Chatterjee S, Pal JK. Role of 5′- and 3′-untranslated regions of mRNAs in human diseases. Biol Cell. 2009;101(5):251–62.

46. Reif A, Herterich S, Strobel A, Ehlis AC, Saur D, Jacob CP, Wienker T, Topner T, Fritzen S, Walter U, et al. A neuronal nitric oxide synthase (NOS-I) haplotype associated with schizophrenia modifies prefrontal cortex function. Mol Psychiatry. 2006;11(3):286–300.

47. Fallin MD, Lasseter VK, Avramopoulos D, Nicodemus KK, Wolyniec PS, McGrath JA, Steel G, Nestadt G, Liang KY, Huganir RL, et al. Bipolar I disorder and schizophrenia: a 440-single-nucleotide polymorphism screen of 64 candidate genes among Ashkenazi Jewish case-parent trios. Am J Hum Genet. 2005;77(6):918–36.

48. Rujescu D, Giegling I, Mandelli L, Schneider B, Hartmann AM, Schnabel A, Maurer K, Moller HJ, Serretti A. NOS-I and -III gene variants are differentially associated with facets of suicidal behavior and aggression-related traits. Am J Med Genet B Neuropsychiatr Genet. 2008;147B(1):42–8.

17

Toward the precision breast cancer survival prediction utilizing combined whole genome-wide expression and somatic mutation analysis

Yifan Zhang[1], William Yang[2], Dan Li[1], Jack Y Yang[1], Renchu Guan[1] and Mary Qu Yang[1*]

From Selected articles from the IEEE BIBM International Conference on Bioinformatics & Biomedicine (BIBM) 2017: medical genomics
Kansas City, MO, USA. 13-16 November 2017

Abstract

Background: Breast cancer is the most common type of invasive cancer in woman. It accounts for approximately 18% of all cancer deaths worldwide. It is well known that somatic mutation plays an essential role in cancer development. Hence, we propose that a prognostic prediction model that integrates somatic mutations with gene expression can improve survival prediction for cancer patients and also be able to reveal the genetic mutations associated with survival.

Method: Differential expression analysis was used to identify breast cancer related genes. Genetic algorithm (GA) and univariate Cox regression analysis were applied to filter out survival related genes. DAVID was used for enrichment analysis on somatic mutated gene set. The performance of survival predictors were assessed by Cox regression model and concordance index(C-index).

Results: We investigated the genome-wide gene expression profile and somatic mutations of 1091 breast invasive carcinoma cases from The Cancer Genome Atlas (TCGA). We identified 118 genes with high hazard ratios as breast cancer survival risk gene candidates (log rank $p < 0.0001$ and c-index = 0.636). Multiple breast cancer survival related genes were found in this gene set, including *FOXR2*, *FOXD1*, *MTNR1B* and *SDC1*. Further genetic algorithm (GA) revealed an optimal gene set consisted of 88 genes with higher c-index (log rank $p < 0.0001$ and c-index = 0.656). We validated this gene set on an independent breast cancer data set and achieved a similar performance (log rank $p < 0.0001$ and c-index = 0.614). Moreover, we revealed 25 functional annotations, 15 gene ontology terms and 14 pathways that were significantly enriched in the genes that showed distinct mutation patterns in the different survival risk groups. These functional gene sets were used as new features for the survival prediction model. In particular, our results suggested that the Fanconi anemia pathway had an important role in breast cancer prognosis.

(Continued on next page)

* Correspondence: mqyang@ualr.edu
[1]MidSouth Bioinformatics Center and Joint Bioinformatics Ph.D. Program of University of Arkansas at Little Rock and Univ. of Arkansas Medical Sciences, 2801 S. Univ. Ave, Little Rock 72204, USA
Full list of author information is available at the end of the article

(Continued from previous page)

Conclusions: Our study indicated that the expression levels of the gene signatures remain the effective indicators for breast cancer survival prediction. Combining the gene expression information with other types of features derived from somatic mutations can further improve the performance of survival prediction. The pathways that were associated with survival risk suggested by our study can be further investigated for improving cancer patient survival.

Keywords: Breast Cancer, Somatic mutations, Whole genome-wide expression, Survival analysis, Precision survival prediction

Background

Breast cancer is the most commonly occurring female cancer in developed countries. Over 40,000 breast cancer deaths and approximately 250,000 new cases were reported in 2016 [1]. The survival rate in HER2+ breast cancer patients [2] has been remarkably increased through targeted therapies including tyrosine kinase inhibitors. Adjuvant treatments such as chemotherapy also improved the 5-year survival rate of the breast patients [3, 4]. However, the significant side effects of chemotherapy can shorten the lifespan of cancer patients in some cases [5]. Additionally, due to potential metastasis and invasion of cancer, the overall outcome for breast cancer patients remains bleak. An effective survival predictor, which is capable of helping cancer treatment and foreseeing the clinical outcomes, can improve life quality and lifespan of cancer patients. Thus, better prognostic biomarkers of survival risk prediction are needed.

In clinical practice, clinicopathological prognostic indicators, such as tumor size, lymph node (LN) status and pathological grade [6, 7] have been widely used in prognostic analysis models. However, in some cases, the treatment responses vary greatly even with similar prognoses. Recently, single cell genomics analysis have shown that ostensibly similar tumor defined by traditional pathological analysis could be distinct diseases at the cell levels [8–10]. Due to the highly heterogeneous nature of cancer cells, the predictive ability of some traditional indicators can be less effective for over 50% of patients [11].

Multiple survival analysis models have developed mainly based on gene expression profiles. The cox regression model and machine learning algorithms have been widely used to reveal molecular signatures related to survival. Bair et al. [12] used semi-supervised methods to cluster patients with different survival risk based on gene expression profiles and clinical data. Sun et al. [13] applied univariate Cox regression analysis and identified nine long noncoding RNAs (lncRNAs) that were highly associated with their metastasis-free survival for breast cancer patients. Zhang et al. [14] developed a two-stage method, using Bayesian hierarchical Cox model and the penalized Cox model, and incorporated pathway information with gene expression profiles to predict survival.

Most survival prediction methods mainly utilize gene expression profiles. Somatic mutations are involved in the cancer development [15]. Several studies showed that genetic mutations are associated with cancer survival, such as BRCA1- and BRCA2-related mutations, and HER2 somatic mutations [16, 17]. Thus, identifying survival related mutations are meaningful for prognosis and treatment. However, it is difficult to detect mutation patterns in a patient cohort for survival analysis since most commonly mutated genes are found in less than 10% of patients. Consequently, using common mutations alone to predict survival is less effective. To address this issue, we integrated somatic mutations with pathway, function annotation and gene ontology (GO) analysis. We then synergistically used the significantly mutated gene sets as predictors coupled with gene expression for survival analysis. Our results suggested that combining somatic mutations improved the performance of survival risk prediction.

Results

Gene differential expression and survival risk detection

We identified 4327 differentially expressed genes (adjust P-value < 0.01 and $|logFC| > 2$) based on the gene expression profile for 1091 breast cancer patients (151 deceased and 940 living) and 113 normal tissue samples, using the software tools developed in our laboratory (http://mqyang.net) along with other existing tools. Next, we applied univariate cox regression analysis to select the differential expressed genes that were also associated with survival. Out of 4327 genes, 330 were significantly associated with survival time (P-value $<$ 0.05). The patients were clustered into two distinct groups, high survival risk and low survival risk, using k-means according to the expression levels of 330 survival-related genes. Then, a Cox proportional hazards model was fitted to the patient survival data for the two groups (Fig. 1a). We calculated the Concordance index (C-index) to assess the predictive ability of our survival model. The C-index measures the concordance between the observed survival times and predicted survival times. The C-index of 330 gene signature-based model was 0.584 (P-value = 0.0011).

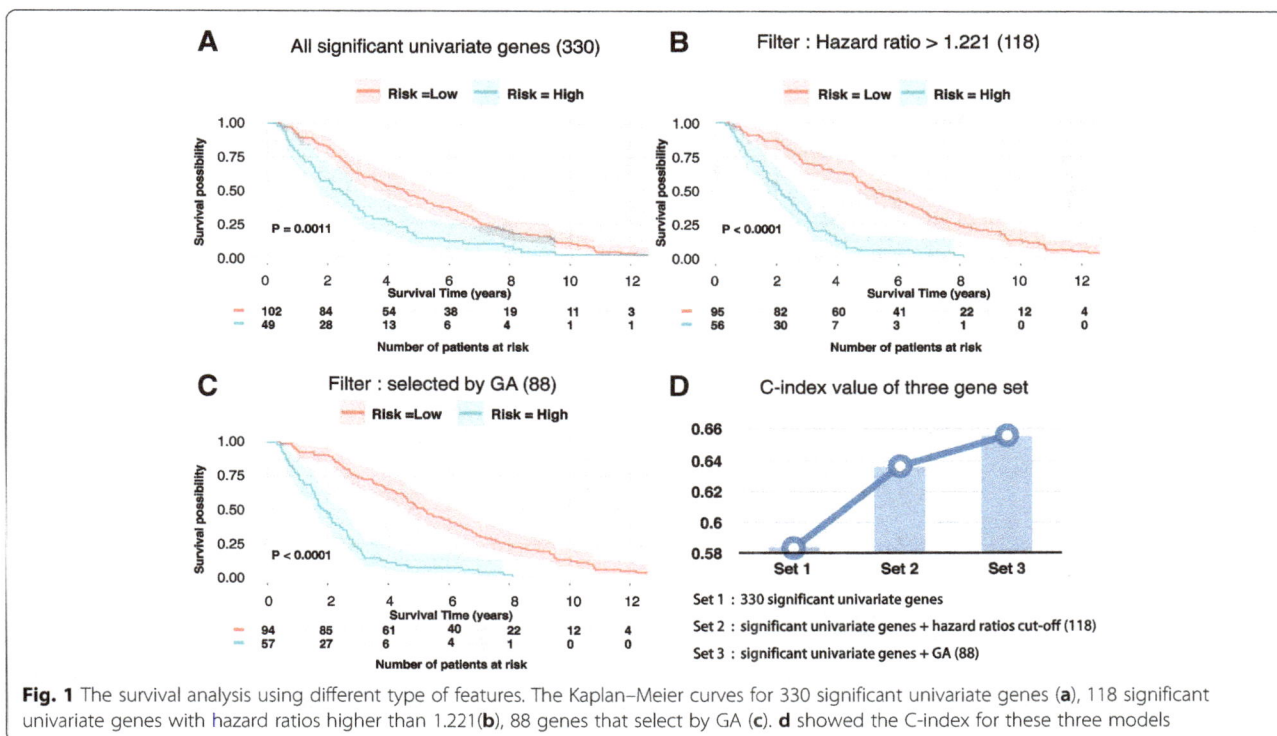

Fig. 1 The survival analysis using different type of features. The Kaplan–Meier curves for 330 significant univariate genes (**a**), 118 significant univariate genes with hazard ratios higher than 1.221(**b**), 88 genes that select by GA (**c**). **d** showed the C-index for these three models

Out of the 330 genes, we further selected 118 genes with hazard ratio > 1.221. The resulting new prediction model yielded a higher C-index, 0.636.(P-value < 0.001). According to Kaplan–Meier curve (Fig. 1b), the survival rate of 1500 days (4 years and 1 month) was 63.2% and 12.5% for patients in the low risk group and high risk group, respectively (Fig. 1b). The 118 genes contained several well-known breast cancer survival related genes or oncogenes, including *FOXR2*, *FOXD1*, *MTNR1B* and *SDC1* [18–24]. Additionally, PANTHER [25] pathway analysis revealed 17 biological processes that were significantly enriched in the 118 genes (Additional file 1). Some are known biological process related to cancer, such as: DNA replication (P-value = 0.037), structural molecule activity (P-value = 0.00035), system development (P-value =0.00047), and cytoskeleton (P-value 0.000062) [26–28], while some others have not been well studied (Additional file 1), such as peptide cross-linking (P-value=0.00027).

Survival-related genes selected by genetic algorithm
We developed a genetic algorithm (GA)-based method to further optimize gene selection from original 330 significant univariate genes. The method is able to assess the combinatorial effects of multiple genes on survival. As a result, 88 genes were revealed as the optimal gene set which maximized the C-index. Using this gene set, we conducted survival analysis (Fig. 1c) and achieved a better c-index 0.656 compared to 0.636 yielded by the model constructed based on the 118

genes selected by hazard ratio. We found that 67 of 88 (75.3%) genes were overlapped with the 118-gene set. Hence, hazard ratio from the univariate test may not be the only factor that determines the prediction accuracy. Nevertheless, genes with higher hazard ratio tend to have higher possibility to generate more accurate survival prediction. (Fig. 2a).

We obtained an independent data set from Molecular Taxonomy of Breast Cancer International Consortium (METABRIC) [29] to validate our models. This dataset includes the expression profile and clinical data for 2509 breast cancer tissue samples. We found 61 genes in the 88-gene set and 64 genes in the 118-gene set shown in the expression profile of this patient cohort. Similar data normalization and survival analysis were performed. The models based on both gene sets were able to separate the high-risk and low-risk survival groups (P-value < 0.0001, Fig. 2b and Additional file 2). The C-index was 0.614 and 0.6004 for the models based on 61 GA-selected genes and 64 hazard-ratio-selected genes, respectively. Consistent with the result for the TCGA dataset, the gene set that was identified by GA searching yielded higher prediction accuracy.

Survival-related somatic mutations
A total of 105,425 single-nucleotide variances (SNVs) were identified in 1044 breast cancer patient samples (1044 of 1091 patients have mutation data). The maximum and median SNV mutation rate was 10.4% and

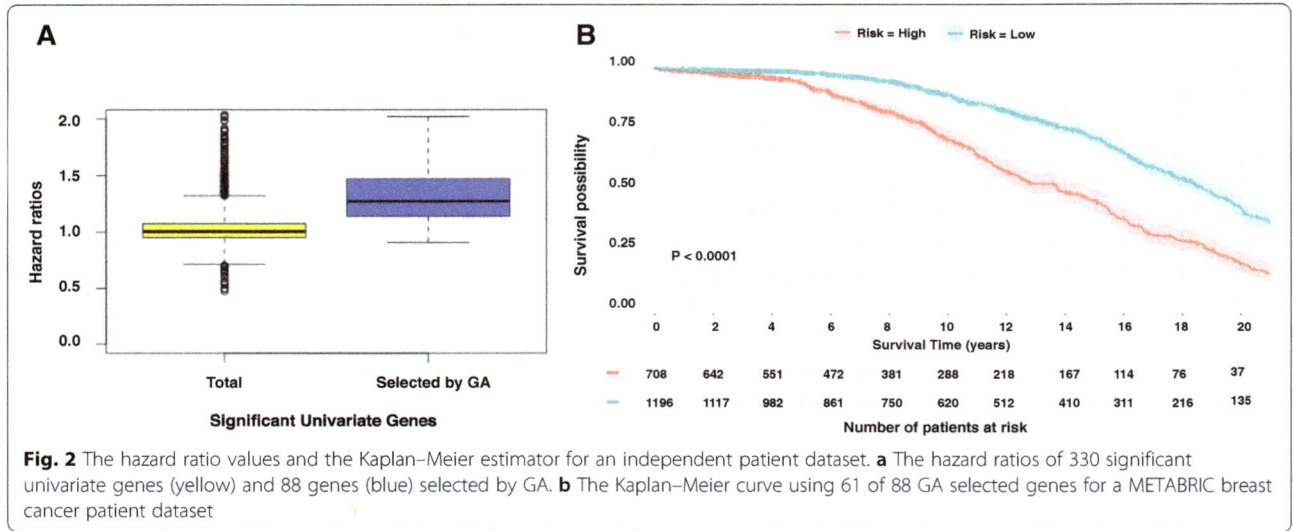

Fig. 2 The hazard ratio values and the Kaplan–Meier estimator for an independent patient dataset. **a** The hazard ratios of 330 significant univariate genes (yellow) and 88 genes (blue) selected by GA. **b** The Kaplan–Meier curve using 61 of 88 GA selected genes for a METABRIC breast cancer patient dataset

0.095%, respectively (Fig. 3a), while the maximum and median gene mutation rate was 32.95% and 0.48%, respectively. rs121913279 was the most frequent SNP, which was located at the *PIK3CA* gene. *TP53*, *PIK3CA*, *TTN*, *CDH1*, *GATA3*, *MUC16*, *KMT2C* and *MAP3K1* were the top frequently mutated genes (Fig. 3a). The gene pairs consisting of these eight genes have differential mutation patterns, four pairs tend to mutual exclusively, while six pairs tend to be co-occurred (P-adjust <= 0.008) (Table 1). The C-index and *P*-value of the survival model based on these eight top mutated genes were 0.539 and 0.085. We expanded the mutated gene list to 88, 118, 330, which matched the number of differential genes used in the survival models. The resulting c-index for these different gene signature set was 0.565, 0.522

and 0.567, and corresponding P-value was 0.035, 0.23 and 0.028. Thus, the top mutated genes were not necessarily effective gene signatures for survival prediction; the correlation coefficient of gene mutation rates and P-values of the univariate tests was − 0.22 (Fig. 3b).

To combine gene expression and mutation for survival analysis, we first clustered the breast cancer patients into two groups (high survival risk and low survival risk) based on the expression levels of 118 genes. Then we analyzed the corresponding somatic mutation profiles for the patients in the distinct groups. We found that 48,404 and 57,024 SNVs were found for the patients in the high-risk group and the low risk group, respectively.

We compared the percentage of different types of SNVs in the two groups (Fig. 4a). The C- > G and G- > C SNVs

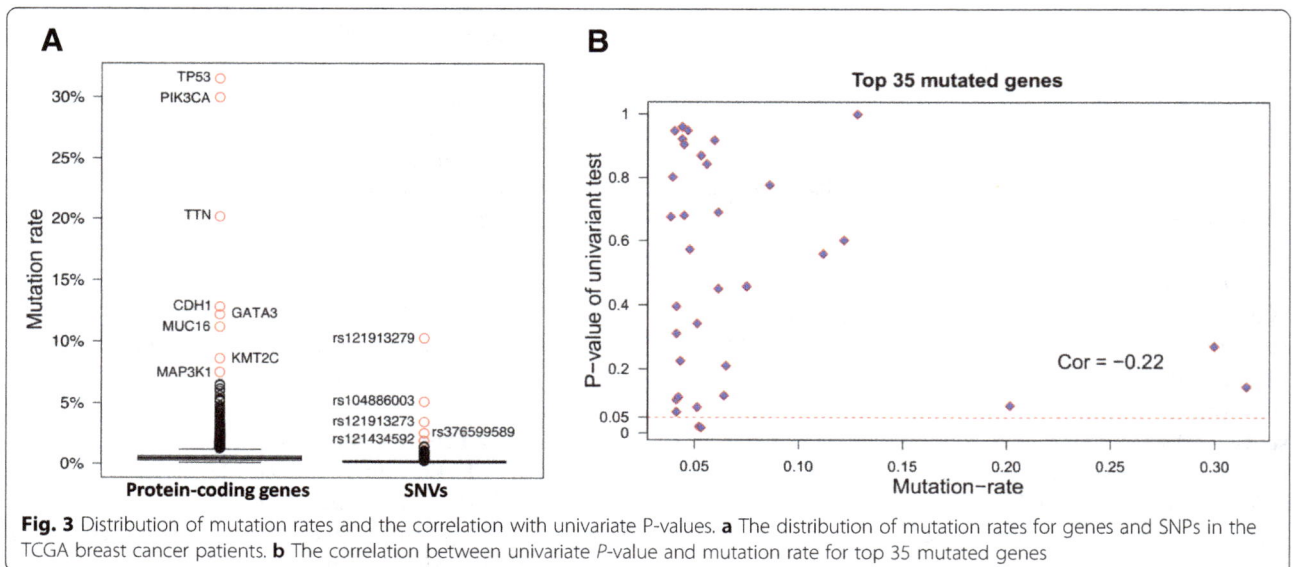

Fig. 3 Distribution of mutation rates and the correlation with univariate P-values. **a** The distribution of mutation rates for genes and SNPs in the TCGA breast cancer patients. **b** The correlation between univariate *P*-value and mutation rate for top 35 mutated genes

Table 1 The top mutated genes in the TCGA 1044 breast cancer dataset

Gene A	Gene B	A Not B	B Not A	Both	Log Odds Ratio	Adjusted *p*-Value	Tendency
TP53	*CDH1*	338	125	9	−2.067	< 0.001	Mutual exclusivity
TP53	*GATA3*	336	116	11	−1.771	< 0.001	Mutual exclusivity
TP53	*MAP3K1*	336	79	11	−1.327	< 0.001	Mutual exclusivity
TP53	*PIK3CA*	265	266	82	−0.641	< 0.001	Mutual exclusivity
PIK3CA	*CDH1*	284	70	64	0.735	0.002	Co-occurrence
TP53	*TTN*	264	104	83	0.62	0.004	Co-occurrence
PIK3CA	*KMT2C*	296	55	52	0.75	0.006	Co-occurrence
TTN	*KMT2C*	154	74	33	0.846	0.007	Co-occurrence
PIK3CA	*MAP3K1*	303	45	45	0.798	0.008	Co-occurrence
TTN	*MUC16*	146	68	41	1.209	< 0.001	Co-occurrence

frequencies in the high-risk group were significantly higher than these SNVs (13.1% versus 8.31%, 12.6% versus 7.82%) in the low risk group (t-test, P-value = 5.5e-14, P-value = 1.3e-14). We thus used C- > G and G- > C SNP frequencies as the two features to perform survival analysis. The survival risk curves showed a noticeable yet insignificant difference (P-value= 0.36). Combining the 118 gene expression with C- > G and G- > C SNP frequencies, we conduct another survival analysis. We obtained similar prediction accuracy as using the gene expression alone (Fig. 4b). Our results suggested that GC SNV frequencies were weaker features for survival prediction.

We also calculated the mutation rates of all genes in the high-risk and low-risk groups. The mutation rate here refers to the percentage of the patients who harbored somatic mutation(s) in a specific gene in the patient group. Then we computed the mutation rate differential scores (MRDS)(Method) for each individual genes.

Some genes showed quite distinct mutation rates in the different groups. For example, the mutation rates of *TP53* in the high and low risk group were 0.634 and 0.208, respectively. We selected the top 2000 genes ranked by MRDS. Multiples genes in this list present in breast cancer related pathways. For example, *ATM, ATR, TP53, PTEN, CASP8, and IGFBP3* participate in p53 signal pathway, while *MMP, EGFR, CREP, PLC, and RAS* participate in estrogen signaling pathway.

Based on DAVID analysis [30, 31], we identified 30 pathways, 114 functional annotations and 38 Gene Ontology (GO) terms that were significantly enriched of the 2000 mutated genes (P-value < 0.05). We then build new features using these molecular function gene sets. If a patient carried mutation(s) in at least one gene of individual enriched function gene sets, we set the corresponding feature value as 1; otherwise we set the value as 0. Then we performed a univariate Cox regression analysis for each of new features. As a result, we

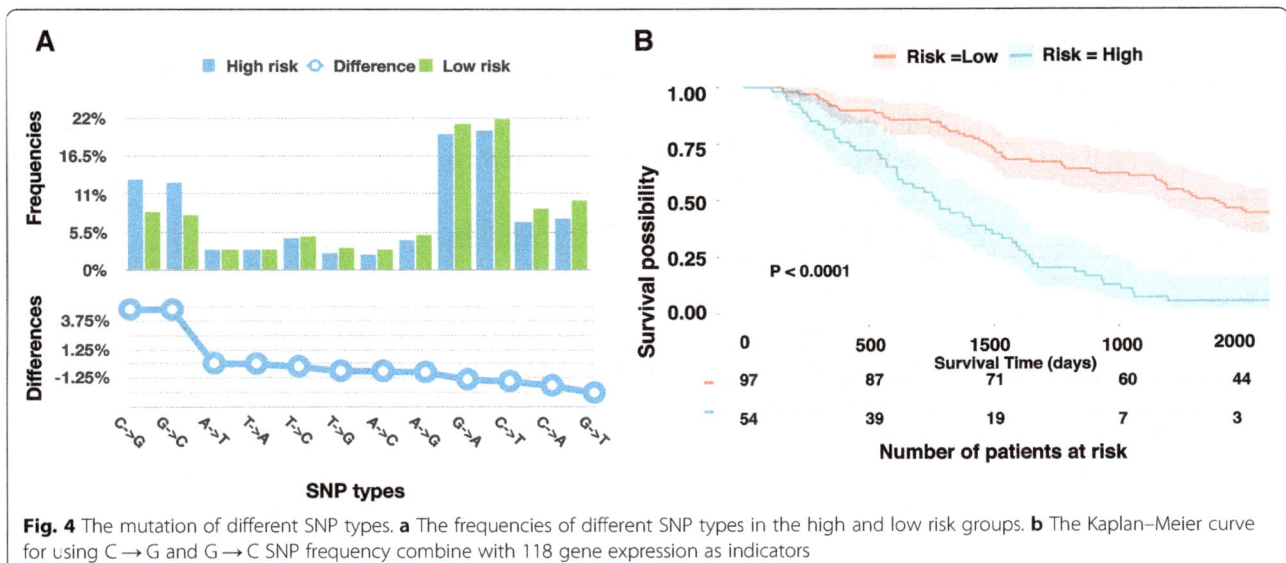

Fig. 4 The mutation of different SNP types. **a** The frequencies of different SNP types in the high and low risk groups. **b** The Kaplan–Meier curve for using C → G and G → C SNP frequency combine with 118 gene expression as indicators

identified 15 function annotations (FA), 15 GO terms and 14 pathways that were significant in the univariate test (*P*-value < 0.05 and hazard ratio > 1.221). Using a total of 54 mutated functional gene set, the C-index survival model was 0.591 (P-value = 0.0016). The C-index of the models that utilized different type of gene set (Table 2) showed that integrating gene expression and mutation analysis generated a survival model with better accuracy (Table 2) (Fig. 4b).

Discussion

The gene signatures derived from expression profiles have commonly been used in survival analysis [18–21, 24]. The survival-related genes are often selected through the univariate regression model. The resulting P-value and/or hazard ratio were used as criteria for gene selection. However, the gene list composed of the gene selected from the univariate tests may not be necessary the optimal gene set for the survival prediction. To address this limitation, we employed a GA searching algorithm to optimize gene set selection for accurate survival prediction. The GA searching enables the assessment of the combinatorial effect of a gene set on the survival analysis. As expected, we identified a set of genes that yielded higher prediction accuracy than the gene list obtained from the univariate regression model. In this study, the GA only searched for the best gene combination of 330 univariate genes, which was the length of initial chromosome. The pre-filtered gene candidate set can reduce the searching space of the GA algorithm and save the computation time, however, the optimal gene set could be overlooked by this strategy.

The cancer survival analysis merely using the gene expression levels shows the limited ability for accurate survival risk prediction [32]. The genetic mutations have an important role in cancer development. Hence, the genetic mutation profiles can provide additional values for survival analysis and lead to uncover genetic variations that are associated with patient survival [27]. We found that the most frequently mutated genes were not necessarily significant in survival analysis. The correlation coefficient of the top eight mutated genes and the *P*-values

from the univariate regression model is – 0.22 in the breast cancer dataset that we studied. The mutated genes selected by the univariate regression test often resulted in very unbalanced survival risked groups (Additional file 3). In addition, it is commonly known that the drive gene mutations in a pathway tend to be mutually exclusive. Here, we proposed a system biology method: first projected the somatic mutations onto the pathways and gene function sets, then used significantly mutated pathways or function gene sets as additional signatures for survival analysis. For example, we found 14 pathways were significant abundance of the mutated genes as well as showed significance in the univariate regression test (Fig. 5). The mutated rates of these pathway-genes were relatively low (Additional file 4).

Despite of low mutation rate of pathway-gene, they tended to be more effective for survival prediction. In the Cox univariate regression, the 14 pathways consistently demonstrated lower *P*-values than the top mutated genes set (Additional file 5). Here, the number of top mutated genes set is the same as the number of mutated genes in the corresponding pathways. We also performed multivariate regression test. In the multivariate test, each individual mutated gene in the pathways or the top mutated genes was considered a feature. We found most pathway-genes tend to have high P-value than the individual top mutated genes, excepting the Fanconi anemia pathway and ECM-receptor interaction pathways. Specially, the Fanconi anemia pathway performed well in both univariate regression and multivariate regression models (Additional file 5), suggest this pathway has an essential role in the breast cancer survival.

In this study, we integrated somatic mutations with gene expression in our survival analysis and built an improved model for survival risk prediction. Further improvement could be achieved when several related issues are solved. First, previous studies showed that somatic mutation identification remains inaccurate [33, 34]. The mutations identified by different mutation callers often have relatively low overlap. Better mutation caller can potentially improve survival prediction accuracy. Second,

Table 2 C-index of the Cox proportional hazards models based on different features

Feature type	Features	C-index	P-value
Gene expression	330 significant univariate genes	0.584	0.0011
	118 significant univariate genes with hazard ratio > 1.221	0.636	< 0.0001
	88 significant univariate genes selected by GA	0.656	< 0.0001
Somatic mutation	25 functional annotations	0.603	0.0012
	15 gene ontology terms	0.567	0.0013
	14 pathways	0.548	0.0037
	54 functional gene sets combining functional annotations, GO terms and pathways	0.591	0.0016
Gene expression & somatic mutation	All 142 features (88 significant univariate genes and 54 functional gene sets)	0.658	< 0.0001

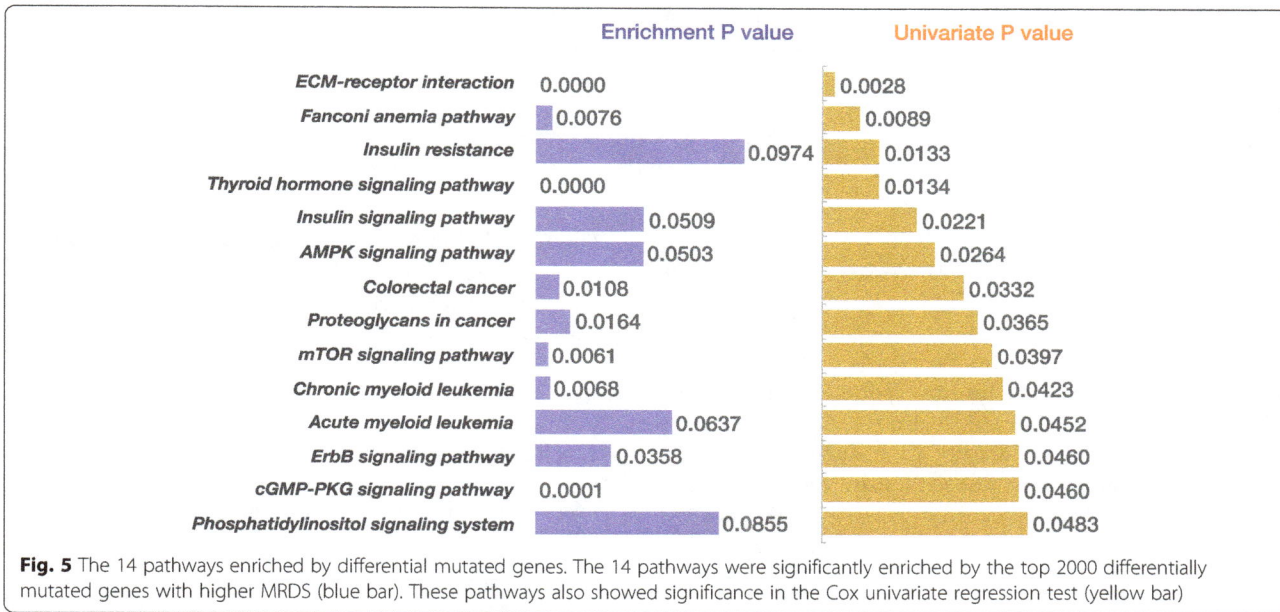

Fig. 5 The 14 pathways enriched by differential mutated genes. The 14 pathways were significantly enriched by the top 2000 differentially mutated genes with higher MRDS (blue bar). These pathways also showed significance in the Cox univariate regression test (yellow bar)

somatic mutations are highly heterogeneous among patients. Identifying survival driver genes could be valuable for survival prediction. In addition, allele frequency, the mutation positions and the other mutation information can be further incorporated into the survival model for survival model enhancement. Unlike gene expression, the quantitative relationship between somatic mutation and phenotypic characteristics are unknown. With better understanding of somatic mutation roles in the patient survival, we can build a better prognosis model for survival analysis.

Conclusions

Our study suggested that expressions of genes were the effective indicators for breast cancer survival prediction. By coupling with somatic mutations, we were able to improve the survival predict model, however, the improvement was marginal. Also, we found that some genes demonstrated significantly distinct mutation rates between high risk and low risk breast cancer patients. Better utilizing the mutation difference for cancer prognostic analysis can be further investigated.

Methods
Breast cancer datasets
We obtained RNAseq datasets including raw counts and FPKM (Fragments Per Kilobase of transcript per Million) counts from TCGA (The Cancer Genome Atlas) project. The RNAseq datasets were generated from 1091 breast tumor tissue samples. We downloaded the somatic mutation profile generated by MuTect2 workflow, for 1044 tumor tissue samples. Out of 1044 cases in the somatic mutation file, 980 were common cases with gene expression profiles. Survival information was

obtained from the metadata for each individual cases. All TCGA datasets used in the study are publicly available at the GDC Portal website (https://portal.gdc.cancer.gov/).

An independent breast cancer datasets including the patient clinical information and the expression profile for 2509 breast cancer patients were downloaded from *cBioportal* (www.cbioportal.org/). The data was generated by the Molecular Taxonomy of Breast Cancer International Consortium (METABRIC).

An R-package 'edgeR' was applied for differential expression analysis. We used adjusted P-value lower than 0.01 and absolute log fold change larger than 2 to define significantly differentially expressed genes.

Feature selection
We first used the univariate Cox regression analysis to choose features for survival analysis. The output of the regression analysis includes three important statistics: statistical significance (p), regression coefficients (coef) (Eq. 1), and hazard ratios (HR) (Eq. 2). These statistics were used to select the significant survival-related features.

$$coef = \frac{n(\sum xy) - \sum x \sum y}{\sqrt{\left[n \sum x^2 - (\sum x)^2\right]\left[n \sum y^2 - (\sum y)^2\right]}} \tag{1}$$

$$HR = \exp(coef) \tag{2}$$

where x and y are two vectors that represent the survival time and one predictor variable. Base on C-index statistics, we chose the thresholds P-value < 0.05 and hazard ratios > 1.221 for selecting survival-related genes.

Survival analysis

We normalized each feature gene-wisely using the following equation:

$$\frac{g_{i,j} - \min\limits_{j \in N} g_{i,j}}{\max\limits_{j \in N} g_{i,j} - \min\limits_{j \in N} g_{i,j}} \qquad i = 1, 2, ..., M \qquad (3)$$

where $g_{i,j}$ represent the value of feature i in the sample j. N is the total number patient samples and M is the total number of features. Then, we used k-means algorithm to identify high survival risk and low survival risk groups. Subsequently, each individual samples were labeled accordingly. Using R package "survival", the Cox proportional hazards model was fitted with the data and the corresponding C-index was calculated. The R package 'survminer' was used to plot the Kaplan–Meier curve.

Genetic algorithm identifies survival indicators

The genetic algorithm (GA) is a heuristic method for searching the global optimum. We employed the GA to reveal a gene set that yields the best survival prediction accuracy. An R package "Genalg" was used for GA searching. [35]. We set the population size as 200. The chromosome is a 0/1 vector with the length of 330. Here, 330 is the total number of significant univariate genes, 1 means the corresponding gene is selected while 0 refer to the unselected gene. Mutate rate was set to 0.01. The fitness score was calculated by (1 - C-index) of each candidate gene set. The number of generation is set to 100.

Building somatic mutation and functional gene set based features

Based on the gene signatures derived from the expression profiles, we divided the patients into high and low survival risk groups. Then, the somatic mutation profiles for patients in each group were extracted from the annotated somatic mutation file accordingly. For SNPs, we calculated and compared the percentage of various types of SNPs in the two groups. The t-test was applied to assess whether a type of SNPs demonstrated significantly different mutation rate between the two survival risk groups.

For mutated genes, we compared the mutation rate of each gene (i) in the two groups. Mutation rate (R) was calculated using the number of the samples containing the mutated gene divided by the total number of samples in the individual groups. Then, we calculated a mutation rate differential score (MRDS) for each gene (Eq. 4). The top 2000 genes

with higher MRDS were selected for enrichment analysis.

$$MRDS_i = \frac{R_{(high,i)}}{R_{(low,i)}} \times e^{R_{(high,i)} - R_{(low,i)}} \qquad (4)$$

The DAVID [30, 31] analysis was used to identify functional annotation sets, gene ontology terms and pathways that were enriched by the top differentially mutated genes.

Additional files

Additional file 1: PATHER significantly enriched terms base on 118 survival related genes.

Additional file 2: The Kaplan–Meier estimator for an independent patient dataset. The survival curve base on 64 of 118 hazard-ratio-selected genes for METABRIC breast cancer patient dataset.

Additional file 3: The Kaplan–Meier estimator using top 35 mutated genes. The Kaplan–Meier curves using 35 mutated genes selected by the univariate regression as predictors displayed two very unbalanced survival risk groups.

Additional file 4: The comparison of mutation rates for top mutated genes and 14 pathway genes. The mutation rates for 15 different gene sets, including one top-35-mutated gene set and 14 pathway-based gene sets. The genes in each set were ordered by their mutation rates.

Additional file 5: The P-value of the Cox univariate regression analysis using different gene sets. (A) The P-values of the Cox univariate regression analysis for pathway-based genes (blue) and top mutated genes (orange). (B) The P-values of univariant test and multivariant test for pathway-based genes (blue and grey) and top mutated genes (orange and purple).

Abbreviations

C-Index: Concordance Index; GA: Genetic Algorithm; GO: Gene ontology; LN: Lymph node; LOOCV: Leave-one-out cross-validated; METABRIC: Molecular Taxonomy of Breast Cancer International Consortium; SNPs: Single-Nucleotide Polymorphisms; TCGA: The Cancer Genome Atlas; TKIs: Tyrosine Kinase Inhibitors

Acknowledgements

This research was supported by United States National Institutes of Health (NIH) Academic Research Enhancement Award 1R15GM114739 and National Institute of General Medical Sciences (NIH/NIGMS) 5P20GM103429, and Arkansas Science and Technology Authority (ASTA) Basic Science Research 15-B-23 and 15-B-38. However, the information contained herein represents the position of the author(s) and not necessarily that of the NIH.

Funding

The publication cost of this article was funded by United States National Institutes of Health (NIH) Academic Research Enhancement Award 1R15GM114739.

Authors' contributions

MQY conceived the project. YZ and MQY designed the experiments. YZ performed the experiments and analysis. WY, DL, JY and RG participate in discussions. All authors have read and approved final manuscript.

Competing interests

The authors declare that they have no competing interests.

Author details

[1]MidSouth Bioinformatics Center and Joint Bioinformatics Ph.D. Program of University of Arkansas at Little Rock and Univ. of Arkansas Medical Sciences, 2801 S. Univ. Ave, Little Rock 72204, USA. [2]Department of Computer Science, Carnegie Mellon University School of Computer Science, 5000 Forbes Ave, Pittsburgh 24105, USA.

References

1. Siegel RL, Miller KD, Jemal A. Cancer statistics, 2016. CA Cancer J Clin. 2016; 66:7–30.
2. Yang Y, Zhou X, Xu M, Piao J, Zhang Y, Lin Z, et al. β-Lapachone suppresses tumour progression by inhibiting epithelial-to-mesenchymal transition in NQO1-positive breast cancers. Sci Rep. 2017;7:2681.
3. Weigelt B, Peterse JL, van't VLJ. Breast cancer metastasis: markers and models. Nat Rev Cancer. 2005;5:591–602.
4. Early Breast Cancer Trialists' Collaborative Group (EBCTCG), Effects of chemotherapy and hormonal therapy for early breast cancer on recurrence and 15-year survival: an overview of the randomised trials. Lancet. 2005;365: 1687–17.
5. Liu B, Yang M, Li R, Ding Y, Qian X, Yu L, et al. The antitumor effect of novel docetaxel-loaded thermosensitive micelles. Eur J Pharm Biopharm. 2008;69:527–34.
6. Li J, Chen Z, Su K, Zeng J. Clinicopathological classification and traditional prognostic indicators of breast cancer. Int J Clin Exp Pathol. 2015;8:8500–5.
7. Gong G, Kwon MJ, Han J, Lee HJ, Lee SK, Lee JE, et al. A new molecular prognostic score for predicting the risk of distant metastasis in patients with HR+/HER2– early breast cancer. Sci Rep. 2017;7:45554.
8. Alizadeh AA, Eisen MB, Davis RE, Ma C, Lossos IS, Rosenwald A, et al. Distinct types of diffuse large B-cell lymphoma identified by gene expression profiling. Nature. 2000;403:503–11.
9. Sørlie T, Perou CM, Tibshirani R, Aas T, Geisler S, Johnsen H, et al. Gene expression patterns of breast carcinomas distinguish tumor subclasses with clinical implications. Proc Natl Acad Sci. 2001;98:10869–74.
10. van de Vijver MJ, He YD, van 't Veer LJ, Dai H, Hart AAM, Voskuil DW, et al. A gene-expression signature as a predictor of survival in breast Cancer. N Engl J Med. 2002;347:1999–2009.
11. Network TCGA. Comprehensive molecular portraits of human breast tumours. Nature. 2012;490:61–70.
12. Bair E, Tibshirani R. Semi-supervised methods to predict patient survival from gene expression data. PLoS Biol. 2004;2:e108.
13. Sun J, Chen X, Wang Z, Guo M, Shi H, Wang X, et al. A potential prognostic long non-coding RNA signature to predict metastasis-free survival of breast cancer patients. Sci Rep. 2015;5:16553.
14. Zhang X, Li Y, Akinyemiju T, Ojesina AI, Buckhaults P, Liu N, et al. Pathway-structured predictive model for Cancer survival prediction: a two-stage approach. Genetics. 2017;205:89–100.
15. Nik-Zainal S, Davies H, Staaf J, Ramakrishna M, Glodzik D, Zou X, et al. Landscape of somatic mutations in 560 breast cancer whole-genome sequences. Nature. 2016;534:47–54.
16. Zhong Q, Peng H-L, Zhao X, Zhang L, Hwang W-T. Effects of BRCA1- and BRCA2-related mutations on ovarian and breast cancer survival: a meta-analysis. Clin Cancer res. 2014;:clincanres1816.2014.
17. Tonghui W, Ye X, Shuyan S, Hua Y, Tao O, Li J, et al. HER2 somatic mutations are associated with poor survival in HER2-negative breast cancers. Cancer Sci. 2017;108:671–7.
18. Pucci F, Rickelt S, Newton AP, Garris C, Nunes E, Evavold C, et al. PF4 promotes platelet production and lung Cancer growth. Cell Rep. 2016;17: 1764–72.
19. Zhao Y-F, Zhao J-Y, Yue H, Hu K-S, Shen H, Guo Z-G, et al. FOXD1 promotes breast cancer proliferation and chemotherapeutic drug resistance by targeting p27. Biochem Biophys Res Commun. 2015;456:232–7.
20. Song H, He W, Huang X, Zhang H, Huang T. High expression of FOXR2 in breast cancer correlates with poor prognosis. Tumor Biol. 2016;37:5991–7.
21. Mathew S, Merdad A, Al-Maghrabi J, Dallol A. Identification of frequent MTNR1B methylation in breast cancer following the application of high-throughput methylome analysis. BMC Genomics. 2014;15:P44.
22. Reis-Filho JS, Pusztai L. Gene expression profiling in breast cancer: classification, prognostication, and prediction. Lancet. 2011;378:1812–23.
23. Fakhraldeen SA, Clark RJ, Roopra A, Chin EN, Huang W, Castorino J, et al. Two isoforms of the RNA binding protein, coding region determinant-binding protein (CRD-BP/IGF2BP1), are expressed in breast epithelium and support Clonogenic growth of breast tumor cells. J Biol Chem. 2015;290: 13386–400.
24. Syndecan-1 in Breast Cancer Stroma Fibroblasts Regulates Extracellular Matrix Fiber Organization and Carcinoma Cell Motility - Am J Pathol http://ajp.amjpathol.org/article/S0002-9440(10)00086-6/abstract. Accessed 9 Apr 2018.
25. Thomas PD, Campbell MJ, Kejariwal A, Mi H, Karlak B, Daverman R, et al. PANTHER: a library of protein families and subfamilies indexed by function. Genome Res. 2003;13:2129–41.
26. Liao L, Kuang S-Q, Yuan Y, Gonzalez SM, O'Malley BW, Xu J. Molecular structure and biological function of the cancer-amplified nuclear receptor coactivator SRC-3/AIB1. J Steroid Biochem Mol Biol. 2002;83:3–14.
27. Jass JR, Do K-A, Simms LA, Iino H, Wynter C, Pillay SP, et al. Morphology of sporadic colorectal cancer with DNA replication errors. Gut. 1998;42:673–9.
28. Hall A. The cytoskeleton and cancer. Cancer Metastasis Rev. 2009;28:5–14.
29. Curtis C, Shah SP, Chin S-F, Turashvili G, Rueda OM, Dunning MJ, et al. The genomic and transcriptomic architecture of 2,000 breast tumours reveals novel subgroups. Nature. 2012;486:346–52.
30. Huang DW, Sherman BT, Lempicki RA. Systematic and integrative analysis of large gene lists using DAVID bioinformatics resources. Nat Protoc. 2009;4:44–57.
31. Huang DW, Sherman BT, Lempicki RA. Bioinformatics enrichment tools: paths toward the comprehensive functional analysis of large gene lists. Nucleic Acids Res. 2009;37:1–13.
32. Gatza ML, Lucas JE, Barry WT, Kim JW, Wang Q, Crawford MD, et al. A pathway-based classification of human breast cancer. Proc Natl Acad Sci. 2010;107:6994–9.
33. Xu H, DiCarlo J, Satya RV, Peng Q, Wang Y. Comparison of somatic mutation calling methods in amplicon and whole exome sequence data. BMC Genomics. 2014;15:244.
34. Krøigård AB, Thomassen M, Lænkholm A-V, Kruse TA, Larsen MJ. Evaluation of nine somatic variant callers for detection of somatic mutations in exome and targeted deep sequencing data. PLoS One. 2016;11:e0151664.
35. Mitchell M. An introduction to genetic algorithms. Cambridge: MIT Press; 1998.

integRATE: a desirability-based data integration framework for the prioritization of candidate genes across heterogeneous omics and its application to preterm birth

Haley R. Eidem[1], Jacob L. Steenwyk[1], Jennifer H. Wisecaver[1,2], John A. Capra[1,3,4], Patrick Abbot[1] and Antonis Rokas[1,3,4]* (iD)

Abstract

Background: The integration of high-quality, genome-wide analyses offers a robust approach to elucidating genetic factors involved in complex human diseases. Even though several methods exist to integrate heterogeneous omics data, most biologists still manually select candidate genes by examining the intersection of lists of candidates stemming from analyses of different types of omics data that have been generated by imposing hard (strict) thresholds on quantitative variables, such as P-values and fold changes, increasing the chance of missing potentially important candidates.

Methods: To better facilitate the unbiased integration of heterogeneous omics data collected from diverse platforms and samples, we propose a desirability function framework for identifying candidate genes with strong evidence across data types as targets for follow-up functional analysis. Our approach is targeted towards disease systems with sparse, heterogeneous omics data, so we tested it on one such pathology: spontaneous preterm birth (sPTB).

Results: We developed the software integRATE, which uses desirability functions to rank genes both within and across studies, identifying well-supported candidate genes according to the cumulative weight of biological evidence rather than based on imposition of hard thresholds of key variables. Integrating 10 sPTB omics studies identified both genes in pathways previously suspected to be involved in sPTB as well as novel genes never before linked to this syndrome. integRATE is available as an R package on GitHub (https://github.com/haleyeidem/integRATE).

Conclusions: Desirability-based data integration is a solution most applicable in biological research areas where omics data is especially heterogeneous and sparse, allowing for the prioritization of candidate genes that can be used to inform more targeted downstream functional analyses.

Keywords: Prematurity, Integrative genomics, Complex disease, Candidate gene ranking, Venn diagram

Background

Biological processes underlying disease pathogenesis typically involve a complex, dynamic, and interconnected system of molecular and environmental factors [1]. Advances in high-throughput omics technologies have allowed for the collection of data corresponding to the genomic, transcriptomic, epigenomic, proteomic, and metabolomic elements that contribute to variation in these biological processes [2]. However, each of these omics approaches, when employed in isolation, can only capture variation within a single layer of a much more complicated biological system [3, 4]. For example, even though the thousands of single nucleotide polymorphisms (SNPs) that have been linked to complex diseases or traits via genome-wide association studies (GWAS) have greatly contributed to our understanding of complex disease, these SNPs may only be tagging the

* Correspondence: antonis.rokas@vanderbilt.edu
[1]Department of Biological Sciences, Vanderbilt University, Nashville, TN, USA
[3]Department of Biomedical Informatics, Vanderbilt University, Nashville, TN, USA
Full list of author information is available at the end of the article

causal genetic element(s), and we still lack in depth knowledge of the molecular mechanisms underlying the vast majority of these associations [5, 6]. Similarly, transcriptomics studies routinely identify hundreds to thousands of differentially expressed genes between diseased and healthy tissue samples, but disentangling the disease-causing changes in gene expression from its byproducts can be far more challenging [7]. Given the limitations of each omics approach and their focuses on different layers of the biological system, integration of different types of omics data to identify the key biological pathways involved in disease has emerged as a promising avenue for research [4].

One integrative study design is to obtain diverse types of omics data from the same tissue samples or patient cohorts. The resulting data can then be vertically integrated (Fig. 1a, top left) to identify candidate genes and pathways involved in complex disease. Alternatively, a single type of omics data can be collected from a variety of tissue samples or patient cohorts, facilitating their horizontal integration across many samples, which can substantially increase the experiment's power (Fig. 1a, top right). In both vertical and horizontal integration study designs, the availability of diverse types of omics data from the same samples enables the use of a variety of statistical integration approaches (Fig. 1a, bottom) [8]. For example, multi-staged integration uses multiple steps to first identify associations between different data types and then identify associations between data types and the phenotype of interest [9], whereas meta-dimensional integration combines data simultaneously based on concatenation, transformation, or model building [10].

Although multi-omics data sets generated using vertical and horizontal study designs are becoming increasingly common, such data sets are lacking for many complex diseases [11–15]. Often, heterogeneous omics data are collected study by study, for a limited set of tissue samples and across only one or two omics data types at a time (Fig. 1b, top). For each study, a long list of genes or genomic regions with associated data is produced and sorted based on effect size (e.g., fold change), significance (e.g., P-value), or some other criterion. Hard thresholds can then be imposed on P-values, for example, to bin the genes or genomic regions and identify significant candidates for further analysis; this type of approach can then be applied across multiple, heterogeneous omics studies.

Several problems exist with the imposition of hard thresholds, however. Including (or excluding) genes or genomic regions as candidates based on P-value, fold change, expression level, and/or odds ratio cutoffs introduces biases and removes information, especially when combining multiple cutoffs from several criteria [16–18]. These cutoffs can sometimes even be arbitrary, like selecting the top n or n% from each data set. Additionally,

statistical significance is not always equivalent to biological significance, meaning that non-statistically significant genes may still be involved in disease pathogenesis, or vice versa. Moreover, while selecting the top n genes might limit the scope of further functional analysis, the alternative approach of selecting all significant hits could mean that thousands of genes are identified as candidates. A final consideration in analyzing heterogeneous omics data is that we sometimes do not know any genes, pathways, or networks that have already been shown to be involved in complex disease. Some integration methods, especially those based on prediction (e.g., machine learning, network analysis), depend on the availability of such knowledge for algorithm training and cannot be performed in their absence [8, 9, 19–22].

Desirability functions provide a way to integrate heterogeneous omics data in systems where gold standards (i.e., genes known to be involved in the complex disease under investigation) are not yet known (Fig. 1b, bottom). Originally developed for industrial quality control, desirability functions have been successfully used in chemoinformatics to rank compounds for drug discovery and have been proposed as a way to integrate multiple selection criteria in functional genomics experiments [23–27]. In the context of integrating diverse but heterogeneous omics data, desirability functions allow for the ranking and prioritizing of candidate genes based on cumulative evidence across data types and their variables, rather than within-study separation of significant and non-significant genes based on single variables in single studies. For example, a 2015 study initially proposed the use of desirability functions to integrate multiple selection criteria for ranking, selecting, and prioritizing genes across heterogeneous biological analyses and demonstrated its use by analyzing a set of microarray-generated gene expression data [23].

To facilitate data integration in the presence of heterogeneous multi-omics data and when prior biological knowledge is limited, we propose a desirability-based framework to prioritize candidate genes for functional analysis. To facilitate application of our framework, we built a user-friendly software package called integRATE, which takes as input data sets from any omics experiment and generates a single desirability score based on all available information. This approach is targeted towards biological processes or diseases with particularly sparse or heterogeneous data, so we test integRATE on a set of 10 omics data sets related to spontaneous preterm birth (sPTB), a complex disease where heterogeneous multi-omics data are the only omics data currently available.

Design
Variable transformation
First, relevant studies need to be identified for integration; this selection can be based on any number of

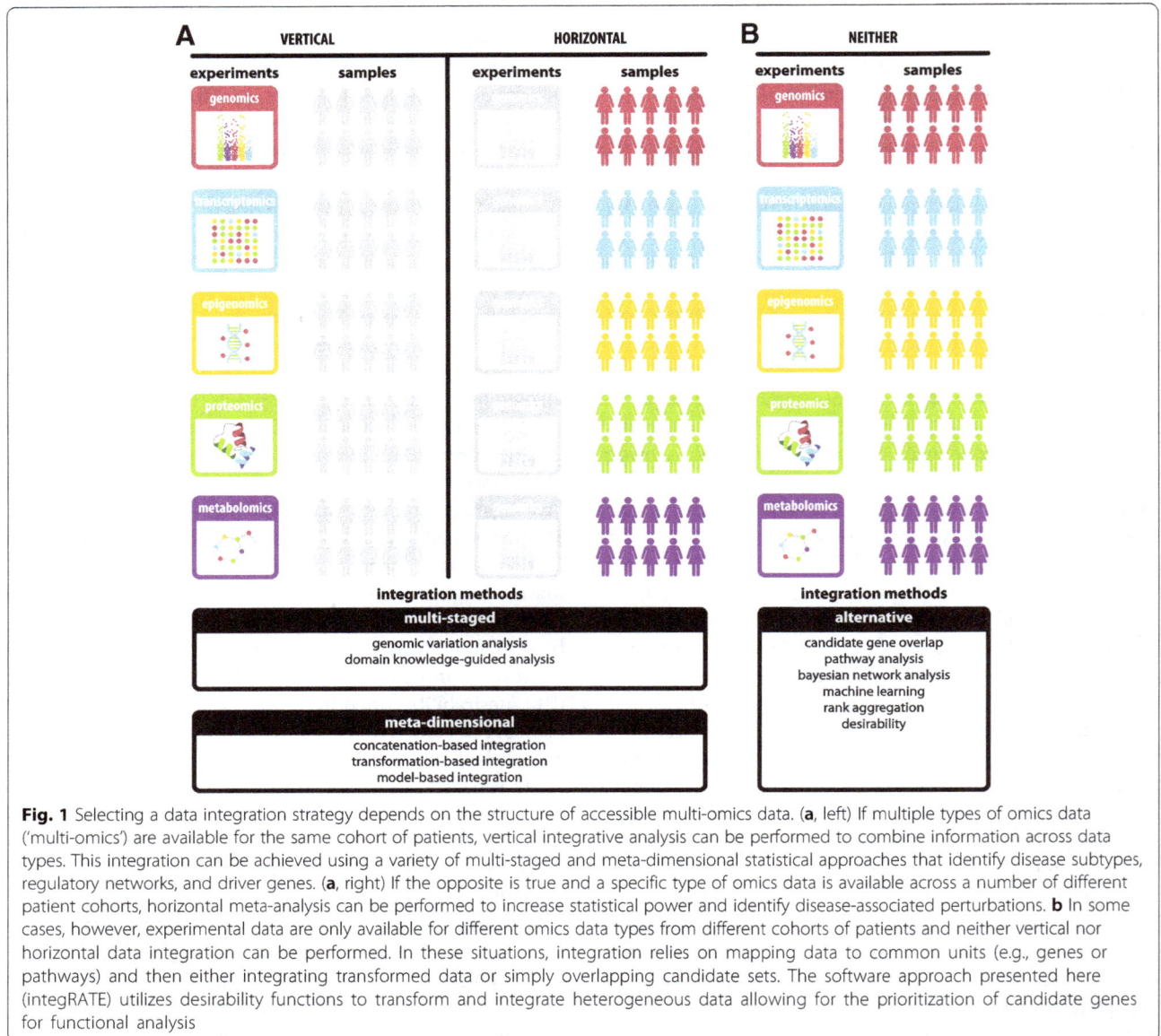

Fig. 1 Selecting a data integration strategy depends on the structure of accessible multi-omics data. (**a**, left) If multiple types of omics data ('multi-omics') are available for the same cohort of patients, vertical integrative analysis can be performed to combine information across data types. This integration can be achieved using a variety of multi-staged and meta-dimensional statistical approaches that identify disease subtypes, regulatory networks, and driver genes. (**a**, right) If the opposite is true and a specific type of omics data is available across a number of different patient cohorts, horizontal meta-analysis can be performed to increase statistical power and identify disease-associated perturbations. **b** In some cases, however, experimental data are only available for different omics data types from different cohorts of patients and neither vertical nor horizontal data integration can be performed. In these situations, integration relies on mapping data to common units (e.g., genes or pathways) and then either integrating transformed data or simply overlapping candidate sets. The software approach presented here (integRATE) utilizes desirability functions to transform and integrate heterogeneous data allowing for the prioritization of candidate genes for functional analysis

characteristics including tissue(s) sampled, disease subtype, or experimental designs (Fig. 2, step 1). The data in each of these studies (e.g., gene expression data, proteomic data, GWAS data, etc.) are typically specific to or can be mapped to individual genetic elements (e.g., genes) in the genome. Furthermore, each study's data contain genetic element-specific values for many different variables (e.g., P-value, odds ratio, fold change, etc.). Then desirability functions are fit to the observations for each variable within a study (e.g., P-value, odds ratio, fold change, etc.) according to whether low values are most desirable (d_{low}, e.g., P-value), high values are most desirable (d_{high}, e.g., odds ratio), or extreme values are most desirable ($d_{extreme}$, e.g., fold change) (Fig. 2, step 2).

The desirability score for each genetic element can be calculated by applying one of the following equations to a given variable:

$$d_{low} = \begin{cases} 0 & Y > B \\ \left[\dfrac{Y-B}{A-B}\right]^s & A \le Y \le B \\ 1 & Y < A \end{cases} \tag{1}$$

$$d_{high} = \begin{cases} 0 & Y < A \\ \left[\dfrac{Y-A}{B-A}\right]^s & A \le Y \le B \\ 1 & Y > B \end{cases} \tag{2}$$

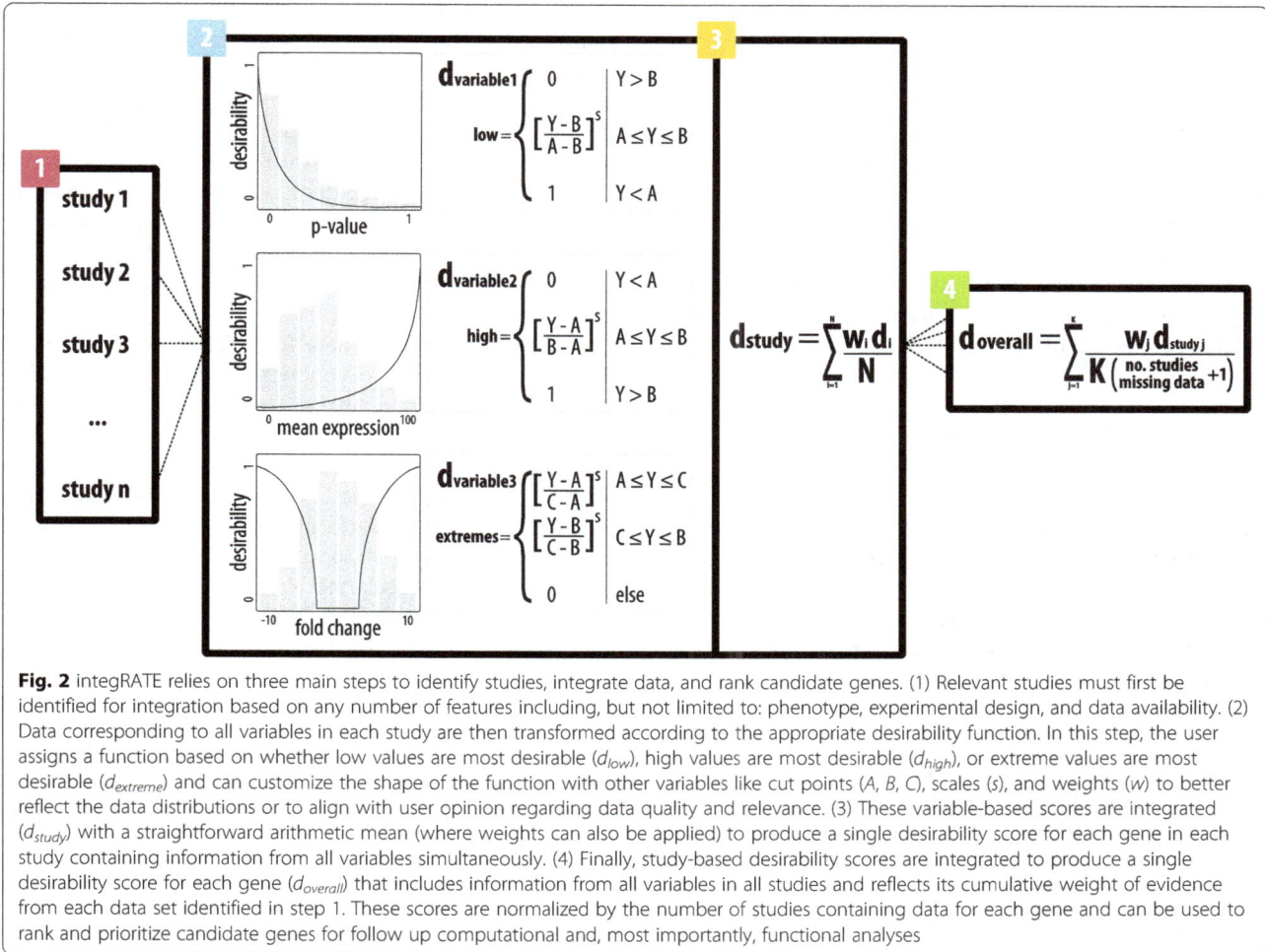

$$d_{variable1} \quad low = \begin{cases} 0 & Y > B \\ \left[\dfrac{Y-B}{A-B}\right]^s & A \leq Y \leq B \\ 1 & Y < A \end{cases}$$

$$d_{variable2} \quad high = \begin{cases} 0 & Y < A \\ \left[\dfrac{Y-A}{B-A}\right]^s & A \leq Y \leq B \\ 1 & Y > B \end{cases}$$

$$d_{variable3} \quad extremes = \begin{cases} \left[\dfrac{Y-A}{C-A}\right]^s & A \leq Y \leq C \\ \left[\dfrac{Y-B}{C-B}\right]^s & C \leq Y \leq B \\ 0 & else \end{cases}$$

$$d_{study} = \sum_{i=1}^{i} \frac{w_i d_i}{N}$$

$$d_{overall} \leq \sum_{j=1}^{k} \frac{w_j d_{study j}}{K \left(\begin{array}{c} no.\ studies \\ missing\ data \end{array} +1\right)}$$

Fig. 2 integRATE relies on three main steps to identify studies, integrate data, and rank candidate genes. (1) Relevant studies must first be identified for integration based on any number of features including, but not limited to: phenotype, experimental design, and data availability. (2) Data corresponding to all variables in each study are then transformed according to the appropriate desirability function. In this step, the user assigns a function based on whether low values are most desirable (d_{low}), high values are most desirable (d_{high}), or extreme values are most desirable ($d_{extreme}$) and can customize the shape of the function with other variables like cut points (A, B, C), scales (s), and weights (w) to better reflect the data distributions or to align with user opinion regarding data quality and relevance. (3) These variable-based scores are integrated (d_{study}) with a straightforward arithmetic mean (where weights can also be applied) to produce a single desirability score for each gene in each study containing information from all variables simultaneously. (4) Finally, study-based desirability scores are integrated to produce a single desirability score for each gene ($d_{overall}$) that includes information from all variables in all studies and reflects its cumulative weight of evidence from each data set identified in step 1. These scores are normalized by the number of studies containing data for each gene and can be used to rank and prioritize candidate genes for follow up computational and, most importantly, functional analyses

$$d_{extreme} = \begin{cases} \left[\dfrac{Y-A}{C-A}\right]^s & A \leq Y \leq C \\ \left[\dfrac{Y-B}{C-B}\right]^s & C \leq Y \leq B \\ 0 & else \end{cases} \quad (3)$$

In these equations, Y is the variable value and s is the scale coefficient affecting the function's rate of change that can be customized according to user preference. Alternatively, the equations could be used without any scaling by setting the scale coefficient to 1. For d_{low} and d_{high}, A is the low cut point and B is the high cut point where the function changes. For $d_{extreme}$, A is the low cut point, C is the intermediate cut point, and B is the high cut point where the function changes. The user can customize these cut points based on numerical values (e.g., P-value < 0.05) or percentile values (e.g., top 10%). The resulting values, ranging from 0 to 1 (or the minimum and maximum values specified) are transformed desirability scores based on information from each variable.

Variable integration

Next, desirability scores for each of the N variables within a study (e.g., P-value, odds ratio, fold change, etc.) are combined using an arithmetic mean so that genetic elements (e.g., genes) with desirability scores of zero for any given variable remain in the analysis (Fig. 2, step 3). Desirability for genetic elements within a study can be calculated by:

$$d_{study} = \sum_{i=1}^{N} \frac{w_i d_i}{N} \quad (4)$$

In this equation, w_i is the weight parameter (assigned to each variable), d_i is desirability score for each genetic element based on the values of each variable derived from Eqs. (1), (2) or (3), and N is the total number of transformed variables. This step produces a single desirability score (d_{study}) for each genetic element in the study containing information from all transformed variables. Here, the user is also able to include variable weights (w_i) when integrating their desirability scores, which can be useful in cases where certain variables are considered more informative or accurate than others.

Study integration
Finally, the d_{study} values can be integrated using the arithmetic mean to produce a single desirability score ($d_{overall}$) for each genetic element, representing its desirability as a candidate according to the weight of evidence from all variables in all K studies that were integrated (Fig. 2, step 4). The overall score used to prioritize candidates can be calculated by:

$$d_{overall} = \sum_{j=1}^{K} \frac{w_j d_{study\ j}}{K(no.studies\ missing\ data + 1)} \quad (5)$$

In this equation, w_j is the weight parameter (assigned to each study), $d_{study\ j}$ is the desirability score for each study, and K is the total number of studies integrated. Importantly, the overall desirability score $d_{overall}$ is normalized by the number of studies missing data for each genetic element to account for the number of values contributing to each overall desirability score. This normalization factor can be used to calculate a soft cutoff for the most desirable candidates that is equivalent or higher than the desirability score that would be achieved by a genetic element with a perfect desirability score of 1 in a single study but missing from all other studies. We call genetic elements achieving desirability scores equal to or above this cutoff 'desirable.'

Software
The methodology described above is implemented in our software, integRATE, available on GitHub as an R package (https://github.com/haleyeidem/integRATE). Although we focus on using desirability functions to integrate heterogeneous omics data corresponding to complex human diseases, integRATE can be applied to data sets from any phenotype, species, and data type (provided that the units can all be mapped to a common set of elements, such as genes). Functionality is provided for the application of customizable desirability functions as well as data visualization.

Implementation
One human complex genetic disease where the omics data available are heterogeneous is preterm birth (PTB). Defined as birth before 37 weeks of completed gestation, PTB is the leading cause of newborn death worldwide [28]. Although 30% of preterm births are medically indicated due to complications including preeclampsia (PE) or intrauterine growth restriction (IUGR), the remaining 70% occur spontaneously either due to the preterm

premature rupture of membranes (PPROM) or idiopathically (sPTB). Further complicating factors are that multiple maternal and fetal tissues are involved (e.g., placenta, fetal membranes, umbilical cord, myometrium, decidua, etc.) as well as multiple genomes (maternal, paternal, and fetal) [29]. Evidence from family, twin, and case-control studies suggests that genetics plays a role in determining birth timing and a recent GWAS identified a handful of genes linked to prematurity [30]. Nevertheless, the pathogenesis of PTB and its many subtypes remains poorly understood [31–33].

The publicly available data for sPTB consist of several different independently conducted omics analyses that would be challenging to analyze with statistical approaches developed for vertical and horizontal integration [30, 34, 35]. Although these omics data have been analyzed in isolation, integration of their information using the desirability-based platform implemented in integRATE may provide unique insights into the complex mechanisms involved in regulating birth timing and, thus, allow for the identification and prioritization of novel candidate genes for further functional and targeted analyses.

Study identification
Studies were initially identified based on the PubMed searches (up to 10/19/2017) using combinations of terms, including "Pregnancy", "Humans", "Preterm birth", "Placenta", "Decidua", "Myometrium", "Cervix Uteri", "Extraembryonic Membranes", "Blood", "Plasma" and "Umbilical Cord". Studies that reported conducting a genome-wide omics analysis of sPTB from a preliminary scan of the abstract were downloaded for full-text assessment. Furthermore, a thorough investigation was conducted of their associated reference lists to identify studies not captured via PubMed. Additionally, each study had to meet the following inclusion criteria:

1) Experimental group consisted of sPTB cases only and was not confounded by other pregnancy phenotypes (e.g., preeclampsia),
2) Analysis was genome-wide and not targeted to any specific subset of genes or pathways, and
3) Full data set was publicly available (not just top n%).

We identified 54 studies through the first phase of our literature search, but only 10 data sets that met all inclusion criteria. All excluded studies are listed in Additional file 1 with reasons for exclusion and the 10 data sets used in our pilot analysis are outlined in Table 1 [30, 34–46].

Data transformation
Each of the 10 data sets was mapped to a gene-based format. This step was necessary because integRATE

Table 1 The 10 sPTB omics data sets identified for desirability-based integration

First author	Year	Experiment	Control	Tissue	omics Type
Zhang	2017	sPTB	term	maternal blood	genomics (GWAS)
Ackerman	2015	sPTB	term	placenta	transcriptomics (RNA-seq)
Heng	2014	sPTB	term	maternal blood	transcriptomics (microarray)
Chim	2012	sPTB	term	maternal blood	transcriptomics (microarray)
Mayor-Lynn	2011	sPTB	term	placenta	transcriptomics (microarray)
de Goede	2017	sPTB	term	cord blood	epigenomics (microarray)
Fernando	2015	sPTB	term	cord blood	epigenomics (microarray)
Parets	2015	sPTB	term	maternal blood	epigenomics (microarray)
Cruickshank	2013	sPTB	term	fetal blood	epigenomics (microarray)
Heng	2015	sPTB	term	maternal blood	proteomics (mass spec)

applies desirability functions both within and across studies and, in order for that integration to be possible, the genetic elements of each study have to match.

Genomics
SNP-based data containing *P*-values and effect sizes were mapped to genes with MAGMA, as outlined in the Zhang et al. supplementary methods (http://ctg.cncr.nl/software/magma) [39, 47, 48].

Transcriptomics
Gene expression data from microarray experiments were accessed via GEO (https://www.ncbi.nlm.nih.gov/geo/) and re-analyzed using the GEO2R plugin (https://www.ncbi.nlm.nih.gov/geo/info/geo2r.html) [40–43]. Raw RNA-seq data from Ackerman et al. were analyzed in-house with custom scripts [34].

Epigenomics
Methylation data were accessed via GEO (https://www.ncbi.nlm.nih.gov/geo/) and re-analyzed using the GEO2R plugin (https://www.ncbi.nlm.nih.gov/geo/info/geo2r.html) [36, 37, 44–46].

Proteomics
Protein expression data were downloaded from supplementary files associated with each publication and the protein IDs were mapped to genes using Ensemble's BioMart tool (https://www.ensembl.org/info/data/biomart/index.html) [35, 38].

Application of integRATE
After mapping results from all 10 omics studies to genes, we used integRATE to calculate desirabilities for all genes across all variables within studies. We ran four different sPTB analyses:

1) In the first analysis (**iR-none**), we ran integRATE with no added customizations (e.g., no cut points, no scales (i.e., scale coefficient = 1), no minimum or maximum desirabilities, etc.) (Figs. 3, 4 and 5, Additional file 2).
2) In the second analysis (**iR-num**), we ran integRATE using numerical cut points ($P = 0.0001$, 0.1 and fold change = 1.5, 0.5, − 0.5, − 1.5) and no scales (Additional files 3, 4, 5, 6).
3) In the third analysis (**iR-per**), we ran integRATE using percentile cut points ($P = 5$, 95%, and fold change = 5, 50, 95%) and no scales (Additional files 7, 8, 9, 10).
4) In the fourth analysis (**HardThresh**), we considered statistically significant genes from each study to represent the results that would have been obtained if the typical approach based on hard thresholds and intersection of significant genes across studies outlined earlier was applied (Additional files 11, 12). All genes with adjusted *P*-values < 0.1 or unadjusted *P*-values < 0.05 were deemed significant in each study and intersected to compare with the results from integRATE [49].

To test whether the analyses described above produced results different from what might occur at random, we performed a permutation test shuffling desirabilities for all 26,868 genes 1000 times.

Results
In total, our sPTB analyses integrated gene-based results from 10 omics studies (1 genomics, 4 transcriptomics, 4 epigenomics, and 1 proteomics; Table 1) and included data sets ranging from 422 genes [35] to 20,841 genes [42]. The null distribution generated by our random permutation test had mean desirability range from 0.056 to 0.062, with an average of 0.059 (95% CI [0.058, 0.061]) (Fig. 3).

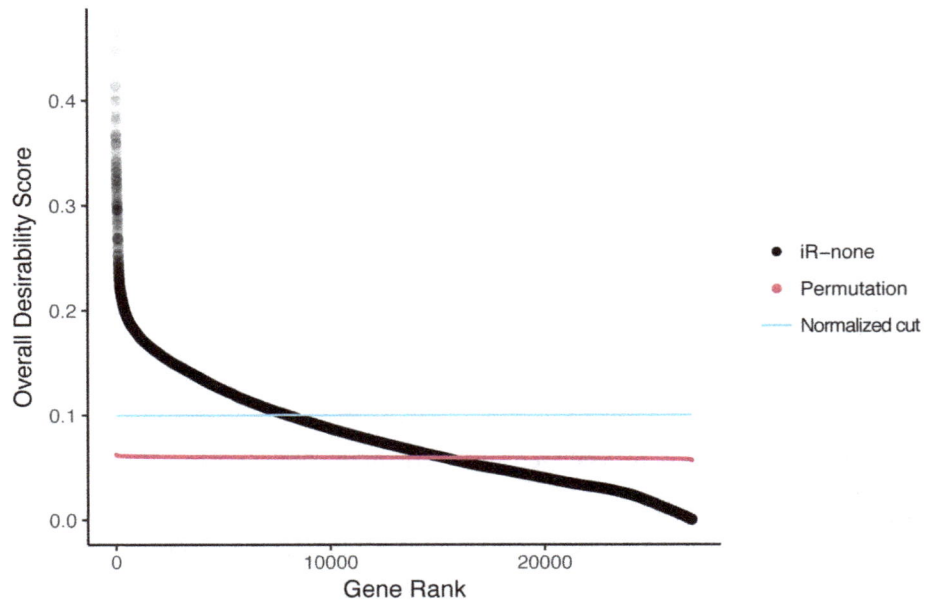

Fig. 3 After integration, 7977/26,868 genes were identified as highly desirable. All genes in the iR-none analysis were sorted from most desirable (rank = 1) to least desirable (rank = 26,868) and plotted according to their overall desirability scores, ranging from 8.04E-16 to 0.46. Because this analysis included 10 omics studies, the normalized lower bound for our set of 'desirable' candidate genes is 0.1 (blue line) and 7977 genes achieved scores greater than or equal to that value. Furthermore, the results of our permutation test are plotted in pink, with a mean of 0.059 (95% CI [0.058, 0.061]). All desirability scores for the entire data set are available in Additional file 2 (and in Additional files 3 and 7 for iR-num and iR-per, respectively)

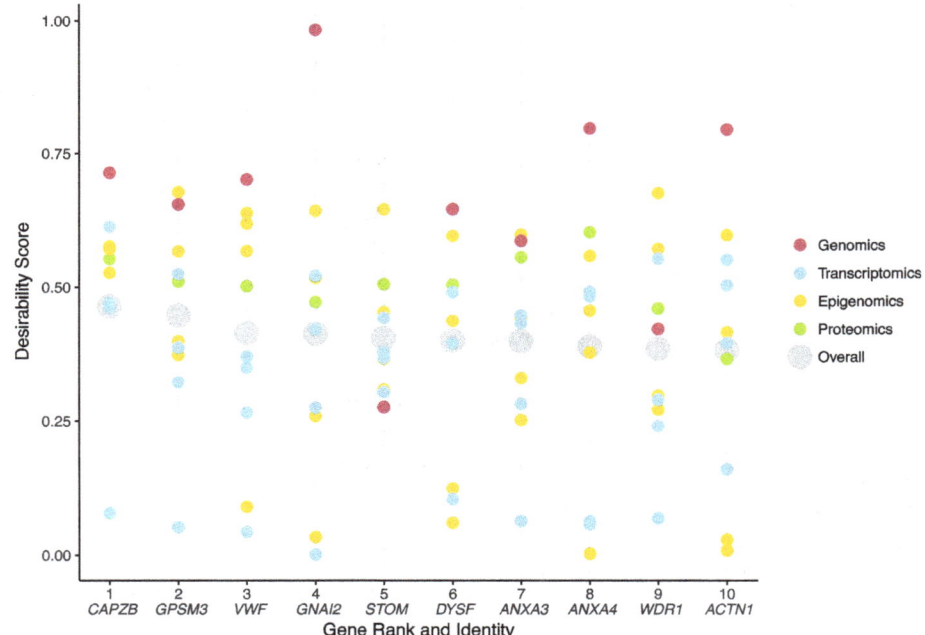

Fig. 4 The top 10 most desirable genes have a wide range of desirabilities across data types. The top 10 genes from our iR-none analysis have overall desirabilities ranging from 0.38 (*ACTN1*) to 0.46 (*CAPZB*), but the d_{study} values range, even when organized by data type. Some genes, like *STOM*, appear to be highly ranked not because of any extremely high d_{study} value, but rather due to a lack of low d_{study} values in any data type. In other words, this gene is likely not identified as particularly important in any individual study but shows a consensus of relatively strong evidence across all 10 studies. Contrastingly, other genes, like *CAPZB*, appear to be highly ranked due to one very high desirability score in a single data type (GWAS) that overpowers underwhelming evidence in other studies

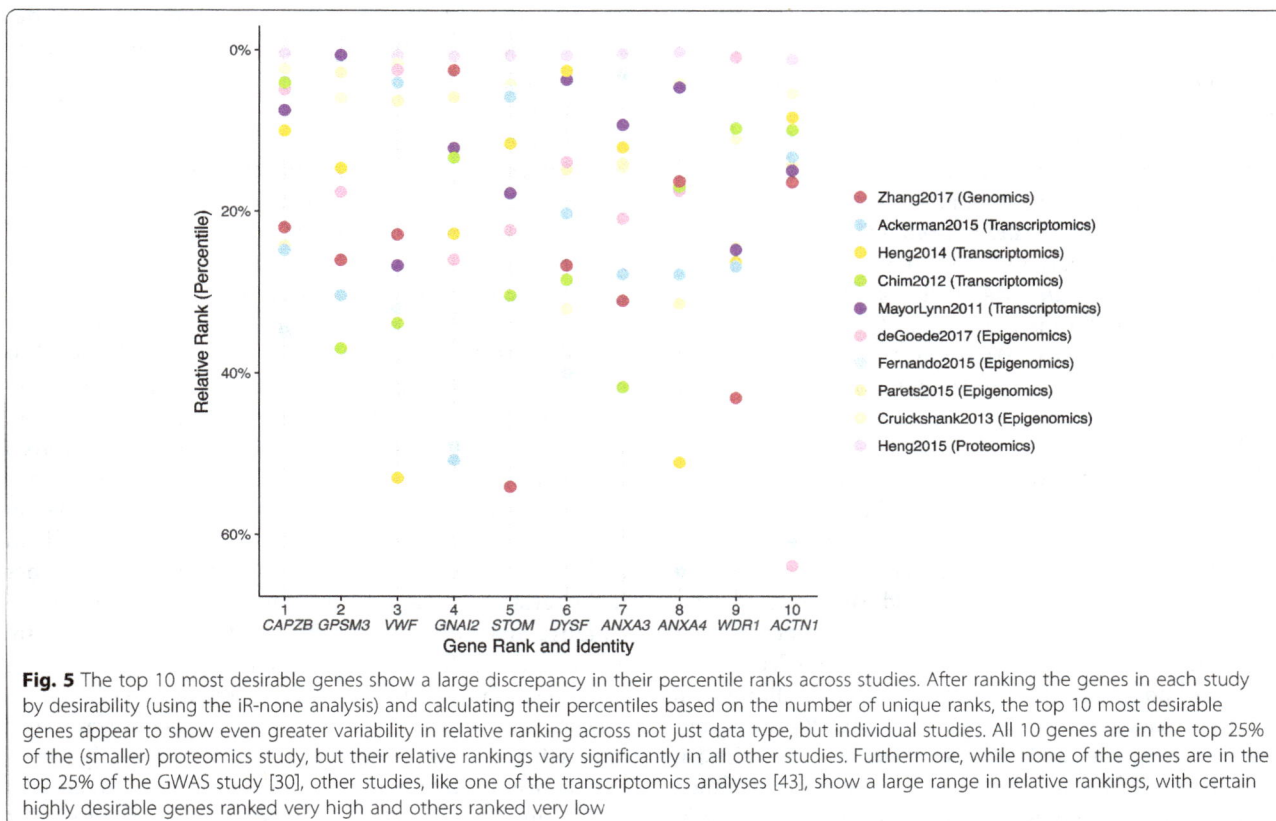

Fig. 5 The top 10 most desirable genes show a large discrepancy in their percentile ranks across studies. After ranking the genes in each study by desirability (using the iR-none analysis) and calculating their percentiles based on the number of unique ranks, the top 10 most desirable genes appear to show even greater variability in relative ranking across not just data type, but individual studies. All 10 genes are in the top 25% of the (smaller) proteomics study, but their relative rankings vary significantly in all other studies. Furthermore, while none of the genes are in the top 25% of the GWAS study [30], other studies, like one of the transcriptomics analyses [43], show a large range in relative rankings, with certain highly desirable genes ranked very high and others ranked very low

iR-none

First, the software was run without any added cuts, weights, or scales, resulting in a list of 26,868 genes with data from one or more of the 10 omics studies (Additional file 2). Normalized desirabilities for these 26,868 genes ranged from 8.04E-16 to 0.46 (mean = 0.08 ± 0.05) (Fig. 3). Furthermore, 7977 genes (29.7%) had desirabilities ≥0.1 corresponding to values equal to or higher than what would be achieved if a given gene achieved maximal desirability in one study but was absent from all others. These top 7977 genes were enriched for 70 unique GO-Slim Biological Process categories, including pathways involved in metabolic processes, immunity, and signal transduction (Additional file 13) [50]. Additionally, 15,285/26,868 (56.9%) genes achieved desirabilities greater than the permutation mean of 0.059. The top 10 genes (Figs. 4 and 5) had desirabilities ranging from 0.46 (*CAPZB*) to 0.38 (*ACTN1*) and were all represented in each of the 10 omics data sets analyzed. This analysis applied integRATE without cut points, allowing for a straightforward, linear transformation of data across all variables and studies.

iR-num

We next applied cut points based on numerical values (Additional file 3). *P*-values such that values smaller than

0.0001 received the maximum desirability score of 1 and values larger than 0.1 received the minimum desirability score of 0. All *P*-values between 0.0001 and 0.1 were transformed according to the d_{low} function. For $d_{extreme}$ functions, 4 cut points were assigned and we chose commonly used values of 0.5 and 1.5 (or their equivalents if the values were log transformed). Therefore, fold changes below − 1.5 or above − 1.5 (or below log2(1/3) or above log2(3)) received the maximum desirability score of 1 and fold changes between − 0.5 and 0.5 (or between log2(1/ 1.5) and log2(1.5)) received the minimum desirability score of 0. Intermediate values were transformed according to the $d_{extreme}$ function. This approach mirrors what was applied in a previous implementation of the desirability framework for omics data, and takes into account prior knowledge of typical *P*-value and fold change distributions [23]. While the top most desirable genes in iR-num appeared to be better candidates in each individual study (Additional file 6), using these cut points corresponding to standard significant *P*-value and fold change cut offs greatly reduced the number of desirable genes identified (Additional file 3). Specifically, only 1386/26,868 (5.1%) genes achieved desirabilities greater than the permutation mean of 0.059 and the top 10 most desirable genes were analyzed by only 4 or 5 studies instead of all 10 (Additional file 5).

iR-per

Finally, we applied cut points based on percentiles (Additional file 7). *P*-values were cut such that those in the top 5% received the maximum desirability score of 1 and those in the bottom 5% received the minimum desirability score of 0, with all values in between transformed according to the d_{low} function. Fold changes were cut such that those in the top 5% and bottom 5% received the maximum desirability score of 1 and those in the middle 50% received the minimum desirability score of 0, with all other values transformed according to the $d_{extreme}$ function. In this analysis, 16,604/26,868 (61.8%) genes achieved desirabilities greater than the permutation mean of 0.059.

HardThresh

For comparison, we also manually selected candidate genes by imposing a hard threshold on *P*-value (*P*-value < 0.05 if unadjusted and *P*-value < 0.1 if adjusted) (Additional file 11). After binning data into 'significant' gene lists, we intersected these lists to pull out genes that would have been identified simply by selecting the intersection of all significant genes. Although 18,727 genes were considered 'significant' in at least one study, no genes were identified as significant in all 10 studies. The top candidate gene (*KIAA0040*) was significant in 6/10 studies and 15 other genes were identified in 5/10 studies (Additional file 12). Interestingly, none of these 16 genes appear in the top 10 of our most desirable candidates after integration and, even more generally, none are specifically discussed in any of the studies, either.

Using integRATE to identify the most desirable sPTB genes

In our sPTB pilot analyses, members of the annexin family (*ANXA3*, *ANXA4* and *ANXA9*) appear in the top 10 most desirable candidate gene sets regardless of analysis approach (e.g., without cut points as well as with numerical *and* percentile cut points). This family is involved in calcium-dependent phospholipid binding and membrane-related exocytotic and endocytotic events, including endosome aggregation mediation (*ANXA6*). In a previous proteomic analysis, *ANXA3* was found to be differentially expressed in cervicovaginal fluid 26–30 days before the eventual onset of sPTB as compared to before healthy, term deliveries [51]. Furthermore, members of the annexin family are known to be involved in coagulation (*ANXA3*, *ANXA4*). Coagulation has been previously suggested to be involved in PTB and, even though the mechanism of such involvement is still a mystery, it is interesting that several genes involved in coagulation or blood disorders appear in our top candidate lists [52]. In addition to *ANXA3* and *ANXA4*, *VWF* (or Von Willebrand Factor) is a gene encoding a glycoprotein involved in coagulation that has been found to be expressed significantly more in preterm infant serum

as compared to term [53, 54]. Finally, another highly desirable candidate, *STOM*, encodes an integral membrane protein that localizes to red blood cells, the loss of which has been linked to anemia [55].

In addition to coagulation, another biological process represented across our results is actin regulation and muscle activity. The most notable gene associated with this biological process is *CAPZB*, which encodes part of an actin binding protein that regulates actin filament dynamics and stabilization and is present in the top 10 most desirable candidate gene list in all three analyses. Although *CAPZB* has never been linked to sPTB or other pregnancy pathologies, its role in muscle function could be linked to myometrial and uterine contractions that, when they occur prematurely, might be directly involved in the development of sPTB [56, 57]. Another one of our top candidates, *ACTN1*, is also involved in actin regulation and, even more interestingly, has also been linked to blood and bleeding disorders [58, 59]. Finally, several other highly desirable genes identified in one or more of our integrative analyses include *GPSM3*, *WDR1*, and *DYSF*, are all involved in the development and regulation of muscle or in the pathogenesis of muscle-related diseases [60–62].

Even outside the top 10 most desirable genes across our integrative analyses, we found genes both previously identified as being involved in pregnancy or sPTB pathology as well as involved in pathways potentially relevant to sPTB (Additional file 2). For example, one gene falling just outside the top 10 most desirable candidates in all analyses is *MMP9*, a matrix metalloproteinase. Interestingly, *MMP9* has been linked not only to sPTB, but also to PPROM and PE across a number of fetal and maternal tissues and at a variety of time points during pregnancy [63–67]. *MMP9* gene expression has been observed as significantly higher during preterm labor than during term labor in maternal serum, placenta, and fetal membranes [68–70]. Even in the first trimester, levels of *MMP9* in maternal serum were higher in PE cases than in healthy controls, suggesting that increased *MMP9* protein expression is linked to the underlying inflammatory processes governing PE pathogenesis [66]. Finally, fetal plasma *MMP9* concentration has been found to be significantly higher in fetuses with PPROM than in early and term deliveries with intact membranes, implicating *MMP9* in the membrane rupture mechanism controlling early delivery due to membrane rupture [67]. We see similar evidence of *MMP9* as a desirable sPTB candidate maintained across omics and tissue types in our integRATE analyses, raising the hypothesis that its role in inflammation and extracellular matrix organization relates to sPTB even in the absence of PPROM or PE.

Discussion

By using desirability functions to rank genes within studies and combine results across studies, integRATE allows for the identification of candidate genes supported across experimental conditions and omics data types. This is especially important when heterogeneous sets of omics data, like those available for sPTB, where the statistical approaches developed for vertical or horizontal integration are challenging to apply. We have shown that integRATE can map any omics data to a common [0, 1] scale for linear integration and produce a list of the most desirable candidates according to their weight of evidence across available studies. These candidates then become promising targets for follow-up functional testing depending on where in the data their desirability signals come from. Analysis of 10 heterogeneous omics data sets on sPTB showed that the gene candidates identified using desirability functions appear to be much more broadly supported than those identified by the intersection of all significant genes across all studies and contain both genes that have been previously associated with sPTB as well as novel ones (Figs. 4 and 5, Additional file 12).

integRATE identifies both known and novel candidate genes associated with a complex disease, including ones that are not among the top candidates in any single omics study but are consistently (i.e., across studies) recovered as significantly (or nearly significantly) associated. For example, genes that are significantly differentially expressed at an intermediate to high level across *many* studies will have high desirability scores. Furthermore, integRATE can identify such genes across omics types, tissues, patient groups, and any other variable condition. Although integRATE allows for this kind of synergistic, desirability-based analysis, it is important to note that integRATE is not a statistical tool nor is it intended to be the end point of any analysis. Rather, it is a straightforward framework for the identification of well-supported candidate genes in any phenotype where true multi-omics data are unavailable and can also serve as a springboard for future functional analysis, an essential next-step in testing whether the candidates are actually involved in the biology of the disease or phenotype at hand.

In our analyses, the genomics data set was typically the one with the highest desirability scores for each of the top 10 genes (Fig. 4) and the proteomics data set was typically the one in which the relative rank of the top 10 genes was the highest (Fig. 5). Both of these trends may appear surprising considering that our analyses contained just one genomics and one proteomics data set compared to four transcriptomics and four epigenomics ones (Table 1). There are three reasons for these two trends. First, there is substantial heterogeneity among the top genes identified by the four transcriptomic studies (see also [71]), as well as among the top genes identified by the four epigenomic studies. As a consequence, there is no common signature of the four

transcriptomic studies or the four epigenomic studies (see Fig. 4). Second, there are many more genes with high desirability scores in the genomics data set than in the other nine data sets (Additional file 1). However, we note that the ranking of the top 10 genes is not driven by the genomics data set; as we discuss below (see last paragraph of the discussion section), only one of the top 10 genes (*EBF1*) is among the candidate genes identified to be significantly associated with preterm birth and gestation length in the genomics data set [47]. Third, the number of differentially expressed proteins (mapped to genes) in the proteomics data set, and as a consequence the number of genes with desirability scores in this data set, was substantially lower than that of all other studies (and included hundreds of genes vs tens of thousands of genes). As a result, the percentile rank of the top 10 genes for the proteomics data set (Fig. 5) was much higher than their percentile rank in other data sets. However, as shown in Fig. 4, the desirability scores of the top 10 genes in the proteomics data set were typically neither very high nor very low, and did not appear to exert a disproportionate influence on the ranking of our top 10 genes.

Importantly, there is no single principled strategy for the selection of cut points. In our sPTB analyses (iR-none, iR-num, and iR-per), we observed that the imposition of cut points corresponding to generally agreed upon values (e.g., *P*-value < 0.0001) has the potential to greatly affect the resulting gene prioritization. On this basis, we propose that desirability functions are best used to integrate highly heterogeneous omics data without imposed numerical cut points for *P*-values, fold changes, and other variables. Implemented this way, one can maximize the information from the analysis of each omics data set used in prioritizing candidate genes. But users may also have reasons to want to put more weight on data sets that are of higher quality or on data types that may be more informative. In such instances, the weight parameter can be used to reflect study quality instead of imposing cut points (e.g., studies that fail to achieve *P*-values as low as others in the integrative analysis can be weighted less to reflect potentially lower experimental quality).

A recent GWAS analysis, the largest of its kind across pregnancy research, identified several candidate genes with SNPs linked to PTB [47]. This study linked *EBF1*, *EEFSEC*, and *AGTR2* to preterm birth and *EBF1*, *EEFSEC*, *AGTR2*, and *WNT4* to gestational duration (with *ADCY5* and *RAP2C* linked suggestively). By analyzing 43,568 women of European ancestry, this large study is the first to identify variants and genes that are statistically associated with sPTB. Interestingly, our integrative analysis identified *EBF1* as a desirable candidate ($d_{overall}$ = 0.15 [top 3%] in iR-none and $d_{overall}$ = 0.23 [top 1%] in iR-per), suggesting that this gene, in addition to GWAS, might also be functionally linked to sPTB pathogenesis across transcriptomics, epigenomics, and proteomics studies. Even when analyzing the 9 other omics studies without this GWAS data set, *EBF1* still achieved a $d_{overall}$ score of 0.17, placing it in the top 2% of all genes (Additional file 14). While our integrative analysis supports the identification of *EBF1* as an interesting candidate gene for follow up, the lack of signal for any of the other GWAS-identified hits also reinforces the need to approach complex phenotypes like sPTB from a variety of omics perspectives, since sequenced-based changes may impact the phenotype in indirect and complicated functional ways.

Conclusions

Desirability-based data integration (and our integRATE software) is a solution most applicable in biological research areas where omics data is especially heterogeneous and sparse. Our approach combines information from all variables across all related studies to calculate the total weight of evidence for any given gene as a candidate involved in disease pathogenesis, for example. Although not a statistical approach, this method of data integration allows for the prioritization of candidate genes based on information from heterogeneous omics data even without known 'gold standard' genes to test against and can be used to inform more targeted downstream functional analyses.

Additional files

Additional file 1: Results of meta-analysis to identify studies for integration. We outline the 10 studies meeting all inclusion criteria for integrative analysis. Furthermore, we list the other 44 studies that we identified through our literature search but we excluded from the data analysis as well as reasons for their exclusion.

Additional file 2: All results from iR-none. All desirability scores across all variables in all studies as well as overall desirabilities and normalized overall desirabilities are presented.

Additional file 3: All results from iR-num. All desirability scores across all variables in all studies as well as overall desirabilities and normalized overall desirabilities are presented.

Additional file 4: Results from iR-num. All genes in the analysis including numerical cut points were sorted from most desirable (rank = 1) to least desirable (rank = 26,869) and plotted according to their overall desirability scores.

Additional file 5: Top 10 genes from iR-num by data type. Desirability scores for the top 10 most desirable genes are plotted according to the type of omics analysis.

Additional file 6: Top 10 genes from iR-num by study. Desirability scores for the top 10 most desirable genes are plotted according to individual study.

Additional file 7: All results from iR-per. All desirability scores across all variables in all studies as well as overall desirabilities and normalized overall desirabilities are presented.

Additional file 8: Results from iR-per. All genes in the iR-per analysis were sorted from most desirable (rank = 1) to least desirable (rank = 26,869) and plotted according to their overall desirability scores.

Additional file 9: Top 10 genes from iR-per by data type. Desirability scores for the top 10 most desirable genes are plotted according to the type of omics analysis.

Additional file 10: Top 10 genes from iR-per by study. Desirability scores for the top 10 most desirable genes are plotted according to individual study.

Additional file 11: Raw data for manual overlap based on significance dichotomization. All 18,727 genes identified as significant in at least 1 study and overlap across the entire data set.

Additional file 12: Genes binned as significant in 4 or more omics studies. Upset plot showing intersections of significant genes across all 10 omics studies.

Additional file 13: GO-Slim gene set enrichment results. The PANTHER output for gene set functional enrichment is provided, including 37 statistically enriched biological pathways.

Additional file 14: All results *without* including the Zhang 2017 data set [30]. All desirability scores across all variables in all studies as well as overall desirabilities and normalized overall desirabilities are presented.

Abbreviations

GWAS: Genome-wide association study; IUGR: Intrauterine growth restriction; PE: Preeclampsia; PPROM: Premature rupture of membranes; PTB: Preterm birth; SNP: Single nucleotide polymorphism; sPTB: Spontaneous preterm birth

Acknowledgements

We thank Dr. Lou Muglia for invaluable discussion and support in designing and applying this approach to data integration and Dr. Ge Zhang for providing access to preprocessed GWAS data.

Funding

HRE was supported by a Transdisciplinary Scholar Award from the March of Dimes Prematurity Research Center Ohio Collaborative. This research was supported by the March of Dimes through the March of Dimes Prematurity Research Center Ohio Collaborative and the Burroughs Wellcome Fund. The funders had no role in study design, data collection and analysis, decision to publish, or preparation of the manuscript.

Authors' contributions

Conceived and designed experiments: HRE, AR. Performed experiments: HRE. Developed scripts: HRE, JS. Analyzed data: HRE. Wrote paper: HRE. Assisted with project development: AR, JHW, PA, JAC. Provided feedback: JHW, PA, JAC, AR. All authors have read and approved the manuscript.

Competing interests

The authors declare that they have no competing interests.

Author details

[1]Department of Biological Sciences, Vanderbilt University, Nashville, TN, USA. [2]Department of Biochemistry, Purdue University, West Lafayette, IN, USA. [3]Department of Biomedical Informatics, Vanderbilt University, Nashville, TN, USA. [4]Vanderbilt Genetics Institute, Vanderbilt University, Nashville, TN, USA.

References

1. Gohlke JM, Thomas R, Zhang Y, Rosenstein MC, Davis AP, Murphy C, et al. Genetic and environmental pathways to complex diseases. BMC Syst Biol. 2009;3:46.

2. Hasin Y, Seldin M, Lusis A. Multi-omics approaches to disease. Genome Biol. 2017;18:83.

3. Chen R, Mias GI, Li-Pook-Than J, Jiang L, Lam HYK, Chen R, et al. Personal omics profiling reveals dynamic molecular and medical phenotypes. Cell. 2012;148:1293–307. https://doi.org/10.1016/j.cell.2012.02.009.

4. Karczewski KJ, Snyder MP. Integrative omics for health and disease. Nat Rev Genet. 2018;19:299–310. https://doi.org/10.1038/nrg.2018.4.

5. Edwards SL, Beesley J, French JD, Dunning AM. Beyond GWASs: illuminating the dark road from association to function. Am J Hum Genet. 2013;93: 779–97.

6. Visscher PM, Wray NR, Zhang Q, Sklar P, McCarthy MI, Brown MA, et al. 10 years of GWAS discovery: biology, function, and translation. Am J Hum Genet. 2017;101:5–22.

7. Casamassimi A, Federico A, Rienzo M, Esposito S, Ciccodicola A. Transcriptome profiling in human diseases: new advances and perspectives. Int J Mol Sci. 2017;18:1652. https://doi.org/10.3390/ijms18081652.

8. Ritchie MD, Holzinger ER, Li R, Pendergrass SA, Kim D. Methods of integrating data to uncover genotype–phenotype interactions. Nat Rev Genet. 2015;16:85–97. https://doi.org/10.1038/nrg3868.

9. Holzinger ER, Ritchie MD. Integrating heterogeneous high-throughput data for meta-dimensional pharmacogenomics and disease-related studies. Pharmacogenomics. 2012;13:213–22. https://doi.org/10.2217/pgs.11.145.

10. Kim D, Shin H, Song YS, Kim JH. Synergistic effect of different levels of genomic data for cancer clinical outcome prediction. J Biomed Inform. 2012;45:1191–8. https://doi.org/10.1016/j.jbi.2012.07.008.

11. Peng C, Li A, Wang M. Discovery of bladder cancer-related genes using integrative heterogeneous network modeling of multi-omics data. Sci Rep. 2017;7:15639. https://doi.org/10.1038/s41598-017-15890-9.

12. Pavel AB, Sonkin D, Reddy A. Integrative modeling of multi-omics data to identify cancer drivers and infer patient-specific gene activity. BMC Syst Biol. 2016;10:16. https://doi.org/10.1186/s12918-016-0260-9.

13. Zhu J, Shi Z, Wang J, Zhang B. Empowering biologists with multi-omics data: colorectal cancer as a paradigm. Bioinformatics. 2015;31:1436–43. https://doi.org/10.1093/bioinformatics/btu834.

14. McLendon R, Friedman A, Bigner D, Van Meir EG, Brat DJ, Mastrogianakis GM, et al. Comprehensive genomic characterization defines human glioblastoma genes and core pathways. Nature. 2008;455:1061–8. https://doi.org/10.1038/nature07385.

15. Verhaak RGW, Hoadley KA, Purdom E, Wang V, Qi Y, Wilkerson MD, et al. Integrated genomic analysis identifies clinically relevant subtypes of glioblastoma characterized by abnormalities in PDGFRA, IDH1, EGFR, and NF1. Cancer Cell. 2010;17:98–110. https://doi.org/10.1016/j.ccr.2009.12.020.

16. Cohen J. The cost of dichotomization. Appl Psychol Meas. 1983;7:249–53. https://doi.org/10.1177/014662168300700301.

17. Streiner DL. Breaking up is hard to do: the heartbreak of dichotomizing continuous data. Can J Psychiatr. 2002;47:262–6. https://doi.org/10.1177/070674370204700307.

18. Barnwell-Ménard J-L, Li Q, Cohen AA. Effects of categorization method, regression type, and variable distribution on the inflation of type-I error rate when categorizing a confounding variable. Stat Med. 2015;34:936–49. https://doi.org/10.1002/sim.6387.

19. Reif DM, White BC, Moore JH. Integrated analysis of genetic, genomic and proteomic data. Expert Rev Proteomics. 2004;1:67–75. https://doi.org/10.1586/14789450.1.1.67.

20. Hamid JS, Hu P, Roslin NM, Ling V, Greenwood CMT, Beyene J. Data integration in genetics and genomics: methods and challenges. Hum Genomics Proteomics. 2009;2009:1–13. https://doi.org/10.4061/2009/869093.

21. Sieberts SK, Schadt EE. Moving toward a system genetics view of disease. Mamm Genome. 2007;18:389–401. https://doi.org/10.1007/s00335-007-9040-6.

22. Hawkins RD, Hon GC, Ren B. Next-generation genomics: an integrative approach. Nat Rev Genet. 2010;11:476–86. https://doi.org/10.1038/nrg2795.

23. Lazic SE. Ranking, selecting, and prioritising genes with desirability functions. PeerJ. 2015;3:e1444. https://doi.org/10.7717/peerj.1444.

24. Bickerton GR, Paolini GV, Besnard J, Muresan S, Hopkins AL. Quantifying the chemical beauty of drugs. Nat Chem. 2012;4:90–8. https://doi.org/10.1038/nchem.1243

25. Harrington E. The desirability function. Ind Qual Control. 1965;21:494–8.

26. Derringer G, Suich R. Simultaneous optimization of several response variables. J Qual Technol. 1980;12:214–9.

27. Derringer G. A balancing act: optimizing a products properties. Qual Prog. 1994;27:51.

28. Romero R, Dey SK, Fisher SJ. Preterm labor: one syndrome, many causes. Science. 2014;345:760–5. https://doi.org/10.1126/science.1251816.

29. Eidem HR, McGary KL, Capra JA, Abbot P, Rokas A. The transformative potential of an integrative approach to pregnancy. Placenta. 2017;57: 204–15.

30. Zhang G, Jacobsson B, Muglia LJ. Genetic associations with spontaneous preterm birth. N Engl J Med. 2017;377:2401–2. https://doi.org/10.1056/NEJMc1713902.

31. Plunkett J, Muglia LJ. Genetic contributions to preterm birth: implications from epidemiological and genetic association studies. Ann Med. 2008;40: 167–9. https://doi.org/10.1080/07853890701806181.

32. Muglia LJ, Katz M. The enigma of spontaneous preterm birth. N Engl J Med. 2010;362:529–35. https://doi.org/10.1056/NEJMra0904308.

33. Lengyel C, Muglia LJ, Pavličev M. Genetics of Preterm Birth. In: eLS. Chichester: Wiley; 2014. https://doi.org/10.1002/9780470015902.a0025448.

34. Ackerman WE, Buhimschi IA, Eidem HR, Rinker DC, Rokas A, Rood K, et al. Comprehensive RNA profiling of villous trophoblast and decidua basalis in pregnancies complicated by preterm birth following intra-amniotic infection. Placenta. 2016;44:23–33. https://doi.org/10.1016/j.placenta. 2016.05.010.

35. Heng YJ, Taylor L, Larsen BG, Chua HN, Pung SM, Lee MWF, et al. Albumin decrease is associated with spontaneous preterm delivery within 48 h in women with threatened preterm labor. J Proteome Res. 2015;14:457–66. https://doi.org/10.1021/pr500852p.

36. Parets SE, Conneely KN, Kilaru V, Fortunato SJ, Syed TA, Saade G, et al. Fetal DNA methylation associates with early spontaneous preterm birth and gestational age. PLoS One. 2013;8:e67489. https://doi.org/10.1371/journal.pone.0067489.

37. Cruickshank MN, Oshlack A, Theda C, Davis PG, Martino D, Sheehan P, et al. Analysis of epigenetic changes in survivors of preterm birth reveals the effect of gestational age and evidence for a long term legacy. Genome Med. 2013;5:96. https://doi.org/10.1186/gm500.

38. Saade GR, Boggess KA, Sullivan SA, Markenson GR, Iams JD, Coonrod DV, et al. Development and validation of a spontaneous preterm delivery predictor in asymptomatic women. Am J Obstet Gynecol. 2016;214:633.e1–633.e24. https://doi.org/10.1016/j.ajog.2016.02.001.

39. Zhang G, Bacelis J, Lengyel C, Teramo K, Hallman M, Helgeland Ø, et al. Assessing the causal relationship of maternal height on birth size and gestational age at birth: a Mendelian randomization analysis. PLoS Med. 2015;12:e1001865. https://doi.org/10.1371/journal.pmed.1001865.

40. Makieva S, Dubicke A, Rinaldi SF, Fransson E, Ekman-Ordeberg G, Norman JE. The preterm cervix reveals a transcriptomic signature in the presence of premature prelabor rupture of membranes. Am J Obstet Gynecol. 2017;216: 602.e1–602.e21. https://doi.org/10.1016/j.ajog.2017.02.009.

41. Heng YJ, Pennell CE, Chua HN, Perkins JE, Lye SJ. Whole blood gene expression profile associated with spontaneous preterm birth in women with threatened preterm labor. PLoS One. 2014;9:e96901. https://doi.org/10.1371/journal.pone.0096901.

42. Chim SSC, Lee WS, Ting YH, Chan OK, Lee SWY, Leung TY. Systematic identification of spontaneous preterm birth-associated RNA transcripts in maternal plasma. PLoS One. 2012;7:e34328. https://doi.org/10.1371/journal.pone.0034328.

43. Mayor-Lynn K, Toloubeydokhti T, Cruz AC, Chegini N. Expression profile of MicroRNAs and mRNAs in human placentas from pregnancies complicated by preeclampsia and preterm labor. Reprod Sci. 2011;18:46–56. https://doi.org/10.1177/1933719110374115.

44. de Goede OM, Lavoie PM, Robinson WP. Cord blood hematopoietic cells from preterm infants display altered DNA methylation patterns. Clin Epigenetics. 2017;9:39. https://doi.org/10.1186/s13148-017-0339-1.

45. Hong X, Sherwood B, Ladd-Acosta C, Peng S, Ji H, Hao K, et al. Genome-wide DNA methylation associations with spontaneous preterm birth in US blacks: findings in maternal and cord blood samples. Epigenetics. 2018;13: 163–72. https://doi.org/10.1080/15592294.2017.1287654.

46. Fernando F, Keijser R, Henneman P, van der Kevie-Kersemaekers A-MF, Mannens MM, van der Post JA, et al. The idiopathic preterm delivery

methylation profile in umbilical cord blood DNA. BMC Genomics. 2015;16: 736. https://doi.org/10.1186/s12864-015-1915-4.

47. Zhang G, Feenstra B, Bacelis J, Liu X, Muglia LM, Juodakis J, et al. Genetic associations with gestational duration and spontaneous preterm birth. Obstet Gynecol Surv. 2017;73:83–5. https://doi.org/10.1097/01.ogx.0000530434.15441.45.

48. de Leeuw CA, Mooij JM, Heskes T, Posthuma D. MAGMA: generalized gene-set analysis of GWAS data. PLoS Comput Biol. 2015;11:e1004219. https://doi.org/10.1371/journal.pcbi.1004219.

49. Conway JR, Lex A, Gehlenborg N. UpSetR: an R package for the visualization of intersecting sets and their properties. Bioinformatics. 2017;33:2938–40. https://doi.org/10.1093/bioinformatics/btx364.

50. Mi H, Huang X, Muruganujan A, Tang H, Mills C, Kang D, et al. PANTHER version 11: expanded annotation data from gene ontology and reactome pathways, and data analysis tool enhancements. Nucleic Acids Res. 2017;45: D183–9. https://doi.org/10.1093/nar/gkw1138.

51. Heng YJ, Liong S, Permezel M, Rice GE, Di Quinzio MKW, Georgiou HM. Human cervicovaginal fluid biomarkers to predict term and preterm labor. Front Physiol. 2015;6. https://doi.org/10.3389/fphys.2015.00151.

52. Velez DR, Fortunato SJ, Thorsen P, Lombardi SJ, Williams SM, Menon R. Preterm birth in Caucasians is associated with coagulation and inflammation pathway gene variants. PLoS One. 2008;3:e3283. https://doi.org/10.1371/journal.pone.0003283.

53. Cowman J, Quinn N, Geoghegan S, Müllers S, Oglesby I, Byrne B, et al. Dynamic platelet function on von Willebrand factor is different in preterm neonates and full-term neonates: changes in neonatal platelet function. J Thromb Haemost. 2016;14:2027–35. https://doi.org/10.1111/jth.13414.

54. Strauss T, Elisha N, Ravid B, Rosenberg N, Lubetsky A, Levy-Mendelovich S, et al. Activity of Von Willebrand factor and levels of VWF-cleaving protease (ADAMTS13) in preterm and full term neonates. Blood Cells Mol Dis. 2017; 67:14–7. https://doi.org/10.1016/j.bcmd.2016.12.013.

55. Zhu Y, Paszty C, Turetsky T, Tsai S, Kuypers FA, Lee G, et al. Stomatocytosis is absent in "stomatin"-deficient murine red blood cells. Blood. 1999;93:2404–10 http://www.ncbi.nlm.nih.gov/pubmed/10090952.

56. Littlefield R, Almenar-Queralt A, Fowler VM. Actin dynamics at pointed ends regulates thin filament length in striated muscle. Nat Cell Biol. 2001;3:544–51. https://doi.org/10.1038/35078517.

57. Caldwell JE, Heiss SG, Mermall V, Cooper JA. Effects of CapZ, an actin-capping protein of muscle, on the polymerization of actin. Biochemistry. 1989;28:8506–14. https://doi.org/10.1021/bi00447a036.

58. Bottega R, Marconi C, Faleschini M, Baj G, Cagioni C, Pecci A, et al. ACTN1-related thrombocytopenia: identification of novel families for phenotypic characterization. Blood. 2015;125:869–72. https://doi.org/10.1182/blood-2014-08-594531.

59. Kunishima S, Okuno Y, Yoshida K, Shiraishi Y, Sanada M, Muramatsu H, et al. ACTN1 mutations cause congenital macrothrombocytopenia. Am J Hum Genet. 2013;92:431–8. https://doi.org/10.1016/j.ajhg.2013.01.015.

60. Zhao P, Chidiac P. Regulation of RGS5 GAP activity by GPSM3. Mol Cell Biochem. 2015;405:33–40. https://doi.org/10.1007/s11010-015-2393-3.

61. Ono S. Functions of actin-interacting protein 1 (AIP1)/WD repeat protein 1 (WDR1) in actin filament dynamics and cytoskeletal regulation. Biochem Biophys Res Commun. 2017. https://doi.org/10.1016/j.bbrc.2017.10.096.

62. Liu J, Aoki M, Illa I, Wu C, Fardeau M, Angelini C, et al. Dysferlin, a novel skeletal muscle gene, is mutated in Miyoshi myopathy and limb girdle muscular dystrophy. Nat Genet. 1998;20:31–6. https://doi.org/10.1038/1682.

63. Athayde N, Romero R, Gomez R, Maymon E, Pacora P, Mazor M, et al. Matrix metalloproteinases-9 in preterm and term human parturition. J Matern Neonatal Med. 1999;8:213–9. https://doi.org/10.3109/14767059909052049.

64. Chen J, Khalil RA. Matrix metalloproteinases in normal pregnancy and preeclampsia. In: Progress in molecular biology and translational science; 2017. p. 87–165. https://doi.org/10.1016/bs.pmbts.2017.04.001.

65. Xu P, Alfaidy N, Challis JRG. Expression of matrix metalloproteinase (MMP)-2 and MMP-9 in human placenta and fetal membranes in relation to preterm and term labor. J Clin Endocrinol Metab. 2002;87:1353–61. https://doi.org/10.1210/jcem.87.3.8320.

66. Poon LCY, Nekrasova E, Anastassopoulos P, Livanos P, Nicolaides KH. First-trimester maternal serum matrix metalloproteinase-9 (MMP-9) and adverse pregnancy outcome. Prenat Diagn. 2009;29:553–9. https://doi.org/10.1002/pd.2234.

67. Romero R, Chaiworapongsa T, Espinoza J, Gomez R, Yoon BH, Edwin S, et al. Fetal plasma MMP-9 concentrations are elevated in preterm premature rupture of the membranes. Am J Obstet Gynecol. 2002;187:1125–30. https://doi.org/10.1067/mob.2002.127312.

68. Tency I, Verstraelen H, Kroes I, Holtappels G, Verhasselt B, Vaneechoutte M, et al. Imbalances between matrix metalloproteinases (MMPs) and tissue inhibitor of metalloproteinases (TIMPs) in maternal serum during preterm labor. PLoS One. 2012;7:e49042. https://doi.org/10.1371/journal.pone.0049042.

69. Sundrani DP, Chavan-Gautam PM, Pisal HR, Mehendale SS, Joshi SR. Matrix metalloproteinase-1 and -9 in human placenta during spontaneous vaginal delivery and caesarean sectioning in preterm pregnancy. PLoS One. 2012;7:e29855.

70. Yonemoto H, Young CB, Ross JT, Guilbert LL, Fairclough RJ, Olson DM. Changes in matrix metalloproteinase (MMP)-2 and MMP-9 in the fetal amnion and chorion during gestation and at term and preterm labor. Placenta. 2006;27:669–77.

71. Eidem HR, Ackerman WE, McGary KL, Abbot P, Rokas A. Gestational tissue transcriptomics in term and preterm human pregnancies: a systematic review and meta-analysis. BMC Med Genet. 2015;8:27.

19

A pan-cancer analysis of driver gene mutations, DNA methylation and gene expressions reveals that chromatin remodeling is a major mechanism inducing global changes in cancer epigenomes

Ahrim Youn[1,2], Kyung In Kim[2], Raul Rabadan[3,4], Benjamin Tycko[5], Yufeng Shen[3,4,6] and Shuang Wang[1*]

Abstract

Background: Recent large-scale cancer sequencing studies have discovered many novel cancer driver genes (CDGs) in human cancers. Some studies also suggest that CDG mutations contribute to cancer-associated epigenomic and transcriptomic alterations across many cancer types. Here we aim to improve our understanding of the connections between CDG mutations and altered cancer cell epigenomes and transcriptomes on pan-cancer level and how these connections contribute to the known association between epigenome and transcriptome.

Method: Using multi-omics data including somatic mutation, DNA methylation, and gene expression data of 20 cancer types from The Cancer Genome Atlas (TCGA) project, we conducted a pan-cancer analysis to identify CDGs, when mutated, have strong associations with genome-wide methylation or expression changes across cancer types, which we refer as methylation driver genes (MDGs) or expression driver genes (EDGs), respectively.

Results: We identified 32 MDGs, among which, eight are known chromatin modification or remodeling genes. Many of the remaining 24 MDGs are connected to chromatin regulators through either regulating their transcription or physically interacting with them as potential co-factors. We identified 29 EDGs, 26 of which are also MDGs. Further investigation on target genes' promoters methylation and expression alteration patterns of these 26 overlapping driver genes shows that hyper-methylation of target genes' promoters are significantly associated with down-regulation of the same target genes and hypo-methylation of target genes' promoters are significantly associated with up-regulation of the same target genes.

Conclusion: This finding suggests a pivotal role for genetically driven changes in chromatin remodeling in shaping DNA methylation and gene expression patterns during tumor development.

Keywords: Pan-cancer analysis, TCGA, somatic mutation, DNA methylation, gene expression, methylation driver gene, expression driver gene, chromatic remodeling

* Correspondence: sw2206@columbia.edu
[1]Department of Biostatistics, Mailman School of Public Health, Columbia University, New York, New York, USA
Full list of author information is available at the end of the article

Background

Cancer arises through accumulation of somatically acquired genetic and epigenetic aberrations that lead to malignant transformation [1, 2]. Comprehensive characterization of somatic mutations in cancer genomes using next-generation sequencing technology has led to discoveries of cancer driver genes (CDGs) in human cancers [2]. The interplay between genetic and epigenetic alterations was only recently revealed through genome-wide scale genomic and epigenomic analyses. Specifically, genome-wide change of DNA methylation was observed in patients with mutations in epigenetic regulators [2–4], affecting both the global levels of 5-methyl-cytosine (5mC) and the precise DNA methylation patterns in diverse regulatory sequences across the genome [2, 3]. A recent study investigated associations between driver gene mutations and DNA methylation alterations across many cancer types [5], and identified associations between mutated driver genes and site-specific methylation changes as well as some genome-wide trends in specific cancer types. They further used these mutation-methylation associations to better define cancer subtypes. However, it remains largely unknown how the CDG mutations contribute to changes in cancer cell epigenomes on a pan-cancer level [6]. A better understanding of the connections between CDGs and altered cancer cell epigenomes is an important goal, particularly since mutations in epigenetic regulators could be novel targets for anti-cancer therapies [6].

Studies have integrated multi-scale omics data, including somatic mutation data, epigenomes, and transcriptomes across various cancer types to improve the mechanistic understanding of the interplay between cancer genome and cancer epigenome and transcriptome. An integrative analysis of DNA methylation data and gene expression data of various cancer types identified pan-cancer hypo- and hyper-methylated genes that are predictive of transcription as well as methylation-driven subgroups with clinical implications [7]. Another integrative analysis on a set of known epigenetic regulators with DNA methylation data and gene expression data from various cancer types identified key epigenetic regulators whose deregulation patterns are associated with genome-wide DNA methylation changes, which transcend cancer types [8].

Here we aim to improve our understanding of the connections between CDGs and altered cancer cell epigenomes and altered cancer cell transcriptome on pan-cancer level, and how these connections contribute to the known association between cancer epigenome and transcriptome. We used somatic mutation, DNA methylation, and gene expression data of 20 cancer types from The Cancer Genome Atlas (TCGA) project to identify CDGs that, when mutated, have strong associations with genome-wide methylation or expression changes across cancer types, which we refer as methylation driver genes (MDGs) or expression driver genes (EDGs). We identified 32 MDGs and found that most of them are either chromatin regulators (genes involved in chromatin remodeling) or ones that regulate the expression of or physically interact with chromatin regulators. We also identified 29 EDGs and found that 26 of them overlap with the 32 MDGs. We further investigated target genes' methylation and expression alteration patterns that are associated with mutation status of these 26 overlapping driver genes and found that hyper-methylation of target genes' promoters are significantly associated with down-regulation of the same target genes and hypo-methylation of target genes' promoters are significantly associated with up-regulation of the same target genes. This finding shows that dysregulation of chromatin regulators is potentially an important mechanism that induces global change of DNA methylation and gene expression in tumor development.

Methods

We downloaded somatic mutation data, DNA methylation 450K array data, and gene-level RNA-seq data of 20 tumor types with at least 100 samples available in all three data types from TCGA. For DNA methylation 450K array data, we conducted standard quality control steps removing CpG sites that overlap with known single nuclear polymorphisms (SNPs), sites on the sex chromosomes and sites with missing values for more than 5% of the tumor samples within a tumor type. After these steps, 370,877 CpG sites remained. We then corrected for the type I/II probe bias using the BMIQ algorithm [9]

Selection of candidate CDGs

We obtained level 2 somatic mutation data of the above-mentioned 20 tumor types from Broad Institute TCGA Genome Data Analysis Center Firehose [10] and selected candidate CDGs using the MutSIG [11] algorithm that tests how frequently a gene is mutated in a tumor type comparing to the background mutation rate. We used the false discovery rate (FDR) < 0.1 to select candidate CDGs. We then assessed the functional impact of mutations at gene levels using the MutationAssessor [12] algorithm to further remove mutations classified as neutral. Additional steps were done for COAD and STAD when an abnormally large number of candidate CDGs remained (1,433 and 553, respectively) after these steps to avoid potential high false positive discovery rate of CDGs. Specifically, we only kept the genes that were identified in any of the other 18 tumor types as well as identified in the Cancer Gene Census [13] and the numbers of candidate CDGs in COAD and STAD then dropped to 193 and 67. The number of candidate CDGs selected in all 20 tumor types is provided in Additional file 1: Table S1.

To conduct pan-cancer analysis associating mutation and methylation/expression, within a tumor type, we selected CDGs that have mutations in at least 5 samples with matched methylation data or expression data in order to have not-too-sparse numbers in the mutated group. For matched mutation and methylation data, 445 CDGs were selected across the 20 tumor types. Here we analyzed somatic mutations at the gene level and a gene is considered mutated in a tumor sample as long as there is any mutation in this gene. Within these driver genes, the number of tumor types in which a driver gene was mutated in at least five samples varies from 1 to 15 (Additional file 2: Table S2) where most of the CDGs were mutated in only one or two tumor types. *TP53* was mutated in 15 tumor types and *PTEN* was mutated in 14 tumor types. For matched mutation data and expression data, 422 CDGs were similarly selected. Of them, 403 CDGs overlap with the CDGs selected for matched mutation data and methylation data. For the 422 CDGs, the number of tumor types in which a CDG is mutated in at least five samples varies from 1 to 14 (Additional file 2: Table S2), where *TP53* and *PTEN* were mutated in 14 tumor types.

Pan-cancer analysis to identify MDGs

We described the details in the pan-cancer analysis associating driver genes and genome-wide methylation alterations across cancer types. Similar procedures with necessary modifications to associate driver genes and gene expression changes were described in the Additional file 3: Text S1.

Associate CDGs and DNA methylation in one cancer type

For CDG i, let A_i denote the set of tumor types in which CDG i is mutated in at least 5 tumor samples with methylation data available. We then determine the hyper- or hypo-methylation status per CpG site by the mutation status of CDG i using the nonparametric Wilcoxon test. Since methylation levels range from 0 to 1 and are often bimodally distributed across tumor samples and the numbers of samples in the mutated and non-mutated groups are extremely unbalanced. With the Wilcoxon test, we define a set of genome-wide hyper-methylated sites $S_{i,k}+$ whose methylation levels are significantly increased at significance level 0.01 in the mutated group comparing to the non-mutated group of CDG i in cancer type k. We similarly define a set of hypo-methylated sites $S_{i,k}-$. Since the goal is not to identify specific CpG sites that are affected by the mutation status but to see how the mutation status is associated with genome-wide methylation changes, no multiple comparisons adjustment is applied to the site-level differential methylation association test.

To determine if mutation status of CDG i is significantly associated with genome-wide methylation changes in cancer type k, we calculate the p-value pi,k, which is the probability of observing the number of differentially (hyper- or hypo-) methylated sites $n_{i,k}^m = | S_{i,k}^+ \cup S_{i,k}^- |$ or more that are associated with the mutation status of CDG i in cancer type k under the null hypothesis that the mutation status of CDG i is not associated with genome-wide methylation changes. To do so, we generate a "methylation null pool", which has the number of differentially methylated sites under the null hypothesis. We first selected genes that were mutated in at least 5 samples with methylation data available within a tumor type. We then further selected only top 500 highly mutated genes within each tumor type for computational efficiency and also excluded the 445 CDGs selected above. We ended up with 7,019 mutation genes (those are considered as passenger mutation genes) across 20 tumor types in the "methylation null pool" (see Additional file 4: Table S3 for the number of mutation genes from each tumor type). The 7,019 mutation genes have similar mutation rate (average number of mutations in a cancer type) with that of the 445 CDGs. The average mutation rate of these 7,019 mutation genes is 0.082 with standard deviation (SD) 0.10 while the average mutation rate of the 445 CDGs is 0.085 with SD = 0.13 (p-value=0.54 from a t-test).

Within each cancer type, we calculated $n_{j_{null}}^m$, the number of differentially methylated sites that are associated with the mutation status of the methylation null gene $jnull$= 1,...,7019, which form the "methylation null pool". The p-value pi,k, is then calculated as the proportion of numbers $n_{j_{null}}^m$ in the "methylation null pool" that is greater than or equal to the observed number of differentially methylated sites $n_{i,k}^m$, that is, $p_{i,k} = \frac{1}{7019} \sum_{j_{null}=1}^{7019} I(n_{i,k}^m \leq n_{j_{null}}^m)$, where $I(.)$ is the indicator function.

To investigate the potential selection bias in the "methylation null pool", we also generated the null distribution of number of genome-wide differentially methylated sites by randomly splitting tumor samples of a tumor type into mutation and non-mutation groups, varying the percentage of mutation from 5 to 40% based on the mutation rate of the TCGA 20 tumor types and calculated numbers of differentially methylated sites between the two groups. We repeated this 10 times for each percentage from 5 to 40%, increasing by 1%. Therefore, we ended up with 360*20 values for the number of differentially methylated sites across 20 tumor types. We found that these numbers are on average much smaller than those from the "methylation null pool" generated using passenger mutations, making the p-values of CDGs more significant. This indicates that there is some association between passenger mutations and global methylation changes that random sampling cannot capture. Therefore, the methylation null pool generated by using the passenger mutations rather than randomly splitting may represent a better null distribution. The MDGs identified this way are those associated with methylation changes beyond what is expected for passenger mutations.

We classify the effect of CDG i on genome-wide methylation in tumor type k as:

CDG i in tumor type k

$$= \begin{cases} \text{genome-wide hyper-methylated if } p_{i,k} < 0.05 & \left(|S_{i,k}^{+}| > |S_{i,k}^{-}|\right) \\ \text{genoem-wide hypo-methylated if } p_{i,k} < 0.05 & \left(|S_{i,k}^{+}| \leq |S_{i,k}^{-}|\right). \end{cases}$$

Associate CDGs and DNA methylation across multiple cancer types

To calculate the p-value, pi, testing if CDG i is significantly associated with genome-wide methylation changes across multiple cancer types, we compare $\sum_{k \in A_i} n_{i,k}^{m}$, the observed total number of differentially methylated sites associated with CDG i summed over Ai cancer types, to B resampled values generated from the "methylation null pool" where we set B=one million. More specifically, for CDG i that was mutated in $|Ai|$ number of tumor types, the null distribution is generated using the B sets of sum of $|Ai|$ random samples from the "methylation null pool". We then calculate pi as follows:

$$p_i = \sum_{b=1}^{B} I\left(\sum_{k \in A_i} n_{i,k}^{m} \leq \sum_{j=1}^{|A_i|} n_{r_{b,j}}^{m}\right)/B,$$

where $r_{b,\ j}$ is a random number between 1 and 7,019 from the bth resampling. We use Benjamini-Hochberg procedure to adjust for multiple comparisons on p_i, which is done within groups of CDGs that were mutated in the same number of tumor types. The MDGs are then identified as those CDGs with adjusted $pi < 0.05$.

Results

TCGA 20 Cancer Types

We assembled somatic mutation data, HM450 DNA methylation data and gene-level RNA-Seq data (upper-quantile-normalized count data) of 20 tumor types with at least 100 samples available in all three data types from TCGA. This includes breast invasive carcinoma (BRCA), bladder urothelial carcinoma (BLCA), cervical squamous cell carcinoma (CESC), colon adenocarcinoma (COAD), glioblastoma (GBM), head and neck squamous cell carcinoma (HNSC), kidney renal clear cell carcinoma (KIRC), kidney renal papillary cell carcinoma (KIRP), acute myeloid leukemia (LAML), lower grade glioma (LGG), liver hepatocellular carcinoma (LIHC), lung adenocarcinoma (LUAD), lung squamous cell carcinoma

(LUSC), pancreatic adenocarcinoma (PAAD), pheochromocytoma and paraganglioma (PCPG), prostate adenocarcinoma (PRAD), sarcoma (SARC), stomach adenocarcinoma (STAD), thyroid carcinoma (THCA), testicular germ cell tumor (TGCT), and uterine corpus endometrial carcinoma (UCEC)). For detailed steps on processing DNA methylation data and selecting candidate CDGs, see Methods. We refer candidate CDGs as CDGs from now on for notation simplicity.

The Pan-Cancer Analysis

We conducted a pan-cancer analysis to identify methylation driver genes (MDGs)/expression driver genes (EDGs) that, when mutated, have strong associations with genome-wide methylation/expression changes across multiple cancer types through integrating somatic mutation and DNA methylation/gene expression data of 20 TCGA tumor types (Fig. 1a, b).

We then showed that some of the identified MDGs are chromatin regulators that directly affect the genome-wide methylation patterns and some are connected to chromatin regulators through either regulating their transcription or physically interacting with them as potential co-factors (Fig. 1c).

We first tested whether mutations in a CDG are significantly associated with changes in genome-wide methylation patterns in one cancer type. For this, we performed CpG-site-level association analysis within a cancer type, where a nonparametric Wilcoxon test was used since the numbers of samples in the mutated and non-mutated groups are extremely unbalanced and methylation measures were usually enriched at 0 and 1 [14]. We then used the number of genome-wide differentially methylated sites as the test statistic to measure degree of genome-wide methylation changes associated with the mutation status of a CDG for one cancer type. Note that we used significance level 0.01 to determine site-level association without multiple comparisons adjustment since the goal is to measure genome-wide degree of differential methylation due to mutation status but not to claim any associated CpG sites. To assess the significance of the genome-wide methylation changes by a CDG in one cancer type, we first generated an empirical null distribution with numbers of genome-wide differentially methylated sites by mutations of non-CDGs and then calculated the p-value pi,k for CDG i in cancer type k by comparing the number of genome-wide differentially methylated sites by the mutation of CDG i in cancer type k with the empirical null distribution. We then classify the effect of CDG i in tumor type k as hyper-methylated if $pi,k<0.05$ and the number of genome-wide hyper-methylated sites is greater than that of hypo-methylated sites or hypo-methylated if $pi,k<0.05$ and the number of genome-wide hypo-methylated sites

A Methylation driver genes (MDGs) associated with differential methylation

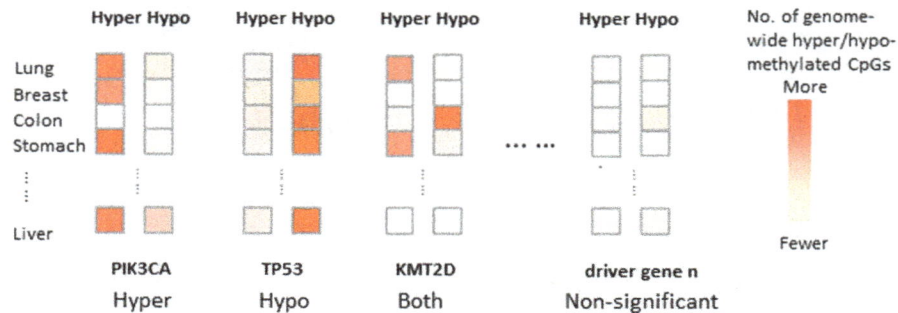

B Expression driver genes (EDGs) associated with differential expression

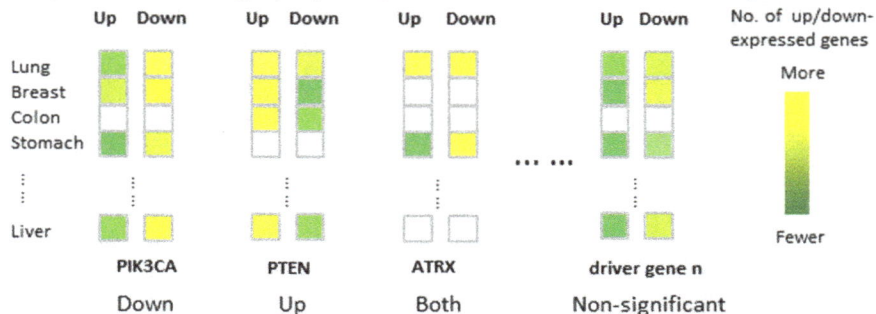

C MDGs change DNA methylation directly or via interacting with chromatin regulators

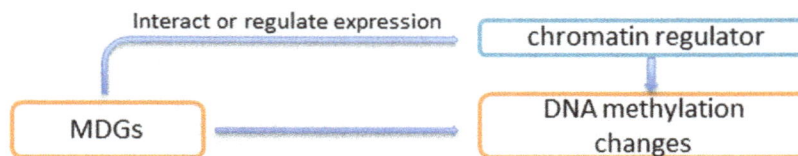

Fig. 1 Rationale underlying the pan-cancer analysis to identify (**a**) MDGs that are associated with genome-wide methylation changes across cancer types and (**b**) EDGs that are associated with genome-wide expression changes across cancer types, with further analysis that reveals (**c**) MDGs mostly consist of chromatin regulators that directly affect the genome-wide methylation patterns or genes that regulate expression of or physically interact with chromatin regulator.

is greater than that of hyper-methylated sites. Finally, to determine the significance of genome-wide methylation changes across multiple cancer types by a CDG, we compare the observed total number of differentially methylated sites associated with a CDG summed over all cancer types with its null distribution to calculate the p-value pi. We use Benjamini-Hochberg procedure to adjust for multiple comparisons for pi, where the adjustment is done within the group of CDGs that were mutated in the same number of cancer types. The MDGs are then identified as those CDGs with adjusted p-values < 0.05. Similar steps are applied to mutation and expression data to identify EDGs. Detailed steps of how to identify MDGs/EDGs are provided in the Methods.

Thirty-two MDGs were identified that, when mutated, have strong association with genome-wide methylation changes across 20 cancers

The pan-cancer analysis of the 20 TCGA cancer types identified 32 MDGs (Table 1). For the complete list of CDGs whose mutation states were significantly associated with genome-wide methylation changes within each cancer type (gene i with $pi,k<0.05$ in the cancer type k), see Additional file 5: Table S4. The genes in Table 1 and Additional file 5: Table S4 highly overlap with the genes identified as the CDGs whose mutation states are associated with genome-wide methylation changes by Chen et al. [5]. They used Principal Component Analysis (PCA) to identify driver genes whose mutations are

Table 1 The identified 32 MDGs

MDGs	$|A_i|$	$|T_i|$	P_i	D_i	T^-_i	T^+_i
_TP53_	15	8	< e-06	both[a]	BLCA BRCA HNSC LIHC LUAD STAD UCEC	LGG[a]
PTEN	14	3	0.00147	both	LGG	STAD UCEC
_RB1_	11	2	0.00861	both	LGG	BLCA
PIK3CA	11	1	0.0277	hyper		STAD
ARID1A	10	1	0.0401	hyper		STAD
KRAS	8	1	1.2e-05	hypo	TGCT	
KMT2D	8	2	0.00575	both	BLCA	STAD
NF1	6	2	0.000227	hypo	LGG PCPG	
CTNNB1	6	2	0.00185	hypo	LIHC UCEC	
SETD2	5	2	0.00351	hyper		KIRC KIRP
KMT2C [b]	5	1	0.00681	hyper		STAD
EGFR	4	1	9.5e-05	hypo	LGG	
HRAS	4	2	0.000266	both	PCPG	HNSC
BRAF	4	2	0.00474	both	THCA	COAD
IDH1	3	2	< e-06	hyper		GBM LGG
CIC	3	1	1.3e-05	hyper		LGG
NRAS	3	2	1.4e-05	both	TGCT	THCA
RNF43	3	2	5.1e-05	both	STAD	COAD
ATRX	3	1	0.000487	hyper[a]		LGG[a]
ZBTB20	3	2	0.00151	hyper		COAD STAD
NOTCH1	3	1	0.00189	hyper		LGG
CDH1	3	2	0.00213	hyper		BRCA STAD
KEAP1	3	1	0.00578	hypo	LUAD	
SMARCA4	3	1	0.00687	hypo	LUAD	
FOXA1[b]	3	1	0.00953	hypo	PRAD	
EPHA2[b]	3	1	0.0104	hyper		STAD
KIT	2	1	< e-06	hypo	TGCT	
KMT2B	2	2	0.000511	both	STAD	COAD
FGFR3[b]	2	1	0.000697	hypo	BLCA	
STK11[b]	2	1	0.00193	hypo	LUAD	
NSD1	1	1	< e-06	hypo	HNSC	
BAP1[b]	1	1	0.000142	hyper		LIHC

$|Ai|$: number of tumor types in which CDG _i_ is mutated in ≥ 5 samples with available methylation data;

$|Ti|$: number of tumor types whose genome-wide methylation levels are significantly associated with the mutation status of CDG _i_;

p_i: p-value testing if CDG _i_ is significantly associated with genome-wide methylation changes across tumor types;

Di: direction of methylation changes associated with mutation status of CDG _i_;

T^+_i: tumor types that are hyper-methylated by CDG _i_;

T^-_i: tumor types that are hypo-methylated by CDG _i_;

[a]: Further stratified analysis by _IDH1_ mutation status in LGG tumor samples suggests an opposite direction from hyper- to hypo-methylation;

[b]: genes that are not overlapping driver genes

___ : genes that are identified as associated with genome-wide patterns of aberrant methylation by Chen et al. [5]

associated with the top five PCs within each cancer. Although the two methods used different approaches, the identified genes are very similar, providing further validation of the results.

The 32 MDGs were mutated with different frequencies in each cancer types (Additional file 6: Figure S1) and the mutation status of the 32 MDGs is associated with different genome-wide number of hyper- and hypo-methylated sites (Fig. 2a). Cancer types COAD and STAD have the highest mutation rate with many of the identified MDGs being mutated. KIRP, PCPG, TGCT and THCA have the smallest number of mutated MDGs. In CESC, LUSC,

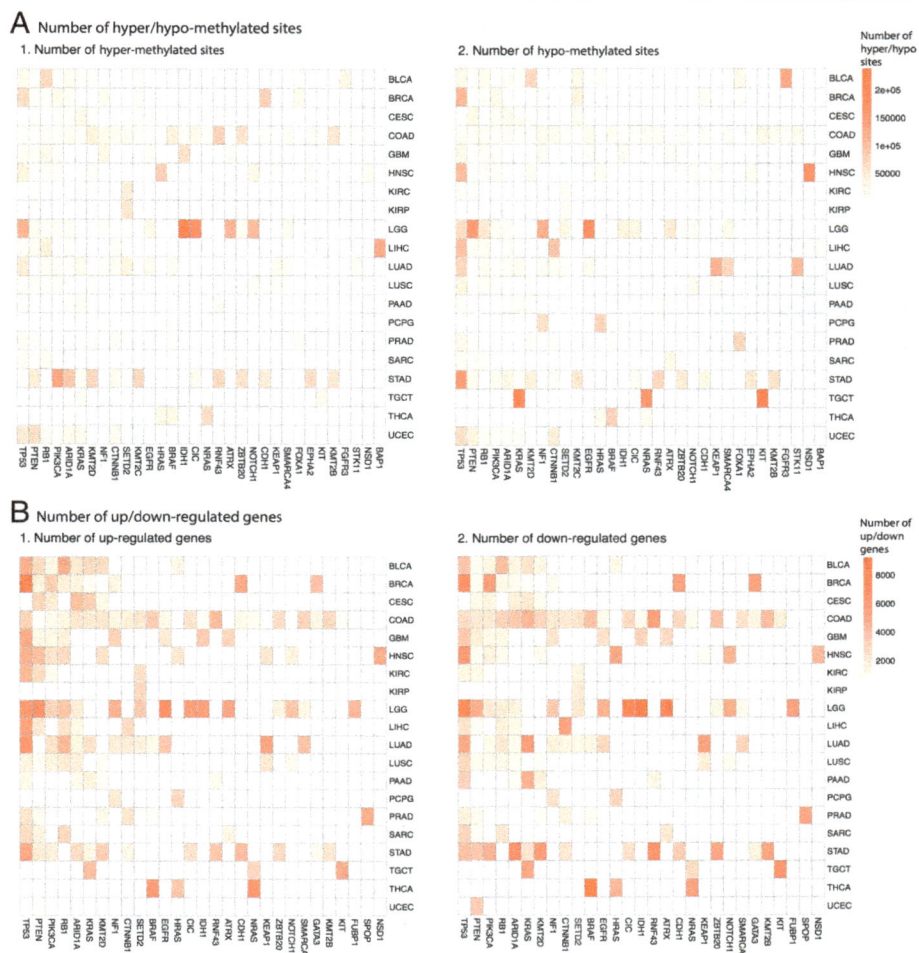

Fig. 2 a Number of genome-wide hyper- (1) and hypo-methylated (2) sites that are associated with the mutation status of the 32 identified MDGs (columns) for each of the 20 TCGA tumor types (rows). (**b**) Number of genome-wide up-regulated- (1) and down-regulated- (2) genes that are associated with the mutation status of the 29 identified EDGs (columns) for each of the 20 TCGA tumor types (rows). The color code represents the number of differentially methylated sites/differentially expressed genes. Only driver genes that were mutated in ≥ 5 samples for the given tumor type were colored

PAAD, and SARC tumor types, genome-wide methylation patterns were not significantly affected by mutations of any of the identified 32 MDGs, potentially due to small sample sizes or fewer number of CDGs. *TP53* mutations are associated with significant genome-wide methylation changes in 8 out of the 15 tumor types in which it was mutated in more than 5 samples (Table 1). Among these 8 tumor types, more CpG sites were hypo-methylated in all but LGG. Instead, in LGG, *TP53* mutations are associated with more hyper-methylated CpG sites. However, almost all LGG tumors with *TP53* mutations also have *IDH1* mutations (Additional file 6: Figure S1), which are known to lead to hyper-methylation in LGG [15–17]. *IDH1* is also identified as one of the 32 MDGs, where in GBM and LGG, it is associated with more CpGs to be hyper-methylated. Given the prominent role of *IDH1* in LGG, we stratified LGG tumor samples by the *IDH1* mutation status and further

examined the effect of the other 31 MDGs within the *IDH1* mutation stratum and the *IDH1* wild-type stratum and found that *TP53* mutations are now significantly associated with more hypo-methylation genome-wide in each stratum (Additional file 3: Text S1). Similar stratified analyses were conducted in all other tumor types whose genome-wide methylation patterns were significantly associated with mutations of the identified MDGs. Similar patterns as in the non-stratified analysis were observed (Additional file 7: Table S5).

Many MDGs are known chromatin regulators or the ones that regulate the expression of or physically interact with chromatin regulators

Among the identified 32 MDGs, 8 are known chromatin regulators that are either histone modification enzymes (*KMT2D, KMT2C, KMT2B, NSD1*, and *SETD2*), or part of ATP-dependent chromatin remodeling complexes (*ARID1A*, *ATRX*, and *SMARCA4*, all from the SWI/SNF family [18]).

We hypothesize that among the remaining 24 MDGs, some are "epigenetic modulators" in that these genes change genome-wide methylation patterns by regulating the expression of chromatin regulators/DNA methyltransferases, or through physically interacting with these epigenomic regulators as cofactors. To test this hypothesis, we examined whether mutations of these 24 MDGs are associated with the expression changes of known epigenomic regulator genes across the 20 tumor types, where we used the exon level RNA-Seq data of the 20 tumor tissue types from TCGA. We also investigated if epigenomic regulator genes are over-represented among genes that physically interact with these 24 MDGs.

We created two lists of known chromatin regulator genes. List A has 720 DNA/RNA, histone and chromatin-modifying enzymes and their co-factors from the EpiFactors database [19]. List B has 18 epigenetic regulators that were identified as the master regulators of global DNA methylation by Yang *et al.* [8], including *EYA4*, *SETBP1*, *PRDM2*, *PRDM5*, *CBX7*, *DUSP1*, *KAT2B*, *RAD54L*, *WHSC1*, *EZH2*, *UHRF1*, *PCNA*, *TTF2*, *KDM1A*, *SUV39H2*, *HDAC1*, *TDG* and *TET3*, plus the DNA methyltransferase *DNMT1*, *3A*, *3B* that were not identified as master regulators by Yang *et al.* [8].

Among the remaining 24 MDGs that are potentially new "epigenetic modulators", 12 are associated with genome-wide methylation changes in more than one cancer type (Table 1), including *TP53*, *PTEN*, *RB1*, *NF1*, *CTNNB1*, *HRAS*, *BRAF*, *IDH1*, *NRAS*, *RNF43*,*ZBTB20*, and *CDH1*. To focus on pan-cancer effects, we worked on only these 12 driver genes that are associated with genome-wide methylation changes in more than one cancer types. For each of these 12 genes, we first identified genome-wide target genes whose expression levels were dysregulated by the mutation status commonly across tumor types. We compared the expression levels of all genes between mutated and non-mutated groups of a MDG using a two-sample t-test and identified target genes that show significantly differential expressions (p-value <0.05) in all tumor types whose methylation patterns are associated with the mutation status. Similarly, since the goal here is not to identify specific target genes that are affected by the MDGs but to quantify degree of dysregulation by MDGs through number of target genes that are commonly dysregulated across cancer types, we used a loose p-value cutoff without considering multiple comparisons. We then examined if known chromatin regulators in lists A and B were over represented among the genome-wide dysregulated target genes by a MDG. The expression data were only available for 717 out of the 720 genes in list A, but were

available for all 21 genes in list B. We used a hypergeometric distribution to calculate p-values for the enrichment of known chromatin regulators and described the procedure to examine this mechanistic hypothesis in more details in Fig. 3.

We found that among the genome-wide dysregulated target genes by each of the 12 MDGs, known chromatin regulators were clearly enriched (Table 2). In addition, 7 out of the 12 MDGs are associated with differential expression of the *DNMT* genes. Additionally, the results in Table 2 confirm some previously known interactions between MDGs and chromatin regulators. For example, *TP53* mutations are associated with upregulated *KDM1A* expression levels across all tumor types whose genome-wide methylation patterns are also significantly associated with *TP53* mutations. *KDM1A* is known to physically interact with *TP53* [20] and it demethylates histone lysine residues 9 of histone 3, which in turn leads to extensive hypo-methylation in that region [21]. This analysis suggests that *KDM1A* may play a role in the association between *TP53* mutations and genome-wide hypo-methylation changes across tumor types. Other notable associations that were confirmed by results in Table 2 include interactions between *RB1* and *DNMT1*, and between *RAS* genes (*HRAS*, *NRAS*) and *HDAC1* [22].

We next investigated if the epigenomic regulator genes in lists A and B are over represented among genes that physically interact with these 12 MDGs. To do so, we first obtained a list of genes that physically interact with each of them from the HumanMine database [23]. We then tested if the epigenomic regulator genes in lists A and B are over-represented among them. Since the number of physically interacting genes was too small for some MDGs, the enrichment analysis was only conducted for the genes in list A that had enough overlap with the interacting genes. We found that known epigenomic regulator genes in list A were highly enriched in the lists of interacting genes of the 12 MDGs (Table 3). These results support our hypothesis that these 12 MDGs that are not known chromatin regulators but are associated with changes in epigenomes either through regulating expression of epigenomic regulators or through physically interacting with them.

We also investigated whether differential expression of target genes in list B of 21 epigenetic regulators are directly or indirectly associated with differential methylation of the same genes. We found only a small fraction of genes in list B whose expression and methylation levels are both associated with the mutation status of the MDGs (Table 2), which suggests that the differential expression of these target genes may be directly associated with mutations of these MDGs instead of being indirectly associated through changes in their

8 known chromatin regulators:
KMT2D KMT2C KMT2B NSD1 SETD2
ARID1A ATRX SMARCA4

We hypothesize that these 12 MDGs *regulate* chromatin regulators or physically interact with them.

24 candidates of new "epigenetic modulators":

TP53 PTEN RB1
PIK3CA KRAS NF1
CTNNB1 EGFR
HRAS BRAF IDH1
CIC NRAS ZBTB20
NOTCH1 CDH1
KEAP1 FOXA1 KIT
FGFR3 STK11
BAP1

12 out of 24 affect > 1 tumor types:

TP53 PTEN
RB1 NF1
CTNNB1
HRAS BRAF
IDH1 NRAS
RNF43
ZBTB20
CDH1

We test if genes from lists A and B are enriched among dysregulated genes D_i by MDG i.

	listA (listA)^C	
D_i	N_2	N_1
$(D_i)^C$		
	717	Total N=20,531

	listB (listB)^C	
D_i	N_3	N_1
$(D_i)^C$		
	21	Total N=20,531

Gene enrichment analyses using hypergeometric($N_2, N, N_1, 717$) and hypergeometric($N_3, N, N_1, 21$).
N_1, N_2, N_3 : number of genes in D_i, D_i & listA, D_i & listB.

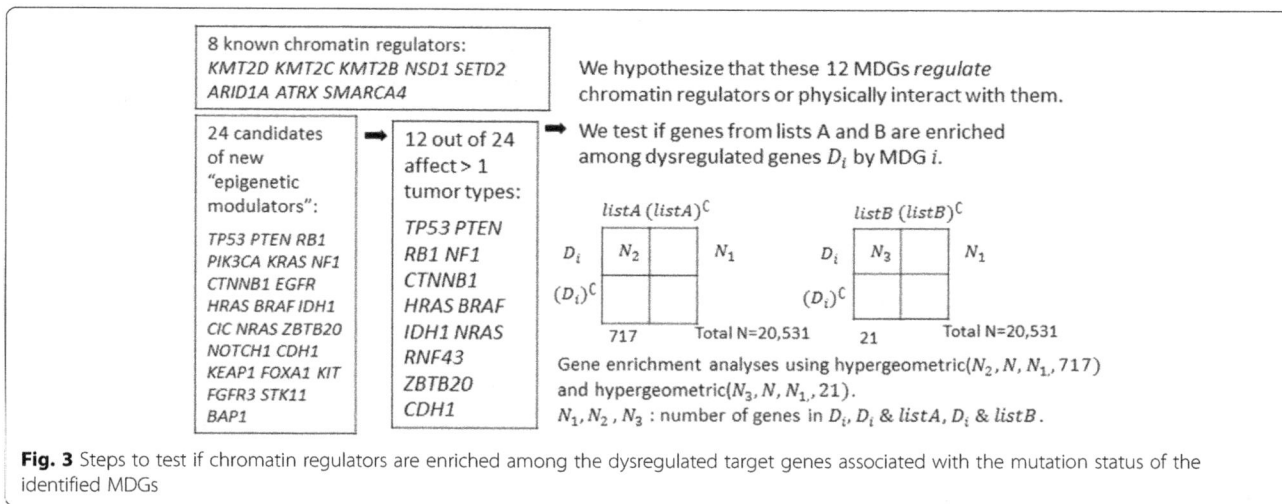

Fig. 3 Steps to test if chromatin regulators are enriched among the dysregulated target genes associated with the mutation status of the identified MDGs

methylation patterns. We further investigated mutation status of genes in list B to examine if the mutations affect their expression or methylation levels directly and found that the majority of genes in list B were rarely mutated across tumor types (Additional file 8: Table S6).

Although *CIC* was not included in the above analyses since it was mutated only in LGG, due to its important role in LGG tumors, we examined how *CIC* regulates expressions of target genes and found that chromatin remodeling genes in list A were significantly enriched

Table 2 MDGs dysregulate expression levels of chromatin regulators

MDGs	$|T_i|$	N_1 (# of dysregulated genes)	N_2 (# of dysregulated genes in list A)	Enrichment Pvalue$_A$	N_3 (# of dysregulated genes in list B)	Enrichment Pvalue$_B$	Genes in list B that are dysregulated[a]	Genes in list B that are differentially methylated[b]
TP53	8	233	19	0.00056	5	3.2e-06	CBX7 RAD54L TTF2 KDM1A SUV39H2	
PTEN	3	1,534	81	0.00012	9	9.1e-06	DNMT1 DNMT3A SETBP1 PRDM5 CBX7 RAD54L EZH2 PCNA HDAC1	DNMT3A PRDM5 HDAC1
RB1	2	1,447	83	5.2e-06	4	0.056	DNMT1 EYA4 EZH2 PCNA	PCNA
NF1	2	766	36	0.044	0	1		
CTNNB1	2	5,515	207	0.12	12	0.0033	DNMT1 SETBP1 PRDM2 PRDM5 CBX7 KAT2B RAD54L WHSC1 EZH2 UHRF1 TDG TET3	PRDM2 CBX7
HRAS	2	1,137	63	2.0e-04	3	0.11	PRDM2 RAD54L HDAC1	PRDM2
BRAF	2	3,128	133	0.008	8	0.0091	DNMT1 DNMT3A DNMT3B KAT2B WHSC1 EZH2 UHRF1 KDM1A	DNMT3A UHRF1
IDH1	2	3,560	208	2.8e-15	2	0.9	SUV39H2 TET3	
NRAS	2	1,609	87	2.8e-05	1	0.82	HDAC1	
RNF43	2	3,212	157	4.4e-06	8	0.011	DNMT3A DNMT3B PRDM2 RAD54L WHSC1 UHRF1 HDAC1 TET3	DNMT3A DNMT3B PRDM2 WHSC1
ZBTB20	2	1,563	78	0.00088	6	0.0039	DNMT3A RAD54L WHSC1 UHRF1 TTF2 HDAC1	DNMT3A WHSC1 UHRF11
CDH1	2	2,792	136	2.7e-05	14	3.3e-08	DNMT3B SETBP1 PRDM2 CBX7 DUSP1 RAD54L WHSC1 EZH2 PCNA KDM1A SUV39H2 HDAC1 TDG TET3	PRDM2 CBX7 WHSC1 KDM1A

$|Ti|$: number of tumor types whose genome-wide methylation levels are significantly associated with the mutation status of CDG i;
N_1: number of genes whose expression levels are dysregulated by MDG i in all $|Ti|$ tumor types;
N_2: number of genes in list A that are dysregulated in all $|Ti|$ tumor types;
N_3: number of genes in list B that are dysregulated in all $|Ti|$ tumor types;
Enrichment Pvalue$_A$ and Pvalue$_B$ are calculated using hypergeometric distributions testing if genes in lists A and B are enriched among genome-wide differentially expressed target genes;
[a]Genes in list B that are dysregulated in all $|Ti|$ tumor types;
[b]Genes in list B that are differentially methylated in all $|Ti|$ tumor types.

Table 3 Chromatin regulators are enriched in genes that physically interact with MDGs

MDGs	|Tᵢ|	N₄ (# of physically interacting genes)	N₅ (# of physically interacting genes in list A)	Enrichment Pvalueₐⁱ
TP53	8	923	192	0
PTEN	3	224	19	0.00035
RB1	2	250	64	0
NF1	2	29	3	0.079
CTNNB1	2	364	63	0
HRAS	2	86	6	0.08
BRAF	2	54	8	0.00053
IDH1	2	49	7	0.0015
NRAS	2	36	3	0.13
RNF43	2	18	7	1.4e-06
ZBTB20	2	17	1	0.45
CDH1	2	144	18	2.9e-06

$|Ti|$: number of tumor types whose genome-wide methylation levels are significantly associated with the mutation status of CDG i;

N_4: number of genes physically interact with MDG i;

N_5: number of genes physically interact with MDG i that are also in list A;

Enrichment Pvalueₐⁱ is calculated using a hypergeometric distribution testing if genes in list A are enriched among selected physically interacting genes.

among dysregulated target genes, in both full LGG tumor samples and in stratified samples by *IDH1* mutation status (Additional file 9: Table S7).

Twenty-nine EDGs were identified, out of which, 26 overlaps with the identified 32 MDGs

We conducted similar pan-cancer analysis to associate driver genes and gene expression across the 20 TCGA cancer types. We identified 29 CDGs as the expression driver genes (EDGs) that, when mutated, are significantly associated with genome-wide expression changes across multiple cancer types (Table 4). The mutation status of these 29 EDGs is associated with different genome-wide number of up- and down-regulated genes (Fig. 2b). For the complete list of CDGs whose mutation states were significantly associated with genome-wide expression changes within each cancer type, see Additional file 10: Table S8.

Of the 29 EDGs, 26 overlap with the 32 MDGs. To understand this high rate of overlap, within each cancer type, we examined the overlap between CDGs that are significantly associated with genome-wide methylation changes and CDGs that are significantly associated with genome-wide expression changes, and found they overlap highly. Moreover, there is a high correlation between the number of differentially methylated sites and the number of differentially expressed genes by each CDG (Additional file 11: Table S9), which implies a close connection between genome-wide methylation changes and genome-wide expression changes.

We further investigated patterns of target genes' methylation in promoter regions and target genes' expression changes of the 26 overlapping driver genes. A target gene is hyper-methylated if the number of hyper-methylated sites is larger than that of hypo-methylated in the promoter region of the gene (1,500 base pairs upstream of the transcription start site) and hypo-methylated otherwise. If there are the same numbers of hyper-/hypo-methylated sites or no hyper/hypo-methylated sites in the promoter region, the gene is considered not differentially methylated. The signature patterns of target genes' methylation and expression changes by the overlapping driver genes could be hyper-methylated and up-regulated, the "++" pattern; hyper-methylated and down-regulated, the "+-" pattern; hypo-methylated and up-regulated, the "-+" pattern; and hypo-methylated and down- regulated, the "--" pattern. We used a hypergeometric distribution to calculate p-values for the enrichment of each pattern in a cancer type and combined per tumor type p-values using the Fisher's method (Additional file 12: Figure S2, Table 5).

It is clear that across the 26 overlapping driver genes, target genes' hyper-methylation are significantly associated with their down-regulation ("+-" pattern) and target genes' hypo-methylation are significantly associated with their up-regulation ("-+" pattern). A specific example of a target gene that is hypo-methylated and up-regulated by the mutation of *TP53* is *HSF1* gene. It is hypo-methylated and up-regulated by *TP53* mutations across 9 tumor types. Dysregulation of chromatin regulators induces global change of chromatin architecture, which is highly interconnected with DNA methylation. DNA methylation and histone modification interact with each other to determine the chromatin state as an euchromatic (on) or heterochromatic (off) state, where euchromatic state is associated with hypomethylation and active gene expression

Table 4 Identified 29 EDGs

EDGs	$|A'_i|$	$|E_i|$	p'_i	B_i	E_i^-	E_i^+
TP53	14	11	< e-06	both	HNSC LGG SARC	BLCA BRCA COAD GBM KIRC LIHC LUAD STAD
PTEN	14	1	0.00299	up		LGG
PIK3CA	11	2	0.00536	down	BRCA STAD	
RB1	10	3	9e-05	up		BLCA LGG LUAD
ARID1A	10	2	0.00557	both	STAD	CESC
KRAS	8	4	4e-06	down	COAD LUAD PAAD TGCT	
KMT2D	8	1	0.0265	down	STAD	
NF1	6	1	0.00274	up		LGG
CTNNB1	5	1	0.00572	down	LIHC	
†SETD2	5	0	0.00833	NA	NA	NA
BRAF	4	2	1.1e-05	down	COAD THCA	
EGFR	4	2	5.3e-05	up		LGG LUAD
HRAS	4	3	7e-05	down	HNSC PCPG THCA	
CIC	3	1	< e-06	down	LGG	
IDH1	3	2	< e-06	both	LGG	GBM
RNF43	3	2	1e-06	down	COAD STAD	
ATRX	3	2	2e-06	both	LGG	GBM
CDH1	3	2	7e-06	both	BRCA	STAD
NRAS	3	2	0.000199	up		TGCT THCA
KEAP1	3	1	0.000809	down	LUAD	
ZBTB20	3	2	0.00119	down	COAD STAD	
NOTCH1	3	2	0.00182	down	HNSC LGG	
SMARCA4	3	1	0.0108	up		LUAD
GATA3[a]	3	1	0.0138	down	BRCA	
KMT2B	2	2	0.000317	down	COAD STAD	
KIT	2	1	0.000889	down	TGCT	
FUBP1[a]	1	1	< e-06	down	LGG	
SPOP[a]	1	1	< e-06	down	PRAD	
NSD1	1	1	0.000432	up		HNSC

$|A'_i|$ = number of tumor types in which EDG i is mutated in ≥ 5 samples with expression data;
$|E_i|$ = number of tumor types whose genome-wide expression levels are significantly associated with CDG i;
p'_i = p-value testing if CDG i is significantly associated with genome-wide expression changes across tumor types;
B_i is the direction of change of expression levels associated with the mutation status of CDG i;
E_i^+ = tumor types that are up-regulated by CDG i, E_i^- = tumor types that are down-regulated by CDG i;
[a] : genes that are not overlapping driver genes.
†Note that SETD2 gene has a significant p-value p'_i for testing association of genome-wide expression changes across multiple tumor types, but there is not a specific tumor type in which SETD2 mutation is significantly associated with genome-wide expression changes.

and heterochromatic state is associated with hypermethylation and repressed gene expression [24].

We also investigated the consistency of the differential gene expression and DNA methylation patterns across tumor types. For each CDG, for every pair of tumor types in which it is mutated in more than five samples, we tested using a hypergeometric distribution if the number of overlapping target genes that are differentially methylated by the mutation of the CDG is larger than expected. We then reported the median p-values (Table 5) from all pairs of two tumor types and repeated the same analysis

for differential expression. Both median p-values for differential expression and methylation are '0' or close to '0' for most CDGs, which indicates that the differential expression or methylation associated with CDGs are consistent across tumor types. Note that NSD1 gene was only mutated in one tumor type.

Our findings on how CDG mutations contribute to pan-cancer-associated epigenomic alterations and transcriptomic alterations suggest that there are potentially three mechanisms (Fig. 4): 1) genome-wide methylation and expression changes are associated with changes in

Table 5 Patterns of target genes' promoter regions methylation and expression changes by mutations of the overlapping driver genes across tumor types

Overlapping driver genes	$\lvert T_i \rvert$	$\lvert E_i \rvert$	$\lvert T_i \cap E_i \rvert$	$\lvert DM \rvert$	$\lvert DE \rvert$	$\frac{\lvert DM \cap DE \rvert}{\lvert DE \rvert}$ (%)	$p(DM \cdot DE)$	$p(--)$	$p(+-)$	$p(-+)$	$p(++)$	p.methyl	p.exp
TP53	8	11	7	10389	10066	52	2.8e-32	1	9.7e-95	7.1e-65	1	0	0
PTEN	3	1	1	12259	10293	61	0.014	1	1e-15	1e-15	1	2.98e-10	0
RB1	2	3	1	9049	8062	46	0.0066	0.81	0.05	1e-15	1	0	0
PIK3CA	1	2	1	13933	5822	73	5e-12	1	1e-15	5.4e-05	1	1.93e-11	0
ARID1A	1	2	1	9487	8573	53	1e-15	0.98	1e-15	0.29	1	0	0
KRAS	1	4	1	15041	8427	73	1	1	7.5e-12	1	0.87	0	0
KMT2D	2	1	1	9802	8485	52	4.3e-14	1	1e-15	0.014	1	7.37e-10	0
NF1	2	1	1	10288	7435	53	9e-07	1	1e-15	1e-15	1	0	0
CTNNB1	2	1	1	7583	7591	37	0.64	1	1e-15	1	1	0	0
EGFR	1	2	1	13156	10606	66	0.0096	1	1e-15	1e-15	1	7.63e-07	0
HRAS	2	3	2	8758	6300	47	3.7e-19	0.97	7e-29	8.1e-20	1	0	0
BRAF	2	2	2	9120	10092	47	1.3e-06	0.96	1.3e-14	7e-29	1	0	9.99e-16
IDH1	2	2	2	10596	10134	55	6.6e-16	1	7e-29	7e-29	1	0	0
CIC	1	1	1	14066	12718	71	1.2e-08	1	1e-15	1e-15	1	0	0
NRAS	2	2	1	8413	10581	43	5.6e-06	1	1e-15	1e-15	1	0	0
RNF43	2	2	2	9978	9292	51	4.9e-08	1	3.9e-29	2e-14	1	0	0
ATRX	1	2	1	11646	12114	60	2.2e-16	1	1e-15	1e-15	1	0	0
ZBTB20	2	2	2	8415	6667	43	1.1e-10	0.94	8.6e-19	2.1e-09	1	0	0
NOTCH1	1	2	1	10225	7849	55	1e-15	1	1e-15	1e-15	1	0	0
CDH1	2	2	2	8634	8254	45	3.6e-16	1	1.1e-23	3.5e-26	1	0	0
KEAP1	1	1	1	10060	10030	50	0.4	1	1e-15	0.017	1	1.25e-12	0
SMARCA4	1	1	1	6118	6234	30	0.86	1	1e-15	0.93	1	1.11e-16	3.56e-11
KIT	1	1	1	15035	10164	74	0.87	1	4.4e-16	0.029	0.95	2.54e-09	1.07e-06
KMT2B	2	2	2	8066	6649	44	1.7e-24	1	7e-29	2.3e-24	1	0	0
NSD1	1	1	1	13052	8233	67	1.2e-10	0.55	1.9e-14	3.1e-10	1	NA	NA

$\lvert DM \rvert$: number of differentially methylated genes averaged across $T_i \cap E_i$ tumor types;

$\lvert DE \rvert$: number of differentially expressed genes averaged across $T_i \cap E_i$ tumor types;

$\frac{DM \cap DE}{DE}$ (%): percent of differentially methylated target genes out of differentially expressed target genes, averaged across tumor types $T_i \cap E_i$

$p(DM \cdot DE)$: p-value testing if number of target genes that are differentially methylated and expression is larger than expected using a hypergeometric distribution combined across tumor types $T_i \cap E_i$ using the Fisher's method.

$p(--)$, $p(+-)$, $p(-+)$, $p(++)$: p-values that test if number of target genes with "--","+-","-+","++" pattern of methylation and expression changes is larger than expected a using hypergeometric distribution combined across tumor types using the Fisher's method.

p.methyl: median p-value from testing if the number of overlapping target genes that are differentially methylated by the mutation of the CDG between any pair of two tumor types is larger than expected using a hypergeometric distribution.

p.exp: median p-value from testing if the number of overlapping target genes that are differentially expressed by the mutation of the CDG between any pair of two tumor types is larger than expected using a hypergeometric distribution.

chromatin states induced by malfunctions of chromatin regulators directly through mutations of these genes; 2) or indirectly through mutations of other genes that regulate the expression of chromatin regulators; 3) or indirectly through mutations of other genes with which chromatin regulators physically interact with for epigenomic regulation.

Discussion

We conducted a pan-cancer analysis to identify CDGs whose somatic mutations are associated with genome-wide methylation/expression changes across multiple cancer types. We used a straightforward method to compare methylation/expression levels between mutated and non-mutated groups of each CDG. The MDGs identified highly overlap with the driver genes identified whose mutation states are associated with genome-wide methylation changes by Chen et al. [5] (these overlapping genes are underlined in Table 1), where they used a different method, the Principal Component Analysis (PCA). This provides further validation of the MDGs results. However, our method also identified several MDGs that were not identified by Chen et al. [5] including well-known chromatin regulators KMT2B, KMT2C, KMT2D and SMARCA4.

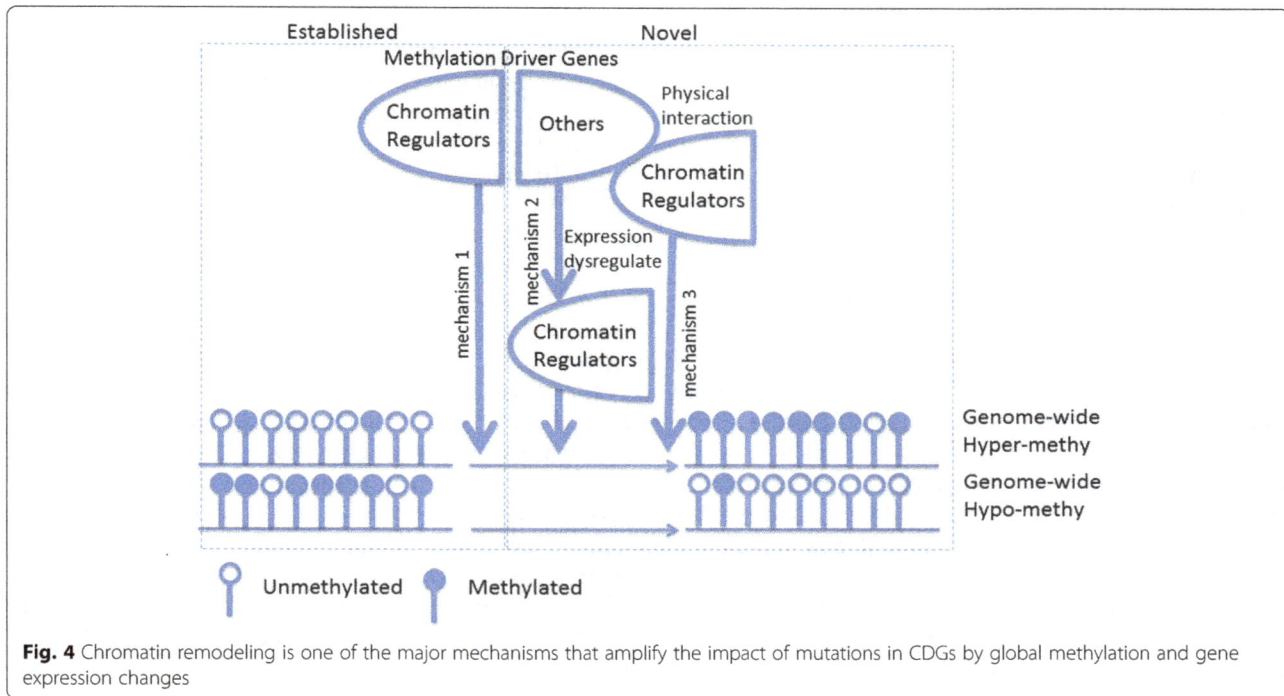

Fig. 4 Chromatin remodeling is one of the major mechanisms that amplify the impact of mutations in CDGs by global methylation and gene expression changes

The MDGs that we identified do not overlap the 18 master regulators identified by Yang *et al.* [8]. This is because they did not consider mutation data and focused only on epigenetic enzymes, which exhibit consistently differential expression and DNA methylation instability correlation patterns across cancer types. However, as Table 2 shows, the deregulation of the 18 master regulators in list B are correlated with the mutation status of the MDGs.

Interestingly, the MDGs and EDGs also include genes that are associated with telomere length (TL) elongation in cancers. Telomeres shorten with each cell division, therefore, maintenance of telomere length is critical in tumorigenesis. While telomere shortening is often prevented by activation of telomerase reverse transcriptase (TERT), it is also prevented by a homologous recombination-based process known as alternative lengthening of telomeres (ALT), where remodeling of the telomeric architecture may play a key role [25]. Floris *et al.* [26] recently performed a comprehensive analysis of association between TL and somatic alterations in cancers. To identify TERT-independent TL regulation, they associated somatic alterations of 196 telomere-associated genes to TL ratio between matching tumor and normal samples and found alterations of *ATRX, IDH1, TP53, BCOR,* and *RB1* were significantly associated with relative TL elongation under FDR<0.05. Our MDGs include four out of these five genes, suggesting that chromatin remodeling plays an important role in ALT.

In a recent review by Feinberg *et al.* [27], an epigenetic functional classification system was introduced that classifies epigenetic genes into three categories 1) "epigenetic mediators", which correspond to tumor progenitor genes that are targets of epigenetic modification; 2) "epigenetic modifiers", which modify DNA methylation or chromatin structure; and 3) "epigenetic modulators", which influence activities of epigenetic modifiers to destabilize epigenetic states.

Among the 32 MDGs, 8 are well-known chromatin regulators that fall in the category of "epigenetic modifiers". The remaining 24 genes are considered as new candidates of "epigenetic modulators" that are associated with genome-wide methylation changes through regulating or interacting with chromatin regulators. Further analysis that examined whether mutations of 12 MDGs out of these 24 MDGs are associated with the expression of known epigenetic modifiers across cancer types supports our mechanistic hypothesis that some of these MDGs are the ones that regulate expression of chromatin regulators. Similarly, analysis that examined whether chromatin regulators are enriched among genes that physically interact with the 12 MDGs supports our mechanistic hypothesis that some of these MDGs are the ones that physically interact with chromatin regulators.

Seven out of the 24 MDGs: *PTEN, PIK3CA, KRAS, HRAS, BRAF, NRAS,* and *KIT* belong to the PI3K/AKT signaling pathway which is known to target and change the function of chromatin-modifying enzymes in SWI/

SNF family members [28]. Previous studies provide strong evidence that all these 7 genes are involved in chromatin remodeling. *BRAF* mutation is known to be tightly associated with a CpG island methylator phenotype (CIMP) and alteration of SWI/SNF chromatin remodeling pathway [29]. *RAS* genes which were classified as epigenetic modifiers in the review by Feinberg *et al.* induce global and local chromatin modifications [27]. There is also evidence for direct or indirect interactions between chromatin regulators or chromatin themselves and *KIT* [30], *PIK3CA* [31], and *PTEN* [32].

Another highly enriched function among the identified MDGs is DNA repair. Eight of the 24 MDGs: *TP53*, *PTEN*, *RB1*, *FOXA1*, *BAP1*, *IDH1* and *NF1* are known to play a role in DNA repair, when DNA repair is known to interact with chromatin remodeling. Studies of DNA repair have uncovered that many histone modifications occur after induction of a double-strand break [33]. *TP53* binds to and regulates chromatin regulators, including the methyltransferases *KMT2A* and *KMT2D* and acetyltransferase *KAT6A*, resulting in genome-wide increases of histone methylation and acetylation [34]. *RB1* is also known to bind to and regulate DNA methyltransferase, histone methyltransferases and histone acetyltransferase [35]. *FOXA1* is a pioneer transcription factor whose recruitment to enhancers is associated with DNA demethylation and induction of histone H3 lysine 4 methylation at these enhancers [36, 37]. It was recently uncovered that *FOXA1* interacts with components of DNA repair complexes and that the FOXA1-associated DNA repair complex is implicated in active DNA demethylation [38]. *BAP1*, which is critical for promoting DNA repair by homologous recombination [39], plays a key role in chromatin remodeling by mediating deubiquitination of histone H2A and HCFC1 [40]; *IDH1* is classified as an epigenetic modifier in the review by Feinberg *et al.* [27] and its mutation is known to induce the genome-wide alterations in DNA methylation by inhibiting function of histone and DNA demethylases [41], which also impairs DNA repair [42]. *NF1* is also known to participate in chromatin remodeling activities [43].

For the rest of the MDGs, there is evidence supporting many of their involvement in chromatin modification either by interacting with histone modification enzymes or chromatin remodeling complexes or with chromatin directly, such as *CDH1* [44], *CTNNB1* [45], *EGFR* [46], *KEAP1* [47], *NOTCH1* [48], *STK11*[49], and *ZBTB20* [50]. Especially gene *CIC*, a transcription repressor in the central nervous system identified as the MDG in LGG, physically interacts with a histone methyltransferase *KMT3A* [51]. Note that *CIC* mutations are associated with hyper-methylation in LGG both among *IDH1* wild-type tumors and *IDH1* mutated tumors. Further

studies are needed to investigate if the observed clinical and biological impact of *CIC* mutations in LGG is through hyper-methylation of the epigenome.

In this study, we identified CDGs whose somatic mutations are associated with pan-cancer genome-wide methylation/expression changes by using a simple and straightforward method to compare methylation or expression levels between mutated and non-mutated groups of each CDG. We acknowledge that the difference between the two groups may be confounded by other factors, such as mutations in other genes as we observed for *TP53* and *IDH1* in LGG tumors. However, multivariate approaches such as regression models to control for other gene mutations may not be feasible for our purpose due to highly non-normal distribution of methylation levels and sparseness of mutations. Although we focused on associations of somatic mutations with genome-wide methylation and expression changes in this study, this approach can be readily modified to examine association between copy number variations or structural variations with genome-wide methylation and expression changes.

Conclusions

Our pan-cancer analysis examining connections between somatic mutation and DNA methylation/gene expression identified CDGs (32 MDGs and 29 EDGs) whose somatic mutations are associated with genome-wide methylation/expression changes across multiple cancer types. Many of the identified MDGs are either chromatin regulators or the ones that regulate the expression of or physically interact with chromatin regulators. Twenty-six out of the 29 EDGs overlap with the 32 MDGs. We further confirmed the enrichment of target gene patterns being hyper-methylated and down-regulated or hypo-methylated and up-regulated, by the 26 overlapping genes. These findings highlight that the dysregulation of chromatin regulation is an important mechanism that amplifies the impact of mutations in CDGs by global methylation and gene expression changes.

Additional files

Additional file 1: Table S1. Selection of candidate CDGs across tumor types.

Additional file 2: Table S2. A. Number of CDGs mutated in at least 5 samples with methylation data in one tumor type; B. Number of CDGs mutated in at least 5 samples with expression data in one tumor type.

Additional file 3: Text S1. Details with some modified steps for identifying EDGs.; Results of MDGs in LGG; Results from stratified analysis in all other cancers other than LGG.

Additional file 4: Table S3. Number of genes in the methylation null pool.

Additional file 5: Table S4. CDGs associated with significant genome-wide methylation changes in one cancer type. Hyper-methylation is defined as CDGs with pi,k <0.05 and the number of hyper-methylated sites is larger than the number of hypo-methylated sites ($| S_{i,k}^+ | > | S_{i,k}^- |$). Hypo-methylation is defined as CDGs with pi,k <0.05 and the number of hyper-methylated sites is smaller than the number of hypo-methylated sites ($| S_{i,k}^+ | \leq | S_{i,k}^- |$).

Additional file 6: Figure S1. Mutation patterns of the identified 32 MDGs across 20 TCGA tumor types. Each row represents a tumor sample and each column represents a MDG. Light color indicates no mutation and dark color indicates mutations.

Additional file 7: Table S5. Results from stratified analysis for the rest of the 15 cancer types (other than LGG) whose genome-wide methylation patterns were affected by one of the identified 32 major MDGs.

Additional file 8: Table S6. Number of tumor samples with mutations in each of the 21 chromatin regulator genes in list B.

Additional file 9: Table S7. Chromatin regulators dysregulated by *IDH1* and *CIC* in LGG. $|Ti|$ is number of tumor types whose genome-wide methylation levels are significantly associated with the mutation status of CDG *i*; N_1 is number of genome-wide genes whose expression levels are dysregulated by MDG *i* in all $|Ti|$ tumor types; N_2 is number of genes in list A that are dysregulated in all $|Ti|$ tumor types; N_3 is number of genes in list B that are dysregulated in all $|Ti|$ tumor types; Enrichment Pvalue$_A$ and Pvalue$_B$ are calculated using hypergeometric distributions testing if genes in lists A and B occur more frequently than expected by random chance among genome-wide differentially expressed target genes.

Additional file 10: Table S8. CDGs associated with significant genome-wide expression changes in one cancer type. Up-regulation is defined as CDGs with $p'_{i,k}$ <0.05 and the number of up-regulated genes is larger than the number of down-regulated genes ($| G_{i,k}^+ | > | G_{i,k}^- |$). Down-regulation is defined as CDGs with $p'_{i,k}$ <0.05 and the number of up-regulated genes is smaller than the number of down-regulated genes ($| G_{i,k}^+ | \leq | G_{i,k}^- |$).

Additional file 11: Table S9. Correlation between methylation and expression changes in each cancer type. K_1 is number of CDGs mutated in ≥ 5 samples with expression data available; K_2 is number of CDGs mutated in ≥ 5 samples with methylation data available; E is set of CDGs with $p_{i,k}$ <0.05, that is, CDGs whose mutation status are significantly associated with f differentially expressed genes; M is set of CDGs with $p_{i,k}$ <0.05, that is, CDGs whose mutation status are significantly associated with differential methylation; 'cor' stands for correlation between the number of differentially methylated sites and the number of differentially expressed genes by the CDG mutation.

Additional file 12: Figure S2. Significance of overlap between genome-wide up/down-regulation and hyper/hypo-methylation associated with the mutation status of the overlapping driver genes. (a) We examined signature patterns of target genes' promotor regions methylation and expression changes by the overlapping driver genes, i.e., target genes that are hyper-methylated and up-regulated by overlapping driver gene *i*, the "++" pattern; target genes that are hyper- methylated and down-regulated by overlapping driver gene *i*, the "+-" pattern; target genes that are hypo-methylated and up-regulated by overlapping driver gene *i*, the "-+" pattern; and target genes that are hypo-methylated and down- regulated by overlapping driver gene *i*, the "--" pattern. (b) We calculated a p-value that tests if number of target genes that are differentially methylated and expressed is larger than expected using a hypergeometric distribution, and a p-value that tests if number of target genes with one of the 4 pattern of methylation and expression changes is larger than expected using a hypergeometric distribution, where we combined per tumor type p-values across tumor types using the Fisher's method.

Abbreviations
BLCA: Bladder urothelial carcinoma; BRCA: Breast invasive carcinoma; CDG: Cancer driver genes; CESC: Cervical squamous cell carcinoma; COAD: Colon adenocarcinoma; EDG: Expression driver gene; GBM: Glioblastoma; HNSC: Head and neck squamous cell carcinoma; KIRC: Kidney renal clear cell carcinoma; KIRP: Kidney renal papillary cell carcinoma; LGG: Acute myeloid leukemia (LAML), lower grade glioma; LIHC: Liver hepatocellular carcinoma; LUAD: Lung adenocarcinoma; LUSC: Lung squamous cell carcinoma; MDG: Methylation driver gene; PAAD: Pancreatic adenocarcinoma; PCPG: Pheochromocytoma and paraganglioma; PRAD: Prostate adenocarcinoma; SARC: Sarcoma; STAD: Stomach adenocarcinoma; TCGA: The Cancer Genome Atlas; TERT: Telomerase reverse transcriptase; THCA: Thyroid carcinoma; TL: Telomere length; UCEC: Uterine corpus endometrial carcinoma

Acknowledgements
Not applicable.

Funding
This research was supported by the Departmental fund.

Authors' contributions
AY, YS, and SW conceived and designed the study. AY and KK performed the analysis. SW supervised the study. AY, YS, SW wrote the manuscript. KK, RR and BT contributed to the interpretation of data, reviewed and edited the manuscript. All authors approved the final manuscript for publication.

Competing interests
The authors declare that they have no competing interests.

Author details
[1]Department of Biostatistics, Mailman School of Public Health, Columbia University, New York, New York, USA. [2]The Jackson Laboratory For Genomic Medicine, Farmington, Connecticut, USA. [3]Department of System Biology, Columbia University, New York, New York, USA. [4]Department of Biomedical Informatics, Columbia University, New York, New York, USA. [5]Division of Genetics & Epigenetics, Hackensack University Medical Center, Hackensack, New Jersey, USA. [6]Columbia Genome Center, Columbia University, New York, New York, USA.

References
1. Martincorena I, Campbell PJ. Somatic mutation in cancer and normal cells. Science. 2015;349(6255):1483–9.
2. Watson IR, Takahashi K, Futreal PA, Chin L. Emerging patterns of somatic mutations in cancer. Nat Rev Genet. 2013;14(10):703–18.
3. Shen H, Laird PW. Interplay between the cancer genome and epigenome. Cell. 2013;153(1):38–55.
4. Gonzalez-Perez A, Jene-Sanz A, Loprez-Bigas N. The mutational landscape of chromatin regulatory factors across 4,623 tumor samples. Genome Biol. 2013;14(9):r106.
5. Chen YC, Gotea V, Margolin G, Elnitski L. Significant associations between driver gene mutations and DNA methylation alterations across many cancer types. PLoS Comput Biol. 2017;13(11):e1005840.
6. Hanahan D, Weinberg RA. Hallmarks of cancer: the next generation. Cell. 2011;144(5):646–74.
7. Gevaert O, Tibshirani R, Plevritis SK. Pancancer analysis of DNA methylation-driven genes using MethylMix. Genome Biol. 2015;16:17.
8. Yang Z, Jones A, Widschwendter M, Teschendorff AE. An integrative pan-cancer-wide analysis of epigenetic enzymes reveals universal patterns of epigenomic deregulation in cancer. Genome biol. 2015;16:140.
9. Pidsley R, Y Wong CC, Volta M, Lunnon K, Mill J, Schalkwyk LC. A data-driven approach to preprocessing Illumina 450K methylation array data. BMC genomics. 2013;14:293.
10. Center BITGDA: Firehose stddata__2015_08_21 run. Broad Institute of MIT and Harvard; 2015. https://doi.org/10.7908/C18W3CNQ.
11. Lawrence MS, Stojanov P, Polak P, Kryukov GV, Cibulskis K, Sivachenko A, Carter SL, Stewart C, Mermel CH, Roberts SA, et al. Mutational heterogeneity in cancer and the search for new cancer-associated genes. Nature. 2013; 499(7457):214–8.
12. Reva B, Antipin Y, Sander C. Determinants of protein function revealed by combinatorial entropy optimization. Genome biol. 2007;8(11):R232.
13. Forbes SA, Beare D, Gunasekaran P, Leung K, Bindal N, Boutselakis H, Ding M, Bamford S, Cole C, Ward S, et al. COSMIC: exploring the world's knowledge of somatic mutations in human cancer. Nucleic Acids Res. 2015;43(D1):D805–11.

14. Wang S. Method to detect differentially methylated loci with case-control designs using Illumina arrays. Genet Epidemiol. 2011;35(7):686–94.

15. Dimitrov L, Hong CS, Yang C, Zhuang Z, Heiss JD. New developments in the pathogenesis and therapeutic targeting of the IDH1 mutation in glioma. Int J Med Sci. 2015;12(3):201–13.

16. Turcan S, Rohle D Fau-Goenka A, Goenka A, Fau-Walsh LA, Walsh LA, Fau-Fang F, Fang F, Fau-Yilmaz E, Yilmaz E, Fau-Campos C, Campos C Fau-Fabius AWM, Fabius AW, Fau-Lu C, Lu C, Fau-Ward PS, Ward PS, Fau-Thompson CB, et al. IDH1 mutation is sufficient to establish the glioma hypermethylator phenotype. Nature. 2012;483(7390):479-83.

17. Bolouri H, Zhao LP, Holland EC. Big data visualization identifies the multidimensional molecular landscape of human gliomas. Proc Natl Acad Sci U S A. 2016;113(19):5394–9.

18. Teif VB, Rippe K. Predicting nucleosome positions on the DNA: combining intrinsic sequence preferences and remodeler activities. Nucleic Acids Res. 2009;37(17):5641–55.

19. Medvedeva YA, Lennartsson A, Ehsani R, Kulakovskiy IV, Vorontsov IE, Panahandeh P, Khimulya G, Kasukawa T, Consortium TF, Drabløs F. EpiFactors: a comprehensive database of human epigenetic factors and complexes. Database. 2015;2015:bav067.

20. Tsai W-W, Nguyen TT, Shi Y, Barton MC. p53-targeted LSD1 functions in repression of chromatin structure and transcription in vivo. Mol Cell Biol. 2008;28(17):5139–46.

21. Hon GC, Hawkins RD, Caballero OL, Lo C, Lister R, Pelizzola M, Valsesia A, Ye Z, Kuan S, Edsall LE, et al. Global DNA hypomethylation coupled to repressive chromatin domain formation and gene silencing in breast cancer. Genome Res. 2012;22(2):246–58.

22. Kobayashi Y, Ohtsuki M, Murakami T, Kobayashi T, Sutheesophon K, Kitayama H, Kano Y, Kusano E, Nakagawa H, Furukawa Y. Histone deacetylase inhibitor FK228 suppresses the Ras-MAP kinase signaling pathway by upregulating Rap1 and induces apoptosis in malignant melanoma. Oncogene. 2006;25(4):512–24.

23. Smith RN, Aleksic J, Butano D, Carr A, Contrino S, Hu F, Lyne M, Lyne R, Kalderimis A, Rutherford K, et al. InterMine: a flexible data warehouse system for the integration and analysis of heterogeneous biological data. Bioinformatics. 2012;28(23):3163–5.

24. Ballestar E, Esteller M. The impact of chromatin in human cancer: linking DNA methylation to gene silencing. Carcinogenesis. 2002;23(7):1103–9.

25. Conomos D, Pickett HA, Reddel RR. Alternative lengthening of telomeres: remodeling the telomere architecture. Front Oncol. 2013;3:27.

26. Barthel FP, Wei W, Tang M, Martinez-Ledesma E, Hu X, Amin SB, Akdemir KC, Seth S, Song X, Wang Q, et al. Systematic analysis of telomere length and somatic alterations in 31 cancer types. Nat Genet. 2017;49(3):349–57.

27. Feinberg AP, Koldobskiy MA, Göndör A. Epigenetic modulators, modifiers and mediators in cancer aetiology and progression. Nat Rev Genet. 2016; 17(5):284–99.

28. Badeaux AI, Shi Y. Emerging roles for chromatin as a signal integration and storage platform. Nat Rev Mol Cell Biol. 2013;14(4):211–24.

29. Simpson DA, Lemonie N, Morgan DS, Gaddameedhi S, Kaufmann WK. Oncogenic BRAF(V600E) Induces Clastogenesis and UVB Hypersensitivity. Cancers. 2015;7(2):1072–90.

30. Chaix A, Lopez S, Voisset E, Gros L, Dubreuil P, De Sepulveda P. Mechanisms of STAT protein activation by oncogenic KIT mutants in neoplastic mast cells. J Biol Chem. 2011;286(8):5956–66.

31. Chandler RL, Damrauer JS, Raab JR, Schisler JC, Wilkerson MD, Didion JP, Starmer J, Serber D, Yee D, Xiong J, et al. Coexistent ARID1A-PIK3CA mutations promote ovarian clear-cell tumorigenesis through pro-tumorigenic inflammatory cytokine signalling. Nat Commun. 2015;6:6118.

32. Chen ZH, Zhu M, Yang J, Liang H, He J, He S, Wang P, Kang X, McNutt MA, Yin Y et al: PTEN interacts with histone H1 and controls chromatin condensation. Cell Rep 2014, 8(6):2003-2014.

33. Nealia CMH, Melissa RK, Catherine HF. Chromatin modifications and DNA repair: beyond double-strand breaks. Front Genet. 2014;5:296.

34. Zhu J, Sammons MA, Donahue G, Dou Z, Vedadi M, Getlik M, Barsyte-Lovejoy D, Al-awar R, Katona BW, Shilatifard A, et al. Gain-of-function p53 mutants co-opt chromatin pathways to drive cancer growth. Nature. 2015; 525(7568):206–11.

35. Vandel L, Nicolas E, Vaute O, Ferriera R, Ait-Si-Ali S, Trouche D. Transcriptional Repression by the Retinoblastoma Protein through the Recruitment of a Histone Methyltransferase. Mol Cell Biol. 2011;21(19):6484–94.

36. Taube JH, Allton K, Duncan SA, Shen L, Barton MC. Foxa1 functions as a pioneer transcription factor at transposable elements to activate Afp during differentiation of embryonic stem cells. J Biol Chem. 2010;285(21):16135–44.

37. Sérandour AA, Avner S, Percevault F, Demay F, Bizot M, Lucchetti-Miganeh C, Barloy-Hubler F, Brown M, Lupien M, Métivier R, et al. Epigenetic switch involved in activation of pioneer factor FOXA1-dependent enhancers. Genome Res. 2011;21(4):555–65.

38. Zhang Y, Zhang D, Li Q, Liang J, Sun L, Yi X, Chen Z, Yan R, Xie G, Li W, et al. Nucleation of DNA repair factors by FOXA1 links DNA demethylation to transcriptional pioneering. Nat Genet. 2016;48(9):1003–13.

39. Yu H, Pak H, Hammond-Martel I, Ghram M, Rodrigue A, Daou S, Barbour H, Corbeil L, Hébert J, Drobetsky E, et al. Tumor suppressor and deubiquitinase BAP1 promotes DNA double-strand break repair. Proc Natl Acad Sci U S A. 2014;111(1):285–90.

40. Mashtalir N, Daou S, Barbour H, Sen NN, Gagnon J, Hammond-Martel I, Dar HH, Therrien M, Affar EB. Autodeubiquitination protects the tumor suppressor BAP1 from cytoplasmic sequestration mediated by the atypical ubiquitin ligase UBE2O. Mol cell. 2014;54(3):392–406.

41. Duncan CG, Benjamin GB, Jin G, Rago C, Kapoor-Vazirani P, Powell DR, Chi J-T, Bigner DD, Vertino PM, Yan H. A heterozygous IDH1R132H/WT mutation induces genome-wide alterations in DNA methylation. Genome Res. 2012; 22(12):2339–55.

42. Inoue S, Li WY, Tseng A, Beerman I, Elia AJ, Bendall SC, Lemonnier F, Kron KJ, Cescon DW, Hao Z, et al. Mutant IDH1 Downregulates ATM and Alters DNA Repair and Sensitivity to DNA Damage Independent of TET2. Cancer cell. 2016;30(2):337–48.

43. Hebbar PB, Archer TK. Nuclear factor 1 is required for both hormone-dependent chromatin remodeling and transcriptional activation of the mouse mammary tumor virus promoter. Mol Cell Biol. 2003;23(3):887–98.

44. Jia YM, Xie YT, Wang YJ, Han JY, Tian XX, Fang WG. Association of Genetic Polymorphisms in CDH1 and CTNNB1 with Breast Cancer Susceptibility and Patients Prognosis among Chinese Han Women. PLos One. 2015;10(8):e0135865.

45. Barker N, Hurlstone A, Musisi H, Miles A, Bienz M, Clevers H. The chromatin remodelling factor Brg-1 interacts with beta-catenin to promote target gene activation. EMBO J. 2001;20(17):4935–43.

46. Wang M, Kern AM, Hülskötter M, Greninger P, Singh A, Pan Y, Chowdhury D, Krause M, Baumann M, Benes CH, et al. EGFR-mediated chromatin condensation protects KRAS-mutant cancer cells against ionizing radiation. Cancer Res. 2014;74(10):2825–34.

47. Hussong M, Börno ST, Kerick M, Wunderlich A, Franz A, Sültmann H, Timmermann B, Lehrach H, Hirsch-Kauffmann M, Schweiger MR. The bromodomain protein BRD4 regulates the KEAP1/NRF2-dependent oxidative stress response. Cell death Dis. 2014;5:e1195.

48. Yamaguchi M, Tonou-Fujimori N, Komori A, Maeda R, Nojima Y, Li H, Okamoto H, Masai I. Histone deacetylase 1 regulates retinal neurogenesis in zebrafish by suppressing Wnt and Notch signaling pathways. Development (Cambridge, England). 2005;132(13):3027–43.

49. Yoo LI, Chung DC, Yuan J. LKB1--a master tumour suppressor of the small intestine and beyond. Nat Rev Cancer. 2002;2(7):529–35.

50. Engelen E, Akinci U, Bryne JC, Hou J, Gontan C, Moen M, Szumska D, Kockx C, van Ijcken W, Dekkers DHW, et al. Sox2 cooperates with Chd7 to regulate genes that are mutated in human syndromes. Nat Genet. 2011;43(6):607–11.

51. Lim J, Hao T, Shaw C, Patel AJ, Szabo G, Rual JF, Fisk CJ, Li N, Smolyar A, Hill DE, et al. A protein-protein interaction network for human inherited ataxias and disorders of Purkinje cell degeneration. Cell. 2006;125(4):801–14.

Permissions

The contributors of this book come from diverse backgrounds, making this book a truly international effort. This book will bring forth new frontiers with its revolutionizing research information and detailed analysis of the nascent developments around the world.

We would like to thank all the contributing authors for lending their expertise to make the book truly unique. They have played a crucial role in the development of this book. Without their invaluable contributions this book wouldn't have been possible. They have made vital efforts to compile up to date information on the varied aspects of this subject to make this book a valuable addition to the collection of many professionals and students.

This book was conceptualized with the vision of imparting up-to-date information and advanced data in this field. To ensure the same, a matchless editorial board was set up. Every individual on the board went through rigorous rounds of assessment to prove their worth. After which they invested a large part of their time researching and compiling the most relevant data for our readers.

The editorial board has been involved in producing this book since its inception. They have spent rigorous hours researching and exploring the diverse topics which have resulted in the successful publishing of this book. They have passed on their knowledge of decades through this book. To expedite this challenging task, the publisher supported the team at every step. A small team of assistant editors was also appointed to further simplify the editing procedure and attain best results for the readers.

Apart from the editorial board, the designing team has also invested a significant amount of their time in understanding the subject and creating the most relevant covers. They scrutinized every image to scout for the most suitable representation of the subject and create an appropriate cover for the book.

The publishing team has been an ardent support to the editorial, designing and production team. Their endless efforts to recruit the best for this project, has resulted in the accomplishment of this book. They are a veteran in the field of academics and their pool of knowledge is as vast as their experience in printing. Their expertise and guidance has proved useful at every step. Their uncompromising quality standards have made this book an exceptional effort. Their encouragement from time to time has been an inspiration for everyone.

The publisher and the editorial board hope that this book will prove to be a valuable piece of knowledge for researchers, students, practitioners and scholars across the globe.

Contributors

Kira Groen and Vicki E. Maltby
School of Medicine and Public Health, University of Newcastle, Callaghan, NSW 2308, Australia
Centre for Information Based Medicine, Level 3 West, Hunter Medical Research Institute, 1 Kookaburra Circuit, New Lambton Heights, NSW 2305, Australia

Jeannette Lechner-Scott
School of Medicine and Public Health, University of Newcastle, Callaghan, NSW 2308, Australia
Centre for Information Based Medicine, Level 3 West, Hunter Medical Research Institute, 1 Kookaburra Circuit, New Lambton Heights, NSW 2305, Australia
Department of Neurology, John Hunter Hospital, New Lambton Heights, NSW 2305, Australia

Rodney A. Lea
Centre for Information Based Medicine, Level 3 West, Hunter Medical Research Institute, 1 Kookaburra Circuit, New Lambton Heights, NSW 2305, Australia
Institute of Health and Biomedical Innovations, Genomics Research Centre, Queensland University of Technology, Kelvin Grove, QLD 4059, Australia

Rodney J. Scott
Centre for Information Based Medicine, Level 3 West, Hunter Medical Research Institute, 1 Kookaburra Circuit, New Lambton Heights, NSW 2305, Australia
Division of Molecular Genetics, Pathology North, John Hunter Hospital, New Lambton Heights, NSW 2305, Australia
School of Biomedical Sciences and Pharmacy, University of Newcastle, Callaghan, NSW 2308, Australia

Katherine A. Sanders
Centre for Anatomical and Human Sciences, Hull York Medical School, Hull HU6 7RX, UK

J. Lynn Fink
Diamantina Institute, University of Queensland, Woolloongabba, QLD 4102, Australia

Lotti Tajouri
Faculty of Health Sciences and Medicine, Bond University, QLD, Robina 4229, Australia

Gordon K C Leung, Christopher C Y Mak, Jasmine L F Fung, Wilfred H S Wong, Mandy H Y Tsang, Mullin H C Yu, Steven L C Pei, K S Yeung, Gary T K Mok, Anthony P Y Liu and Wanling Yang
Department of Paediatrics and Adolescent Medicine, LKS Faculty of Medicine, The University of Hong Kong, Room 103, 1/F, New Clinical Building, Hong Kong, Hong Kong Special Administrative Region, China

Brian H Y Chung
Department of Paediatrics and Adolescent Medicine, LKS Faculty of Medicine, The University of Hong Kong, Room 103, 1/F, New Clinical Building, Hong Kong, Hong Kong Special Administrative Region, China
Department of Obstetrics and Gynaecology, Queen Mary Hospital, The University of Hong Kong, Hong Kong, Hong Kong Special Administrative Region, China
Prenatal Diagnostic Laboratory, Department of Obstetrics and Gynaecology, Tsan Yuk Hospital, Hong Kong, HKSAR, China

C P Lee and Amelia P W Hui
Department of Obstetrics and Gynaecology, Queen Mary Hospital, The University of Hong Kong, Hong Kong, Hong Kong Special Administrative Region, China

Mary H Y Tang, Kelvin Y K Chan and Anita S Y Kan
Department of Obstetrics and Gynaecology, Queen Mary Hospital, The University of Hong Kong, Hong Kong, Hong Kong Special Administrative Region, China
Prenatal Diagnostic Laboratory, Department of Obstetrics and Gynaecology, Tsan Yuk Hospital, Hong Kong, HKSAR, China

P C Sham
Department of Psychiatry, LKS Faculty of Medicine, The University of Hong Kong, Hong Kong, HKSAR, China

Elisabeth De Smit, Amy Wong Ten Yuen, Linda Clarke, Isabel Lopez Sanchez, Sandy S. C. Hung and Alice Pébay
Centre for Eye Research Australia, The University of Melbourne, Royal Victorian Eye and Ear Hospital, 32 Gisborne Street, East Melbourne 3002, Australia

Alex W. Hewitt
Centre for Eye Research Australia, The University of Melbourne, Royal Victorian Eye and Ear Hospital, 32 Gisborne Street, East Melbourne 3002, Australia
School of Medicine, Menzies Research Institute Tasmania, University of Tasmania, Hobart 7000, Tasmania, Australia

Samuel W. Lukowski, Anne Senabouth, Kaisar Dauyey and Joseph E. Powell
Institute for Molecular Bioscience, The University of Queensland, Brisbane 4072, Queensland, Australia

Lisa Anderson, Sharon Song, Bruce Wyse, Lawrie Wheeler and Matthew A. Brown
Institute of Health and Biomedical Innovation, Queensland University of Technology, Translational Research Institute, Princess Alexandra Hospital, Brisbane 4102, Queensland, Australia

Christine Y. Chen and Khoa Cao
Ophthalmology Department at Monash Health, Department of Surgery, School of Clinical Sciences at Monash Health, Melbourne 3168, Victoria, Australia

Neil Shuey
Department of Neuro-Ophthalmology, Royal Victorian Eye and Ear Hospital, Melbourne 3002, Victoria, Australia

David A. Mackey
Centre for Ophthalmology and Visual Science, The University of Western Australia, Lions Eye Institute, Perth 6009, Western Australia, Australia

Dana C. Crawford and Nicole A. Restrepo
Department of Population and Quantitative Health Sciences, Institute for Computational Biology, Case Western Reserve University, 2103 Cornell Road, Wolstein Research Building, Suite 2-527, Cleveland, OH 44106, USA

Kirsten E. Diggins
Cancer Biology, Vanderbilt University School of Medicine, Nashville, TN, USA

Eric Farber-Eger
Vanderbilt Institute for Clinical and Translational Research, Vanderbilt University Medical Center, Nashville, TN, USA

Quinn S. Wells
Departments of Medicine and Pharmacology, Vanderbilt University Medical Center, Nashville, TN, USA

Silke Schultz and Hans J. Neubauer
Department of Obstetrics and Gynaecology, Life-Science-Center, Heinrich-Heine University, Merowingerplatz 1A, 40225 Duesseldorf, Germany

Tanja Fehm
Department of Obstetrics and Gynaecology, Life-Science-Center, Heinrich-Heine University, Merowingerplatz 1A, 40225 Duesseldorf, Germany
Department of Obstetrics and Gynaecology, Heinrich-Heine University, Duesseldorf, Moorenstr. 5, 40225 Duesseldorf, Germany

Harald Bartsch, Karl Sotlar and Karina Petat-Dutter
Institute of Pathology, Department of Pathology, Ludwig Maximilians University, Thalkirchner Straße 36, 80337 Munich, Germany

Michael Bonin
Microarray Facility, Department of Medical Genetics, Eberhard Karls University, Tuebingen, Germany
IMGM Laboratories GmbH, Bunsenstr. 7a, 82152 Martinsried, Germany

Steffen Kahlert and Nadia Harbeck
Department of Obstetrics and Gynaecology, Ludwig Maximilians University, Marchioninistr. 15, 81377 Munich, Germany

Ulrich Vogel
Institute of Pathology, Eberhard Karls University, Tuebingen, Germany

Harald Seeger
Department of Obstetrics and Gynaecology, Eberhard Karls University, Liebermeisterstr. 8, 72076 Tuebingen, Germany
Department of Obstetrics and Gynaecology, Eberhard Karls University, Calwerstr. 7, 72076 Tuebingen, Germany

Lingyan Wang, Xiaoling Yu, Chao Wu, Teng Zhu, Wenming Wang, Xiaofeng Zheng and Hongzhong Jin
Department of Dermatology, Peking Union Medical College Hospital, Chinese Academy of Medical Sciences and Peking Union Medical College, Beijing, China

Kristjan Eerik Kaseniit, Gregory J Hogan, Kevin M D'Auria, Carrie Haverty and Dale Muzzey
Myriad Women's Health (previously Counsyl), 180 Kimball Way, South San Francisco, CA 94080, USA

Nicole A. Restrepo and Dana C. Crawford
Department of Population and Quantitative Health Sciences, Institute for Computational Biology, Case Western Reserve University, 2103 Cornell Road, Wolstein Research Building, Suite 2-527, Cleveland, OH 44106, USA

Sarah M. Laper
Eastern Virginia Medical School, Norfolk, VA, USA

Eric Farber-Eger
Vanderbilt Institute for Clinical and Translational Research, Vanderbilt University Medical Center, Nashville, TN, USA

Dan Li and Renchu Guan
Key Laboratory of Symbolic Computation and Knowledge Engineering of Ministry of Education, College of Computer Science and Technology, Jilin University, Changchun 130012, China
MidSouth Bioinformatics Center and Joint Bioinformatics Ph.D. Program of University of Arkansas at Little Rock and Univ. of Arkansas Medical Sciences, 2801 S. Univ. Ave, Little Rock, AR 72204, USA

Dong Xu
Key Laboratory of Symbolic Computation and Knowledge Engineering of Ministry of Education, College of Computer Science and Technology, Jilin University, Changchun 130012, China
Department of Electrical Engineering and Computer Science, Informatics Institute, and Christopher S. Bond Life Sciences Center, University of Missouri, Columbia, MO 65211, USA

Yifan Zhang, Jack Y Yang and Mary Qu Yang
MidSouth Bioinformatics Center and Joint Bioinformatics Ph.D. Program of University of Arkansas at Little Rock and Univ. of Arkansas Medical Sciences, 2801 S. Univ. Ave, Little Rock, AR 72204, USA

William Yang
Department of Computer Science, Carnegie Mellon University School of Computer Science, 5000 Forbes Ave, Pittsburgh, PA 15213, USA

Xing-Cheng Zhao, Lin Zhang, Bo Jiao, Shuai Jiang and Zhi-Bin Yu
Department of Aerospace Physiology, Fourth Military Medical University, Changle West Road 169#, Xi'an 710032, People's Republic of China

Yi-Quan Yan
Department of Aerospace Physiology, Fourth Military Medical University, Changle West Road 169#, Xi'an 710032, People's Republic of China
Department of Traditional Chinese Medicine, Xijing Hospital, Fourth Military Medical University, Xi'an 710032, China

Shao-Hua Yang and Xin Zhang
Lintong Aviation Medical Evaluating and Training Center of Air Force, Xi'an 710600, China

Lili Ding and Mekibib Altaye
Division of Biostatistics and Epidemiology, Department of Pediatrics, Cincinnati Children's Hospital Medical Center, Cincinnati, OH, USA

Dan Li
Alzheimer's Therapeutic Research Institute, Keck School of Medicine, University of Southern California, San Diego, CA, USA

Michael Wathen and Tesfaye B. Mersha
Division of Asthma Research, Department of Pediatrics, Cincinnati Children's Hospital Medical Center, University of Cincinnati, 3333 Burnet Ave, Cincinnati, OH 45229, USA

Pei-Yuan Zhou, Antonio Sze-To and Andrew K. C. Wong
Kansas City, MO, USA

Madhusudan Grover, Simon J. Gibbons, Cheryl E. Bernard, Adeel S. Zubair, Seth T. Eisenman and Gianrico Farrugia
Enteric NeuroScience Program, Division of Gastroenterology and Hepatology, Mayo Clinic, 200 1st Street SW, Rochester, MN 55905, USA

Asha A. Nair
Biomedical Statistics and Informatics, Mayo Clinic, Rochester, MN, USA

Laura A. Wilson, Laura Miriel and James Tonascia
Johns Hopkins University Bloomberg School of Public Health, Johns Hopkins University, Baltimore, MD, USA

Pankaj J. Pasricha
Johns Hopkins University School of Medicine, Baltimore, MD, USA

Henry P. Parkman
Temple University, Philadelphia, PA, USA

Irene Sarosiek and Richard W. McCallum
Texas Tech University, El Paso, TX, USA

Kenneth L. Koch
Wake Forest University, Winston-Salem, NC, USA

Thomas L. Abell
University of Louisville, Louisville, KY, USA

William J. Snape
California Pacific Medical Center, San Francisco, CA, USA

Braden Kuo
Massachusetts General Hospital, Boston, MA, USA

Robert J. Shulman
Baylor College of Medicine, Houston, TX, USA

Travis J. McKenzie, Todd A. Kellogg and Michael L. Kendrick
Department of Surgery, Mayo Clinic, Rochester, MN, USA

Frank A. Hamilton
National Institute of Diabetes and Digestive and Kidney Diseases, Bethesda, MD, USA

Aliz R. Rao
Department of Human Genetics, University of California, Los Angeles, California, Los Angeles, USA

Stanley F. Nelson
Department of Human Genetics, University of California, Los Angeles, California, Los Angeles, USA
Department of Psychiatry and Biobehavioral Sciences at the David Geffen School of Medicine, University of California, Los Angeles, California, Los Angeles, USA
Department of Pathology and Laboratory Medicine, University of California, Los Angeles, California, Los Angeles, USA

Ye Zhu and Xiang Gu
Clinical Medical College, Yangzhou University, Yangzhou 225001, Jiangsu, China
Department of Cardiology, Northern Jiangsu People's Hospital, Yangzhou 225001, Jiangsu, China

Chao Xu
Department of Biostatistics and Epidemiology, University of Oklahoma Health Science Center, Oklahoma City, OK 73134, USA

Ting Yu and Yangong Wang
Children's Hospital and Institutes of Biomedical Sciences, Fudan University, Wanyuan Road 399, Minhang District, Shanghai 201102, China

Qinghe Xing
Children's Hospital and Institutes of Biomedical Sciences, Fudan University, Wanyuan Road 399, Minhang District, Shanghai 201102, China
Shanghai Center for Women and Children's Health, Shanghai 200062, China

Lei Xia, Dan Bi, Dengna Zhu, Juan Song and Yong Wang
Henan Key Laboratory of Child Brain Injury, Third Affiliated Hospital of Zhengzhou University, Kangfuqian Street 7, Zhengzhou 450052, China

Xiaoyang Wang
Henan Key Laboratory of Child Brain Injury, Third Affiliated Hospital of Zhengzhou University, Kangfuqian Street 7, Zhengzhou 450052, China
Perinatal Center, Institute of Neuroscience and Physiology, University of Gothenburg, Gothenburg 40530, Sweden

Changlian Zhu
Henan Key Laboratory of Child Brain Injury, Third Affiliated Hospital of Zhengzhou University, Kangfuqian Street 7, Zhengzhou 450052, China
Center for Brain Repair and Rehabilitation, Department of Clinical Neuroscience, Sahlgrenska Academy, University of Gothenburg, Gothenburg 40530, Sweden

Qing Shang
Department of Pediatrics, Zhengzhou Children's Hospital, Zhengzhou 450053, China

Yifan Zhang, Dan Li, Jack Y Yang, Renchu Guan and Mary Qu Yang
MidSouth Bioinformatics Center and Joint Bioinformatics Ph.D. Program of University of Arkansas at Little Rock and Univ. of Arkansas Medical Sciences, 2801 S. Univ. Ave, Little Rock 72204, USA

William Yang
Department of Computer Science, Carnegie Mellon University School of Computer Science, 5000 Forbes Ave, Pittsburgh 24105, USA

Haley R. Eidem, Jacob L. Steenwyk and Patrick Abbot
Department of Biological Sciences, Vanderbilt University, Nashville, TN, USA

Jennifer H. Wisecaver
Department of Biological Sciences, Vanderbilt University, Nashville, TN, USA
Department of Biochemistry, Purdue University, West Lafayette, IN, USA

John A. Capra and Antonis Rokas
Department of Biological Sciences, Vanderbilt University, Nashville, TN, USA
Department of Biomedical Informatics, Vanderbilt University, Nashville, TN, USA
Vanderbilt Genetics Institute, Vanderbilt University, Nashville, TN, USA

Shuang Wang
Department of Biostatistics, Mailman School of Public Health, Columbia University, New York, New York, USA

Ahrim Youn
Department of Biostatistics, Mailman School of Public Health, Columbia University, New York, New York, USA
The Jackson Laboratory For Genomic Medicine, Farmington, Connecticut, USA

Kyung In Kim
The Jackson Laboratory For Genomic Medicine, Farmington, Connecticut, USA

Raul Rabadan
Department of System Biology, Columbia University, New York, New York, USA

Department of Biomedical Informatics, Columbia University, New York, New York, USA

Yufeng Shen
Department of System Biology, Columbia University, New York, New York, USA
Department of Biomedical Informatics, Columbia University, New York, New York, USA
Columbia Genome Center, Columbia University, New York, New York, USA

Benjamin Tycko
Division of Genetics and Epigenetics, Hackensack University Medical Center, Hackensack, New Jersey, USA

Index